# A MANUAL
# OF
# FAMILY MEDICINE AND HYGIENE
# FOR INDIA

# A MANUAL
# OF
# FAMILY MEDICINE AND HYGIENE
# FOR INDIA

BY

**SIR WILLIAM MOORE, K.C.I.E.**

HONORARY PHYSICIAN TO H.M. THE QUEEN
FORMERLY SURGEON-GENERAL WITH THE
GOVERNMENT OF BOMBAY

Published under the Authority of the Government of India

SIXTH EDITION

GYAN

*Published by*

Gyan Publishing House
5, Ansari Road
Daryaganj, New Delhi-110002
Phone: 011-47034999, 9811692060
E-mail: books@gyanbooks.com

*Distribution Network*
gyanbooks.com
India, USA, Canada, UK, Australia, France



ISBN : 978-81-212-1484-1 (PB)
First Published, 1893

2nd Impression 2021

*Printed at:* Gyan Press, Delhi.



**A Manual of Family Medicine and Hygiene for India**
Author: Sir William Moore

# A MANUAL
OF
# FAMILY MEDICINE
# AND HYGIENE
## For India

BY

SIR WILLIAM MOORE, K.C.I.E.

HONORARY PHYSICIAN TO H.M. THE QUEEN
FORMERLY SURGEON-GENERAL WITH THE GOVERNMENT OF BOMBAY

---

Published under the Authority of the Government of India

---

*SIXTH EDITION*

LONDON
J. & A. CHURCHILL
11 NEW BURLINGTON STREET
1893

CASES containing the European Medicines recommended for use in the large type of this work (*vide* page 1) can be obtained from the GENERAL APOTHECARIES' COMPANY, Berners Street, London, Messrs BURROUGHS, WELLCOME, & Co., Snow Hill Buildings, London,

Messrs BATHGATE & Co. . . . . Calcutta,

Messrs SCOTT, MASCURINE, & Co. . Madras,

Messrs KEMP & Co. . . . . . . . Bombay,

Messrs PHILLIPS & Co. . . . . Bombay.

# PREFACE

THE origin of this work was the offer of a prize by the Government of India (awarded to the author in 1873) for a manual suitable for the numerous individuals, families, and office establishments, necessarily scattered over India in positions more or less remote from medical and surgical aid: also containing general instructions for preserving health in circumstances of exposure, and of residence in unhealthy localities; and adapted to a small economical medicine case, carrying as few medicines as possible. When the remedies most desirable for a malady are not in the case, the course recommended indicates the general treatment and dietary to be pursued, and the use of the most fitting medicines or applications available, either from the case, or *secondly*, as may be generally obtained in an Indian village bazaar. Where necessary a paragraph in small type is added to the treatment of diseases, advising what medicines should be procured, as soon as practicable, from a chemist. In some places less important information, but still information which will doubtless be sought for in the book, is also given in small type.

The whole text has been attentively reconsidered; various alterations, tending to simplification, have been made in the wording; and several additions have been inserted, the alterations and additions having in most instances been determined upon in consequence of communications expressing doubt as to meaning, or disappointment at the absence of certain information. As before, special attention has been given to the maladies of children, and to the treatment of infants.

It is therefore hoped this sixth edition will prove even more useful than preceding volumes.

15 PORTLAND PLACE, W.
LONDON: *September*, 1893.

# CONTENTS

# LIST OF WOOD ENGRAVINGS

# INDIAN DOMESTIC MEDICINE

## CHAPTER I

### *CONTENTS OF THE INDIAN MEDICINE CASE, AND DESCRIPTION OF MEDICINES RECOMMENDED FOR USE*

THE MEDICINES CONTAINED in the small case designed to accompany the *Manual of Family Medicine for India*, and which *are referred to in the large type* on the treatment of the various diseases (Chapters II. and III.), are fourteen in number. They have been selected with special regard to economy of means and space, and to efficiency, as being the medicines most useful in non-professional hands, *until other remedies, as mentioned in the small type, or professional aid*, may be procurable. The list of the contents of the small medicine case is as follows. The English or more common names are first given, opposite which the Latin terms are inserted; so that, in procuring the medicines, both names being used, there cannot be a mistake.

| | |
|---|---|
| 1. AMMONIA, AROMATIC SPIRITS OF, OR SAL VOLATILE . . | *Spiritus Ammoniæ Aromaticus* |
| 2. BROMIDE OF POTASSIUM . . | *Bromidum Potassii* |
| 3. CHLORAL . . . . . . . . | *Chloral Hydras* |
| 4. CHLORODYNE . . . . . . . | *Chlorodyne* |

| | |
|---|---|
| 5. Dover's Powder, or Compound Powder of Opium and Ipecacuanha . . . | *Pulvis Ipecacuanhæ Compositus* |
| 6. Ether, Nitrous Spirits of; or Sweet Spirits of Nitre . . . . . . . . | *Spiritus Ætheris Nitrosi* |
| 7. Ginger, Tincture of, Strong | *Tinctura Zingiberis Fortior* |
| 8. Ipecacuanha Powder. . . | *Pulvis Ipecacuanhæ* |
| 9. Ipecacuanha Wine . . . | *Vinum Ipecacuanhæ* |
| 10. Magnesia, Citrate of, Granular Effervescent . . | *Magnesiæ Citras* (*Granular*) |
| 11. Opium, Camphorated Tincture of; or Paregoric . | *Tinctura Camphoræ Composita cum Opio* |
| 12. Podophyllum Resin Pills Compound . . . . . . | *Podophylli Resinæ Pilula, composita* |
| 13. Quinine, Sulphate of . . | *Quiniæ Sulphas* |
| 14. Soda, Sulphate of . . . | *Sodæ Sulphas* |

*Note.—No.* 12, *Podophyllum, is not carried in the case in the pure form, but it is recommended made into pills of which it forms the most active ingredient ; vide p.* 16, *and Recipe* 1.

The medicine case also carries a minim measure, a box of scales and weights, and a small knife, or spatula.[1]

*Various other medicines*, ordinarily procurable in the Indian bazaars, have been also recommended in the *large type* for use on emergency. The list of these medicines is as below, and the Hindustanee name is given opposite the English one:—

| | |
|---|---|
| 1. Alum . . . . . . . . . . . . . | *Phitkarree* |
| 2. Ammonium, Chloride of, or Hydrochlorate of Ammonia; also commonly called Sal-Ammoniac . . | *Naushadur or Nissadal* |
| 3. Assafœtida . . . . . . . . . | *Hing* |
| 4. Bael, or Ægle Marmelos . . . | *Bael* |
| 5. Castor Oil . . . . . . . . . | *Rindee ka Tail* |
| 6. Camphor. . . . . . . . . . | *Kafoor* |

[1] The instruments mentioned at the commencement of Chapter III., for use in surgical cases, should also be provided.

| | |
|---|---|
| 7. IRON, SULPHATE OF; also COPPERAS, OR GREEN VITRIOL . . . . . | *Hera-kusees* |
| 8. POMEGRANATE . . . . . . . . . | *Anar* |
| 9. POTASH, NITRATE OF, OR SALT-PETRE . . . . . . . . . . . | *Shora* |
| 10. SENNA . . . . . . . . . . . | *Senna Mukki* |
| 11. STRAMONIUM . . . . . . . . . | *Dhatura* |
| 12. SULPHUR. . . . . . . . . . . | *Ghunduk* |

The appearance, use, action, and doses of the medicines above enumerated are detailed at pages 8 to 28.

It has not been considered necessary to describe the medicines which are recommended for use in the *small type*, which must be obtained from the chemists, as the person using the Manual will not be required to manipulate them.

*It should be clearly understood that the treatment of illness by the medicines in the case, or by medicines obtainable from the bazaar, as advised in Chapters II. and III., is not intended to take the place of medical assistance and advice; but it is offered as a substitute when such aid is not obtainable, and as the method by which improper treatment may be avoided.*

## COMPOUNDING OF MEDICINES

### Weights and Measures used in Compounding Medicines

*Weight for Solids*

| | |
|---|---|
| 20 grains make . . . . . . . | 1 scruple |
| 3 scruples ,, . . . . . . . | 1 drachm |
| 8 drachms ,, . . . . . . . | 1 ounce |
| 12 ounces ,, . . . . . . . | 1 pound |

The grain weights, except the half-grain, are stamped with as many dots or circles ○ as they weigh grains; one mark on the one-grain, two on the two-grain weight, and so on. On the half-grain weight are the figures ½. The larger weights are marked in English, and in the old symbolical characters.

*Measure for Fluids*

| | | |
|---|---|---|
| 60 minims make | . . . . . . | 1 drachm |
| 8 drachms „ | . . . . . . | 1 ounce |
| 20 ounces „ | . . . . . . | 1 pint |
| 8 pints „ | . . . . . . | 1 gallon |

Glass measures as sketched below are placed in all medicine chests large enough to admit them:—

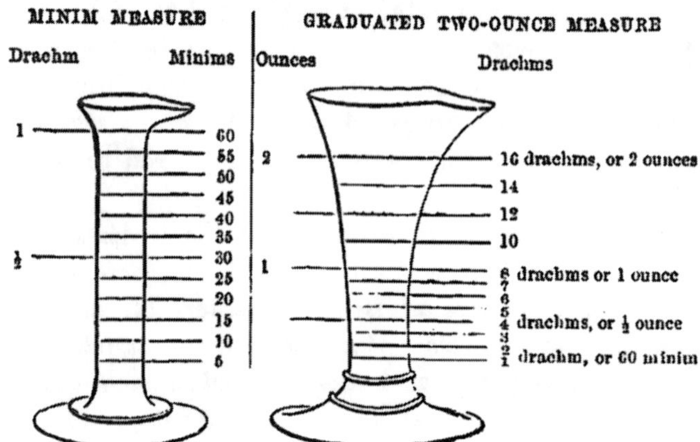


When the quantity of fluid medicines is so small that it cannot be measured by minims, *drops* are ordered, which should be poured from the bottle accurately. The bottle should be held obliquely, with the lower part of the lip resting against the stopper. The bottle should then be carefully tilted, when the contents will drop from the lower edge of the stopper. A little practice will enable any person to drop one or more drops with exactness (*vide* p. 5).

It should be remembered that drops do not necessarily equal minims, as fluids vary in density; as, for instance, oil and water. The size of the mouth of the bottle, and the manner in which the fluid is manipulated, may also vary the size of the drops. The best plan is, therefore, to obtain a *glass medicine dropper*, by which greater accuracy is insured. Measurement of fluids by the minim glass should, however, always be adopted, unless the medicine is required in very small quantities.

The following is a rough measurement of fluids approximating to the apothecaries' measure for fluids (*vide*

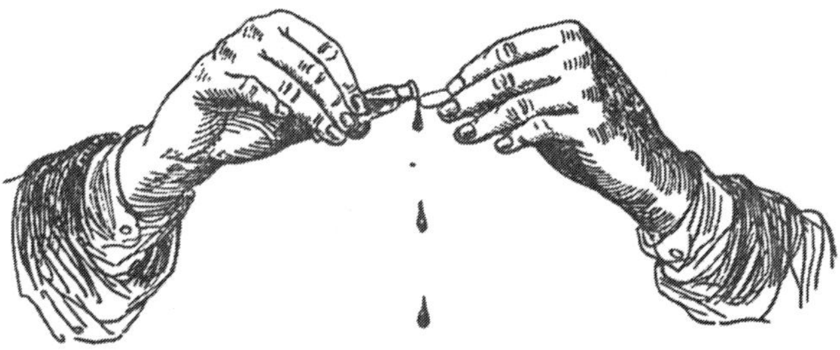

p. 4). This rough measurement is sufficiently accurate for giving out doses of ordinary mixtures, the active ingredients in which are diluted by water; but it should *not* be used to compound medicines, or to measure them in the undiluted condition, as the size of spoons, even of the same class, is liable to vary.

| | |
|---|---|
| 1 tea-spoonful . . . | = one drachm |
| 1 dessert-spoonful . . | = two drachms |
| 1 table-spoonful . . | = four drachms, or half an ounce |
| 1 small wine-glassful . | = about two ounces |

In Compounding Medicines distilled water should be used. If this cannot be procured, water which has been purified by boiling and filtering (*vide* Chapter VI., *Water, or refer to Index*) should always be used, and the measures, knives, &c., should be kept perfectly clean.

## DOSES OF MEDICINES

Unless expressly stated to the contrary, the doses mentioned in the account of diseases, and in the collection of prescriptions (*vide* Appendix), are those adapted for an ordinary strong adult. The younger and less robust the child the smaller is the dose necessary, and delicate females usually require a less powerful agent than stronger women, or than those of the other sex.

The following table shows the approximate doses of medicines for different ages. For solids the scales and weights must be used, according to apothecaries' weight (*vide* p. 3). For fluids the measures must be used (*vide* p. 4), and *minims* must be substituted for grains, according to apothecaries' measure (*vide* p. 4). Below five minims drops should be given (*vide* p. 4).

| Age above | Maximum dose one ounce | Maximum dose one drachm | Maximum dose one scruple |
|---|---|---|---|
| 1 month | 24 grains | 3 grains | 1 grain |
| 6 months | 2 scruples | 5 grains | 1¾ grain |
| 1 year | 1 drachm | 8 grains | 2½ grains |
| 2 years | 1¼ drachm | 9 grains | 3 grains |
| 3 „ | 1½ drachm | 12 grains | 4 grains |
| 5 „ | 2 drachms | 15 grains | 5 grains |
| 7 „ | 3 drachms | 20 grains | 7 grains |
| 10 „ | ½ ounce | ½ drachm | ½ scruple |
| 12 „ | 5 drachms | 40 grains | 14 grains |
| 15 „ | 6 drachms | 45 grains | 16 grains |
| 20 „ | 7 drachms | 50 grains | 18 grains |
| 21 „ | 1 ounce | 1 drachm | 1 scruple |

It appears by the table that, if the dose of any medicine for a man of twenty-one years of age is 1 ounce (maximum dose), then the dose of the same medicine for a child above one month is 24 grains, or 24 minims if a fluid; for a child above five years of age, 2 drachms; and for a child above ten, half an ounce. Or, if 1 scruple, or of fluid 20 minims, is the maximum dose for a full-grown man, then the dose of the same medicine for a child seven years old will be 7 grains of a solid medicine, and 7 drops of a fluid medicine; and for a child one month old 1 grain, or 1 drop.

The above may be accepted as for ordinarily strong children; but when dealing with weakly children it may be advisable to lessen the quantities by one-sixth up to one year of age, and by one-eighth from one year to ten years of age.

Independent of the differences which exist between the doses suited for an adult male and a delicate female, as mentioned above, other circumstances, as *habit, disease, climate, mind, temperament, race, and idiosyncrasy*, must often be considered when regulating the dose. Thus children are peculiarly susceptible to the influence of opium, very minute quantities having proved fatal to infants; and unfortunately opium is the powerful agent in various 'soothing syrups' and 'cordials' sold for children. In this book preparations containing opium are rarely, and always most cautiously, prescribed for children. Habit will enable certain people to consume large quantities of opium, arsenic, and of some other substances: in certain maladies—as, for instance, *senile gangrene*—large doses of opium produce little effect. In a tropical climate it is sometimes undesirable to use purgatives with the freedom with which they may be given in other latitudes; and especially so if cholera prevails. Mercury is borne best in hot climates, as the more free perspiration carries it out of the system; while opium is not so well tolerated, because the heat increases the determination to the head. Alcoholic stimulants follow the same rule, being more injurious in hot than in cold climates. A peculiar temperament often forbids an energetic treatment proper for other persons. Natives of India, as a rule, require smaller doses than Europeans. Lastly, idiosyncrasy is illustrated by the smallest particle of mercury sometimes producing salivation (*vide note to* Recipe 23), by iodide of potassium occasionally exciting symptoms of *coryza* (*vide note to* Recipe 21), by quinine causing sore-throat and eruptions on the skin (*vide* p. 18), by assafœtida sometimes causing faintness (*vide* p. 22), by ipecacuanha producing cough, sneezing, and watering of the eyes and nose (*vide* p. 14), by santonin occasioning red-coloured urine, and green or yellow vision (*vide* p. 486), and by pollen exciting hay asthma (*vide*

p. 64). It is not, however, medicines only which produce extraordinary effects on peculiar constitutions. There are persons who cannot eat celery, shell-fish, oatmeal cakes, strawberries, apples, mushrooms, or cucumber without suffering from nettle-rash or colic. There are persons with whom neither milk, eggs, nor mutton agrees. Others cannot take sherry without suffering from acidity, and the slightest quantity of port wine sometimes excites gouty pains.

## DESCRIPTIONS OF MEDICINES

The appearance, action, principal uses, and doses of the various medicines carried in the case are now noted. The prescriptions referred to by number in the account of medicines, and in the treatment of diseases, will be found in the Appendix of Prescriptions at the end of the volume.

1. **AMMONIA, AROMATIC SPIRITS OF; or SAL VOLATILE** (*Spiritus Ammoniæ Aromaticus*).—Aromatic spirits of ammonia is a nearly colourless liquid, with strong ammoniacal odour and pungent taste. It is a strong stimulant, producing a sensation of warmth at the pit of the stomach, and an agreeable glow throughout the body. It is used in hysteria, headache, nervous disorders, giddiness, palpitation, fainting, and in some forms of dyspepsia, as heartburn, flatulence, and acidity of the stomach. It is also very useful for children; especially for infants, who, generally owing to bad or over feeding, may be tormented by wind, or by colicky pains in the bowels. The dose for an adult is half a drachm to a drachm, in half an ounce to an ounce of water. To children of from one to three months old, from 1 to 2 drops may be given; from three to six months old, 2 to 5 drops; from six to twelve months old, 5 to 8 drops in a tea-spoonful of water; or in sufficient water to reduce the strength, so that it may be easily swallowed. It should be kept in a stoppered bottle. Aromatic spirits of ammonia enters in Recipes 26, 38, 39, 40, 51, 55, 56.

2. **BROMIDE OF POTASSIUM** (*Bromidum Potassii*).—It consists of white cubical crystals without odour, of pungent saline taste, and soluble in water. As it is affected by damp it must be kept in a stoppered bottle. It exercises a sedative action on the nerves generally, and especially on those supplying the back part of the mouth, throat, and entrance to the windpipe. It is useful for persons suffering from overwork, worry, despondency, and *insomnia* or inability to sleep, and in delirium tremens. It is given with great benefit in hysteria, epilepsy, for the 'night terrors,' and for the convulsions of children. It is employed advantageously for the vomiting of pregnant women, for spasmodic cough, and for spasmodic asthma, also for nervous headache, or *migraine*. It is also recommended as diminishing the spasms of tetanus and of poisoning by strychnine. Lastly, it is sometimes given for glandular swellings. In too large or too frequently repeated doses, it lessens the force and frequency of the heart's action and causes mental weakness, somnolence, and depression. It also occasions dryness, soreness, and loss of sensibility in the throat. There may also be an eruption of pimples, chiefly on the forehead and face, and which eventually contain matter. To this full effect of the medicine the term 'bromism' is applied. The dose for an adult is from 5 or 6 to 30 grains in an ounce, to two or three ounces of water; the first if given repeatedly, the latter if used to allay sudden convulsive seizures. For a child the dose, if given repeatedly, varies from 1 grain at one year old to 2 grains at four years old in two or three tea-spoonfuls of water; increasing the dose by a quarter of a grain for each year of age. In convulsive seizures three times the quantity may be given. For children, it may be mixed with an equal quantity of salt and given at the meals, without the child being aware that it is taking medicine. Bromide of potassium enters into Recipes 19, 20.

3. **CHLORAL** (*Chloral Hydras*).—It is a white crystalline substance, generally seen in small pieces about the size of a pea, but sometimes in much larger flakes. It has a pungent odour, and a cool acrid taste, rapidly melting on the tongue. In small doses chloral exerts a calmative influence over the system. In larger doses it induces sleep, which usually comes on in less than half an hour after taking chloral, and is generally calm and refreshing, yet not so profound as to prevent waking to cough, take food, &c. It is given in many cases instead of opium to procure sleep, and it differs from opium in its action in not producing any excitement of the system; nor usually any subsequent giddiness, headache, nervous depression, loss of appetite, or constipation, so often following the use of opium. First doses are, however, more likely to be followed by some feelings of the kind than when the person has become accustomed to the medicine. Chloral has also a further advantage over opium, as the dose does not need to be so steadily increased to produce the same effects. It has been used for neuralgia, rheumatism, sea-sickness, convulsions, asthma, cough, tetanus, delirium tremens, nervous irritability, spasmodic complaints, for the wakefulness induced by mental fatigue, and in most other diseases characterised by restlessness and want of sleep.

As cases of poisoning have occurred from chloral, and as the drug acts more strongly on some persons than on others, it must always be used with caution. In diseases of the chest attended with profuse expectoration, especial caution is required in the use of chloral, as, if given in too large quantities, the soporific effect may prevent the patient expectorating, and thus increase difficulty of breathing. The use of chloral is also contra-indicated when the heart is weak. The ordinary dose for an adult is from 5 to 10 grains as a calmative, and from 15 to 40 when required to produce sleep. After 20 grains the dose should be increased *cautiously*, by 5 grains at one time, up to 40 grains if necessary. A person in the habit of drinking spirits will require a larger dose of chloral than one unaccustomed to alcoholic drinks. Those debilitated and enfeebled by almost any cause require a smaller dose than stronger persons. Chloral is best given dissolved in a little sugar and water. A convenient form of chloral is the *Syrup of chloral*, sold by the chemists, of which one fluid drachm contains 10 grains of chloral. The usual dose for children is 1 grain; or 7 drops of the syrup (which should contain 1 grain) for each year of the child's age. Sometimes, especially in children, even one dose of chloral causes a rash resembling *erythema* (*vide* p. 386). It comes on, about half an hour or longer, after taking the medicine, and is of no consequence. Chloral enters into Recipe 54.

Poisoning by Chloral.—Chloral is not a medicine which can be taken habitually with safety. For the habit of chloral-drinking is one which grows upon the person indulging, so that he cannot sleep without the drug, the result being the production of a condition, from chloral-drinking, as pitiable as that arising from either opium or spirits. The person suffers from languor and weakness, the heart's action becomes weakened, and he complains of shortness of breath on walking. The will becomes enfeebled, and there is profound melancholy. Red patches appear on the skin, especially on the face and about the nose, known as the 'chloral rash,' and sometimes there are swellings on other parts of the body, resembling scurvy.

The effects of an over-dose of chloral are swimming in the head, flushed face, closed but blood-shot eyes, and sometimes cramps in the legs. When the dose is still larger, there is insensibility from which the person cannot be roused, the pulse is quick, and the face flushed, afterwards becoming livid, while the pupils of the eyes are contracted, and the breathing is of a snoring character. The treatment is a mustard emetic (Recipe 54) if the patient can swallow, otherwise the throat should be tickled with a feather to excite vomiting. Mustard plasters should be applied to the calves of the legs; the feet, hands, and arms should be well rubbed; the warmth of the body should be maintained by blanket covering, and artificial respiration (*vide* p. 642) should be used.

A medical man would probably inject solution of atropia beneath the skin.

4. **CHLORODYNE** (*Chlorodyne*).—A dark-coloured thick fluid containing morphia, chloroform, Indian hemp, hydrocyanic acid, peppermint, and spirit. It is agreeable to the taste, and very useful in slight disorders, such as stomach spasms, flatulency, griping, also for simple bronchial and asthmatic affections. In the use of chlorodyne reference must be had both to the age of the patient and to the urgency of the symptoms, also to the effect desired to be produced. The following scale of doses may be adopted for adults :—

*Anodyne and Diaphoretic, 5 to 15 drops.*—In Coughs, Colds, Influenza, Agues.

*Sedative and Anti-Spasmodic, 10 to 25 drops.*—In Asthma, Bronchitis, Spasms, Cramp, Sea-sickness.

*Astringent, 15 to 30 drops.*—In Cholera, Dysentery, Diarrhœa, Colics.

FOR CHILDREN

| Age | Dose | Age | Dose |
|---|---|---|---|
| 1 month to 3 | 1 drop to 2 | 3 years to 5 | 3 drops to 8 |
| 3 months to 6 | 2 drops to 4 | 5 „ 8 | 4 „ 10 |
| 6 „ 12 | 2 „ 5 | 8 „ 12 | 8 „ 12 |
| 1 year to 3 | 3 „ 6 | 12 „ 16 | 10 „ 20 |

Chlorodyne may be taken in water, tea, or any convenient fluid, or in small quantities dropped on sugar, and repeated in diminished doses every two or three hours, until the desired effect is produced. Chlorodyne enters into Recipe 33.

*Caution.*—The chlorodyne bottle should be kept well corked, and be well shaken previous to use ; otherwise the thick portion falls, and an unequal dose results.

5. **DOVER'S POWDER**; **OPIUM AND IPECACUANHA POWDER, COMPOUND**, commonly called **DOVER'S POWDER** (*Pulvis Ipecacuanhæ Compositus*).—This medicine is placed under its popular name, 'Dover's Powder,' to render the

difference between ipecacuanha powder (*vide* p. 14) and *compound* ipecacuanha powder (ipecacuanha powder with opium—*Dover's powder*) more apparent. Compound ipecacuanha powder is of a light yellowish-grey colour. Containing both ipecacuanha and opium, also a considerable proportion of sulphate of potash, it is useful in a great variety of complaints, particularly in chest affections, and in maladies such as rheumatism, when action on the skin is desirable; the ipecacuanha and the opium mutually aiding the separate influence which is induced by each medicine. In malarious seasons or localities, when the bowels are disturbed with a feverish condition of system, a combination of Dover's powder and quinine is often very beneficial. After taking Dover's powder the patient should be kept warm, and to prevent nausea, which may arise from the ipecacuanha, nothing should be drunk for some little time. The dose for adults is 5 grains if given repeatedly; 10 grains if given at long intervals. For a child three months old, from a quarter to half a grain; after a year old, 1 grain; increasing the dose by a quarter of a grain for each year of age. Compound ipecacuanha powder contains 1 grain of opium and 1 grain of ipecacuanha in every 10 grains of the powder. When required for use the quantity must therefore be carefully weighed. Compound ipecacuanha powder enters into Recipes 17, 18.

6. **ETHER, NITROUS, SPIRITS OF,** or **SWEET SPIRITS OF NITRE** (*Spiritus Ætheris Nitrosi*).—A transparent liquid, with slight yellow tinge, affording an apple-like odour, and of sweet, sharp, cooling taste. It stimulates the skin, leading to increase of perspiration, and it acts on the kidneys, promoting the secretion of urine. It is thus useful in complaints such as colds, fevers, and inflammations, when there are dryness of the skin and scanty urine. The dose for an adult is from 30 to 60

minims. For a child six months old, 3 to 4 drops; one year old, 6 to 8 drops. Spirits of nitrous ether enter into Recipes 20, 30, 38, 50, 51, 52, 53, 55, 57.

7. **GINGER, TINCTURE OF, STRONG** (*Tinctura Zingiberis Fortior*).—Strong tincture of ginger, sometimes called *essence of ginger*, is of a bright, slightly yellowish colour. The principal use of tincture of ginger is as a warm stomachic, in diarrhœa, flatulence, and colicky pains, especially if accompanied by hysterical or nervous symptoms. It is also given with other medicines of a cold nature, as acids. It is useful, diluted with about 30 parts of water, as a gargle for sore-throat. The dose is from 5 to 20 drops for an adult. For a child one year old, from 1 to 4 drops. Tincture of ginger enters into Recipes 2, 32, 34, 37, 38, 43, 49, 55, 69, 101.

8. **IPECACUANHA POWDER** (*Pulvis Ipecacuanhæ*).—Powdered ipecacuanha is the pulverised root of the ipecacuanha plant. It is a pale brown powder, with faint nauseous odour. It is of importance that the powder should be fresh, as it soon deteriorates by keeping. In large doses ipecacuanha powder is the most valuable and safe of all vegetable emetics. In smaller doses it acts on the skin, exciting perspiration, and on the wind-pipe and tubes leading to the lungs, promoting expectoration. Ipecacuanha is used chiefly as an emetic; in large doses in the treatment of dysentery; and in smaller quantities in cough, bronchial, and lung affections. It is often useful in checking the vomiting of pregnancy. In exceptional instances ipecacuanha, or even the smell of it, excites cough, sneezing, and watering of the eyes and nose, pain in the forehead, and a feeling of oppression at the chest. The dose of powdered ipecacuanha for an adult is, as an emetic, from 20 to 30 grains; for a child of one year old, from 2½ to 3 grains. As an expectorant, or to act on the skin, 1 grain for an adult, and the twelfth

of a grain for a child. Powdered ipecacuanha enters into Recipes 12, 13, 17, 24, 58.

9. **IPECACUANHA WINE** (*Vinum Ipecacuanhæ*).—Ipecacuanha wine resembles sherry in appearance, and has a vinous, slightly bitter taste. Its action is the same as powdered ipecacuanha, viz. emetic in large doses, diaphoretic and expectorant (that is, increasing perspiration and expectoration) in small doses. Mixed with an equal quantity of water and converted into spray by an ordinary spray-producer, it is often found useful in chronic, bronchial, and asthmatic affections. Ipecacuanha wine, being a liquid, is better adapted for children than the powder. The dose of ipecacuanha wine *as an emetic* for an adult is from 6 to 8 drachms in a pint of warm water. For a child six months old, half a drachm in one ounce of water; at one year old, 1 drachm in two ounces of water, increasing the dose by a quarter of a drachm of tincture, and half an ounce of water, for each year of age; the dose to be repeated every quarter of an hour till vomiting results. To act on the skin, or to promote expectoration, from 10 to 20 minims for an adult. For a child 1 drop at one month old; 2 drops at six months old, increasing the dose by 1 drop for each year of age. Twenty minims of ipecacuanha wine are reputed to contain one grain of ipecacuanha, but the strength of the preparation varies, being often more powerful than the officinal computation. Ipecacuaha wine enters into Recipes 51, 57, 60.

10. **MAGNESIA, CITRATE OF, GRANULAR EFFERVESCENT** (*Magnesia Citras* [*Granular*]).—Is composed of light, white, rough-looking granules, of agreeable, slightly acid taste. Placed in water it effervesces briskly. One or two dessert-spoonfuls or more, put into a tumbler half full of water, will prove a mild but efficient aperient. For feeble persons, 20 drops of tincture of ginger may be added. A small tea-spoonful taken in a wine-glassful of

water will act both as an antacid and as a cooling draught. Half a tea-spoonful with twenty minims of spirits of nitric ether, in one ounce and a half of water, forms a cooling febrifuge draught which may be taken during the hot stage of fevers. A cooling and refreshing drink may be made by adding to a tumblerful of cold water, sweetened with sugar, a small quantity of the citrate. The absence of nauseous taste renders it a favourite aperient and febrifuge for children. At one year old the dose would be one-eighth of the above-mentioned quantities.

11. **OPIUM, CAMPHORATED TINCTURE OF**, commonly called **PAREGORIC** (*Tinctura Camphoræ composita cum Opio*).—A light-coloured liquid, made by macerating opium, benzoic acid, camphor, and anise, in spirits of wine. The combination of other drugs with opium renders this a very useful preparation for cough, bronchial irritation, hooping cough, and chest complaints generally, especially when a cough is hacking and wearisome, and expectoration scanty. It contains two grains of opium in every ounce of the tincture, and therefore must be carefully measured. The dose for an adult is from 30 minims to 1 drachm, and if used alone it may be taken on white sugar. It is, however, more efficacious in combination with other remedies, as spirits of nitrous ether, and ipecacuanha wine. The dose for a child one month old is 1 drop; at six months old, 3 drops; at one year old, 6 drops; 1 drop being added for each year of age up to twelve, and 2 drops afterwards up to twenty years of age. Camphorated tincture of opium enters into Recipes 56, 57, 59, 60, 62.

12. **PODOPHYLLUM RESIN PILLS, COMPOUND.**—As podophyllum is not carried in the medicine case (*vide* p. 2) it need not be described. Its action is aperient, exerting a special influence on the liver. Hence it is useful for constipation, for torpor of the liver, and for other chronic liver affections. It is seldom given alone, but

generally in combination with other medicines which add to its efficiency. Podophyllum resin has been chosen as the active ingredient of the only aperient pills carried in the small medicine case to accompany this volume, as being on the whole better adapted to the purpose than any other agent. (*Vide* p. 2, and the remarks attached to Recipe No. 1, Appendix.)

13. **QUININE, SULPHATE OF** (*Quiniæ Sulphas*).—Sulphate of quinine is made by submitting cinchona bark to a chemical action by sulphuric acid. Pure sulphate of quinine presents the appearance of silky, snow-white crystals of an intensely bitter taste, sparingly soluble in water, and imparting to it a peculiar bluish tint.

The following tests determine whether a specimen of quinine is pure or adulterated: It dissolves in pure sulphuric acid with a feeble yellowish tint. Ten grains, with 10 minims of dilute sulphuric acid and an ounce of water, should form a perfect solution. A reddish tiut with sulphuric acid indicates adulteration with salicin; a black tint evidences sugar. Heated to a red heat on the blade of a knife held over a spirit-lamp, it is entirely destroyed and disappears, leaving only a black mark.

The precise manner in which quinine acts is not thoroughly understood; but as a substance very much resembling quinine has been found in the healthy blood, it is possible quinine supplies some constituent to that fluid which is deficient, particularly in malarious febrile diseases. It dulls the sensibility of the nervous system, and renders the nerves less susceptible to malarious influences. It exerts a certain power in reducing the temperature of the body. It has also an antiseptic power and arrests putrefaction. In addition to the influences exerted on the general system, quinine has also a well-ascertained influence over the digestive organs. It gives rise to a slight increase of the flow of gastric juice into the stomach, and of other secretions into the intestines.

Quinine will sometimes act on the womb, so that it should be given with caution to pregnant women; and not at all if there is any peculiar susceptibility (as noted below) to the influence of quinine.

Quinine acts very differently on various constitutions, some persons taking large doses without appreciable effect, others suffering more or less from various unpleasant effects after taking very small doses. These effects are: singing in the ears, noises in the head, deafness, headache, flushed face, bloodshot eyes, dimness of sight, eruptions on the skin resembling 'nettle-rash,' sore-throat, difficulty of breathing. In exceptional cases even a grain of quinine has been known to excite such results. Or, one too large dose may act as a succession of smaller, and cause such unpleasant symptoms. These effects of large or repeated doses of quinine are known as 'cinchonism.' They generally pass off altogether in a few days, but sometimes permanent singing in the ears or slight deafness remains.

The principal uses of quinine are as a remedy for so-called malarious fevers; for neuralgic or rheumatic affections, especially when they assume a periodical form, recurring at intervals of hours or days; and as a general and digestive tonic, in various forms of debility and dyspepsia. The influence excited on the digestive organs, together with the power of retarding putrefaction, before alluded to, renders quinine serviceable in various forms of dyspepsia marked by flatulence and acidity, and in all cases of weak digestion, especially during the convalescence from acute diseases.

Quinine is also useful as a prophylactic, or preventive of malarious diseases. During unhealthy seasons, or in malarious localities, persons would do well to take a grain or two of quinine daily, either as Recipes 67, 69, 76, or in a little sherry wine.

As a rule, quinine should not be given until the bowels, if costive, have been cleared by laxative medicine.

Regarding the employment of quinine in fevers, the rule that the bowels should be previously opened holds good. Also, quinine should not be ordinarily given during either the cold or hot stages of fever. Except under medical advice, it will only be right to prescribe quinine when the fever has abated, when perspiration has commenced, and when the pulse is soft and the skin cool. It should not be given (except under medical advice) when there is headache, high fever, quick pulse, and dry skin. But as soon as perspiration occurs, presuming the bowels in proper condition, quinine may be administered with advantage. It is usually given in solution with lemon-juice or sulphuric acid (Recipes 67, 69). But when the taste is very objectionable to the patient, or when irritability of the stomach exists, it may be used in the form of pills made up with a little gum-arabic. But quinine pills should always be freshly made, as if kept more than a week or so they become hard and useless. It sometimes happens that quinine will not produce its full effect until the whole system has been alkalised, and it is therefore advisable to give, as well as quinine, during fevers, some alkaline medicine, as Recipe 35 or 36, or citrate of magnesia (*vide* p. 15). Sufficient quinine will have been taken when singing, or other noises in the ears, or slight deafness occurs, when the medicine should be reduced in quantity, or altogether stopped. The dose of quinine given repeated during fevers is for adults from 5 to 10 grains, or a larger amount may be given at one time, up to 15 or 20 grains, when it is desired to attempt to check a fever. For children, from half a grain upwards is the dose, according to the table of proportions (*vide* p. 6), counting the maximum adult dose at 10 grains or half a scruple. When quinine is given to aid digestion, or as a tonic for debility, 2 or 3 grains will be the suitable dose for an adult.

Quinine enters into Recipes 3, 17, 18, 66, 67, 69, 76.

Cinchona bark contains other matters, besides quinine, which have an influence over malarious fevers. A preparation called *Cinchona febrifuge*, or *mixed cinchona alkaloids*, is manufactured at the Government cinchona plantations in India, which may be used in most cases when quinine is required, the only objection being that in some people nausea follows taking it in large doses. It is best given with sulphuric acid, and may be substituted for the quinine in Recipe 60 when quinine is not available.

**14. SODA, SULPHATE OF** (*Sodæ Sulphas*).—Sulphate of soda, better known as 'Glauber's salt,' usually occurs in the form of oblique, rhombic, transparent prisms; but sometimes it is seen in a less pure condition in the shape of small acicular crystals. Sulphate of soda is a saline purgative, producing watery stools, and acting, to a slight degree, on the kidneys. Like many other salines, when given in large doses, it slightly lowers the pulse, weakens the blood, and depresses the system. Hence it is termed a cooling purgative, and is adapted for use in inflammations, excepting inflammation of the bowels, and in fevers. With senna it may be used, instead of the more nauseous and powerful purgative *sulphate of magnesia* or 'Epsom salts,' to form a combination in common use known as 'black draught.' Being less powerful in its action and less nauseous than Epsom salts, it is more fitted for use by delicate persons, and in all cases where a mild aperient is desirable. By increasing the quantity it acts as energetically and less unpleasantly than 'salts,' and is therefore prescribed in this manual instead of the latter medicine. The success of Carlsbad, Friedrichshall, and Hunyadi Janos water, in the treatment of various diseases, depends much on the sulphate of soda contained in these mineral waters; and, if available, they may often be used instead of sulphate of soda, the water last mentioned having the advantage of being nearly tasteless. The dose of sulphate of soda for an adult is from half an ounce to one ounce in water.

and the taste may be much disguised by a tea-spoonful of lemon-juice, or by 8 or 10 drops of *dilute* sulphuric acid. It should be kept in a stoppered bottle. Sulphate of soda enters into Recipes 2, 3, 4, 26, 73.

The appearance, properties, doses, and principal uses of the medicines which are recommended as procurable in the bazaars are now noted.

1. **ALUM.** Hindustanee: *Phitkari.*—When pure, alum is a colourless, crystalline, semi-transparent mass, having an acid, sweetish, astringent taste. The bazaar alum, when not pure, may be rendered fit for medicinal purposes by dissolving it in distilled water, straining, and evaporating the solution so as to obtain crystals of alum, which form as the water evaporates or 'dries up.' If distilled water cannot be obtained, water which has been boiled should be used. Alum is a powerful astringent causing the tissues with which it comes in contact to shrink and contract, and thus closing the orifices of bleeding or secreting vessels and ducts. It is used as a lotion for ulcers when there is fear of 'proud flesh'; as a gargle for sore or ulcerated throats; as an application to the eyes in ophthalmia; as a wash for sore nipples; and as an injection. It is seldom used internally, but it is beneficial in diarrhœa and other chronic discharges. Alum enters into Recipes 42, 48, 97, 100.

2. **AMMONIUM, CHLORIDE OF**; or **HYDROCHLORATE OF AMMONIA**, commonly called *Sal-Ammoniac.* Hind.: *Naushadur* or *Nissadel.*—It occurs in the form of colourless, inodorous, translucent, tough, fibrous masses, difficult to pulverise, but soluble in water, and of a salt cold taste. When taken internally in eight- or ten-grain doses daily, it exerts an alterative effect. In large doses it is stimulant, acting chiefly on the glandular structures. It has been used with advantage in chronic affections of

the liver and spleen, in neuralgic affections of the head, in rheumatic affections, and in amenorrhœa. Locally, it is applied as a lotion to enlarged glands or swellings. Its principal use is the formation with nitre of a cooling lotion or a freezing mixture. (*Vide* Recipe 83.)

3. **ASSAFŒTIDA** (*Assafœtida*). Hind.: *Hing.*—Assafœtida is the gum resin of a plant growing in Persia and Northern India. It occurs in the form of irregular masses partly composed of 'tears,' of a dark pink, or, if long kept, of a dull yellow colour. Assafœtida is stimulant and antispasmodic, and is useful in hysteria, flatulence, and in the nervous affections of females. The dose is from 5 to 10 grains, but it is generally given in combination with other remedies, and is mostly used as an injection. In exceptional instances, assafœtida excites giddiness or even fainting. It is rarely used for children. Assafœtida enters into Recipe 105.

4. **BAEL** (*Ægle Marmelos,* called also *Stone Apple*). Hind.: *Bael geerie.*—A tree growing in India, the fruit of which is used medicinally. The fruit is about the size of an orange, with a hard woody rind, divided inside into ten or fifteen cells, containing a quantity of seeds and tenacious transparent pulp. It has a mild turpentine-like smell and taste. It contains tannic acid, and therefore acts as an astringent to the bowels, and is also slightly aperient; a union of qualities not found in other astringents. It is useful in chronic diarrhœa and dysentery. Also in that irregularity of the bowels so often presenting in children, marked by alternations of diarrhœa and constipation. The decoction and the syrup are the best forms for taking bael.

*The decoction* is made as follows: Boil 3 ounces of the dried fruit—or, if obtainable, 1½ ounce of the half-ripe fruit, discarding rind and seeds—in a pint of water until it evaporates to one half-pint. The dose is a wine-glassful for an adult three or four times daily. *Syrup of bael* is prepared by adding a wine-glassful of water and a tea-spoonful of sugar to the soft juicy part of half a moderate-sized bael, rejecting the stringy pieces. This may be taken three times a day.

5. **CASTOR OIL** (*Oleum Ricini*). Hind.: *Rindee ka Tail.*—Castor oil is prepared by pressure from the seeds of the castor-oil plant. It is a mild but efficient purgative. But care should be taken that the oil used is fresh, as if at all rancid, it causes irritation, griping, and sometimes troublesome diarrhœa. As it rarely, when fresh and good, causes griping or irritation, it is preferred for delicate persons and pregnant women, or for those labouring under disease of internal organs, forbidding the use of any powerful cathartic. In ordinary constipation it is also a good aperient, for the dose, when repeated, may be gradually lessened; whereas other purgatives become less active the longer they are used, and increased quantities are necessary. The nauseous taste of castor oil may be much disguised by taking a little lemon-juice into the mouth beforehand, or by taking it in peppermint water, or by mixing with an equal quantity of glycerine and flavouring with cinnamon. The dose is half an ounce to an ounce for adults, and from half a drachm to 2 drachms for children. It is also used as an injection. Castor oil enters into Recipes 105, 106.

6. **CAMPHOR** (*Camphora*). Hind.: *Kafoor.*—Camphor is the concrete volatile oil of a tree growing in China and Japan. It occurs as white translucent masses, of a crystalline structure, powerful odour, and pungent taste, followed by a sensation of cold. It has a stimulating effect on the system, also increasing the action of the skin, and thereby promoting perspiration. In larger doses it acts as a sedative antispasmodic. It has been given for a number of diseases, as hysteria, asthma, rheumatism, gout, cholera, cold in the head, hooping-cough, palpitations, but with doubtful efficacy in some.

The dose of camphor for an adult is from 2 to 3 or 4 grains. Camphor enters into Recipes 40, 41, 58, 76.

*Preparations of camphor*, which may be made as required, are CAMPHOR WATER (*Mistura Camphoræ*) and SPIRITS OF CAMPHOR (*Spiritus Camphoræ*). *Camphor water* is prepared by putting a few lumps of camphor into a bottle of distilled water and allowing it to stand for a few hours. Camphor is but slightly soluble in water, so that the latter will only absorb a certain quantity of the former. Camphor water is not used as a medicine by itself, but it is useful in compounding medicines, when camphor water may be employed instead of plain water. By compounding medicines with camphor water, attention to the purity of the water is additionally secured. *Spirits of camphor* is prepared by dissolving 1 drachm of camphor in 1 ounce and 1 drachm of rectified spirits of wine. Spirits of camphor, taken hourly in 5-drop doses, will, if used at the commencement, often arrest a cold in the head. It is also very useful in a variety of maladies, when a stimulant is required, as in the latter stages of fever, in palpitation of the heart, in hooping-cough, in asthma, in hysteria, and in painful menstruation. It is also a good external application to sprains, bruises, and for chronic rheumatism. Applied frequently, and allowed to dry on sluggish boils, it will often check their progress. The dose for an adult is from 10 to 30 minims in half a wine-glassful of water. When added to water, a white deposit forms.

7. **IRON, SULPHATE OF** (*Ferri Sulphas*), commonly known as *Copperas* or *Green Vitriol.* Hind.: *Hera Kusees.*— Sulphate of iron has the appearance of green crystalline masses, with faint odour and ink-like taste. All the compounds of iron, though they differ in strength, possess nearly the same medicinal properties; but some are more astringent than others. The principal use of iron preparations is in cases of debility accompanied by pallor, especially occurring in the female sex, and particularly in young girls. The red colour of the blood is due to a certain proportion of red corpuscles or granules which that fluid should contain, and which have iron as one of their chemical constituent parts. When these red corpuscles, which may be seen under the microscope, sink in quantity below the normal proportion, they are increased by giving iron as a medicine, and with their increase there is return-

ing colour, health, and strength. Iron has also an influence, indirectly, over the monthly discharges of women, and is therefore often useful in irregularities of this kind. As a rule, before giving any preparation of iron, the bowels should be acted upon by purgative medicines. It should be recollected that all preparations of iron colour the stools more or less black. It is also well to know that from peculiar idiosyncrasy (*vide* p. 7) some *few* persons cannot take iron in any form without suffering from indigestion, or pain and fulness in the head. Such symptoms following the use of iron would indicate its employment in smaller doses, or, if necessary, the stopping of the medicine altogether. After taking iron the móuth should be well washed, to prevent discoloration of the teeth.

Sulphate of iron, besides possessing the ordinary action of iron salts, is also powerfully astringent; but it may be given in most cases when iron is required. The dose for an adult is from 2 to 5 grains in 2 or 3 ounces of water; for a child, from one-sixth to half a grain in a little water. It is sometimes used externally, as an application to indolent sores, when there is a growth of flabby, pale-looking 'proud flesh,' on which it acts if applied in substance as an 'escharotic' or caustic; if used in solution it acts less strongly, or as a stimulant. Sulphate of iron is also used for disinfecting purposes (*vide* Appendix No. 128). Sulphate of iron enters into Recipes 3, 15, 72, 73.

8. **POMEGRANATE** (*Punica Granatum.*) Hind.: *Anar.*—Two parts of the pomegranate tree are used medicinally, in the form of decoctions—viz. the root bark, and the rind of the fruit, both fresh and dried. The dried root bark occurs in the form of quills or fragments of a greyish yellow colour externally, and yellow internally, without odour, but of an astringent, slightly bitter taste. The dried rind appears as more or less curved fragments of a

dark brown colour, and taste similar to that of the bark. The principal uses of the root bark decoction are for the destruction of tape-worm, as an astringent in chronic diarrhœa and dysentery, and as a gargle for ulcerated mouth. A decoction of the pomegranate rind is, however, a better remedy for dysentery or diarrhœa, and is also a good astringent for relaxed or sore throat.

The decoctions are made as follows: Take of fresh pomegranate root bark, sliced, 2 ounces (or dried, 3 ounces). Water, 2 pints. Boil down to a pint and strain. To be used for tape-worm, as mentioned under that heading. For bowel complaints, 1 ounce three times a day. Decoction of pomegranate rind is made in the same manner, and the dose is 1 to 1½ ounce thrice daily. A decoction made with milk instead of water is sometimes efficacious in bowel complaints. The decoction may be rendered more palatable by the addition of cloves or other aromatics. These decoctions of pomegranate root bark and fruit rind are especially efficacious in the bowel complaints of the natives of India.

9. **POTASH, NITRATE OF,** commonly called **SALT-PETRE** (*Potassæ Nitras*). Hind.: *Shora*.—Nitrate of potash consists of white crystalline masses, possessing a saline cooling taste. It exists in a natural state in the soil of many parts of India. Specimens found in the bazaars are sometimes not sufficiently pure for internal medicinal use, but it may be readily cleansed by dissolving it in hot water, straining, and setting the solution aside to crystallise. It stimulates the skin and kidneys, increasing perspiration and flow of urine, and so cooling the body. It is very useful in fevers, in inflammatory affections, in common colds, in rheumatism, in bronchitis, and in many other diseased conditions. The dose for an adult is from 8 to 20 grains; for a child, according to the table at p. 6, taking 20 grains as the maximum. A good cooling drink for fever may be composed of nitre 2 drachms, the juice of two limes, and water 2 pints, with a little sugar. Nitrate of potash enters into Recipes 37, 50, 52, 53, 83, 92.

10. **SENNA LEAVES** (*Sennæ Alexandrinæ Folia.*)

Hind.: *Senna Mukkee.*—The Alexandria or Egyptian senna is the best; the leaf is about one inch in length, greyish-green in colour, unequal at the base, of faint odour, and of sweetish taste. The leaf of the Indian senna (Tinnevelly) is nearly two inches long, acute in shape, also unequal at the base, green in colour, and of sweet taste. Senna is often adulterated with a very similar-looking leaf of the *Solenostemma Argel* (native name, *Argel*). But these leaves are thicker and stiffer than senna; they are equal at the base and bitterish, in taste. Both Indian senna and *Argel* are purgative like Egyptian senna, but they gripe, which Alexandria senna rarely does. Senna is a safe and efficient purgative, well adapted for childhood, for old age, for pregnant females and for delicate persons. But it is not so well adapted for nursing women, as it may render the milk purgative, and so cause colic in the child. The taste of senna may be much disguised by sweetening the infusion and adding milk, when it much resembles ordinary tea. Infusion of senna is made by steeping 1 ounce of senna and 30 grains of ginger in 10 ounces of boiling water for one hour, and then straining. The dose for an adult is from 1 to 2 ounces. Infusion of senna with Epsom salts constitutes the once much-used 'black draught.'

A simple, quickly prepared purgative for children may be made thus: Take of senna leaves a tea-spoonful; boiling water 4 ounces. Infuse for ten minutes. Pour off into a teacup and sweeten with sugar, and let the child drink it off, fasting, in the morning. It may be used for a child of three or four years of age.

11. **STRAMONIUM** (*Dhatura Stramonium*). Hind.: *Dhatura.*—The leaves and stems of the dhatura—a plant growing in India—are used medicinally. The seeds are poisonous, and very like capsicum seeds. The leaves are large, ovate, deeply cut, of a heavy odour, and of a

mawkish, faintly bitter, nauseous taste. They are only recommended for smoking to check asthma (*vide* p. 62).

A preparation of dhatura is also used as an antidote to poisoning by opium. But as this requires some time to prepare, it cannot be available except in hospitals or dispensaries where it is kept ready-made.

12. **SULPHUR** (*Sulphur Sublimatum*). Hind.: *Ghunduk*.—Sulphur employed in medicine is called flowers of sulphur, and is used both as an internal and an external agent. As an internal medicine it is laxative and purgative, being principally given to act on the bowels, when there are piles, or blotches and pimples on the skin. The dose for an adult is from 20 to 60 grains; for a child from 2 to 5 grains. Externally it enters into the composition of ointments, particularly for itch. Sulphur enters into Recipe 92.

Of the foregoing medicines, the following are manufactured into a very portable and palatable form termed tabloids by Messrs. Burroughs, Wellcome & Co., Snow Hill Buildings, London, who have prepared a case to accompany this volume. These tabloids may be conveniently substituted for the ordinary remedies:—

| | |
|---|---|
| Bromide of potassium . . . | 5- and 10-grain tablets |
| Chloral . . . . . . | 5-grain tabloids |
| Dover's powder . . . . | 5-grain tabloids |
| Ginger, essence of . . . | 5- and 10-grain tabloids |
| Ipecacuanha powder . . . | 5-grain tabloids; for infants, $\frac{1}{10}$ grain |
| Opium, camphorated tincture of (Paregoric) . . . . | 15-minim tabloids |
| Podophyllum resin pills compound | in tabloid form |
| Quinine . . . . . | 1-, 2-, 3-, and 5-grain tabloids |
| Sal-volatile . . . . . | tabloids of carbonate of ammonia equivalent to 1 drachm of sal-volatile |
| Ammonium chloride . . . | 3-, 5-, and 10-grain tabloids |
| Iron, sulphate of . . . . | 3-grain tabloids |
| Potash, nitrate of . . . | 5-grain tabloids |
| Soda, sulphate of . . . | half-drachm tabloids |

# CHAPTER II

## *DISEASES*

### INTRODUCTORY REMARKS

GREAT ignorance almost necessarily prevails respecting the locality or site within the body of most internal parts;

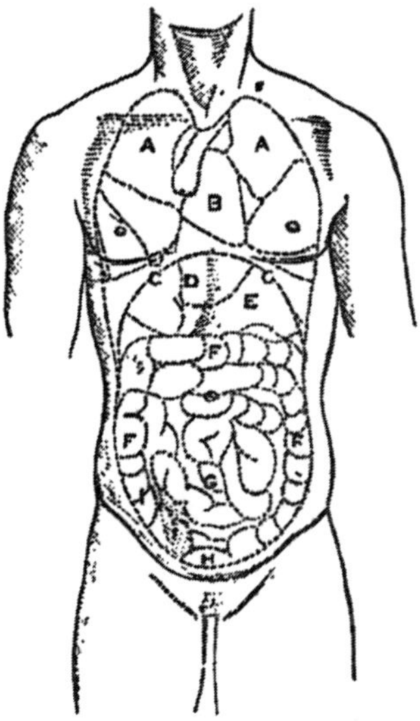


THE FRONT OF THE BODY, SHOWING,

A A, The Lungs, one on each side.
B, The Heart enclosed in its bag, with the great blood-vessels proceeding from the upper part.
C C, The Diaphragm, or division between the chest, and the bowels, liver and stomach.
D, The Liver, partly covered by the Diaphragm.
E, The Stomach, partly covered by the Liver and Diaphragm.
F F F, The Large Intestine, passing across the centre, down the left side, and up the right.
G, The Small Intestines.
H, The Bladder in the Male, and Womb in the Female.
I, The Cæcum.

a knowledge only to be thoroughly acquired by actual dissection, although some useful idea of the interior arrangement of organs may be obtained from plates. Therefore, before proceeding to describe the symptoms and treatment of diseases, the introduction of the accom-

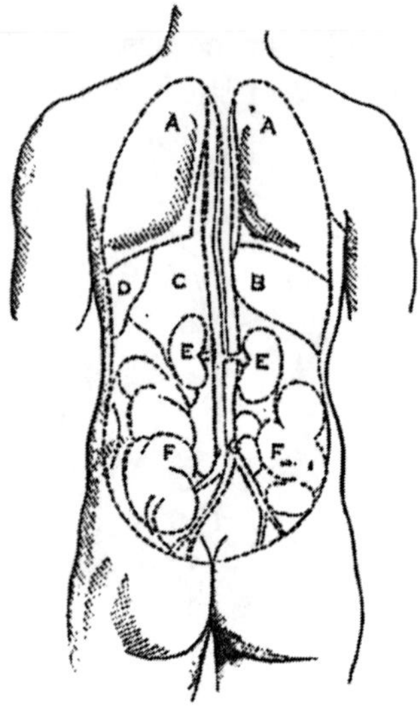


THE BACK OF THE BODY, SHOWING,

A A, The Posterior part of the Lungs.
B, The Back part of the Liver.
C, The Stomach.
D, The Spleen.
The mark or line above B, C, D, is the Diaphragm, which is supposed to be lifted up in order to show the position of the three organs last named, as they appear at the back.
E E, The Kidneys.
F F, The Large Intestines ascending on the right side, descending on the left.
G, The course of the large artery and vein supplying all the organs with blood.

panying rough diagrams, showing the position of the principal internal organs, appears desirable. An examination of the sketches will facilitate the formation of an opinion regarding the locality of any particular pain.

*Certain facts connected with the pulse, with the breathing or respiration, with the temperature of the body, and with the tongue*, are of the utmost importance, and should be borne in mind when attempting to discover the nature of, or to treat disease (*vide* also p. 37).

**THE PULSE.**—The pulse is caused by the beating of the vessels (called *arteries*, *vide* p. 500) conveying the blood from the heart to all parts of the body. For convenience it is generally felt at the wrists, but may be counted in the neck, or at the thigh, or wherever there is an artery near the surface of the body. The number of beats per minute, in the healthy state, varies according to age, but may be generally accepted as follows:—

| | | |
|---|---|---|
| At birth and till end of the first year of age . | 140 | beats per minute |
| Infancy and till end of the third year . | . 120 | „ |
| Childhood or till end of the sixth year . | . 106 | „ |
| Youth or till end of the seventeenth year | . 90 | „ |
| Adult age or till end of the fiftieth year | . 75 | „ |
| Old age . . . . . . . . | . 70 | „ |

The pulse may vary from this standard to some extent, and there are few persons in whom the pulse may be extraordinarily slow, or the reverse, and this naturally, without deviation from health. But as a rule, if the pulse, without previous bodily exertion (which always increases its action), is quicker by eight or ten beats than the standard, or a similar number of beats lower, there is something wrong. If higher, there will be more or less of *feverishness* present; if lower, there will be a want of tone, or *vitality* below *par*.

The educated fingers of the physician also convey, through the sense of touch, much information derived from the peculiar sensation afforded by the pulse, irrespective of the actual frequency of the beats. Thus, a *frequent* pulse, also feeling to the fingers *large and soft*, is indicative of the premonitory stages of febrile diseases. A *frequent, hard, and full* pulse accompanies inflammations. A pulse increasing in frequency after meals, or in the *evening*, indicates hectic fever. Disease of the heart is often signified by an *irregular, jerking,* or *vibrating* pulse. An *intermittent* pulse may also attend heart-disease, but is often caused by indigestion, by drinking too much tea, or by smoking. A weak, *thread-like* pulse occurs in rapidly exhausting diseases, as cholera, or as a consequence of bleeding.

Physicians also judge of the pulse by a small delicate machine, called the *sphygmograph,* which traces the beatings of the pulse on paper.

**THE BREATHING, or RESPIRATORY MOVEMENT.**—Breathing is consequent on the expansion and contraction of the lungs, as the air passes into, and out from, those organs. There should be no difference in the movements of the two sides of the chest. Breathing, like the pulse, is quickened by bodily exertion, and also affected by mental excitement. The number of breaths taken by a healthy adult, in a state of repose both of body and mind, is about one for every four beats of the pulse, but varies in different people from fifteen to eighteen per minute. As with the pulse, there are persons occasionally met with in whom the breathing may be either slower or quicker than the standard; but, as a rule, deviation from the numbers given during a state of rest indicates disease. If higher, there will generally be present some malady either directly or indirectly affecting the lungs; if lower, there will be debility, or loss of vital power, or nervous shock.

The breathing of children differs in some characteristics from that of adults. The bowels move more than in adults, and the breathing is much quicker, corresponding with the more rapid rate of the pulse (*vide* p. 31). Thus, a child up to two years of age breathes 35 times in a minute; from two years old to nine, 18 times during sleep, and about 23 when awake; from nine years to fifteen, 18 times during sleep, and 20 when awake.

Indications of diseased conditions may also be derived from the *smell of the breath.* In diabetes, the breath has a faint, apple-like odour; in gastric disorders, especially of children, there is a sour smell; in some forms of dyspepsia, a smell of sulphuretted hydrogen; in bladder and kidney affections, an ammoniacal or urinous odour; from excess in spirituous liquors, a sour and vitriol-like smell.

**THE TEMPERATURE OF THE BODY.**—The bodily temperature, as affected in disease, is instructive, and may be easily tested by a thermometer constructed for the purpose, and which may be inclosed in a case, to prevent injury to the glass. This instrument, known as the *clinical thermometer*, is self-registering. If it were not so, leaning over the patient's body would be necessary for the purpose of reading the scale while in contact with the skin, which is inconvenient, disagreeable, and, in infectious diseases, dangerous. At the top of the ordinary column of mercury, and separated from it, there is a little piece which has been purposely detached, to serve as an *index*. Before taking the temperature, this index should be *gently* shaken down to about 96°. This may be done by holding the thermometer in the right hand, and then tapping that hand against the other. The constriction at the lower part of the instrument is to prevent the index being accidentally shaken into the bulb. When the mercury rises it drives this index before it, and when the mercury falls the index remains, showing by its *upper* surface the highest temperature reached. The manner in which the clinical thermometer is graduated, and the method of reading it off, are simple. The scale is shown on p. 34. Each of the longer lines indicates a degree, although, as a matter of convenience, only every fifth degree is numbered. The spaces between the degrees are divided into fifths, by smaller lines. It is more easy to read the figures on a thermometer with a flat back.

The average temperature of the surface of the human body in a condition of health and repose is 98·4° Fahr. In the mouth it is 99·5°. The temperature of the blood is 100°. A rising of the temperature of the surface of the body above 99·5°, or a falling below 97·3°, are sure signs of some kind of disease when such variations are persistent. The fall is significant of depressed vitality, either from rapidly exhausting diseases, or from long-continued maladies. The rise is indicative of fever, or of some disease accompanied by fever. All this is shown by the accompanying woodcut of a clinical thermometer.

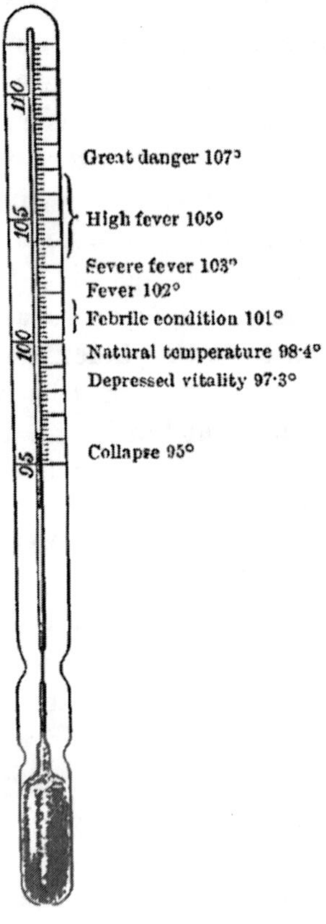


Previously to using it the thermometer should be slightly warmed, but not so much as to send the mercury above the natural temperature of 98·4°. The temperature must not be taken by letting the patient hold the instrument in the hand, as the heat of the palms varies considerably. The hands (of *Indians* especially) are often cold and moist, and would therefore show a lower degree of temperature than that of the body; while under some other conditions, as masked malarious fever (*vide* p. 266), and sometimes from dyspepsia, the palms burn, and would show a higher temperature. As the most convenient place, the thermometer is generally introduced into the armpit. The armpit should be wiped dry, and then the bulb of the instrument should be placed in the centre of the armpit beneath the clothing, and the arm should be held closely to the side, with the hand lying on the chest, pointing towards the opposite shoulder, so that the skin may perfectly surround the bulb of the instrument. It should be kept in this position for three or four minutes, and during the time it should not be exposed to the action of a punkah. It should then be removed, and the point to which the mercury has risen in the graduated tube should be immediately read off. In doing so the observer should not allow the bulb to come in contact with his own hand, which might alter the reading of so sensitive an instrument. For recording the readings it is best to be provided with a chart printed for the purpose. A thermometer should always be washed after being used, and in contagious diseases carbolic acid solution (Recipe 117) should be used for this purpose.

Watch-shaped clinical thermometers have been invented, but, although less liable to break, they are not quite so accurate as the tubular-shaped.

Each disease which runs a definite course, as scarlet fever, measles, small-pox, typhoid fever, rheumatic fever, &c., has a more or less characteristic range of temperature. The observations with a clinical thermometer ought to be continued regularly, and taken at the same hours every day throughout the sickness. The most useful observations are those taken about eight in the morning, and in the evening. The sensations of heat and cold, as felt by patients, do not always coincide with such observations. In fever, chilliness is often complained of when the body is really hotter than natural, and the patient may feel hot when really cold. Hysteria often simulates inflammatory disease; but the temperature of hysterical patients is not increased, whereas that of persons suffering from inflammatory disease is always raised.

*The Temperature of Children* is usually a very little higher than that of adults; and a word of caution is necessary. In children the temperature sometimes increases rapidly, probably from stomach derangement, when there is nothing serious the matter. Care, therefore, should be taken not to form a hasty conclusion of some serious disease simply because the thermometer indicates much heat of surface, which often falls with equal rapidity. If, however, the deviation from the healthy standard continues more than twelve hours, there is almost certainty that an illness is commencing.

RELATION OF THE PULSE, RESPIRATION, AND TEMPERATURE.—An increase of temperature of one degree above the natural standard corresponds with an increase of the pulse of about ten beats per minute, and of two or three respirations per minute. Thus, if the natural pulse and temperature were respectively 75 beats in the minute and 98·4°, while the number of respirations was 18, an elevation of the temperature to 100 would probably bring up the pulse to 90 or 95, and the respirations to about 23.

**THE TONGUE.**—This organ presents peculiarities in many maladies, of which the following are the principal:—

1. *A pale, white, flabby, broad, tremulous tongue, indented by the teeth,* denotes a weak, debilitated condition of system, and a watery state of the blood, as occurs in *anæmia.*

2. *A florid redness of the tongue* denotes *plethora*, or too full a condition of the system. When there are symptoms of dyspepsia present, it denotes a similar condition of the coats of the stomach.

3. *A livid or purplish colour of the tongue* occurs in various diseases of the chest, when there is obstruction to the circulation of blood in the lungs.

4. *A furred tongue* may not indicate disease, some persons always having it even when in good health, particularly in the morning. Or a furred tongue may arise from local causes, as inflammation in the mouth, throat, or gums. When not referable to such causes, a furred

and dry tongue denotes some kind of febrile affection. Thus it is covered with a cream-like fur in severe inflammations, in acute rheumatism, and in fevers. In the advanced stages of these diseases a thick brown or black coating collects, and the tongue is dry, parched, and cracked. When bright red points show through the fur (the tongue looking like a ripe strawberry, or as if sprinkled with cayenne pepper), it indicates scarlet fever, which has been first detected by this symptom. When jaundice is present the tongue is often coloured yellow from bile. When during acute diseases, as fevers, the fur slowly clears away from the tip and edges, and thins on the upper part, it denotes recovery. When the fur separates in flakes, leaving a smooth, red, glossy, and moist surface, it indicates some internal mischief and lingering convalescence.

5. *A tongue with red edges furred in the middle* and at the base indicates dyspepsia. If *tremulous* when protruded from the mouth, it signifies intemperance.

6. *A tongue furred in the centre, with red tip and edges,* is characteristic of hectic fever.

7. *Loss of the power of motion of the tongue,* or its being drawn aside when protruded, are bad symptoms in paralysis, fevers, or other acute disorders.

In addition to the indications of the condition of patients to be obtained from the *Pulse, Breathing, Temperature,* and *Tongue,* various other symptoms occur, having more or less reference to the existence of many diseases of which they are the consequence or signs. These symptoms are :—1. *Loss of appetite* (*vide* p. 59). 2. *Cough* (p. 158). 3. *Delirium* (p. 159). 4. *Fever* (p. 238). 5. *Giddiness* (p. 277). 6. *Headache* (p. 291). 7. *Pain* (p. 342). 8. *Palpitation* (p. 297). 9. *Shivering* (p. 386). 10. *Sore-throat* (p. 442). 11. *Thirst* (p. 442). 12. *Urinary Conditions* (p. 453). 13. *Vomiting* (p. 459).

Although the foregoing symptoms are usually prominent *as indications of the diseases to which they point*, it should be understood that *disease differs in different people*, just as the action of medicines has been shown to vary (*vide* p. 7). Sex, habit, age, climate, temperament, race, and idiosyncrasy exert influences which tend to render similar diseases in different people varied in their characteristics; sometimes one class of symptoms being more prominent, sometimes another. In tropical climates the great characteristics are, the tendency to a remittent form of the accompanying fever, and to rapid failure of the vital powers. From the above it will be evident that the aim of the physician must be the treatment of each individual case in accordance with the peculiar symptoms presenting; and it should be equally evident that the popular idea of *this* medicine for *that* disease must be erroneous, and hence that *patent* medicines vaunted to cure all, or even many maladies in all persons, *must* be unequal to so desirable a result.

**Climacteric Periods.**—There is probably some truth in the popular belief that each seventh day is a critical period in fevers. Also, that the odd numbers, 3, 5, 7, 9, multiplied by 7 are climacteric years, especially 49 in women and 63 in men.

**Signs of Death.**—As there are instances of persons supposed to be dead recovering, it is desirable to note the *signs of death*. These are:—1. *Cessation of the circulation*: the pulse cannot be felt, and the beating of the heart cannot be felt or heard. 2. *Cessation of respiration*: the chest does not move, a feather held to the mouth is not stirred, and a looking-glass is not made dim by the breath. But none of these signs are infallible, as instances are known of persons being able to suspend circulation and respiration, or at least to carry on these processes so slightly that they could not be recognised. 3. *Coldness of the body, commencing at the extremities*: not infallible, as after death from cholera the temperature sometimes rises. 4. *Rigidity of the limbs coming on gradually*: not infallible, as after death from some maladies it is long in appearing, and in the cataleptic condition rigidity may be counterfeited. 5. *Death-like stillness*: not infallible, as after death from cholera startings of the limbs sometimes occur. 6. *Eyes dull, flaccid, and shrunken*: not infallible, as after death from some poisons the eyes remain bright for a long time. 7. *Absence of a red colour in semi-transparent parts*, as, for instance, the sides of the fingers when viewed with a powerful light behind. 8. *Absence of muscular contraction* on an electric or galvanic current being applied. 9. *Absence of a blister* on touching the skin with very hot iron, but not sufficiently hot to destroy the skin. Sufficient heat being applied to the skin during life, or within a few minutes after death, produces a blister containing water with a line of redness round. Heat applied after death produces a blister containing air except in dropsical bodies. 10. *On opening a vein water oozes out instead of blood.* None of these latter tests are to be regarded as infallible, as mistakes may occur in their application and in the appreciation of results. 11. *Commencement of putrefactive changes*, usually first seen over the bowels: certain. It will thus be seen that none of the signs of death, excepting the last, are in themselves certain evidence of life having ceased. But taken altogether, the evidence is conclusive.

## DISEASES

**ABSCESS.**—This term is applied to a painful and inflamed swelling, which, after a certain course—in most instances rapid, in others slow—terminates in a discharge of a yellowish creamy fluid called *pus*, or popularly 'matter.' Abscess may present in any part of the body: a gumboil, a whitlow, and the painful swelling sometimes formed in the female breast during suckling, are all instances of abscess. Abscess may also attack some internal organ, as the brain or liver. Abscess differs from boils in *not* containing dead flesh, or a central hard part, commonly called the 'core.' Abscess often arises from local injury; but it may originate from cold, or without any assignable cause, or be connected with want, scorbutic, scrofulous, syphilitic, or other morbid or debilitated conditions.

It is necessary to *distinguish those swellings which are much inflamed, very painful, and rapid in their course from those which grow slowly and gently, and with little, if any, redness of the skin.* The symptoms of the *first* variety, or of an *acute inflammatory abscess*, are these: A swelling, becoming in the course of two or three days, or often in a few hours, very hot, painful, and tender, the skin assuming a stretched appearance, with a bright red hue, most intense at the centre. As the swelling increases the pain becomes more severe, and has a characteristic *throbbing* peculiarity, which is worse if the part affected is allowed to hang down. The skin and subjacent soft parts become 'puffy,' and retain for a short time the mark made by pressure with the finger. As the centre of the abscess becomes more painful and inflamed it softens and gradually 'ripens,' or turns into matter. The skin at this part becomes thinner, more prominent, and loses its bright red colour, 'pointing,' as it is termed, in the shape of a light yellow or bluish spot. The whole swelling is now soft, and by making gentle pressure, alternately with the fingers of each hand, the sensation may be generally felt of fluid moved from side to side. The abscess finally bursts, and discharges the contained matter through one or more small apertures formed in the thinnest and most distended portion of the skin. The discharge at first is profuse, and consists of a thick yellowish fluid; as the cavity of the abscess contracts and closes, it diminishes and becomes clear and thin. During the progress of healing the superficial layers of skin about the seat of the abscess peel off. The progress of an abscess towards ripening is usually accompanied by constitutional symptoms, proportional in severity to the size of the swelling and the amount of inflammation. These symptoms are, shivering, feverishness, headache, and often pains in the back and joints. *Shivering*, particularly, is regarded as indicating the commencement of the formation of matter. When abscesses form deeply below the surface of the skin, especially where the skin is hard, as on the heel; or when they form beneath tendons and ligaments, as in one form of whitlow, the suffering is more intense, the matter longer in coming to the surface, the parts implicated more important, and professional assistance oftener required.

*The symptoms of the second variety of abscess,* called 'chronic' or 'cold' abscesses, are much less severe. Feverishness and headache are slight, and the sign of matter forming, viz.-*shivering,* may not occur, or be so trivial as to escape notice. The swelling increases very slowly, and with little pain or tenderness. The skin remains for a long time free from puffiness or inflammation. At length there is a slight blush or redness, and the matter is discharged through a small opening, as in acute abscess. Although the commencement of this form of abscess is attended with less fever, the termination of the malady is not so characterised. *Chronic abscesses* are generally large, and when the discharge is profuse and long-continued, hectic fever (*vide* p. 269) is usually excited. Scrofulous individuals are most usually affected, and a chronic abscess may depend on disease of a joint, bone, or gland.

*Treatment.*—In abscess arising from injury all irritating causes, as thorns or splinters, should if possible be removed, and then, if the person is in good health, the parts will usually heal under simple water dressing (Recipe 85). In the early stage of a painful inflamed swelling, an attempt may be made to prevent the formation of matter by applying lint, or a piece of linen wet with cold water or with cold vinegar and water (one-third vinegar), or by using the cold lotion (Recipe 83), which is a preferable application; by keeping the part in perfect rest, and as much as possible in an elevated position; by an aperient (Recipe 2); and by prohibiting the consumption of meat, beer, or spirits. *But if the patient has had shivering, or complains of throbbing pain,* measures calculated to further the *ripening* and *pointing* of the abscess should be adopted. Local application in the shape of hot poultices (Recipes 77, 78, 79), of the variety most easily procurable, should be used, and the poultice should be changed every four or five hours, or as soon as it feels cool; or, as is sometimes more convenient for small abscesses, warm-water dressing (Recipe 85), or spongio-piline, wet with hot water, may be substituted. Or the water-dressing may be used during the day, and a poultice at night. At each change of applications the part should be well bathed with hot water. Nourishing and easily digestible foods, as soups, beef-tea, eggs, and light puddings, should be allowed, a liberal diet being more especially required by feeble or debilitated persons. In most cases a small quantity of wine or malt liquor may be given.

*When abscess occurs without any irritating cause*, it will probably depend on some morbid state of the constitution, and *first* the possibility of a scorbutic taint should be recollected. If the gums, being spongy or inclined to bleed, show evidence of scurvy; or if the person has been in a locality where fresh vegetables could not be procured, such vegetables or other anti-scorbutic remedies (*vide Scurvy*, p. 382) should be taken. If symptoms of *anæmia* (*vide* p. 46) are present, sulphate of iron (*vide* p. 24) may be obtained. If there are indications of a scrofulous condition, or of hectic fever, which is more likely to be the case during the progress of chronic or 'cold' abscess, the remedies mentioned under the head *Scrofula* (p. 379) should be obtained, viz. cod-liver oil, and iodine with iron (Recipe 74); or the treatment required for *hectic fever* (p. 269) should be employed.

*If the constitution of the patient is weakened without evident cause*, tonics will also be required, and quinine (Recipes 66, 67) may be used. A close room is to be avoided, as fresh air will assist in favouring the rapid formation and discharge of matter, and the contraction and healing of the abscess.

If necessary to use iron (as mentioned above), in consequence of symptoms of anæmia, instead of sulphate of iron, it will be preferable to obtain Recipe 70 for children and Recipe 71 for adults. Or the articles mentioned in the note to Recipe 71 may be substituted, in doses according to the table of proportions at p. 6.

After a variable time, generally two or three days in acute abscess, but a much longer period in chronic or cold abscess, matter having formed, the abscess becomes prominent or pointed; then the skin, at the thinnest or most prominent part, should be punctured with a clean, sharp lancet, when the matter will usually flow out, often with a spurt. The part should never be roughly squeezed in order to get the matter out quickly. Having allowed as much matter to flow as will easily escape, put, with the blunt end of a probe, a very thin strip of oiled lint or linen into the aperture, to prevent closure, and apply a poultice. The poultice and lint should be removed after two or three hours. Then with a soft sponge and warm water as much more matter as can be expelled without pain should be pressed away. The poulticing (but not the lint) and gentle pressure should be repeated at longer intervals, until all discharge ceases. If at any time there is a tendency to closure of the opening, the blunt end of a probe should be gently passed from one end of the opening to the other (*vide Sinus*, p. 44). So long as discharge continues the part should be kept in that position which will best favour the outward flow of the matter. When discharge ceases, if the edges of the wound appear to gape and require support, plaster should be applied. Otherwise, water-dressing (Recipe 85).

If obtainable, carbolic oil—or, oil not being at hand, carbolic acid lotion (*vide* Appendix, No. 119)—should be used instead of plain water, as mentioned above, and at p. 42.

The preceding is the simple way of treating an abscess. In hospitals antiseptic dressings would probably be used. And for large abscesses surgeons would insert a drainage tube, which if used should be placed in the most dependent position.

When opening an abscess no plunge should be made, which causes unnecessary alarm. Neither should the lancet be used slowly, which causes prolonged pain. The puncture should be made with confidence, decision, and a moderate degree of rapidity; and if an aperture is required larger than the shoulder of the lancet used (*vide* p. 491), it should be made the necessary length by cutting *outwards*, when withdrawing the instrument.

*When abscess occurs in the neck*, it is important to open it early, and the puncture should be made *longitudinally* (or in a direction with the lines or folds of the skin), and not horizontally, in order to avoid a large scar. *In the female breast*, it prevents much suffering to make a puncture as soon as the presence of matter is ascertained; and to avoid a scar, the puncture should be made from the nipple towards the circumference, *not* across the breast. A similar caution applies to abscess, or *bubo*, in the groin, where the puncture should be made in the direction of the natural skin-folds. When abscesses are near the *anus*, the use of the lancet should not be deferred for a single hour after discovery, or the danger of a fistula resulting will be increased (*vide Fistula-in-ano*, p. 271). An abscess of the *perinæum* (*vide* p. 421) and a *whitlow* (*vide* p. 463) should also be opened early.

*Abscesses are liable to terminate in sinus or fistula*: which means an unsound condition of the parts beneath the skin. This may result from the abscess not being opened sufficiently early, or from the opening being too small for the exit of the matter, which becomes pent up, and burrows under the skin. Or it may arise from want of care in dressing the part, or from an improper position assumed by the patient. *Sinus* is to be prevented by making the opening sufficiently early; by making the opening large enough; by keeping the opening in such a dependent position that the matter may easily flow out; by care in dressing the part, when it is often necessary to place and secure a small pad of lint over any position where there is any tendency of the matter to gravitate or 'bag'; and by not allowing the opening to close up too soon, which is to be effected by the insertion of a thin strip of lint into the wound at first (*vide* p. 43), and afterwards by the daily insertion of the blunt end of a probe (*vide* p. 43) to the depth of less than a quarter of an inch between the lips of the wound, and carrying it through the whole length of the orifice, so as to separate the parts.

ACIDITY.—Acidity of the stomach is a frequent symptom of indigestion, and is often an accompaniment of chronic rheumatism and of gout. It usually arises from articles of food taken—especially those containing sugar—being converted, from error of digestion, into acids of various kinds. When the formation of acid in the stomach is only slight, or temporarily in excess, the symptoms may be limited to slight heartburn or flatulence, or to a little acid rising and sour eructations. There may also be fulness, oppression, uneasiness, or even aching pain *felt in the chest.* In larger quantity acidity causes irregularity or capriciousness of appetite, headache, aching of the limbs, spots before the eyes, sleeplessness, depression of spirits, nausea, pain at the pit of the stomach or behind the ribs of the left side, and skin affections, such as nettlerash and erythema (pp. 386, 387). When the acidity is still more confirmed or long-continued, the sour eructations set the teeth on edge, the nerves of the stomach become more sensitive, and there will be pain at the pit of the stomach, of a burning, gnawing character, temporarily relieved by taking food.

*Treatment* consists in avoiding those articles of diet which produce acidity, as unripe fruit, cabbage, acid wines, sugar, butter, and food containing much starch, as rice, potatoes, and arrowroot; and in taking medicines which will correct acidity. Among the best of these is citrate of magnesia, which may be taken in tea-spoonful doses dissolved in two or three ounces of water, to which a grain or two of quinine and 20 minims of tincture of ginger (*vide* p. 14) may be added; or 40 minims of sal volatile, and a grain or two of quinine in an ounce of water. Effervescing draughts (Recipe 36), aerated water, or draughts of simple cold water, are often temporarily beneficial. In some instances much benefit is experienced from sipping a pint of hot water twice or three times a day between meals, or night and morning. If the bowels are costive, sulphate of soda may be taken as a laxative (Recipe 2).

Acidity of the stomach in children is always combined with *flatulence*, for the treatment of which *vide* p. 273.

[Other antacid medicines which may be procured if the above do not relieve are, bicarbonate of soda, bicarbonate of potash, and bicarbonate of magnesia, each of which may be taken in from 20- to 30-grain doses. But a more convenient method of taking these remedies is by using 'soluble compressed tabloids,' as prepared by Messrs. Burroughs, Wellcome & Co., London. These are made of either bicarbonate of soda or of bicarbonate of potash, or of bicarbonate of soda with carbonate of ammonia and oil of peppermint. The latter are called 'soda-mint' or neutralising tablets, and are especially useful in acidity. When acidity occurs without disordered bowels, 5 drops of tincture of nux vomica, three times a day, before food, often gives relief. There is also a form of acidity characterised by eructations like rotten egg, which is only to be checked by acids, as Recipes 34 and 43, which should be taken after meals; the first being adopted if there is any suspicion of liver-disorder. But in the great majority of cases, acidity of the stomach is a symptom of dyspepsia, and all medicines are only palliative. The great means of cure are careful dieting and moderate exercise. Saccharin tabloids may be tried instead of sugar (*vide* p. 200).]

**ANÆMIA.**—Anæmia really signifies lack of blood, but poorness of blood is a principal characteristic. Healthy blood contains an immense number of red globules, which are seen under the microscope, and which give the blood its red colour. In anæmia these red globules are lessened in number, and are deficient in a constituent known as *hæmoglobin*, which contains iron, and which has the special power of carrying the oxygen taken in by breathing from the lungs to all parts of the body. There is also an excess of water in the blood, and some other of the constituents of the blood are changed in character.

The causes of anæmia are numerous, the principal being as below. Insufficient diet not amounting to actual starvation. Want of sufficient light; the bleaching effect of want of solar light on vegetables is well known, and a similar sinister influence is exerted on animal life. Habitually living in darkened rooms, and want of sufficient fresh air and exercise, lead to loss of appetite and nutrition. Prolonged fatigue, which causes a greater waste of the body than the digestive organs can meet. Habitual constipation, during which the absorption of the products of retained fæcal matter takes place, which act as poisons. Excessive mental work, which involves loss of sleep and digestive derangements. Worry, anxiety, and depressing mental emotions have long been recognised as causing the 'cheeks to grow pale,' and 'gnawing at our life and health.' Living in damp and so-called malarious localities. In short, bad hygienic conditions of all kinds predispose to anæmia. Anæmia may also arise from various diseased conditions. An unsuspected scorbutic or venereal taint, or a tape-worm, may be the concealed cause. It results in women from bearing children too quickly, and from prolonged suckling. Anæmia is also a consequence of most chronic exhausting maladies, such as Bright's disease, bleeding piles, spleen disease, repeated ague, &c.

It is not, however, the anæmia caused by exhausting diseases which is now considered, but the anæmia which arises as a distinct malady, especially in the tropics. For, in addition to the manifold causes of anæmia, which may excite the malady in any climate, *there is in hot climates an additional potent factor in the heat.* Even in extraordinarily hot summers in temperate climates, a greater tendency to languor and debility is generally observed. How heat acts injuriously in the production of blood-deterioration is referred to in Chapter VI. under the heading 'Heat.' One, or several, of the causes of anæmia mentioned above may be in operation in addition to the heat of the climate, thus rendering anæmia, more or less marked, a very prevalent condition among both Europeans and natives in India; while anæmia itself renders the same sufferer more liable to most tropical diseases.

*Symptoms.*—The skin becomes pale, and may in dark complexions present a sallow appearance. In the native and half-caste the skin loses its brilliancy and softness, becoming of a lighter tinge and looking more semi-transparent, while the ordinarily lighter-coloured palms of the hand become much whiter. The whites of the eyes look pearl-coloured, the eyes are encircled by a more or less dark ring, and the interior of the eyelids, of the nose, and of the mouth, the tongue, and the lips, instead of being rosy red, are a pale pink colour. The tongue is also tremulous. The cheeks lose their colour, being bleached 'from the aspect of the rose, to the whiteness of the lily.' The sallowness of countenance in dark people is readily distinguished from the sallowness arising from affections of the liver, as it is never so yellow, and the whites of the eyes do not become yellow as from liver disease. In addition to the bloodless expression of countenance, the face often appears bloated or 'puffy,' although the body loses weight. The patient is habitually chilly, languid, and indisposed to exertion, and the extremities, especially the feet, are usually cold, although the palms of the hands may often burn. The system being so sensitive to cold, sore-throats, catarrhs, bronchial affections, and diarrhœa result from slight atmospheric changes. The appetite becomes variable, and sometimes depraved. The urine is generally pale and the bowels usually costive. There is also headache, mostly felt about the temples, or at the top of the head, and often described as *throbbing*, or as if something were pressing down and out. It is generally relieved by taking food and by lying down, and aggravated by the erect posture or by exertion. Aching of the limbs, coming on suddenly and lasting a variable time, is a frequent symptom. The monthly courses of females become irregular, scanty, thin, watery, and painful; varied sometimes by a profuse flow (*vide* pp. 468, 474). Whites in females is an almost certain complication (*vide* p. 462). As the malady progresses there is shortness of breath, especially on exertion, such as going up hill, or up stairs; palpitation of the heart, pain in the left side, a tendency to fainting, singing in the ears, spots or sparks before the eyes, the sleep is very heavy, and there may be bleeding from the nose. The previous languor and disinclination for exertion now gives place to a feeling of thorough weariness. The appetite becomes more variable and fastidious, while digestion is more and more impaired, and acidity (p. 45) and flatulent dyspepsia (p. 204) become troublesome. The brain, now being also affected by the deteriorated blood, presents various evidences of weakness. There is capriciousness and irritability of temper, impressions too feeble to be perceived by healthy persons harassing the anæmic. There is also loss of memory, and of the power of fixing the attention. The man becomes hypochondriacal, and the woman hysterical. When the malady has lasted some time, the spleen may become enlarged, and swelling of the feet and ankles may be expected.

*It is not to be understood that all the symptoms enumerated appear immediately, or in regular sequence*, for the process of blood degeneration may be one of months or years, and one organ or the other may be first and most affected. Anæmia may present in all degrees of severity, from slight pallor and debility to the condition known as *pernicious anæmia*, when all the symptoms are aggravated, and the person dies, probably from sheer debility, or from apoplexy or paralysis (*vide* pp. 53, 342) resulting from the anæmic condition. A minor degree of the symptoms described is not incompatible with *apparently* fair health and with the pursuit of ordinary avocations. But warnings of anæmia should not be neglected, especially by the European in tropical climates, for the anæmic condition induces dyspepsia, neuralgia, nostalgia (or home craving), boils, abscesses, chronic diarrhœa, fatty degeneration of the heart; it predisposes to apoplectiform attacks, and it renders the person much more liable to the fevers of the tropics.

There are several forms or phases of anæmia, the principal of which are as below.

1. *The form of anæmia known as green sickness or chlorosis.*—When anæmia is connected with the first appearance, or with irregularities of the monthly courses of females, it is commonly called 'green sickness' or *chlorosis*, and it presents some features different to those of ordinary anæmia. There is a greenish-yellow colour of skin different to the pallor of ordinary anæmia; there is a more marked dark halo round the eyes; there is a more frequent depraved appetite, causing such things as slate pencil and dry rice to be greedily eaten; there is a more frequent complaint of throbbing pain at the top of the head and in the left side; the urine is paler and more copious, and hysterical symptoms are more frequent. Constipation is also a more marked feature, and in some instances the anæmia of girls is altogether due to the absorption of the products of the decomposition of retained fæcal matter. This will especially be likely if with

constipation there is also pain or uneasiness in either side of the bowels, particularly the left side. Further green sickness is usually attended with marked pain in the back and loins at the monthly periods, and probably swelling of the feet.

2. *Leucocythæmia, or white cell blood*, is an advanced stage of anæmia, in which there is a large increase of white cells in the blood, enlargement of the glands in various parts of the body, and usually also of the spleen.

3. *Malarious cachexia* is merely another name for anæmia.

4. *Masked malarious fever* (*vide* p. 266) is anæmia accompanied by slight fever.

5. *Melasma*, or *Addison's disease*, the symptoms of which are progressive feebleness without any apparent cause, and often a peculiar change in the appearance of the skin which becomes bronzed. This condition is connected with changes in the structure of attachments to the kidneys, known as the supra-renal capsules.

*Treatment.*—The treatment consists in moderate exercise every day, and of free ventilation of the living, sleeping, or working apartments. The diet should be nourishing, and a moderate amount of animal food should be taken; but anything causing indigestion should be avoided. Stimulants should be resorted to sparingly, a small allowance of malt liquor being the most advisable. Cold or tepid bathing is often of great service, and change of air and scene is always useful. Tonic medicines, especially iron, are of great value. The red globules of the blood, as previously explained, contain iron, and iron given as a medicine tends to increase their quantity. It must, however, be understood that anæmia is dependent as much on scanty absorption of iron into the system as on a deficiency of the supply of iron; hence, unless combined with well-regulated sanitary conditions, as mentioned above, iron will do little good. These being attended to, sulphate of iron may be used (*vide* p. 24). Sulphate of iron will be found especially useful when the tongue is flabby, pale, broad, and indented by the teeth. Should the bowels be confined, citrate of magnesia may be used, or, if a stronger aperient is wanted, Recipe 2. If disorders of the monthly flow exist, the treatment recommended for *amenorrhœa* or *dysmenorrhœa* should be pursued (*vide* pp. 468, 472). What is said at p. 50 regarding the anæmia of girls being caused by constipation should be recollected, for which Recipes 1, 2 may be used. In such cases tight-lacing must be avoided and regular habits insisted upon.

When anæmia is long confirmed change of climate should be taken, the European to Europe, the Indian to the hills. For the European, short sea-voyages or the hill climates are not sufficient. But the change to Europe should not be made in the winter, and the greatest care should be taken to avoid chill.

[Better medicines for anæmia are, the iron mixtures (Recipes 71, 73): No. 73 when delayed menstruation exists; Recipe 71 when there is not this complication. Or for simple uncomplicated anæmia, the medicines mentioned in the note to Recipe 71 may be substituted for the iron mixture by those disliking the taste of the latter. When the colour begins to return, Recipe 75. If constipation exists, it is also desirable to use aloetic laxatives, as Recipe 13; if the motions are light in colour, or it is supposed the liver is not acting freely, acid baths may also be taken (*vide* Recipe 113). If there is no suspicion of inactive liver, Recipe 15, which contains iron. If the appetite is bad, pepsine may be taken with the food, and Fairchild's 'pepsine tabloids' are to be recommended. The Burroughs & Wellcome pills, containing the one-fiftieth part of a grain of phosphorus, taken night and morning, are also advisable under almost any circumstances. For the anæmia of young and rapidly growing children, phosphate of lime in 1- to 2-grain doses three times daily. The Burroughs 'beef and iron wine,' which is a highly concentrated stimulating and strengthening food, with an agreeable flavour liked by children, is very valuable in anæmia. When the disease is long-continued, a visit to the mineral springs, or at least drinking the mineral waters containing iron, is often beneficial.]

**APOPLEXY.**—The disease attacks in three ways.

1st, suddenly, the patient falling down without warning, as if from a blow. In this *first* form of the disease, the patient falls to the ground, deprived of sense and motion, and lies like a person in a deep sleep; the face flushed, the breathing laboured, and the pulse full and slow. The pupils of the eyes may be dilated, or one may be dilated and the other contracted. The mouth may be drawn to one side, and there may be convulsions, also often confined to one side of the body. When convulsions occur at the onset there is often some kidney affection.

2ndly, and more usually, after *premonitory* symptoms or 'warnings,' which may be of days', weeks', or even months' duration. Such *premonitory* symptoms may be giddiness, especially on stooping, nausea, sickness, and fainty feelings, headache, a sense of pressure, constriction or heat in the head, constipation, scanty urine, confusion of ideas, faltering speech, flushing of the face, bleeding from the nose, flashes of light in the eyes, double vision, noises in the ears, numbness of the extremities, loss of memory, or the anæmic condition generally (*vide* p. 46). In this *second* form of the malady, the *first symptoms of the actual fit* are more like those of fainting, viz. feeble pulse, sighing respiration, pallid face, cold surface, and attempts to vomit.

3rdly, with sudden paralysis of one side of the body, or of one leg only. In this *third* form, the person cannot move the affected part, or the limb is dragged with difficulty. In more serious cases the face is also drawn to one side; the tongue cannot be put out straight; the speech is impaired, so that the person endeavours to express himself by signs; and the intellect may be confused.

In whatever way it may commence, the fit, especially after beginning in either of the first two manners, is usually ultimately characterised by insensibility, accompanied by slow, noisy, *puffing* breathing, and frothy saliva about the mouth. The teeth are clenched, and the person is unable to swallow; often, fluids put into the mouth run out at the corners; or swallowing is performed with difficulty; the countenance becomes flushed or livid; the eyes are dull and glassy, and the pupils of the eyes are contracted, or one remains dilated and the other contracted; the mouth is drawn to one side; the limbs are motionless and rigid, but sometimes convulsed, or the latter conditions present only on one side of the body. The extremities are cold, and the body is bathed in cold sweat; the bowels are either obstinately confined, or motions may be passed involuntarily. The urine may also be passed involuntarily, or retained till the bladder is full, when it dribbles away. The pulse, at first slow, becomes quicker, fuller, and stronger as the system recovers from the first shock, although it often remains less frequent than natural, and may be irregular. Falling to 60 beats per minute, or rising to 110, are both unfavourable signs. Slight alteration of the natural temperature of the body is a favourable indication, but a persistent depression or rise is unfavourable.

The duration of an apoplectic fit varies from two to three hours to as many days. The longer the apoplectic condition continues without improvement, the less is the prospect of recovery. It may terminate by gradually passing off, leaving the person *apparently* little the worse, or it may terminate in incomplete recovery, the mind remaining impaired, or some part of the body being paralysed; or, the person not regaining sensibility, the increasing stupor may end in death.

The *predisposing* causes of apoplexy are—age, from the fiftieth year upwards; sex, men being more liable to it than women; make of body, combining a short thick neck, large chest, florid complexion and stoutness; hereditary tendency, the malady often running in families; indulgence in eating and drinking; a gouty condition of system; prolonged constipation; the anæmic condition; and disease of the liver, heart, or kidneys. The *immediate* causes are whatever unduly impedes or accelerates the circulation of the blood within the brain, or exerts a certain degree of pressure on it—such as violent exercise; straining, as in lifting heavy weights, or as at stool; sudden mental emotions, and violent passions; intense heat; overloading the stomach; tight stocks round the neck; the sudden cessation of any accustomed discharge, as from piles.

[*The immediate attack* of apoplexy depends generally on the sudden escape of blood beneath the skull on the surface of the brain, or on or between its investing membranes. This occurs from the rupture of a blood-vessel (probably diseased from fatty degeneration, *vide* p. 235). Or it may depend on the formation of a blood-clot in the blood-vessels of some part of the body, which is conveyed by the circulation into the brain, there blocking, and eventually causing rupture of a blood-vessel. *Secondly*, the apoplectic seizure may be caused by filtration of watery fluid into the cavities of the brain, without actual rupture of a vessel and escape of blood. This occurs from a congested or too full condition of the vessels, which results in filtration of the water of the blood from them. Or it may depend on an anæmic condition or thinness of blood (*vide* p. 46), which results in similar filtration.]

Attacks resembling apoplexy and resulting from a condition known as URÆMIA are liable to occur when, from any cause, there is interference with the secretion or discharge of urine. Uræmia signifies the retention in the blood of material which ought to be expelled with *the urine*. This condition often occurs, and terminates in an apoplectiform attack, in the latter stages of albuminuria or diabetes. The attack is usually preceded by warnings as mentioned above, and is often characterised by convulsions.

Apoplexy requires to be distinguished *from fainting*,

*from the effects of spirituous liquors, and from the results of narcotic poisons, as opium, and from epilepsy.*

*Fainting* occurs principally to young, nervous, or hysterical females; apoplexy to elderly people. As a rule persons fainting recover in a few minutes, the pulse becoming more distinct, and intelligence being gradually restored. The apoplectic attack continues as described at p. 53.

*Apoplexy is best distinguished from the effects of spirituous liquors*: 1st, by the history of the case; 2ndly, by the smell of liquor in the person's breath—although it must be recollected that this is not a certain sign that the patient has been drinking, for someone may, in mistaken kindness, have given the person struck by apoplexy some kind of liquor; 3rdly, in the 'drunken fit' the size of the pupils is equal, while in apoplexy one is often contracted and the other dilated; 4thly, the person 'dead drunk,' as it is termed, may generally be roused, when he babbles incoherently—from apoplexy the person cannot be roused; 5thly, if the patient be carefully watched, any movements which occur will be usually found to be restricted to one side of the body in apoplexy, while movements occur on both sides in drunkenness.

*Apoplexy is to be distinguished from poisoning by opium*: 1st, by the history of the case; as apoplexy may have been preceded by premonitory symptoms, and opium-poisoning is not so preceded. Apoplexy may come on during or immediately after a meal; while if opium is given during a meal symptoms do not present for from ten to thirty minutes; 2ndly, by the absence or presence of the smell of opium in the breath; 3rdly, by the equal contraction of both pupils caused by opium; 4thly, in apoplexy the patient cannot be roused, while in opium-poisoning he may generally be roused for a moment if shaken or spoken roughly to, or even by tapping the forehead, although he does not then babble as in drunkenness, but lapses at once into sleep again; 5thly, in apoplexy what are called 'reflex actions' may usually be induced,—that is, if the patient's foot or leg is pinched or tickled, there will be an effort made to draw the foot away—in opium-poisoning such movements cannot ordidarily be induced, the patient apparently not feeling pinching or tickling; 6thly, apoplexy chiefly attacks persons in advanced life, while opium-poisoning is most usual in the young, especially young females; 7thly, apoplexy is most usual in either fat or thin people, opium-poisoning occurs in all varieties; 8thly, apoplectic symptoms often occur abruptly, opium-poisoning symptoms always come on gradually.

*Apoplexy is known from epilepsy* by the presence of *puffing* breathing, which is absent in the latter malady. In epilepsy also there is struggling of the limbs; the eyes are turned up under the lids, so that the whites only are visible; and the person generally falls down with a loud cry, none of which are symptoms of apoplexy.

*Treatment.*—The first thing in all cases is to loosen the patient's neckerchief and shirt-collar, to *slightly* raise his head, and give free access of air. The forehead should be bathed with cold water, or, if available, a bladder of pounded ice should be applied; the feet should be put in hot water; and mustard poultices should be applied to the calves. But while this is being done the patient should be kept in the horizontal posture, which may be effected by drawing him down towards the foot of the bed until, the knees being bent, the legs hang over. The feet should be kept in hot water about ten minutes, after which bottles filled with hot water should be applied to them; the mustard poultices being allowed to remain on the calves for an hour. If mustard poultices are not available, the limbs should be well rubbed with the hand;

and in any case they should afterwards be warmed by friction. The head and shoulders should be propped towards the right side (to prevent the tongue falling back). Perfect quiet should be maintained, and the blinds should be drawn down so as not to let too much light into the room, and only one or two people should be allowed by the bedside. Bleeding should not be undertaken, except under medical advice. As soon as the patient can swallow, 1 ounce of sulphate of soda dissolved in 4 ounces of water may be given as a purgative. But until the patient is able to swallow, no attempt should be made to induce him to take either medicines or anything else. Stimulants should not be used under any circumstances. In all cases an assafœtida injection (Recipe 105) should be given as soon as possible. If the person lies insensible more than six or seven hours, without making water, the catheter should be used (*vide* p. 493). If the water is retained till the bladder is full, and then *dribbles* away, it is a sign that the urine should have been drawn off before.

If the fit happens *immediately* after a full meal, the patient may make attempts to vomit; and if this is the case the action of vomiting may be assisted by tickling the throat with a feather. But if there is no spontaneous attempt to vomit, emetics and all excitants to vomiting must be avoided, as the action of vomiting may increase the determination of blood to the head and do mischief.

When there is reason to suppose, from the previous ailments of the person, that the attack depends on *uræmia* (*vide* p. 55), every endeavour should be made to renew the flow of urine and to excite the action of the skin. The loins should be fomented. If the patient can swallow, Recipe 50 should be given; and the bowels should be opened, as detailed above.

After a variable time the patient generally recovers

from a first or even a second apoplectic fit, but it is then often found that he has lost the use of an arm or a leg, or of one side of the body. The power of speech may also be lost and the muscles of the face may be affected.

[It is always desirable to act on the bowels as soon as possible; but as the patient cannot in the majority of cases swallow, it will be desirable to obtain from the chemist's a little croton oil, of which *two or three drops* may be placed on the back of the patient's tongue with a feather. If the croton oil does not operate freely (Recipe 11) followed in three hours by Recipe 5, should be given as soon as the patient can swallow, and the latter should be repeated every six hours until the bowels have been freely moved. An enema (Recipe 106) should also be injected.]

When convalescence commences, the bowels should be regulated, and a generous or a low diet must be given, according to the condition of the patient. As a general rule, the latter will be required; and in some instances, when there is a gouty tendency, nothing but vegetables to eat, and milk and water to drink, will be advisable. All strong medicines, excitement, and mental occupation should be avoided.

*Prevention of Apoplexy.*—Temperate and active habits, with moderation in food and drink, may prevent apoplexy, or at least postpone the seizure; and the 'warnings' noted (*vide* p. 53) as frequently preceding a fit should never be neglected. While the bowels are kept moderately open, bromide of potassium (Recipe 19) may usually be given with advantage. Although any one of the warning symptoms detailed, occurring singly, would probably be of minor significance, a combination of them in a person who is a likely subject for apoplexy, especially if there is any kidney or gouty affection, may be regarded as a sure precursor of an attack, unless abstinence and preventive remedies in the shape of laxative medicines are adopted.

**APPETITE, LOSS OF.**—Loss of appetite occurs in indigestion, fever, debility, and inflammations, and must be regarded as a symptom of disease rather than a disease itself (*vide* p. 37). The appetite is almost always lost in serious illness, and when good it is usually a sign that there is not much the matter. Exceptions are, during some forms of dyspepsia and in 'diabetes.'

**ASTHMA.**—Asthma signifies attacks of difficulty of breathing, of a spasmodic character, occurring in paroxysms. It is often spoken of as *humid* and *dry*, according as it is or is not attended with much expectoration. The wind-pipe divides into two tubes at the upper part of the chest, one passing to each lung. These two tubes divide and subdivide into smaller tubes, which convey the air to and from the cells of the lungs. All the tubes are surrounded by circular muscular fibres, and the cause of asthmatic difficulty of breathing is the contraction of these muscular fibres, which thus reduce the calibre of the tubes. This spasmodic contraction may be excited by *direct* and *indirect* causes. The *direct* are dust, vegetable irritants such as pollen, chemical vapours, animal emanations, climatic influences, especially rapid changes of temperature. The *indirect* are emotions, such as anger or fright, costive bowels, heavy suppers, flatulence, and other forms of dyspepsia, a gouty condition of system (*vide* p. 282), fatty heart, emphysema of the lungs (*vide* p. 330), and hereditary predisposition. Some persons are peculiarly liable to asthma, and their appearance is characterised by thinness, round shoulders, anxious expression of countenance, hollow cheeks, rather hoarse voice, and habitual slight cough.

A fit of asthma generally comes on in the night, the reason being, that the slower circulation, or congestion, which takes place during sleep, or when the body is recumbent, sets up an irritation leading to spasm. But the seizure is often preceded by languor, flatulency, headache, heaviness over the eyes, sickness, pale urine, disturbed rest, and a sense of oppression about the heart.

Yet it often comes on suddenly, without such warnings, the patient waking from his first and deepest sleep labouring for breath. When the fit is fully formed there is intense difficulty of respiration, the patient sitting up in bed, or standing holding on to a table or chair, breathing hard with a wheezing noise. The face becomes livid or bluish, the eyes look prominent, the body is covered with cold perspiration, suffocation appears impending, the sufferer often struggles to the window, which he desires may be open, and there may be cramp in the legs. A paroxysm may last minutes or hours, and when subsiding there is often expectoration of little pellets of thick phlegm or mucus, and perhaps a copious discharge of pale urine. The length of time between successive fits of asthma varies much, during which the person, if he takes care, usually enjoys fairly good health; unless the condition known as emphysema (*vide* p. 330) also exists, when the health is not so good.

*Treatment.*—During a paroxysm the patient should be kept sitting up. If the fit is severe he should be placed in an arm-chair in front of a table, with a pillow on which he may rest his elbows. The spine may be rubbed with equal parts of salad oil and brandy, or, if available, with soap and opium liniment. Pressure with the thumbs on the large (axillary) arteries of the arms, as they issue from the chest (*vide* p. 501), has been found to lessen the difficulty of breathing. To plethoric persons ipecacuanha wine may be given, in 20-drop doses, in an ounce of water. For weaker persons camphorated tincture of opium, combined with a stimulant, as ammonia (Recipe 56), is more advisable. If the attack has followed an injudicious meal, as a late supper or dinner, a mustard emetic (Recipe 54) should be administered. If the attack has been preceded by constipation, sulphate of soda (Recipe 2) should be taken as a purgative. Sometimes a glass of hot brandy and water will relieve a fit of asthma; at other times a cup of hot strong coffee without sugar or milk. Other easily procurable and popular remedies are: 10 grains of powdered alum placed on the tongue; a full dose, as 20 grains, of chloral; spirits of camphor (*vide* p. 24) in 10-drop doses every ten minutes; the inhalation of the fumes from burning straw or blotting-paper previously soaked in strong solution of saltpetre, and dried ready for burning. All these means may be successively tried, for what does not benefit one may do good to another; and what does not ease one attack may afford relief at another time.

Smoking *dhatura stramonium leaves* (*vide* p. 27) sometimes relieves asthma, especially if the smoking is commenced *before* the fit is fully formed. From ten to thirty grains of the dried leaves may be smoked in a common pipe, which will often, if taken in time, prevent an expected paroxysm. It is desirable to commence with the smaller quantity, and gradually to increase it as required. Another way of using the stramonium is by puffing the fumes into an inverted tumbler, which, when full, should be placed over the patient's mouth, who should inhale the contents by a deep breath. This method often excites cough, but is occasionally very beneficial.

[If the above measures do not succeed, Recipes 58 and 60 may be obtained *for use during the fit*; or for plethoric persons, Recipe 59. The following prescription sometimes acts like a charm. Compound spirit of ether (Hoffman's anodyne), half a drachm; acetate of morphia, half a grain; camphor water, one ounce. Bromidia may also be tried. This preparation contains in each tea-spoonful 15 grains of chloral, 15 grains of bromide of potassium, $\frac{1}{8}$ grain of cannabis indica, and $\frac{1}{8}$ grain of hyoscyam. Dose, a tea-spoonful. Burroughs & Wellcome's 'valoid fluid extract of stramonium seeds' is a valuable remedy in spasmodic asthma. Five minims of tincture of lobelia in an ounce of water every half-hour, continuing the medicine until either relief is obtained or the patient feels a little sick or faint, when it should be *immediately* stopped. If lobelia relieves, as it often does, the amount of the divided doses may be taken at once up to forty minims on the next occasion. Many patients are benefited by chloroform, *half a drachm* of which may be placed on a handkerchief, which should be held two or three inches from the nose and mouth. This may be repeated three or four times, at intervals of a quarter of an hour. *Cigars de Joy* or anti-asthmatic cigarettes (both of which are composed principally of stramonium leaves), or *ozone* cigarettes may also be procured and tried. But as with the smoking of stramonium above recommended, it is desirable that the cigars should be smoked *before* the paroxysm of asthma has been fully formed, or the effect is not so powerful. Ozone and nitre paper, and chlorate of potash and nitre paper, are also prepared by the chemists, the fumes from burning which may be inhaled. The inhalation of the spray, produced by a common hand-spray instrument, of equal parts of ipecacuanha wine and water, is also often very beneficial. To relieve the distressing flatulence often preceding or accompanying a fit of asthma, 10 grains of alum, 5 of ginger, and 4 of powdered rhubarb may be taken with advantage.]

Treatment is equally important during the intervals between the fits; and it is found by experience that more is to be done for asthmatic patients by careful dietetic management than in any other direction. However well the person may feel during the intervals between the fits, he should never exceed in diet. Breakfast, which should be the chief meal, should consist of an egg, or chop, or cold chicken; tea is better than coffee, and milk and water better than either. Mutton ought to be the staple dinner diet, with green vegetables and potatoes in moderation, provided they do not cause flatulence. No pastry should be used, and there should be no dessert, but stewed fruits or light pudding may generally be taken with impunity. Sausages, kidneys, salt boiled beef, pickles, or toasted cheese should never be eaten. It has been stated, 'There is as much asthma in a mouthful of Stilton as in a whole dinner.' Water, or very weak brandy-and-water, is the best drink. Late dinners are to be avoided, and the asthmatic should never eat as much as he can. A person subject to asthma cannot eat and drink with the impunity of other people, and it is only by the exercise of self-denial in this respect that he will be able to live in comparative ease and comfort. Similarly, he should avoid excitement, fits often arising from mental emotions.

[*After the fit*, in conjunction with a strict system of diet, as mentioned above, Recipes 14 and 6 should be used on alternate nights and mornings, for three or four days, or until the bowels are freely moved, to be followed by Recipe 41. Iodide and bromide of potassium (Recipes 21 and 19) and arsenic (Recipe 75) are also among the most approved preventives. Wearing a Pulvermacher's galvanic chain is often beneficial.]

Asthma is sometimes more relieved by change of climate than by medical treatment, although it cannot be said with certainty what climate will suit each individual case. Sometimes a dry, at others a moist climate, affords most relief; sometimes town, sometimes country. A very slight change, as from one street to another, or from one house to another, has been known to check the attacks. As a rule, elevated regions, as hill stations, do not suit asthmatics, on account of the greater rarefaction of the air.

When a fit of asthma occurs, especially if the patient is in a strange place, inquiry should be made as to the existence of locally tainted air; as from a neighbouring brick-kiln, from works where sulphur is used, &c., and the asthmatic will do well to leave such a locality immediately. With reference to asthma being sometimes caused by the aroma from hay, as mentioned below, it may be well to state that asthma has been known to be excited by the smell of ipecacuanha, also by the effluvium from horses, wild beasts, guinea-pigs, rabbits, cats, dogs, or even from the skins of animals. The fact that asthmatics of peculiar idiosyncrasy may be thus affected should be borne in mind when searching for a cause of recurring attacks.

**ASTHMA, HAY.**—This malady is known by various

names, as *hay fever*, *pollen fever*, *rose cold*, *grape cold*, *peach cold*, *Roman wormwood cold*, *spasmodic sneezing*, *spasmodic catarrh*, and scientifically *vaso-motor coryza*. Some persons possess a peculiar ill-understood nervous irritability of constitution; or at least local irritability of the nasal passages to particular atoms floating in the atmosphere. It is in fact an idiosyncrasy, several of which have been noted at p. 7. For while some persons are affected when hay is ripening, others are not affected from hay, but suffer when certain other vegetable productions bloom. It is perhaps most frequently excited by hay pollen floating in the air, and it thus occurs, in England and India, more especially during the hay-harvest. There is, however, reason to believe that it may be excited in those predisposed by exposure to heat and dust. The symptoms are spasmodic sneezing (which is sometimes the chief or only symptom), watering of the eyes, feverishness, often cough and expectoration, and sometimes spasmodic attacks of difficulty of breathing.

*Treatment.*—Removal from the locality where the attack takes place is the most certain cure. If this cannot be accomplished, the person may use snuff occasionally and take Recipe 55; and 2 drachms of a solution of quinine (2 grains in 1 ounce of water) may be injected twice daily into the nostrils. Or if the instrument is available, the patient should inhale the quinine solution through the nose from an ordinary hand-spray producer as used for scents, taking care that a spray reaches the back part of the nostrils, which will be known by the taste. A mixture of quinine 1 grain, camphor 2 grains, with starch 3 grains, used as snuff, is sometimes very beneficial.

[An ointment, composed of 1 grain of morphia, 10 grains of quinine, and 3 drachms of spermaceti ointment, smeared on the outside of the nostrils, may also be used. A cocaine tablet (Burroughs & Wellcome), containing one-sixth of a grain slightly moistened and introduced into each nostril, has been found to give immediate relief. The tablets adhere and cause no pain. Or a solution of cocaine (strength from 5 to 15 per cent.) may be applied with a camel's-hair brush, or used with the hand-spray. As internal medicine iodide of potassium 3 drachms; arsenical solution (Liquor Potassæ Arsenitis) minims 30; water 6 ounces. A tea-spoonful every four or six hours.]

**ATROPHY.**—This term signifies wasting, and is the name generally applied to the wasting of children. For the maintenance of a healthy state of the body, a certain supply of nutrition is required to meet the waste which is constantly going on. When from any cause the supply of nutrition is not able to meet this waste, the natural dimensions are reduced. Atrophy may therefore arise from a variety of causes. It may be caused by merely withholding the necessary supply of nutritious food without any actual disease, as occurs from feeding too exclusively on farinaceous food. In children up to twelve months old or thereabouts it may generally be referred to unsuitable food. Atrophy of children sometimes leads to a habit of eating dirt or lime plaster from walls; the habit probably originating from a craving of the child for other food than that supplied. Between one and three years old, atrophy is often associated with a rickety condition of system, or with worms. After the age of three, especially in children having an hereditary scrofulous taint, atrophy is usually associated with tubercular enlargement of the glands of the bowels, known as *the mesenteric glands*, or with worms, or with tubercular affection of the brain, commonly called 'water on the brain.' After six, with scrofula and phthisis. When atrophy occurs to adults it is usually in connection with consumption, kidney diseases, or from climatic or malarious influences. Should unsanitary conditions of life be superadded, such as impure air, confinement in crowded buildings, exposure to emanations from sewers, the course of atrophy from any cause is more rapid. Atrophy, therefore, unless it arises from bad feeding, can only be combated by treating the maladies or conditions of the system of which it may be the early indication, or with the progress of which it may be associated.

The *symptoms* of atrophy when caused by bad feeding, or when originating from an undeveloped condition of the diseases named, are as follows. The approach is insidious, and consists of languor, drooping, lassitude, and loss of flesh. Sometimes the face remains full while the body and limbs waste. Although at first there may be no strongly marked fever, close observation will show heat of skin in the evening, perspiration in the night, and languor and debility in the morning, while the child looks pale and listless, and the appetite is lost. Then, if the atrophy arises from bad feeding, vomiting, diarrhœa, or dysentery occurs. If the atrophy depends on a rickety condition of system, the symptoms given under Rickets (p. 371) gradually develop. If the atrophy depends upon worms, the child will be constantly picking the nose, lips, or fundament, and other symptoms noted under Worms (p. 483) will present. If the atrophy depends on enlargement of the glands of the bowels, known as the *mesenteric glands*, the malady is called *tabes mesenterica.* The belly grows large, and the glands of the bowels being diseased, constipation alternates with diarrhœa, and fever of a hectic character (*vide* p. 269) and night perspirations become more apparent. The bowels now grow hot and tender to the touch, and the enlarged glands may be distinctly felt hard and knotty underneath the skin. There may be frequent vomiting, and the feet may swell. As the disease advances the evacuations change, becoming slimy, bloody, and sour-smelling; the breath is very offensive; and the urine is scanty, depositing a whitish sediment. The appetite is very capricious; the skin is extremely irritable; and the child, instead of being plump and rosy, presents the aspect of shrivelled old age. The more the child wastes, the more restless and irritable does it become, until it dies from diarrhœa and exhaustion. If the atrophy is dependent on scrofula, consumption, or Bright's disease, the symptoms noted under such headings gradually develop. If atrophy depends on malarious influences, the secondary conditions are anæmia, masked malarious fever, or spleen affections (pp. 46, 266, 412). In addition to the above, atrophy may be complicated with attacks of *infantile remittent fever* (p. 263), with swelling and abscess of the glands of the neck, and with skin diseases, all of which are more likely to occur when the condition of atrophy is present, especially if arising from improper feeding.

*Treatment.*—The treatment of atrophy is rather dietetic and hygienic than medicinal, especially when it arises from improper feeding. And when it arises from other causes, the treatment of such other causes is required. But in any case pure air must be ensured, particularly in sleeping apartments. The nature of the food must be scrutinised, and care be taken that the patient is not suffering from the effects of a too exclusively farinaceous diet (*vide Remarks on the Feeding of Children*, Chapter V.) Much of the wasting and accompanying dysentery from which children in India, and particularly the children of soldiers in barracks, suffer arises wholly or partly from want of proper food, which the parents are either unable to obtain, or regarding which, from ignorance or carelessness, they do not take sufficient care. But while attending to diet other matters must not be neglected. Worms if present must be expelled (*vide Worms*, p. 482). Diarrhœa must be treated by appropriate remedies (*vide Infantile Diarrhœa*, p. 172). If the teeth are troublesome the gums must be lanced (*vide* p. 434). Tonics, especially quinine, in doses according to the child's age (*vide* p. 19), should be given. When the bowels are large the abdomen should be gently rubbed daily, for some minutes, with equal parts of brandy and salad oil. Lastly, change of air, milk, baths, and sea-bathing, or at least bathing in sea-water, are important adjuvants in the treatment of lingering cases.

[One of the various malt foods will generally be desirable, regarding which remarks will be found in Chapter V., *On the Feeding of Children.* For the atrophy of children 'Kepler's Extract of Malt' may be specially recommended. Or still better, if available, a fresh infusion of malt. This is made by steeping 1 ounce of bruised malt for two hours in a pint of cold water. Of the strained solution from 4 to 6 ounces daily may be given to a child three years old. Burroughs & Wellcome's 'beef and iron wine' is also generally advisable.]

**BED-SORES.**—When patients, whether from disease or from injury, have to lie long in bed, and especially when they are obliged to lie long in one position, sores are apt to form on those parts of the body subjected to the greatest pressure. It is really the death of the part from long-continued pressure. Thus the back, hips, buttocks, heels, and elbows are liable to suffer, and when a patient is likely to lie long in bed, the commencement of bed-sores should be guarded against from the first. The pressure producing the sore diminishes the sensibility of the part affected, so that the patient himself may be unaware of the formation of a sore. It is therefore necessary that his word should not be accepted on the point, and that examination should be frequently instituted. Want of cleanliness and moisture, especially moisture from urine or fæces, irritates the skin, and renders bed-sores much more likely, and therefore, as preventive measures, great care must be given to these points. In all cases close attention should be paid to keep the bed smooth and the sheets free from 'rucks' or folds. Corded or feather beds should not be used. The best is a horse-hair mattress placed on a second or spring bed. The parts most subjected to pressure should be from the first bathed twice daily with a wash, composed of a drachm of alum dissolved in four ounces of water, which will tend to harden the skin. Plasters should never be used, as they are liable to wrinkle, and thus cause irritation, and they prevent the condition of the parts being seen. Small pads, or pillows, or air-pillows, or water-cushions, should be made use of to relieve the parts most exposed to pressure. Frequently a pillow of circular shape, with a hole in the centre, will be found very useful. When a bed-sore is about forming the skin becomes reddened. If the pressure is not relieved, the part assumes a dusky appearance, afterwards becoming blistered. Then a grey or blackish slough forms, with discharge of thin matter. In such a condition, a poultice made of powdered charcoal should be applied, until the slough separates, after which water-dressing (Recipe 85). No application will, however, be of service unless *pressure* is removed from the part by the use of pads and pillows, as above mentioned. As the condition is attended by great debility, nourishing broths, stimulants and tonics, as quinine (Recipe 66), will be required. In all cases of bed-sores the apartment must be kept well ventilated, and disinfectants should be used (*vide Appendix*, No. 120); the smell from the affected part being always very offensive.

[Instead of water-dressing, if procurable, one part of carbolic acid to 50 parts of salad oil; or *antiseptic cotton wool* specially prepared for such cases, should be used. The use of the artificial sponge mentioned at p. 497 is also desirable.]

**BLADDER, INFLAMMATION OF THE.**—Inflammation of the bladder may be caused by injuries, by exposure to cold, by irritation from a stone, or it may be connected with stricture, or arise from the extension of a gonorrhœal attack. It may be excited by an over-dose of copaiba or of cantharides. It may result from the unskilful use of instruments. It may be a consequence of prolonged labour, or arise from females, after delivery, neglecting to empty the bladder. Shivering often occurs at first, followed by mental depression, fever, thirst, and pain with soreness on pressure over the bladder, or in the lower part of the belly. Pressure in the fork between the legs is also very painful, where there is generally a sense of weight or burning. The urine is voided frequently and in small quantities, often with great straining, followed by aggravation of the pain and burning. The urine also contains a mucous deposit, and sometimes blood. Females often void flakes of mucus much larger than can pass from males. In exceptional cases the inflammation may extend to the bowels, causing peritonitis (*vide* p. 79), or to the kidneys, causing interference with the secretion of urine, when the patient may become delirious and sink into a typhoid condition (*vide* p. 242) or suffer from *Uræmia* (*vide* p. 55).

*Treatment.*—A hot bath will generally be advisable, and fomentations (*vide Appendix*, No. 80) should be afterwards applied over the lower part of the bowels. Barley-water (*vide Addendum*) should be prescribed *ad libitum* as a drink, and for thirst and feverishness effervescing draughts of citrate of magnesia (*vide* p. 15) should be taken. The bowels should also be opened by sulphate of soda draughts (Recipe 2), and clysters of warm water (Recipe 104) will probably be required to relieve pain. At night an opiate, as 10 grains of Dover's powder, or 15 grains of chloral, will be generally advisable; the Dover's powder being most useful when the skin is hot and dry. The patient should be kept in bed, and be restricted to low diet, such as milk, broths, and light puddings.

**BLADDER, CHRONIC INFLAMMATION OF THE.**—Acute inflammation of the bladder sometimes subsides into a minor degree, which may be long continued, becoming, as it is then called, *chronic*. Or it may arise very gradually without the more marked symptoms referred to above. This condition mostly occurs as a result of gonorrhœa or gravel; or in elderly persons in connection with enlargement of a gland situated round the neck of the bladder (*vide* p. 366). It may also be a sequence of stone or of stricture, or of disease of the rectum or kidneys, or it may follow accidents to the spine (*vide* p. 557). It also occurs when the bladder participates in attacks of paralysis (*vide* p. 342). It may result from atony of the bladder in old people who are unable to expel their urine. In chronic inflammation of the bladder the symptoms are those of the acute form, but in a minor degree; and there is, in addition, a discharge of thick ropy mucus with the urine, which adheres to the side of the vessel, smells ammoniacal, and often presents whitish-looking lines or streaks, which are caused by the *phosphate of lime* formed from the urine within the bladder. The urine is also sometimes bloody.

*Treatment.*—Medical aid should be obtained as soon as possible, in order to ascertain if there is stricture (*vide* p. 419), or enlarged prostate (*vide* p. 366), or stone or tumour in the bladder (*vide* pp. 73, 74), or any affection of the kidneys (*vide* p. 101) or of the rectum (*vide* p. 272). In the meantime, the patient should keep himself in the recumbent posture as much as possible. Pain and irritation may be allayed by warm hip baths, or by enemas of warm water (Recipe 104). The bowels should be maintained open by mild aperients (Recipe 2). The diet should be nourishing but plain, with weak gin-and-water or sound sherry in small quantities.

[For chronic inflammation of the bladder not depending on organic changes, as stricture, stone, or enlarged prostate gland, Recipes 27, 28, 31 may be tried in the order named. No sugar should be used with the diet, but 'saccharin tabloids' may be substituted.]

**BLADDER, STONE IN THE.**—Stone in the bladder is in consequence of a diseased condition of the urine, and is most prevalent in localities where the water contains lime. It is often one of the results of *gravel* (*vide* p. 285). When stone is present there is acute pain, aggravated by motion, and worse after making water. There is also frequent desire to make water, with itching and smarting at the end of the penis. This induces children to pull the foreskin continually, which becomes elongated, and often red and inflamed. There is also frequently sudden stoppage of the stream of urine, owing to the stone rolling in front of the passage, and the fluid passed is sometimes bloody. In children especially there is much straining at stool, and usually protrusion of the lower bowel outside (*vide* p. 84). The early symptoms of stone often resemble those of enlargement of the prostate (*vide* p. 366), or of stricture (*vide* p. 419), or of tumour (*vide* p. 74), and instrumental examination is frequently necessary to decide the point. There are various kinds of stone, and the only remedy is surgical operation. Sometimes a small stone passing out of the bladder lodges in the urethra or urinary passage, requiring surgical operation also.

**BLADDER, OTHER DISEASES OF THE.**—Other maladies to which the bladder is liable are as below:—

Irritability of the Bladder is marked by frequent desire to make water without evident cause. This may depend in elderly persons on incipient disease of the prostate gland (*vide* p. 366); or at any age on stone (*vide* p. 73); or on gravel (*vide* p. 285); or on fissure of the anus (*vide* p. 272). It may arise from constipation, when hard fæcal matter in the lower bowel presses against the bladder (*vide* p. 137). The irritation caused by worms is also a cause (*vide* p. 483). It sometimes occurs to children who are overworked. But irritability of the bladder may arise *temporarily* from cold as experienced at the commencement of the cold season, or on change to a colder climate. It may also follow various drinks, especially of an acrid nature, or it may be due altogether to nervousness. When inability to hold the urine occurs to adults, and there is no evident disease, or cause as above, explaining the defect, 15 to 20 grains of chloral given at night will prove an effectual remedy. As the malady grows less the quantity of chloral should be diminished, till the person is able to do without it. A drop of creosote made into a pill with bread, and taken at night, is beneficial.

NEURALGIA OF THE BLADDER is marked by periodic pain, and is benefited by quinine (Recipe 67), or arsenic (Recipe 75).

PARALYSIS OF THE BLADDER is marked by inability to pass urine. If not relieved the bladder becomes full, when the urine dribbles away. Paralysis of the bladder may be *temporary* from cold, or from retaining the urine too long, or from hysteria (*vide* p. 306). Or it may be permanent from injury or disease of the spine (*vide* pp. 343, 557) or as a consequence of apoplexy (*vide* p. 53). Temporary inability to pass urine may usually be relieved by a hot bath and a dose of chloral. Permanent paralysis requires the treatment mentioned under the headings causing it.

TUMOURS OF THE BLADDER.—The bladder is subject to several kinds of morbid growths, the principal of which are *polypus*, chiefly occurring in children; a growth known as *papilloma* (meaning small conical eminences); and *malignant* or *cancerous* growths. The symptoms are at first only a little frequency of making water, and eventually blood in the urine, which may first occur after exercise. The blood is often passed at the end of micturition, the urine at first flowing clear and natural. Pain is not much complained of unless the flow of urine is interfered with by clots of blood. As the disease progresses it causes weakness and exhaustion. Some forms of tumour may be removed by surgical operation, but medicine is not of much benefit.

**BOILS.**—Boils differ from abscess by containing a *core* (*vide Abscess*, p. 39). They are common in India, either occurring singly, or several at one time, or in successive crops. They may be of various sizes, from that of a pea to the bulk of an egg, or larger. Large boils most frequently occur on the limbs, on the back of the neck, in the armpit, or about the buttocks, and are often long before coming to a head. In some instances after pain and swelling have occurred they gradually subside without the formation of matter, and are then popularly termed 'blind boils.' Small boils frequently present on the scalp, when hundreds may sometimes be counted. The cause of these Indian boils is in most instances blood-deterioration, caused by length of residence, heat, scurvy, impure atmosphere, improper food, overwork, or attacks of fever, or *anæmia* (*vide* p. 46). In persons predisposed by such influences, accidental local injury, or irritation, will often excite them. Boils may also result from poisoning of the blood (*vide* p. 587). In children boils may attend teething. Boils sometimes attack new comers, or persons who have suddenly changed their residence from one part of India to another. For instance, after a long period spent in the Upper Provinces, change to the moister climates of the sea-coasts is often followed by boils. Boils are sometimes erroneously attributed to eating mangoes; the fact being that the mango season, or shortly after the mango season, is the period of the year when, owing to the intensity of the heat, and the resulting blood-deterioration (*vide* Chapter VI., *Heat*), boils are most common. Occasionally boils present in persons who declare they 'never felt better in their lives.' But notwithstanding this, the occurrence of boils must always be accepted as evidence of something wrong in the system. Very large boils are termed carbuncles (*vide* p. 113).

*Treatment.*—In all cases of boils the condition of the general health must be attentively considered, and the patient treated accordingly. If the tongue is furred and the digestive organs out of order, aperient doses, as Recipes 1 and 2, or for weakly persons citrate of magnesia (p. 15), will be required. If there is reason to suspect scorbutic taint, evidenced by tender, spongy, or bleeding gums; or even if these signs are not recognised, if the person has been in a locality where fresh vegetables were scarce, two or three ounces of lime-juice should be taken daily, and any green vegetables procurable. If syphilitic taint (evidenced probably by eruptions on the skin) is present, Recipe 19 should be taken, until the medicine mentioned in the small type can be procured. If malarious or anæmic taint (p. 47) exists, quinine (Recipe 66). If no particular taint is evident, Recipe 3, with or without the sulphate of soda, according as the bowels are constipated or the reverse, may be taken with advantage.

Local treatment consists in poultices, which may be of linseed meal, or of flour, or of figs—the latter remedy being as ancient as the Book of Kings. When matter forms, the most prominent part should be pricked with a clean lancet. In short, the whole surgical treatment should be that recommended for abscess (*vide* p. 41). Or if the boil is small, sluggish, and long in coming to a head, the old-fashioned remedy of yellow soap and sugar mixed in equal parts into a thick paste, and spread on wash-leather, may be applied. The piece of leather should be sufficiently large to cover the whole of the boil, and should be kept in place by a bandage. Or a paste of honey and flour may be used instead. Spirits of camphor (*vide* p. 24), applied every three hours and allowed to dry on the part, if used sufficiently early, will sometimes disperse sluggish boils. Ulcers or sores, remaining after a boil ceases to discharge matter, should be treated by water-dressing (Recipe 85), or by simple ointment (Recipe 86).

[Iodine paint (*Liniment of Iodine*) is a better remedy for dispersing boils. It should be applied with a feather or brush over, and for an inch or two round, the boil, three times the first day, and less frequently afterwards, so as to maintain an irritation of, but *not* to blister, the skin. Equal parts of belladonna liniment and glycerine, smeared over the boil *before* the poultice is applied, tends to subdue the inflammation. If there is reason to suspect a scorbutic taint of the blood, while the diet should be arranged as recommended under *Scurvy* (p. 382), Recipe 46 should be procured and used. If a syphilitic taint is suspected, Recipe 74 will be desirable. If no particular taint is evident and boils still present, Recipe 75 should be taken as a tonic. A tenth of a grain of sulphide of calcium, given every two or three hours, generally prevents the formation of fresh boils, while it lessens the inflammation, and reduces the area of the existing boils, and quickly liquefies the core, so that its separation is much more speedy. This may be taken in addition to any other of the remedies noticed.]

*Boils presenting somewhat varied characters*, and occurring in different parts of the East, are often spoken of as if peculiar to that part of the country; as, for example, Aden boils, Scinde boils, Gwalior boils, Delhi boils, Panjdeh sore, Persian ulcer, and Bagdad boils. The Bagdad boil, commonly called the 'date mark,' is the counterpart of the 'Aleppo bouton,' and disfigures, generally in the face, nearly every child born at Bagdad, but attacks adults on some other part of the person. But there is nothing radically different in these boils from any others. What is called the Delhi boil, for instance, is not confined to the city of that name. Neither is it a new disease. For it has been known for many generations under the native name of Arungzebe—after the Emperor of Delhi so called, who suffered from it. A similar boil is common at Muttra, at Agra, at Moultan, and throughout the semi-desert districts of Western

India. The Delhi and similar sores commence as a pimple, and may continue in that condition for some months; then, gradually increasing in size, they break on the surface, becoming unhealthy-looking ulcers or sores, which often leave disfiguring scars. The parts most frequently attacked are the elbows, fore-arms, backs of the hands, ankles, legs, face, and thighs; rarely the trunk, and never the scalp.

Delhi and other similar sores have been thought due to the presence of a parasite, but the evidence is not conclusive. They are, however, always connected with blood-deterioration, and are especially associated with that condition, perhaps at first latent and undetected, arising from the combined effects of scorbutic taint, of malarious influences, of exposure to long-continued heat, of residence in insanitary localities, aided sometimes by a syphilitic taint. The treatment should be decided upon after due inquiry as to which of the influences mentioned has been most powerfully in action. If a scorbutic taint is suspected, fresh vegetables and Recipe 67 will be indicated. If malarious influences are prominent, Recipe 66. If heat appears the cause of debility, removal to a hill station, or the journey home, is the desirable measure. While of course all insanitary conditions must be remedied, particular attention should be given to the water, which should be filtered and prepared for drinking, as recommended under the head *Water*, Chapter VI. The comparative immunity now enjoyed by the residents of Delhi from so-called Delhi boils is doubtless due to the hygienic improvements which have been gradually introduced during the past few years.

Local applications should in the first instance consist of water-dressing (Recipe 85); and when it is concluded, from throbbing pain, or increasing size if pain is absent, that matter is forming, poultices should be applied, of whichever variety is most readily procurable (of the Recipes 77, 78, 79). When, after the discharge of matter, sores form, stimulating applications will generally be required, and a lotion, composed of 20 grains of sulphate of iron (the *Hera-kusees* of the bazaars), dissolved in six ounces of water, may be employed in the same manner as water is to be used in the water-dressing application (Recipe 85). When the sores become healthy and are inclined to heal, simple water-dressing will be the most suitable application.

[If during the process of Delhi or other sore, as mentioned above, scorbutic taint is suspected, Recipe 46 should be procured. When, after the discharge of the matter, the remaining sore requires stimulating, the ointment (Recipe 93) should be obtained and used instead of the sulphate of iron lotion given above.]

**BONES, DISEASE OF THE.**—The bones are subject to numerous diseases, the principal of which are scrofulous affections. Fixed, dull pain in a bone, as the shin bone, for instance, increased at night, is generally the first sign, which is eventually followed by redness, swelling, and abscess, either in the bone itself, or in a neighbouring joint (*vide* p. 312). The first symptom mentioned should lead to early application to a surgeon. In the meantime the part should be kept at rest, and chloral may be given to relieve pain.

**BOWELS, INFLAMMATION OF THE.**—In this term are included the different distinctions, as *peritonitis* and *enteritis*, drawn by physicians. Inflammation of the bowels or of their covering (the peritoneum) is marked by fever, and severe continuous burning pain in the belly, *increased by pressure.* The patient lies on his back in bed with the *knees drawn up,* afraid to increase the pain by movement. If the breathing is watched it will be seen that the belly is nearly motionless, whereas in health it rises and falls. But when inflammation is present, movement of the part is so painful that breathing is performed altogether by the muscles of the chest. There is generally costiveness, nausea, or vomiting, great prostration of strength, and an anxious expression of countenance. The pulse is frequent, and *wiry* to the touch, and the urine is highly coloured. In fatal cases pain increases, the bowels become swollen and *tympanitic* or drum-like from accumulation of gas within, the extremities grow cold, the skin is bathed in cold perspiration, the features are sharpened, pain suddenly ceases, and the patient dies. Inflammation of the bowels must be carefully distinguished from *colic*, in which there is intermitting twisting pain, *relieved* by pressure, the patient often rolling about to obtain ease (*vide Colic*, p. 131).

The *causes* of inflammation of the bowels are various. It may arise from cold, as, for instance, from sleeping with the bowels exposed to a current of cold air. It may be caused by injuries over the bowels, or by some substance lodged in, irritating and inflaming the bowels. In this manner it may be a sequel of colic. It may occur in the course of certain fevers, or as an extension of inflammation of the womb or bladder.

*Treatment.*—Continued fomentations with hot water over the whole of the bowels (*vide Appendix*, No. 80). A cradle (*vide* p. 555), to support the weight of the bedclothes from the tender bowels, is generally required. Placing the hands above the head renders the breathing easier. Clysters of warm water and soap (Recipe 104) should be injected every day; but purgatives should *not* be administered, unless costiveness prevailed previous to the attack, when a dose of castor oil will be proper at the outset. For the relief of pain and to procure sleep, a chloral draught (Recipe 64) may be taken at night. Fluid diet *only*, as weak tea, beef-tea, chicken-tea, and broths (*vide Addendum*), should be given. Iced water or iced barley-water may be allowed.

[In a case of decided inflammation of the bowels or their coverings, in an adult, as evidenced by the symptoms above detailed, calomel and opium pills (Recipe 23) should be procured if possible, and should be given until the gums are slightly tender, or until a metallic taste is experienced in the mouth, when the medicine should be immediately stopped.]

**BOWELS, INFLAMMATION OF THE CÆCUM OF THE, OR TYPHLITIS.**—Portions of the bowels known as the CÆCUM, and APPENDIX VERMIFORMIS, are sometimes affected, independently of the other part of the intestines. The *cæcum* is the commencement of the larger portion of the bowels, or the point of union between the large and small intestines, and the *appendix vermiformis* is a short blind tube attached thereto. They are situated on the right side above the groin (*vide* plate, p. 29), and are the parts of the intestinal tube in which *obstruction* often commences (*vide* p. 82). The peculiar shape and formation of the parts is more favourable than that of any other portion of the intestines to the lodgment of such things as fruit-stones, gall-stones, portions of unripe apples, worms, or even pieces of hard fæcal matter, round or above which other fæcal matter stagnates. When only the cæcum and appendix are inflamed the pain and tenderness are limited to the part, and there are no symptoms of obstruction (*vide* p. 82). But inflammation commencing in the cæcum may spread to the whole of the belly, when the symptoms are as previously detailed. In both cases the treatment is the same as for inflammation of the bowels, fomentations being applied to the most tender part. Recurring attacks of typhlitis, probably excited by something lodging in the parts, may lead to abscess, and the propriety of an operation should be considered.

[The *cæcum* is also liable to a *chronic* or slow form of inflammation, which may arise without any evident cause, or which may be the sequel of an attack of *obstruction*. The symptoms are at first apparently trifling, and the malady may therefore remain for some time unrecognised, and unattended to. There is a vague failing of the general health, comparative weakness, gradual loss of flesh, and occasional transient, colic-like pain, in the position indicated above. Or these slight transient pains may occur at first, without any decided deterioration of the general health. As the malady progresses there is loss of appetite, much flatulence, diarrhœa alternating with constipation, and more decided and permanent local pain. At length the internal coat of the bowel ulcerates and there is an increase of all symptoms, with mucus or slimy discharge streaked with blood as in dysentery, and sometimes large quantities of pure blood are passed.

A malady of the kind always demands skilled advice. Broadly speaking, the treatment consists in nourishing and easily digested food; in the frequent application of some counter-irritant, as iodine paint or mustard leaves; in the administration of tonics, of which the mineral acids with quinine will be best (Recipe 69); and in the prevention of constipation or of diarrhœa—whichever condition may prevail—by the appropriate remedies.]

**BOWELS, OBSTRUCTION OF THE.**—This affection, in which the patient is unable to pass stool, may commence suddenly as an attack of colic (*vide Colic, p.* 131). Or it may commence gradually, probably after dyspeptic symptoms, with inflammation of the cæcum as described above. The constipation not being relieved by medicine, vomiting, first of the contents of the stomach as partially digested food, then of sour bilious material, and lastly of fæcal material (as described in *Rupture*, p. 591), occurs, accompanied by much tenderness, pain, and distension of the bowels. Very often a hard lump may be felt somewhere in the bowels, most frequently on the right side, over the *cæcum* (*vide* plate, p. 29). The neighbourhood of this lump, which should be searched for, is always most painful; the tenderness and distension radiating from this position to other parts, until perhaps the condition above described as inflammation (of portions, or of the whole) of the bowels may be set up; or, the acute symptoms being relieved, chronic inflammation of the cæcum (*vide* p. 81) or an abscess may occur as an insidious and distant result.

*Treatment.*—In the first place, remedies calculated to

remove constipation should be given, and castor-oil or sulphate of soda (Recipe 2) may be used. The action of the purgative should be aided by an injection (Recipe 105), and the belly should be well fomented (*vide Appendix*, No. 80). A hot bath should also be taken. If the part is not too tender, gentle pressure or kneading with the fingers may be used, but it must not be continued if it causes pain. If these remedies do not succeed, 20 grains of chloral (Recipe 64) should be given three times a day, and a large quantity of warm water (about two quarts) should be injected several times daily. The patient should be kept perfectly quiet, and *fluid diet only* should be allowed, in small quantities; for the more freely food and fluid are partaken of, the greater will be the distension, pain, and danger. The best diet will be extract of beef, or strong soup, thickened with flour or eggs, or, still better, raw-meat soup (*vide Addendum*). Thirst may be relieved by sucking ice or frozen milk, or by washing the mouth with cold water. The continued giving of purgatives is useless, as often some part of the gut is twisted, or tied into a knot, or otherwise slipped inside itself, as the finger of a glove is when folded back on itself. In such cases the best chance of recovery is from opiates and perfect rest. Surgical operations have been performed for the relief of obstruction of the bowels, the propriety of which would require the sanction of a medical consultation. During convalescence, and for long afterwards, much care in diet, and particularly measures to avoid constipation, are necessary; otherwise affection of the *cæcum*, as described at page 76, may result.

[In young and robust persons, at the early period of the disease, instead of castor-oil or Recipe 2, as recommended in the large type, give, if procurable, one-tenth of a grain of tartar emetic, and 1 drachm of sulphate of magnesia in 2 ounces of water every hour, up to eight doses, which often aids in breaking up and removing the obstruction. In cases of obstruction of the bowels, after purgatives and choral have failed, 1 grain of hydrochlorate of morphia with 5 grains of extract of belladonna should be given twice a day. A drop of chloroform or of creosote taken on a lump of sugar will often relieve the distressing vomiting present in these cases.]

**BOWELS, PROTRUSION OF THE.**—This affection, which occurs principally to children, but sometimes to old people, is met with in every degree, from the mere protrusion of a ring to the protrusion of half a foot or more. At first the tumour is bright red, and mothers, seeing this for the first time, are often much alarmed without due cause, as it is not a dangerous affection. If the bowel often comes down, it gradually becomes thickened and callous and more like skin. Children who have been much relaxed, as from dysentery or diarrhœa, or from the too frequent use of purgatives, are very subject to the affection. Or it may be a consequence of the irritation excited by stone in the bladder (*vide* p. 73), or by threadworms (*vide* p. 486), or by phimosis (*vide* p. 346). Or the malady may arise from nurses allowing children to sit on their chairs too long. Often it occurs from pure debility; a cough even in feeble children being sufficient to bring the gut down. The gut, when it at first presents, returns by its own elasticity. Afterwards, although thus returning, it comes down again immediately. In old cases, the tumour requires to be replaced.

*Treatment.*—To find out the cause of the affection is the first aim, as on removal of the cause the effect will generally cease. The presence or absence of worms, or of stone, must be assured. Constipation or diarrhœa, if present, must be first treated (*vide* pp. 138, 172). The child should not be allowed to sit on the chair for more than two or three minutes, and if the bowels are unrelieved, the patient should be placed on it again after some little interval. The protrusion of the bowel may often be prevented thus. When the child is about to have a stool, let the nurse with her fingers draw the skin of the buttocks outwards, so as to render it quite tight over the fundament, and hold it in this position till the motion is finished. If the bowel comes down, the child should be laid on its face, the legs should be widely separated, and the protrusion should be lubricated with salad oil. Then it should be gently grasped with the points of the fingers enveloped in a damp, soft, oiled cloth or handkerchief, and steadily but gently squeezed for about half a minute to empty it of blood. Then it should be gently pushed up. But the utmost gentleness must be observed; for with pain from rough handling resistance is produced, and with it increased difficulty of replacement. In cases of *recurring* protrusion, before applying oil as above described the part should be sopped with alum water (Recipe 42). In all cases when much of the bowel has descended the child should not be allowed to sit up for an hour or two afterwards, but should be kept in the horizontal posture, which will admit of the parts recovering strength and elasticity to retain their natural place.

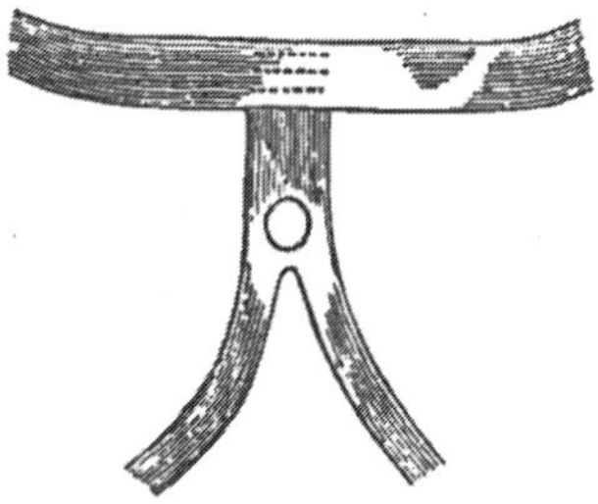

If the protrusion cannot be easily returned, it will be best to apply a bread poultice for a few hours, after which the gut will probably return, or it may be replaced by pressure with the damp oiled cloth. If the protrusion will not remain up, a band should be put round the waist, and another band dividing into two past the anus (*vide* sketch) should be brought from this band at the middle of the back, between the legs, and the ends should be separately fastened in front. Where this latter band passes over the anal orifice, a large cork rounded at the end should be attached, the pressure of which, if rightly adjusted, will prevent the falling down of the bowel. Various belts are sold for the purpose, but the home-made belt as figured is efficacious. In bad cases the sitting posture at stools should be wholly prohibited, and motions should be passed while the child is lying down. Children subject to this affection generally require tonics, and salt-water bathing is often advantageous. Whatever improves the general health will also give increased strength to the parts which naturally support and retain the bowel in its position.

**BRAIN, CONGESTION AND INFLAMMATION OF THE.** —These serious disorders may be the result of injuries, may occur during fevers, may be caused by exposure to heat, may arise from excessive mental toil and anxiety, or from the extension of *erysipelas* (*vide* p. 220) to the inside of the head.

*Symptoms.*—Congestion or fulness of the brain is ordinarily the first condition of subsequent inflammation. It is marked by dull oppressive pain in the head, restlessness, feverishness, intolerance of light, and nausea. If the malady goes on to, or commences as inflammation, all the symptoms are exaggerated. There are shivering, flushes of the face alternating with pallor, great pain in the head, and especially of the forehead of a burning character, vomiting, high fever, intolerance of light, sleeplessness, delirium of a violent character (*vide* p. 159). In the second stage of the malady there is an effusion of the products of the inflammation on the surface of the brain, or in its substance or cavities. The pulse then becomes slow, the pupils become dilated, there is deep insensibility, and sometimes convulsions. Death, palsy, or perfect recovery may result.

*Treatment.*—When there is simply congestion, purgatives and quiet are the remedies, by the judicious use of which many cases have been prevented from passing into inflammation, or into apoplexy or paralysis, of which congestion of the brain may be the warning (*vide Apoplexy*, p. 53). But if there are shivering and flushes, vomiting and high fever, with burning pain in the head, the hair should be shaved off, and a bladder of pounded ice should be applied to the forehead and scalp. Or if ice is not obtainable, cold evaporating lotions (Recipe 83), or vinegar and water, should be used. The bowels should be freely acted upon daily by sulphate of soda (Recipe 2). The patient should be kept in a darkened room, and perfect silence and quiet enjoined. No stimulants should be given, and the diet should consist entirely of beef-tea, broth, and milk-and-water. No opiate or sleeping-draught should be given without medical advice. It is a disorder urgently requiring the assistance of a skilful physician.

[If the bowels are not freely opened, a little croton oil should be obtained if possible, and two drops should be given rolled up with a little gum and water into a pill or pills. If the patient is delirious and will not swallow, the oil should be placed on the back of the tongue with a feather.]

**BRAIN, SOFTENING OF THE.**—This disease is in many instances caused by the want of a proper supply of nourishment to the brain-substance, and may arise secondarily from affections of the vessels supplying the brain with blood. A condition of softening of the brain may be caused by alcohol. It may also occur as a result of sunstroke. It is most usually met with in advanced life, and there is little doubt that the exposure of Europeans to the effects of continued tropical heat during a series of years produces a debilitated condition of system, consequent on blood-degeneration, favourable to brain-softening. Great anxiety and excessive study are also accessory predisposing causes. The malady is characterised by lowness of spirits, headaches, giddiness, loss of memory, confusion of ideas, and at length imbecility and paralysis. Medicinal treatment is of little value, especially if the malady depends on disease of the arteries supplying the brain with blood. Rest, tonics, and removal to a temperate climate would, however, be desirable in any case.

**BRAIN, TUBERCLES ON THE.**—This malady, popularly but erroneously often called '*water on the brain*,' is also frequently termed *Brain-fever*. It is known technically as *hydrocephalus*, but more correctly as *tubercular meningitis*. It depends on the formation of small tubercles on the surface of the brain, or in the investing membranes, in the shape of small yellowish spots, and the subsequent production of a watery effusion into the cavities of the brain. But sometimes the tubercular deposit is not confined to the brain, but also takes place in the lungs and the glands of the bowels. When this occurs the disease is termed *acute general tuberculosis*.

[Recent researches tend to the conclusion that tuberculosis is a specific disease, due to the introduction into the body of a microbe or *bacillus*, which is followed by the formation of tubercle in the part affected. If in the brain, the disease under consideration arises. If in the lungs, consumption occurs. If in the bowels, mesenteric disease happens. Persons of scrofulous habit are most likely to become the subjects of tuberculosis of any part.]

*Tubercular meningitis* generally occurs in young children of scrofulous constitution, and is rare after seven years of age. In children thus predisposed it often follows the convalescence from small-pox, scarlet fever, or hooping-cough, or it may be excited by forcing the mental faculties. It is often preceded for some time by loss of general health, the child taking food freely, but not thriving, and suffering from alternating constipation and diarrhœa. There is loss of flesh in the body and limbs, but the face is less affected. The child is fretful and drowsy ; there are sudden startings during sleep, and often grinding of the teeth. The tongue becomes furred, the breath offensive; there is also headache, and often a peculiar staggering gait. Except the last-mentioned, the early symptoms are very much like those of atrophy (*vide* p. 66) and of worms (*vide* p. 483). After a variable period, during which these early symptoms may have been so strongly marked as to suggest danger, or so trivial as to have escaped notice, either one or other series of 'head symptoms' present. The child may become the subject of *true hydrocephalus*, or *tubercular meningitis*, or *brain fever*, as described below, or it may suffer from a condition which has been termed *spurious hydrocephalus*, as described at p. 92. The symptoms of these two conditions are different; they arise from different causes, and they require different treatment. While *true hydrocephalus* depends on a congested and tubercular condition of the brain, *spurious hydrocephalus* arises from the brain being deprived of sufficient nourishment in consequence of a poor and deteriorated state of the blood. *Spurious hydrocephalus* may occur from this cause, before the condition mentioned above as the cause of *true hydrocephalus* has had time to mature; or spurious hydrocephalus may present in a debilitated child in whom there is no real hydrocephalic condition.

*The first symptoms of true hydrocephalus*, or *tubercular meningitis*, or *brain fever* of children, are, after more or less of the premonitory symptoms noted above, the child being seized with high fever and *obstinate vomiting*, which continues whether the stomach is full or empty. One of the most characteristic symptoms of *hydrocephalus* is *obstinate vomiting*; and whenever obstinate vomiting shows itself in a vaccinated child, hydrocephalus may be suspected; if in an unvaccinated child, it may be premonitory of smallpox (*vide* p. 404). The peculiar gait becomes more staggering, and there is a tendency to cling to surrounding objects. There is squinting, and marked aversion to light, from which the child turns the head away; there is alternate flushing and paleness of the face, which is sometimes sad and frowning, at others vacant and stupid. The skin is harsh and dry, the temperature rising to 102° or 103° every evening. There is severe pain in the forehead, coming on in darting paroxysms and causing the child to scream with a characteristic piercing cry, to which the term *cri hydrocéphalique* has been given. The pain causes the child to put its hands to the head, which is incessantly rolled from side to side. As the disease advances the belly looks shrunken and hollow, but is not tender, the obstinate vomiting continues, the eyes squint, there is delirium, and often repeated convulsions. When not convulsed, the child is generally picking at the bed-clothes, or boring the fingers into the ears or nostrils. When the malady occurs in infants before the bones of the head have united, there is prominence and strong pulsation visible at the *fontanelles*, or where the bones of the head join. In some cases occurring in very young children, before the bones of the skull are consolidated, the head is visibly swollen. Often a fallacious remission of symptoms takes place; but at a later period, or from one week to three after the commencement of the disease, the face assumes an aged expression, vomiting ceases, diarrhœa sets in, the pulse becomes slower, the breathing has a sighing or moaning character, the pupils of the eyes are dilated or they may oscillate, the child becomes drowsy, insensibility ensues, and the child dies. Or death may take place during an attack of convulsions.

When, as previously mentioned as sometimes occurring, the disease attacks the lungs and bowels, symptoms referable to those organs will also arise. When the lungs are implicated there will probably be cough and also expectoration. When the bowels are affected there will be enlargement of the glands and other symptoms, described as *tabes mesenterica* (*vide* p. 67).

Hydrocephalus may be mistaken for *gastric* disorders, or for *typhoid* fever. The distinguishing features are given under *Disorders of the Stomach* (p. 415).

*Treatment.*—The sick-room should be darkened, if possible, with green blinds. The air should be maintained as fresh and pure as can be, only the necessary attendants being admitted, and the utmost quiet being observed. When the child has to be moved, it should be raised in the most careful manner, without shaking. All sources of irritation must be sought for and removed as soon as possible. Thus, if the child is teething, and the gums are anywhere swollen and tender, they must be freely lanced (*vide* p. 434). If the child is being fed by hand, a wet-nurse should, if possible, be obtained. If there is any suspicion that the mother's or nurse's milk does not agree with the child (when at the breast), a fresh and healthy nurse whose milk is a little older than the patient should be obtained. If the bowels have not been previously loose, a purgative dose of castor-oil should be given. If this does not act freely, the necessity of moving the bowels being urgent, sulphate of soda may be used every four hours (half a drachm at six months, one drachm at one year old) until the bowels are well purged. If the child has been ordinarily healthy and robust, and has not been debilitated by previous illness, one leech for each year of the child's age should be applied to the sides of the head behind the ears. But the bleeding from the leech bites should be stopped (*vide* p. 512) immediately the leeches come off. Cold applications, as powdered ice in a bladder or india-rubber bag, or, this not procurable, evaporating lotions (as Recipe 83), should be constantly applied to the head, and every day a mustard poultice (half flour, half mustard) or leaf protected by muslin (Recipe 109) may be used to the nape of the neck. When drowsiness or convulsions come on, it may be also desirable to put mustard poultices on the soles of the feet and calves of the legs, alternately. The diet of the child, if weaned, should at first be restricted to milk-and-water and bread jelly (*vide Addendum*), but as the disease advances the strength of the patient should be supported, and raw-meat soup, essence of beef and chicken broth, or panada (*vide Addendum*) may be used. Eventually a little wine-and-water may also be desirable. But notwithstanding all endeavours, this malady frequently ends fatally.

When a child of a family has died of this disease, every hygienic condition should be brought to bear on the next. In most cases it will be better for the child to be nursed by a stranger. Food, climate, and exercise must be carefully considered, and forcing the intellect must be interdicted.

*Spurious or false hydrocephalus* has the following characteristics. A weakly child becomes heavy and drowsy-looking, but it does not sleep. It moans and whines, occasionally starting with a louder cry. The eyes are half open; there is a *pale* cheek, a *cool* skin, an expression of languor, an absence of any continued febrile symptoms, and in infants a sunken or depressed instead of a swollen and prominent *fontanelle*. A child in this condition will generally be found to have suffered from some loss of blood from long-continued diarrhœa, or from some other exhausting discharge. The treatment of this so-called *spurious* water on the brain must not be that of the true disease. Bromide of potassium (Recipe 20) should be given at once, aided by warmth, nourishing diet, or raw-meat soup, an allowance of wine, careful nursing, and, when the urgent symptoms have passed away, iron (Recipe 70).

As the matter is important the principal characteristics of the two conditions are contrasted below.

| REAL BRAIN-AFFECTION | SPURIOUS BRAIN-AFFECTION |
|---|---|
| Often no previous prolonged illness. | Always some exhausting previous malady, or perhaps premature weaning. |
| Always fever, as shown by the thermometer (*vide* p. 34). | No fever. |
| Flushed face. | Pallid face. |
| Intolerance of light. | Not. |
| Constipation. | Diarrhœa. |
| Rolling of the head. | Not. |
| Prominence and pulsation at the fontanelle. | Depressed or sunken fontanelle. |
| Vomiting constant. | Vomiting only occasionally present. |
| Depends on a congested or tubercular condition of the brain. | Depends upon want of nutrition of the brain. |

If there is any doubt as to the nature of the disease, the fact of other children of the family having suffered from the true affection will indicate that the malady is probably the more dangerous description.

**BRAIN, WATER ON THE.**—This is a chronic malady coming on slowly and insidiously, so that its origin can scarcely be dated from any particular time. Children are sometimes born with the disease, which slowly developes after birth. But sometimes *water on the brain* is a result or continuance of tubercular meningitis, as previously described. The head often becomes of an immense size (known as the *hydrocephalic head*), but the child may survive for months or even for years. Such cases are always accompanied by wasting languor, drowsiness, irritability, frequent attacks of diarrhœa alternating with constipation, and often tendency to convulsions. Such cases rarely terminate favourably, and medicines are useless.

Parents often express anxiety about the large size of their children's heads, and fear the enlargement, real or supposed, may be due to water on the brain. It is therefore mentioned that the disease is not nearly so common as is popularly supposed, and that the large size of any child's head is not to be attributed to water therein, unless accompanied by other decided symptoms of the disease.

**BREAST, INFLAMMATION OF THE.**—This occurs most frequently to nursing-women, but it may present in other females. It may arise from injury, from cold, from too sudden weaning of an infant, or from permitting the breasts to become over-distended with milk during nursing, or in consequence of the death of the infant. It thus frequently follows sore nipples (*vide* p. 97), the pain from the nipple preventing the mother allowing the child to draw off the milk as often as necessary. Sitting up in bed to suckle, and allowing the distended breast to hang down without support; exposing the breast to cold while suckling; imperfectly developed nipples, causing the child to suck or drag too forcibly; the fruitless sucking of a child at a breast containing no milk, are all fertile causes of inflammation. When inflammation happens towards the end of suckling, it is probably the result of over-suckling and weakness. Inflammation of the breast is most common after a first confinement, and is accompanied by sharp shooting pains, fever, and probably shivering, with hardness, heat, redness, and swelling some part of the organ, which is very tender. The pain and tenderness are much aggravated by moving the arm. The secretion of milk is often stopped, but not always, if the inflammation is partial. This may subside, or go on to the formation of abscess in the breast, or it may be cut short by appropriate treatment.

*Treatment.*—Hot fomentations should be applied, and the breasts should be occasionally but not too frequently emptied by suckling or drawing the nipple. This is best accomplished by the child, or, if the infant has died, by another child, or by the mouth of the nurse. Otherwise, it may be effected by an instrument sold for the purpose, consisting of a tube with a mouthpiece fastened to a shield to press over the nipple, and which may be used by the patient or by the nurse. Or by cutting off the bottom of a soda-water bottle, applying the mouth of the bottle to the nipple, and then sucking the cut end, when the milk will flow into the interior. The milk should, however, only be drawn when the breast becomes hard, swollen, and painfully distended. Too much drawing promotes further secretion, and tends to aggravate the inflammation. At the same time, too much distension by milk must be guarded against. The feelings of the patient are perhaps the best guide as regards the frequency with which the breast should be emptied. During the intervals between the change of fomentations, the part may be *gently* rubbed, from the circumference towards the nipple, with salad oil, or, if procurable, with soap liniment; but the rubbing must be *gentle*, as abscess is often induced by strong friction, as sometimes employed by nurses to 'rub the milk away,' or to 'break the string of the nipple;' phrases which are meaningless, and not applicable to facts. Pressure by a thin towel or piece of diaper, with a hole for the nipple, fixed round the body over the opposite shoulder, is often very beneficial. But if this causes pain the breast should be well supported by a handkerchief passed *over* the shoulder and *under* the breast in the manner of a sling, so that the breast may not hang down with the full force of its own weight. The patient should also lie as much as possible, by which the breast is prevented from hanging down. A cushion between the arm and chest often affords relief. Castor-oil should be given to open the bowels, and cooling medicine, as citrate of magnesia (*vide* p. 15), may be taken to lessen feverishness. In India, when the breast is inflamed, 5 grains of quinine should be given every six hours. If inflammation occurs towards the end of suckling the diet should be generous.

[If obtainable, use *belladonna liniment* in all cases. The liniment should be *gently* rubbed on the breast, especially for two or three inches round the nipple. If the breast is merely distended, and the milk cannot be satisfactorily drawn off, the *belladonna* liniment will tend to diminish the formation of milk. If the stage of distension is passed, and the breast has become tense, shining, hard, and acutely painful, showing the existence of inflammation, the application of belladonna liniment every two or three hours, during from one to two days, will often remove the inflammation and arrest impending abscess. *Belladonna liniment would be poisonous to an infant, so that the breast may not be sucked while this remedy is in use.*]

**BREAST, ABSCESS OF THE.**—If the inflammation as above described is not subdued, matter forms in the breast, constituting *abscess of the breast.* After feelings of feverishness, shooting pains, and shivering, the breast enlarges at one particular part with *throbbing* pain, the skin becomes red, and afterwards whitish-coloured, and prominent. If not pricked with a lancet, the surface becomes very prominent and pointed, and ultimately bursts, permitting the *pus* or matter to flow out. As soon as this prominence or pointing is perceived, the matter should be let out by lancing, the puncture being made large, and in a direction *from* the nipple towards the circumference, and *not* across the breast, by which an unsightly scar would result.[1] An early use of the lancet in abscess of the breast will probably prevent much suffering, which may arise from the burrowing of matter (unable to find an exit) in the substance of the breast. If a lancet is not at hand, it will be better to puncture with a sharp penknife than to risk the evil of matter burrowing. Afterwards a bread poultice, or a soft towel moist with warm water, should be applied until the discharge of matter ceases, when the wound should be plastered. If the abscess is small the child may be put to the

[1] For directions how to open an abscess, *vide* p. 44.

breast with advantage. If the abscess is large the breast should not be sucked, but the milk should be drawn off periodically. Sometimes, when abscess of the breast has been neglected, the whole organ is implicated, or even destroyed, by the burrowing of matter throughout its texture. Then canals or *sinuses* form, which require free incisions, often leading to a severe surgical operation requiring professional skill and chloroform.

Milk abscess is often associated with a poor condition of health. As soon, therefore, as matter has formed, the patient should have liberal diet, with a moderate allowance of wine or porter, and strengthening medicines, as Recipe 66; or if the patient was previously pale and debilitated, sulphate of iron (*vide* p. 24).

[If iron is required Recipe 70 will be preferable.]

**BREAST, SORE NIPPLES OF THE.**—Cracks about the nipples, occurring during suckling, not only cause great pain, but are frequently the precursors of inflammation and abscess of the breast. All nipples are liable to crack, especially if not washed and dried after nursing; but the dark-coloured nipple is less liable to become sore than the pink one. The nipple should never be left in the child's mouth after the process of suckling is completed, as it soddens the part, and renders it more liable to crack. It should also be recollected that sore nipples may arise from *aphthæ*, or sores of the child's mouth (*vide* p. 446), which, if present, should be treated as well as the mother's nipple. *When nipples are simply tender but not cracked*, a little sweet oil or glycerine is the best application, and care should be taken that the dress does not press upon and irritate the tender part. Some means by which the milk may be conveyed to the child without the mouth of the latter coming in contact with the nipple should also be adopted. The india-rubber teat, or cork nipple, may be used for this purpose. After suckling, the parts should be bathed with brandy and water in equal proportions, or alum-water (Recipe 42) may be used, and a little salad oil should be afterwards applied. *When cracks exist*, it is a good plan for the mother to draw out the nipple by means of the old-fashioned feeding-bottle before giving it to the infant, the mother's nipple being put into the central opening and her mouth drawing the other one. Another method is the application to the nipple of the mouth of a wide-necked empty bottle that has been heated by hot water. The nipple, as the bottle cools, is pressed into the bottle and rendered prominent without pain. If the abrasion is small, collodion may be used to seal up the crack. *When there is a deep fissure or crack* in the nipple, it should be washed with alum-water *after* every time the child suckles, taking care to wash the nipple *before* the child next sucks. But the best means is the use of a well-made nipple-shield through which the child sucks. For prevention *vide Diseases of Pregnancy*, Irritation of the Breasts, p. 360.

**BREAST, IRRITABLE.**—An irritable breast may be caused by the influences exciting inflammation (*vide* p. 94); or from various maladies affecting the womb, or by profuse painful and irregular monthly periods, or by whites, when the breasts become sympathetically irritable and painful. Or sometimes the pain is purely neuralgic, and is thus recognised by its *periodical* character, and probably by accompanying neuralgia of other parts. The pain is of a wearying aching description, being more violent prior to the monthly periods, and most acute when of a neuralgic character. The pain often radiates to the back, neck, and arms. Sometimes the breast is very sensitive and the person cannot bear it to be touched. There is often a hard and tender lump deep in some part of the breast, and this may give rise to a suspicion of *cancer*. This lump is best felt when the part is pressed sideways between the fingers and thumb. When the breast is pressed gently against the chest the hardness is not felt at all, or very slightly; whereas cancers and tumours are felt in whichever way they are manipulated, and the swelling (of cancer especially) is harder, and directly under the skin, the pain being more acute and lancinating. Also, irritable breast is common in young women, and often occurs to girls about the period of the establishment of the monthly courses, and sometimes in boys about the age of puberty; whereas cancer usually happens to females of middle age. Warm poppy-head fomentations (Recipe 81) will generally relieve the pain and swelling. But the general health must be attended to, and if the monthly courses are irregular, the treatment for *Amenorrhœa* or *Dysmenorrhœa* must be employed (*vide* pp. 468, 472). If the pain is of a neuralgic, intermittent character, quinine, as Recipe 66, will be required.

**BREAST, CANCER OF THE.**—Cancer of the breast mostly occurs to females past middle life. The more usual form of cancer commences as a small hard swelling under the skin, at first painless, but in which attacks of *acute lancinating* pain are eventually experienced. It gradually spreads, involving the substance of the breast and drawing down the skin of the nipple. So long as the mass can be moved and the glands in the armpit are not swelled, there is hope of cure by excision with the knife. When it becomes an open sore the chances are less favourable. Although several remedies for cancer have recently been commended, it is believed that nothing but surgical operation will eradicate the disease, and even after operation it is liable to return, either in the breast or in some other part of the system. Women often imagine they have cancer in the breast, when the malady is not anything of the kind. Until middle life it is rare.

and even then it does not occur so often as is popularly imagined.

BREAST, OTHER DISEASES OF THE.—Other diseases which develop as tumours in the breast are principally: 1. ADENOMA OR FIBROMA, generally met with in women between the ages of twenty and thirty. The growth commences as a hard nodule. When small it is freely movable. The veins under the skin become enlarged, but there is little or no pain. The skin is movable over the tumour, and rarely ulcerates. 2. CYSTS. Cysts are composed of a bag or wall containing fluid. They are most common in women between twenty and forty years of age. A cyst commences as a small globular hard lump, which may attain a large size, affording to the fingers the sensation of a fluid moving from side to side. All such maladies require surgical operation.

The diagnosis of cancer or malignant tumour of the breast from other tumours is a matter of great importance for the mental peace of the patient. The distinctive features are therefore placed in contrast below.

| OTHER TUMOURS | CANCER |
| --- | --- |
| 1. Appear generally before thirty-five. | 1. After thirty-five. |
| 2. May appear shortly after puberty. | 2. Never so. |
| 3. Growth slow. | 3. Often rapid. |
| 4. No tendency to become adherent to the skin or subjacent parts. | 4. Marked tendency to do so. |
| 5. No retraction of the nipple. | 5. Retraction common. |
| 6. Severe pain exceptional, and rarely of a stabbing kind. | 6. Pain a very common symptom, and of a severe darting kind. |
| 7. Little tendency to ulcerate. | 7. Great tendency to ulcerate. |
| 8. No infection of the glands of the armpit. | 8. Infection common. |
| 9. Does not affect the general health. | 9. Affects the general health. |
| 10. Recurrence extremely rare. | 10. Recurrence the rule. |

**BRIGHT'S DISEASE** (*Degeneration of the Kidneys, or Albuminuria*).—Several forms of kidney disease are included under these names. One form originates from inflammation of the kidneys (*vide* p. 314). Another form originates from a gouty condition of system, or from the abuse of alcoholic drinks. A third form accompanies consumption, or other exhausting diseases. Whatever form presents, certain changes in the structure of the kidneys occur, which lead to a number of different symptoms. The most prominent early sign is the occurrence in the urine of a substance called *albumen.* This is not visible, but may be rendered so by boiling a little urine in a test-tube, or in an iron or silver spoon, when, if albumen is present, the urine turns more or less white. If by the addition of a drop or two of *strong nitric acid* the urine does not become clear, it is certain proof that albumen is present. But the fact of albumen being found in the urine is *not* always demonstrative of Bright's disease. Albumen occurs in the urine of some persons as the result of certain articles of diet—cheese, pastry, and eggs being the principal offenders, although they do not appear otherwise to disagree. It also presents in the urine of some people whenever dyspeptic from any cause. It may also depend on defective action of the liver, causing the passage of irritating acid through the kidneys, which acid the liver, if in a healthy condition, decomposes. Albumen not unfrequently occurs after an attack of ague. In some persons it presents after any great muscular exertion. In all these cases there is no real disease of the kidneys. But if, in addition to albumen, casts of the tubes which secrete the urine (and which form part of the structure of the kidneys) are found in the urine, it is evidence of kidney disease. But to discover these casts the urine must be examined with a microscope. In addition to albumen in the urine, the early symptoms of Bright's disease are diminution in the amount of urine passed, having to rise several times in the night to make water, a dull uneasiness in the lower part of the back, indigestion, and debility without any evident cause. When such symptoms occur and albumen is also found permanently in the urine, there is grave cause for uneasiness. But oftentimes Bright's disease comes on so gradually and imperceptibly, that it is only discovered by the condition of the urine. As the disease progresses it is further marked by increasing debility with headache, drowsiness, pallor, puffiness about the eyes, shortness of breath, frequent disposition to make water, especially at night, dyspeptic symptoms, and sometimes nausea, or even vomiting. At a later stage the heart usually becomes implicated, and dropsy almost always occurs (*vide* p. 186). There is also a great tendency in those suffering from Bright's disease to bronchial affections, headache, convulsions, epileptiform and apoplectic attacks, as mentioned under Uræmia (*vide* p. 55). The various forms of Bright's disease require high medical skill both in diagnosis and treatment, and it is only described here with the desire of guarding against the error often committed, of persons supposing comparatively trivial ailments to be the disease. If anyone is afraid he may have Bright's disease, he may test his urine in the manner previously indicated, and if he finds, notwithstanding leaving off cheese, pastry, eggs, and spirits, the urine turning white day after day, for ten or twelve days, he will do well to seek medical advice. In the meantime he should avoid brain work, he should treat any dyspeptic symptoms (*vide* p. 205) which may be present, he should use Recipes 1, 2, and 67, and he should take only very moderate exercise.

**BRONCHITIS.**—This is the term applied to inflammation of the lining membrane of the air-passages or tubes leading to the lungs. These tubes are described at p. 60, under Asthma. Bronchitis is generally caused by chill, and commences with symptoms of a common cold. There is first running at the nose, and a feeling of chilliness and aching pains in the limbs; the patient is thirsty and feverish, and there is languor, headache, furred tongue, loss of appetite, and restlessness. There is also a feeling of soreness behind the breast-bone, and of constriction or tightness of the chest. At first there is a dry hacking cough, the breathing is oppressed and difficult, and very little phlegm is brought up. The fever is often considerable, and the pulse may rise to 120 or higher. In favourable cases, in three or four days the cough becomes looser, and the expectoration more abundant. The expectoration during the earlier period of the malady is frothy when first coughed up, but becoming glairy, like unboiled white of egg, when allowed to remain in the receptacle. After some days the expectoration becomes thicker, and of a greenish-yellow colour, and the feeling of soreness and constriction of the chest then passes away. Throughout the attack, wheezing sounds may be heard with the breathing, and a thrill may be felt when the hand is placed on the chest or back. These signs will partly disappear after phlegm has been coughed up, but occur again with reaccumulation of mucus in the air-passages. The sounds and thrill are due to the air passing through the viscid mucus which more or less fills the bronchial tubes. Exertion or exposure to cold air increases both the cough and difficulty of breathing. In favourable cases, the disease abates about the eighth day, the difficulty of breathing subsides, the expectoration is expelled with less difficulty, and the fever declines. In unfavourable cases the expression of countenance becomes anxious, the patient makes more painful efforts to breathe, the lips become purple, and the cheeks pale and livid; delirium may ensue, and the patient, unable to cough up the tenacious mucus, dies suffocated.

Bronchitis often attacks natives who are suffering from fever during the cold season, especially in the northern districts of India, and on the sea-coasts, which are exposed to great variations of temperature, consequent on the land and sea-breezes and the lulls between. This complication frequently renders the fevers of natives very dangerous. But European adults are less liable to bronchitis in India.

*Treatment.*—Bronchitis may often be cut short at the onset by a warm bath, 8 or 10 grains of Dover's powder taken at night, with half-drachm doses of sweet spirits of nitrous ether in 2 ounces of water every three hours, and the encouragement of free perspiration in bed. A little prepared barley, boiled in half a pint of milk, to which is added half a wine-glassful of brandy or whisky, with nutmeg, lemon-juice, and sugar according to taste, will be found a very useful and agreeable potion, as it both allays thirst and induces perspiration. If the disease is not thus checked, the patient should be kept in bed, and be carefully guarded against cold, the temperature of the apartment being maintained day and night as *equable* as possible. A certain amount of moisture in the air is also advisable, and to effect this the steam from a kettle of water, boiled outside the room, may be allowed to escape into the room by an india-rubber tube attached to the spout. It is of no use keeping a kettle boiling on the fire (if there is one), as the steam passes up the chimney. Burning a charcoal 'sigree' or brazier in the room to boil the kettle is objectionable, as the heat destroys the effect of the moisture, and the fumes of the charcoal are injurious. Mustard poultices should be applied to the chest (*vide* Recipe 109), Dover's powder in 10-grain doses should be given at night, and Recipe 57 every four hours. Bread and milk, rice pudding, arrowroot, beef-tea, and jellies may be given. In unfavourable cases, when the symptoms are as described last, stimulants in the shape of wine or brandy will be required. Although the cough may be troublesome, and the patient may complain much of want of rest, no opiate other than the small proportion of such medicine contained in the above prescriptions should be given without medical advice, as composing or sleeping medicines may increase the danger, by preventing free expectorations.

*In colder countries, and in old people, bronchitis often assumes a chronic form,* when it is frequently termed 'winter cough.' People may have slight bronchial irritation during the cold season of Upper India, which passes off with the return of warmer weather. For this Recipe 56 will be beneficial; or if there is accompanying dyspepsia, Recipe 60 should be procured. But sometimes chronic bronchitis depends on a gouty condition of system, and if this is the case Recipe 52 is required.

**BRONCHITIS OF CHILDREN.**—The acute bronchitis of children is generally of graver importance than when the disease attacks the adult. In children the mischief is more apt to spread down the bronchial tubes, to the smallest branches, or even into the lungs; while in the adult the main branches are, as a rule, the seat of the disorder; and it is in proportion to this downward extension of the inflammation that the relative danger lies. For the more the smaller tubes are effected the less can the blood become properly aerated, and death may take place from suffocation. The disease begins with symptoms of an ordinary cold, and for some days perhaps nothing more serious is apprehended. But by degrees there is more fever and restlessness, while the commencing implication of the bronchial tubes is denoted by short dry cough. Sometimes, again, bronchitis commences with threatenings of croup. The patient may wake in the night with harsh *brassy* cough (as described under *Croup, vide* p. 154), but instead of croup resulting the malady passes into bronchitis. However the disease commences, with increase of fever the cough becomes more noisy, frequent and painful, and the breathing quick and wheezing. The breathing is performed chiefly by the muscles of the belly instead of the chest, which may be seen or felt moving much more forcibly than in a state of health. The child feels as if the chest were stuffed, and wheezing breath may be both heard and felt on one or both sides when the ear or hand is placed on the chest. When the breathing is very difficult, and particularly during the paroxysms of coughing, the veins of the forehead and neck stand prominently out, and the face is flushed. The fever and cough are generally worse at night, and the child is therefore then more irritable and restless. But it will often sleep for several hours, until re-accumulation of phlegm wakens the patient, and causes a paroxysm of suffocative cough. The expectoration, if coughed up, is white and glairy. But often the phlegm secreted by the inflamed bronchial tubes is only coughed into the mouth, when it is swallowed by the child, who cannot understand the desirability of spitting the phlegm out. Often the fits of coughing cause vomiting, which sometimes much relieves the child, by clearing the throat and entrance to the windpipe, and to some extent (from the pressure exerted by the act of vomiting) the bronchial tubes also of accumulated mucus, and thus allowing easier respiration. Although the skin is feverish and warm, it remains moist from perspiration. The mouth and tongue, although warm, are also moist. There is no appetite, but always thirst. If the disease grows worse, the paroxysms of cough become more frequent, until the child has no strength left to cough. Then the face becomes pale, while the lips grow livid and parted, the nostrils dilate with each inspiration, and the breathing is more hurried and difficult. Convulsions sometimes precede a fatal termination, but generally death takes place without much suffering, the child passing gradually into an unconscious state. Favourable symptoms are, lowering of the pulse, diminution of the heat of the skin, less difficulty of breathing, cessation of wheezing, lengthened periods of sound sleep, and return of appetite.

The *cause* of bronchitis in children is usually exposure to cold, and it is more common when north or north-east winds are prevalent. Bronchitis of a mild character sometimes occurs as a result of nervous irritation caused by teething, and therefore the condition of the gums should be inquired into, and if necessary they should be lanced. Children who have recently suffered from hooping-cough or measles are also very liable to bronchitis. Also those who 'drivel' much, if care is not taken to keep their chest dry.

For the distinction between bronchitis and inflammation of the lungs, *vide* the latter disease (p. 329.)

*Treatment.*—When the approach of the malady is feared, the child should be kept in the house, and the temperature of the apartment should be maintained as *equable as possible* both by day and night. The great importance of an *equable* temperature, whatever that temperature may be, cannot be too much insisted upon. In a cold climate the proper temperature of the sick-chamber would be 65° Fahr., but in India it must generally be much higher. But however high it may be, it should be maintained *equable,* and the patient should be guarded against draughts and cold. It is also advisable to moisten the atmosphere of the room in the manner mentioned at p. 104. Recipe 57 should be given, in doses proportionate to the age of the child. If the child is teething the gums should be examined, and lanced if necessary. A warm bath may also be used at the onset, to encourage the action of the skin. If the disease is not thus checked, the child should be put to bed, and a large hot linseed-meal poultice should be applied to the chest. This application may be renewed when it becomes cool, and the same process may be repeated for twenty-four or thirty-six hours. Once daily a little mustard may be mixed with the linseed-meal; but irritating applications, as blisters, cannot safely be used for children. If mustard is used with the linseed-meal, it should be in the proportion of one-tenth part of mustard only; the required effect not being blistering, but simply a degree of warmth. If linseed-meal poultices are used to the chest, great care must be taken that they are not allowed to grow too cold before removal; also, that moisture does not trickle from the poultice into the bed, and that the child is not chilled during the change of applications. A linseed-meal poultice should retain its warmth for three hours, and if made of the proper consistence no moisture will ooze from it. Unless the essentials as above named can be secured, it will be better *not* to use the linseed-meal poultice, but to cover the child's breast with several layers of cotton-wool. The bowels, if confined, should be acted upon by senna or castor oil. If there is much wheezing or stuffing of the chest, an emetic of ipecacuanha wine (*vide* p. 15) should be given once or (if it does good) twice daily, which will often relieve much discomfort. The expectorant mixture (Recipe 57) should be continued during the whole illness. At the same time the strength of the patient must be carefully supported. Milk should be given freely, and beef-tea or mutton broth *offered* alternately. If there is great weakness, a small quantity of brandy or port wine will be necessary. Solid food is not to be given; neither will the child care for it, so long as there is fever. Throughout the illness, the patient should lie with the head rather high, and be encouraged to cough frequently; not being allowed to sleep too long, lest dangerous accumulation should occur. When all severe symptoms have subsided, the patient may return gradually to his usual diet. For some time afterwards care should be taken that the patient is not exposed to cold, as he will remain very susceptible to any influence affecting the chest.

[During convalescence iron and quinine (Recipe 70) will be advisable.]

**BUBO.**—The term bubo is applied to an enlarged and inflamed condition of the glands in the groin. This is often the result of some form of venereal disease (*vide* p. 457). But the glands of the groin may swell and inflame from other causes, especially from the irritation of a sore on the foot or leg, or from a strain of the parts, experienced, perhaps, when riding a restive horse. However bubo arises, the symptoms are, a greater or less degree of heat and swelling of the affected part, with severe throbbing pain, aggravated by pressure or by attempts to walk. Often a bubo results in the formation of matter; but sometimes, after considerable pain and swelling, it gradually subsides. Rest in the horizontal posture is essential, and cold evaporating lotions (*vide Appendix*, No. 83) should be assiduously applied, which may perhaps prevent the formation of matter. If the swelling and tenderness increase, and if the pain becomes of a *throbbing* character, warm applications should be gradually substituted (*vide Appendix, Cooling Applications*), and the case should be treated as an abscess (*vide* p. 41).

[For keeping dressings on the groin the figure of ∞ bandage should be employed. The end of a bandage (*vide* p. 493) should be laid on the front of the thigh of the affected side, and the roller should then be carried round the body, and fixed by a pin where it meets the end. Then it should be carried round the thigh, passing first outside and then inwards, between the legs, across the groin, and so round the body again. If both groins are affected, a double figure of ∞ bandage may be used.]

**BUNION.**—This term is applied to a swelling generally appearing over the joint of the great toe. It principally arises from irritation of the part from the pressure of a tight, ill-fitting shoe, and is in the first instance an effort of nature to afford protection to the part pressed upon. It consists in the formation of a little bag or sac, containing watery fluid, which acts as a pad against pressure. But the pressure soon inflames this bag itself, so that bunions, even when recently formed, are often tender and inflamed, requiring rest and fomentations. When old, the swelling becomes hard, with occasional periods of tenderness. Removal of all pressure is the only certain means of relief. This should be effected by cutting the boot-leather away, when plaster spread on soft leather may be applied over the part as a protection. If a bunion suppurates or 'gathers,' which it sometimes does from irritation and neglect, it must be poulticed and treated as an ordinary abscess (*vide* p. 41).

**BURNING OF THE FEET.**—This is not a very common, although often a very troublesome affection. It may simply be an uneasy sensation of warmth in the soles of the feet; or, in any degree, to the most painful sensation of burning, preventing sleep, and thus destroying the general health. There are usually distinct periods of increase and diminution of the burning pain. In some instances the part affected is moist, in others quite dry. Emaciation and debility accompany the progress of the malady. It more often attacks natives than Europeans. It sometimes occurs unconnected with any other malady; at other times it appears as a sequela of fever, bowel complaint, rheumatism, or beri-beri. Its cause is unknown, some considering it due to malarious influences, others regarding it as rheumatism.

*Treatment.*—As a local application salt, oil of sesamum, and lime-juice in equal proportions. Bathing the feet in strong brine is also efficacious. Chloral may be given at night to relieve pain and procure sleep. Tonics, as quinine, iron, or arsenic, should also be taken. Change of climate is, however, the only certain remedy.

**CANCER.**—Cancer may occur in any part of the body, but is more common in the breasts of women, the lips, the skin, the stomach, the testicle, the tongue, and the womb. The cause of the cancer is not known, but it is believed to be at first a local malady (thought by some to be due to a microbe), and which ultimately leads to a vitiated condition of the blood. It is often hereditary in families.

*Cancer of the Breast.*—*Vide* p. 99.

*Cancer of the Lip.*—Commences as a slight sore or scab which will not heal. But this may also be syphilitic, and the diagnosis requires medical advice.

*Cancer of the Skin.*—Usually commences as a small, hard, and nearly insensible swelling. It may remain in this state for weeks or months, or even longer, but at length it passes into a more active condition. It is then distinguished by shooting or lancinating pains, at first only felt at intervals; by discoloration of the skin, which presents to the touch a knotty uneven surface; by its persistent growth, which cannot be restrained; by its spreading to neighbouring parts; by the adjacent glands becoming swollen, tender, and painful; and by the tendency to form an open and increasing sore.

*Cancer of the Stomach.*—When cancer affects the stomach it causes great pain, vomiting of bloody mucus, emaciation of the body, and a hard tumour, which may be usually felt on examination of the left side below the ribs.

*Cancer of the Testicle.*—Commences as a hard swelling with sense of weight and dragging, and eventually acute lancinating pain, and enlargement of the glands of the groin. The testicle is also subject to a soft variety of cancer.

*Cancer of the Tongue.*—Commences as a small sore or ulcer, generally near the side and behind the middle of the tongue, which will not heal, eventually becoming the seat of lancinating pain. But an obstinate sore on the tongue may be syphilitic.

*Cancer of the Womb.*—Causes much pain, and is accompanied by a badly-smelling discharge, with great weakness and emaciation. It generally occurs after middle life.

*Treatment.*—There is no cure for cancer except removal by the knife. Cancer is only mentioned in this Manual because the brief descriptions may tend to prevent an erroneous impression of cancer being present when the affection is something less important.

**CANCRUM ORIS.**—This is the name given to a very destructive ulcer which attacks the cheeks, lips, or gums, usually of children. It is attributable to debility after small-pox, scarlet-fever, or other exhausting febrile diseases, especially when combined with improper and deficient food, neglect, and living under unsanitary conditions. Or it may arise under such circumstances of life without prior fever. The disease commences as a dark, hard swelling of the cheek, or lips, which soon mortify and slough away. In this manner portions of the cheek, lips, gums, or jaw-bone may be destroyed. There is profuse discharge of both saliva and badly-smelling fluid. It may terminate fatally from exhaustion, or from bleeding from some artery opened during the sloughing process; or the patient may gradually recover, with the loss of some portion of the cheek, lips, or jaw-bone.—*The treatment* consists in keeping the affected parts very clean by frequent washing with alum solution(Recipe 42); in giving tonic medicines (Recipe 66); and in liberal diet, as eggs, beef-tea, wine, milk, or chicken-broth.

[A better application than alum is carbolic acid solution (Recipe 119). If possible, the advice of a medical man should be procured, who would probably endeavour to stay the progress of the disease by the application of strong nitric acid, under chloroform.]

*An allied malady, called noma,* sometimes attacks the private parts of female children, who have been subjected to the predisposing causes described above. The disease when in this part presents very similar progress, and requires a similar treatment.

**CARBUNCLE.**—A carbuncle is an exaggerated boil (*vide Boils*, p. 75), most frequently situated where the tissues underlying the skin are of a dense fibrous character, as the nape of the neck, the back, or buttocks. Carbuncles are usually seen in debilitated people over forty-five years of age, especially if suffering from kidney disease or diabetes. They result from an impure, vitiated, and debilitated condition of the blood, but their appearance at any particular part of the body may be determined by an accidental injury. One variety, known as *anthrax*, arises from contamination from diseased animals, by which a microscopical germ, the *bacillus anthracis*, is conveyed to man. Carbuncles vary in size, sometimes being as large as an orange. They are very hard, dreadfully painful, and cause the skin above to become of a dusky red colour, which gradually fades off into the surrounding skin without any defined border. As the carbuncle forms matter is discharged from several small openings. The progress of the disease is slow, but after a time, generally two or three weeks, the whole of the affected skin and tissues underneath slough away, leaving a deep, irregular cavity, which extends underneath the neighbouring skin. Carbuncles are commonly attended with much constitutional disturbance, such as fever, perspirations, and debility. The strength must be kept up by nourishing diet, port wine, quinine, and iron. The local treatment consists of hot fomentations, poultices, and at the proper period free incision, in order to let the *core* or decayed tissue and matter escape. When the discharge ceases, the part may be dressed with simple dressing or plaster, as an ordinary sore.

**CATARRH.**—Catarrh presents under two forms, viz. a *common cold* and *influenza* (*vide* p. 309). The symptoms of a common cold are lassitude, chilliness, or shivering, a feeling like cold water running down the back, pains in the back and limbs, often sore-throat, sneezing, and a sense of heaviness in the head and eyes, the latter being weak and watery. There is also headache, especially of the forehead, stoppage of the nose, alternating with discharge, while the respiration is impeded from inability to breathe through the nose, the person is feverish, and the taste is perverted. Frequently an eruption of herpes (*vide* p. 395) appears on the lips. At the end of three days the malady begins to subside. The symptoms of a severe cold in the head are very similar to those of the commencement of influenza. But cold in the head is a local complaint, arising from inflammation of the lining membrane of the nose, the result of chill. The satisfaction often expressed by mothers at the running noses of their children is well founded, as it comparatively rarely happens that a catarrh after profuse running at the nose passes into dangerous ailments. This fact, long observed, appears to have given rise to the custom of saluting after sneezing.

*Treatment.*—To escape colds, persons should as much as possible avoid sudden transitions of temperature. When over-heated they should not cool themselves too quickly by throwing off clothing, or suddenly sitting in comparatively cold situations, but cease exercise gradually, and avoid currents of cold air, although grateful to the feelings. Colds may sometimes be taken by passing from a cold atmosphere into a heated one, but such transition is not so apt to occur in India as in colder climates. The remedy for an ordinary cold may be the milk, barley, and spirit mixture, mentioned at p. 104, for slight bronchitis; or, if this cannot be obtained, a stiff glass of spirits and water, taken at night, with the object of inducing sleep and perspiration. For more severe colds a hot bath, or the feet in hot mustard and water, 10 grains of Dover's powder (compound ipecacuanha powder) at night, and half a drachm of sweet spirits of nitre in an ounce of water three or four times a day. If the cold be attended with cough or bronchial irritation, Recipe 57 should be taken. Spirits of camphor (*vide* p. 24) taken every two hours at the very commencement of a catarrh will sometimes arrest it, and is most useful when there is persistent shivering. One drachm of camphor, coarsely powdered and placed in a jug half filled with boiling water, may be used as follows. Make a paper cone sufficiently large for the small end to fit over the jug, and the large end to fit over the mouth and nostrils, and inhale the camphorated fumes three or four times a day. Refraining altogether, or as much as possible, from any kind of liquid for twenty-four hours often affords great relief.

[A mixture, composed of tincture of aconite 1 drachm, water 8 ounces, taken in *teaspoonful* doses every hour, or two hours, according to the severity of the symptoms, is very beneficial, if taken at the commencement of a cold. The patient should go to bed and drink freely of water. The treatment may be continued for six or eight hours, when, the skin becoming moist, the symptoms disappear. If the patient cannot lay up, the following prescription, used frequently *as a snuff*, will afford much relief. Hydrochlorate of morphia 2 grains; acacia powder 2 drachms; subnitrate of bismuth 6 drachms; to be well mixed. To be labelled, 'Poison, not for internal use.' Or carbolic acid and strong liquid of ammonia, of each 5 drachms, rectified spirits of wine 2 ounces. Keep in a stoppered dark glass bottle. When a cold is commencing 10 or 15 drops should be placed on three or four folds of blotting-paper. The eyes should be closed and the patient should inhale as long as any smell is perceptible. To be repeated every two hours.]

Colds, although generally regarded as trivial ailments, should not be neglected, as other intractable diseases may be excited by a succession of colds. Delicate persons who are subject to colds should strengthen their system by regimen and judicious exposure to the external air. Strong persons subject to colds may prevent attacks by care, exercise, free use of the bath, and the flesh-brush.

**CHAPS.**—Chaps and roughness of the skin of the hands chiefly occur from the cold of Northern India, which is sometimes intense, particularly during the nights of the winter season. When the skin cracks over the knuckles or elsewhere, the part is popularly said to be 'chapped.' Protection from the cold winds should be secured by gloves, and cold cream or glycerine may be applied.

**CHILBLAINS.**—Chilblains are seldom seen in India except in the cold weather of the northern districts, when they not unfrequently occur to children. Chilblain is the term commonly applied to inflammation of the skin over the toes, or on some portion of the feet, but it may occur on the hands or ears. Chilblains are caused by sudden alternations of temperature, such as warming the feet and hands when cold and damp by the fire. The skin becomes red in patches, slightly swollen, and there is much irritation and itching, especially in the evening. Sometimes, owing generally to scratching, the parts blister, or even become a sore. Chilblains are most common in delicate women and weakly children, or in persons whose circulation is very languid.

*Treatment.*—On the approach of the cold weather, those liable to chilblains should harden the skin of the feet by rubbing with alum solution (Recipe 42) or with strong brine. The socks should be thick, and the boots roomy, well-fitting, and furnished with strong soles. Sudden exposure to cold and wet should be avoided, and the temptation of bringing a benumbed hand or foot close to the fire should be overcome. When there is a red blush on the skin, and the part is painful, it may be gently rubbed night and morning with brandy and salad oil mixed in equal proportions, or with soap liniment if available. If there are blisters, care must be taken not to break them, and the liniment must be applied lightly with a feather; if ulcers or sores form, poultices will be required, to be followed by simple dressing (Recipe 86). When persons suffer badly from chilblains, tonics and generous diet will generally be indicated; also a moderate degree of exercise sufficient to circulate the blood.

[For chilblains in the unbroken state, either spirits of wine or spirits of camphor (*vide* p. 24) may be used with great advantage, instead of the brine or alum solution mentioned above.]

**CHICKEN-POX.**—Chicken-pox is a contagious eruptive fever of a mild nature, generally occurring in children. It is by some considered to be *modified small-pox* (*vide* p. 408). The period after exposure to infection and appearance of the disease is ordinarily six days. During twenty-four hours there is slight fever, and often catarrh, then an eruption of red pimples appears first on the back, then on the face and other parts of the body, accompanied by slight itching. There may be only one crop, or there may be a succession of crops of such pimples daily, accompanied by an increase of fever, which declines after the spots appear. On the third day the pimples contain a clear fluid, which has led to the term 'Crystalline Pock.' The vesicles break on the fourth day, disappearing about the sixth day, when the thin scabs fall off, without leaving any mark or scar. The vesicles are not 'pitted' or depressed as in small-pox; neither does matter form in them as in the latter malady, and the initiatory and accompanying fever is always much slighter. A gentle aperient, as citrate of magnesia, and care in avoiding catching cold, form all the treatment desirable in most cases. There is no danger of infection three weeks after the first appearance of the eruption.

**CHOLERA.**—Cholera commences in two ways: 1st, *suddenly*; 2ndly, *after 'malaise' and painless diarrhœa,* which may extend from one to ten days, or longer. The choleraic seizure often occurs during the night, or in the early morning, when the atmospheric temperature is coldest, and the vitality of the human system least. There is frequently from the very first great depression and debility. Spasmodic griping in the bowels is first felt, followed by frequent purging, and vomiting, first of the contents of the stomach, then of watery material. These evacuations, which are at first coloured, quickly change to an almost odourless *white-coloured* fluid, resembling water in which rice has been boiled. These 'rice-water' stools may amount to fifteen or twenty in the course of a few hours; and at first they are discharged with great force, and are followed by a sense of relief, although by a peculiar feeling of exhaustion at the pit of the stomach. Vomiting may be equally frequent, and the ease with which the cholera-stricken vomit is remarkable, the rice-water fluid often passing up with scarcely any effort. At the same time severe cramps, commencing in the fingers and toes, occasionally alternating with tingling, rapidly extend to the calves, thighs, and muscles over the bowels. Urine at first is scanty and high-coloured, and ultimately *none* is passed. There is also a burning sensation and a feeling of tightness at the pit of the stomach, which is tender to pressure. The tongue is white and tremulous, and there is a bitter taste in the mouth. Little or no saliva being secreted, the mouth is dry, there is great thirst, and an urgent desire for cool drinks. The pulse is feeble, but more frequent than natural, probably rising to 96°. There is a cool skin and no fever, but the patient often complains of heat and oppression, and prefers to lie uncovered. Noises in the ears may also be complained of. The patient is very restless, and constantly tossing about the bed. Lastly, a rapidly-increasing exhaustion is evident. The patient is now on the verge of *collapse*, or sinking.

Should this condition succeed, the pulse becomes quicker but hardly perceptible, the discharges cease, and so often do the cramps. The skin is covered with cold perspiration, has a sickly smell, and a bluish tinge. The nails and lips especially assume this unnatural appearance. The whole body seems shrunken and withered, the genital organs are shrivelled, and the skin of the fingers is wrinkled like that of a washerwoman. The voice is husky and faint, the tongue is pointed, and both it and the breath are cold. The intelligence is ordinarily clear, but there is apathy as to the result. The countenance assumes the peculiar aspect of the cholera death; the eyes are shrunken and glassy, but the pupils remain of the natural size; the nose is sharpened, the cheeks are hollow, and the jaw falls. The temperature, if tested by the thermometer, is found to have fallen, the pulse becomes imperceptible, there is hiccough, stools may be passed unconsciously, while the whole body becomes bluish-grey. Often two or three hours before death some return of heat in the scalp, forehead, or over the chest may be present. This is an unfavourable sign, being due to a relaxation of minute blood-vessels, caused by the approach of death.

*Favourable symptoms* are the gradual cessation of vomiting and purging, the skin becoming warmer and the pulse fuller, the voice regaining power, urine being voided, colour appearing in the stools, the burning pain in the stomach ceasing, and the patient falling asleep. Even in apparently hopeless cases recovery may take place. So long as the patient has strength to vomit the case is not hopeless. But the immediate danger is not over till urine is passed, and the average time of passing urine in favourable cases is 72 hours after seizure. The duration of the disease may be from several hours to several days, and much longer when secondary results occur (*vide* p. 125).

In some epidemics of cholera the usual cramps have been absent, or much less felt than in the ordinary type of the disease. But in other cases cramps and twitchings have been noted as the principal symptoms. In most great outbreaks persons die suddenly from collapse, without distinctive symptoms—often without vomiting and purging, or after one or two sudden loose stools. Vomiting of worms has often been noticed, both during and after an attack. Sometimes cholera commences with shivering, as an attack of ague. In females there may be a bloody discharge from the privates, even although the monthly 'courses' are not present. The greater or less lividity of the countenance has given rise to such appellations as 'blue' and 'black' cholera. After death a remarkable contraction of the muscles of the limbs sometimes occurs, which has led to stories of persons being removed to the dead-house while yet alive. These contractions are due to *post-mortem* relaxation of blood-vessels, which, as before remarked, also causes the increase of heat noticed previously to, and sometimes after, death. Lastly, more persons always die at the commencement or the middle of an epidemic, in proportion to the number attacked, than towards the termination of an epidemic.

*Causes.*—The precise cause of cholera is not known, but it is generally admitted to be a poison, which may be transmitted from adjacent plaees through the air; which may be conveyed from place to place by human beings, or by other agencies; and which may contaminate drinking-water or food, and may thus be taken into the system. A peculiar *microbe* has been found in the intestines and discharges of cholera patients; but there is not sufficient evidence to show whether this is the cause of the disease. There is, however, evidence tending to prove that the cholera evacuations constitute the principal, if not the only, channel of contagion; and that the great cause of cholera is the contamination of water used for drinking purposes with the dejections of persons suffering from the complaint. There is reason to believe that the contagious principle becomes rapidly multiplied in water, especially if exposed to the heat of the sun. Milk, adulterated with contaminated water, may, it is believed, become a medium of the dissemination of cholera. Or the poison, protected in the clothing or in the soil, may dry, remaining vital in the same way as germs of various fungi are known to remain vital, until brought into activity by favourable circumstances of air, heat, and moisture, as may occur when the dried germs are swallowed or inhaled. The cholera poison has been supposed to have originated in Eastern tropical countries, where, especially in the Delta of Bengal, it is periodically reproduced, spreading thence to an indefinite extent. But there is at least equal reason for the statement that cholera may develop in any country, and that it is not always conveyed from India. Be this, however, as it may, and in whatever manner the poison is produced, experience has demonstrated that whatever tends to lower the vital powers will *predispose* to the disease. Such agencies, for instance, as the depression of the nervous system, following intoxication; long and fatiguing marches, and the exhaustion consequent thereon; sleeping in overcrowded barracks or other crowded apartments, chill from early-morning change of temperature, damp, filth, destitution, drought, famine, and fear of the disease. In most epidemics it is found that the disease is more fatal in those localities notorious for their unsanitary conditions—particularly as regards defective conservancy—and amongst those classes who are rendered feeble and debilitated from want or destitution. Thus three factors are required—the poison germ; the introduction of the germ into the system; and predisposition of the recipient. Therefore, cholera is not contagious in the usual meaning of the term; that is, it is not contracted directly from another person, as small-pox is.

*Diagnosis.*—There are symptoms arising from other causes which in the absence of medical aid may be mistaken for cholera. These causes are principally diarrhœa, arsenic poisoning, impure water, stale fruit, stale fish, fungi mistaken for mushrooms, the fruit of the *luffa echinata*, impure milk and cheese, bad tinned provisions, and colic. *Diarrhœa* may be attended with cramps, and all the early symptoms of cholera excepting rice-water stools and stoppage of urine, which are absent in diarrhœa. But cholera often commences as diarrhœa and gradually develops into cholera. It is often impossible to define with exactness whether the attack should be called cholera or diarrhœa. Moreover, when cholera prevails, diarrhœa, evidently due to similar influences, is also present. The term *choleraic diarrhœa* has been unadvisedly expunged from the official nomenclature of disease, but there is no other term which is applicable to many cases. *Arsenic poisoning* is characterised by vomiting and purging (*vide* p. 586), but there is not ordinarily stoppage of urine, while the stools are not of the rice-water description, but mucus streaked with blood, as in dysentery. *Impure water*, especially brackish water containing mineral water, as so frequently met with in Western India, may excite griping, purging, and vomiting, but the cholera characteristics of rice-water stools and stoppage of urine are absent. Similar remarks apply to the symptoms caused by *stale fruit*. But vomiting, purging, and suppression of urine have been known to follow eating *poisonous fungi*, although no rice-water stools. *Stale fish*, especially *oysters*, particularly if taken from the roots of mangrove trees, or if a shell has opened from some injury and decomposition commenced, sometimes excite all the symptoms of cholera. It should be recollected that a fish which is wholesome when absolutely fresh may become otherwise if kept only a few hours in a moist damp atmosphere, from the formation of a *post-mortem* poison, or *ptomaine*. The fruit or nut of a creeping plant, the *luffa echinata* (native name *deodagri*), is also known to excite symptoms much resembling cholera, but no rice-water stools. *Impure milk*, or milk in which some decomposition has taken place, may, if taken copiously, produce all the symptoms of cholera, for the milk, passing through the intestines more or less unchanged, gives rise to white fluid stools. *Decomposed cheese* and *bad tinned provisions* may also produces choleraic symptoms. The symptoms of *colic* are detailed at p. 131, and a comparison of them with those of cholera will show there is little resemblance, there being no rice-water stools and no suppression of urine, while the pain is of a different character. Yet colic has not unfrequently been mistaken by sufferers and friends for cholera. When a case resembling cholera occurs, especially in the absence of an epidemic, it will be well to inquire into the possibility of these causes of ailment.

*Treatment.*—No certain cure has been discovered. Yet many lives are saved by careful nursing, and by assisting nature's efforts towards reaction by the judicious administration of remedies, and by plenty of fresh air. It is in the premonitory stage of diarrhœa that most good may be done. When cholera prevails the slightest approach to diarrhœa should be at once attended to, otherwise it will probably run on into cholera; and all saline purgatives should be avoided.

Immediately on the first symptoms of diarrhœa the patient should take 30 drops of chlorodyne, with half a wine-glass of brandy in a similar quantity of water, repeating the dose every two hours if necessary. Or, if sickness accompanies the diarrhœa, he should take Recipe 38 hourly. If the above-mentioned medicines are not at hand, 20 drops of spirits of camphor (*vide* p. 24) every half-hour. If purging continues, after two doses of chlorodyne; or four doses of Recipe 38; or eight doses of spirits of camphor; or after four hours have elapsed, ten grains of Dover's powder (vide p. 12) should be given, and repeated after three hours.

To induce the flow of urine, 1 drachm of sweet spirits of nitre, in 2 ounces of water, should be given every three hours, but not at the same time with the Dover's powder. If there is much nausea or vomiting, a mustard poultice should be applied over the pit of the stomach. The patient should be kept in the recumbent posture as quiet as possible, the bed should be protected by a water-proof sheet, and until purging has stopped the diet should consist of tea, arrowroot, or sago, mutton or chicken broth, or Liebig's raw-meat soup (*vide Addendum*), with a little good port wine. But often the patient will not take food, or if he does it is vomited. In such cases, only tea-spoonfuls should be given at half-hour intervals. The thirst may be quenched by plain cold or iced water, or soda-water, and ice, if available, may be kept constantly in the mouth. Filling the stomach with water renders vomiting easy in those cases where it may be the reverse. So long as urine is passed, the case should not be regarded as hopeless, and with the view of encouraging this secretion mustard poultices may be applied over the loins. This measure should be always adopted when cessation of the passage of urine is an early and marked symptom. Cramps and colds are best relieved by friction with the hand, by the application of hot bran bags or of cloths saturated with warm turpentine, or by mustard poultices.

[If obtainable, use Recipe 39 instead of 38 every two hours; also give Recipe 45 every alternate hour, both for four doses.]

This treatment, if commenced early, will often prove successful; but if purging and vomiting continue, the patient becomes as described in the latter stage of the disease, falling into a state of *collapse.* The period for any medicine has now passed. In collapse it is useless giving medicines, as the stomach cannot absorb them. They may accumulate, and become the cause of much mischief by aggravating reactionary fever. *The great desideratum in collapse is to keep up animal heat in every way which will not fatigue the patient.* But while the patient is kept warm, the freest ventilation must be secured. Above all, he must be kept quiet, and *not allowed to assume the erect posture.* If the breathing is difficult, a mustard poultice (Recipe 109) may be applied to the chest. The limbs, especially the legs and feet, should be assiduously rubbed with the hands. Thirst may be checked by a table-spoonful of brandy, or three or four of champagne *in a tumbler of water.* No other stimulants should be given, but broth or raw-meat soup (*vide Addendum*) may be *offered* frequently, but should not be pressed on the patient. Raw-meat soup, in very small quantities, as a tea-spoonful every ten minutes, will often be retained where everything else is vomited, as it requires little digestion.

A cholera patient should be isolated as much as possible, and no one except the attendants actually necessary should be allowed in the apartment. The rules in the *Appendix* regarding the disinfection and disposal of all discharges, the disinfection of the hands of attendants, and of utensils, towels, &c. used, *should be rigidly carried out* during the illness; and afterwards those relating to the disinfection of the bedding, clothing, and rooms (*vide Appendix*, No. 121 to 130).

Great care should be exercised with regard to diet during convalescence. Broths and jellies, farinaceous puddings, sago and arrowroot may be given; but *no solids* whatever, until the stools are of a natural colour, the urine is secreted freely, and all other symptoms have vanished.

SECONDARY RESULTS OF CHOLERA.—When *reaction* or recovery from the collapsed state has commenced, little treatment beyond nourishing diet cautiously given is required in ordinary cases. It sometimes happens, however, and more especially with Europeans, or when much stimulants have been given, that *reactionary fever* succeeds recovery from cholera. This may be mild, terminating in a few hours with an eruption of roseola (*vide* p. 387) or nettlerash (*vide* p. 387). Or the *reactionary fever* may be more severe. For the first few hours after the feverishness commences the tongue is white, but it quickly becomes brown and dry, while black particles form on the teeth; the eyes become red, the cheeks flushed, the pulse rapid, and the surface of the body hot. The patient now often grows delirious, and ultimately becomes insensible, as if suffering from the last stage of typhoid fever (*vide* p. 242). This usually lasts from four to eight days, when the symptoms gradually yield or death ensues.

*Secondly*, a state resembling apoplexy may result, with or without any prior fever, and attended with a second stoppage of urine. This condition is caused by the presence in the blood of material which should be passed off in the urine and bile. (*Vide Uræmia*, p. 55.)

*Thirdly*, persons who have previously suffered from dyspepsia are liable to inveterate hiccough after cholera, rendering them unable to take any nourishment, depriving them of rest, and inducing a very exhausted condition.

*Treatment.*—In the stage of reaction the heat of the skin may be moderated by cold sponging, and the secretion of urine, if not plentiful, may be promoted by a mustard poultice over the loins, or by dry cupping (*vide Appendix*, No. 115), and by sweet spirits of nitre (*vide* p. 13). If there is vomiting, as most frequently happens to patients of intemperate habits, small doses of citrate of magnesia should be given; if sickness prevents food being retained, and the bowels are *not* still loose, digested enemas (*vide Appendix*), or injections of Liebig's raw-meat soup (*vide Addendum*), should be given every four hours. When the tongue becomes brown and dry, the pulse weaker, although not slower, and if delirium occurs, a table-spoonful of port wine should be given every hour. Iced water may be given *ad libitum* according to the patient's desire. Supporting the strength by strong broths and soups, or milk, given frequently but in very small quantities, as a tea-spoonful, or, if so much can be borne, a table-spoonful at a time, is more important in this peculiar condition occurring after cholera, than purely medical treatment.

[When the tongue becomes dry and brown the following mixture should be given: carbonate of ammonia, 2 drachms; sulphuric ether, 4 drachms; spirits of nitrous ether, 6 drachms; camphor water, 12 ounces; 2 table-spoonfuls every three hours.]

When insensibility or a condition resembling apoplexy occurs, the hands and feet should be kept warm, the head cool, and mustard poultices should be again applied over the kidneys and liver. If the person is able to swallow, Liebig's raw-meat soup should be given frequently in small quantities, but no stimulants.

When hiccough is a troublesome result, milk, with one-third lime-water (Recipe 25), will probably be best retained, and otherwise the hiccough should be treated as mentioned under Hiccough (*vide* p. 299).

[If the means mentioned above do not succeed, two or three drops of chloroform in a wineglass of water may be tried for either vomiting or hiccough. Milk treated by Fairchild's peptonising powders (if obtainable) should be substituted for milk and lime-water.]

Cholera in Infants or Children presents the same symptoms as when occurring to older persons.

*Treatment.*—Chlorodyne may be given, in doses corresponding with the age of the child (*vide* p. 12), every two hours for three doses. Equal parts of milk and lime-water (Recipe 25) may be given as a drink, which will tend to moderate the irritability of the stomach and to stop the purging. If no improvement, the pulse being more feeble and exhaustion greater, Recipe 38 may be given in doses according to age; and a little port wine may be used. In some cases very strong infusion of green tea, given in teaspoonful doses with six or eight drops of aromatic spirits of ammonia, has proved of great benefit. The tea often acts energetically on the state of drowsiness, and causes the little patients to revive rapidly, while the ammonia not only stimulates but also acts as an antacid. In all cases, at an early stage, a mustard poultice guarded by muslin (Recipe 109) should be applied over the bowels, while the extremities should be frequently rubbed with brandy and salad oil in equal proportions, or with soap liniment if obtainable. As food, raw-meat soup (*vide Addendum*) is best, and may be offered in small quantities throughout the illness. If not available, good meat broth.

Cholera, Prevention of.—Many preventive measures may be comprised in one word, CLEANLINESS; and especially as regards the matter of *conservancy*. During and after cholera the rules for disinfection (*vide Appendix*), especially of the discharges, and of rooms, should be vigorously pursued. On the *approach* of cholera, increased sanitary vigilance in the vicinity should be enforced; but *after* the disease has appeared, probably more harm than good will be done by opening up foul drains or cesspools (*vide Appendix*, No. 128); but sulphur may be burnt in infected localities. Fires about thirty yards apart should be kept burning for forty-eight hours, sulphur being constantly thrown on the fire. All the fires should be lighted at once, and about four pounds of sulphur will be required for each fire during the period.

When travelling, the neighbourhood of localities in which the disease prevails should be avoided as encamping grounds, or, if necessity compels a stay near such places, tents should be so pitched as to let the wind blow from the tents to the village, instead of the reverse. As little communication as possible should be allowed between the camp and the village people. Neither drinking-water nor food supplies should, if avoidable, be obtained from infected places. Milk especially should not be so obtained, as it may be mixed with contaminated water. If possible, persons should leave infected localities marching against the wind.

What may be regarded as *personal hygiene*, in contradistinction to *general sanitation*, must be attended to. Persons should take especial care not to be chilled by the early-morning change of temperature. Fear of the disease, as predisposing greatly to attacks of cholera, must be guarded against, and it should be recollected that in the worst epidemics exemption is the rule and not attack. Both milk and water should be boiled before being used. Special care should be taken in the use of fish, some varieties being particularly liable to become tainted or even poisonous (*vide* p. 122). The incautious use of unripe fruit, of bad tinned provisions, of badly cooked vegetables, exposure to the midday sun or to cold night dews, great fatigue, and intemperance, all exercise a debilitating effect on the system, or excite irritation in the intestines, and thus render any person a more easy prey to the malady. During cholera seasons, purgative medicines should be avoided if possible altogether, and especially saline purgatives. The best aperient during a cholera season is *pure* and fresh castor oil.

When cholera prevails in a native village, and it may be desirable to send medicines for distribution, or for entrusting to native servants or others, for general use during seasons of cholera epidemic, nothing is a better compound than assafœtida and opium pills. These are composed of one and a half grain of assafœtida, one grain of red pepper, and half a grain of powdered opium or extract of opium, and directions should be given for one pill to be taken by the patient after every loose stool. In the absence of medical aid, these pills will often prove useful in checking the malady, if taken at the commencement of the illness.

**CHYLURIA.**—This term is applied to a milky condition of the urine. Sometimes a milky discharge takes place from the lymph-vessels of the armpit, groin, or scrotum. It may be the forerunner or accompaniment of elephantiasis, and has been thought due to *filaria*, or worms in the blood. Anti-scorbutic remedies (*vide Scurvy*, p. 382) will be advisable, and tonics as Recipe 74.

**CLUB FOOT.**—This affection presents several varieties. The most common are, when the heel is drawn *upwards*, or the foot is turned *inwards*; or, as often happens, when *both* such conditions prevail. When the heel is drawn upwards, the person walks on the sole of the *foot*, and on the toes; or, in bad cases, on the toes only. When the foot is turned inwards, he walks on the outside. Sometimes the foot is turned outwards, and the person walks on the inner edge. Sometimes the toes and front part of the sole are drawn upwards, and he walks on the heel. The deformity arises from *contraction* of some muscle or muscles acting on the foot, or from *paralysis* of some muscle or muscles, in consequence of which the opposing muscle or muscles act uncontrolled. Club foot is commonly congenital, the child being so born; but it may come on gradually after birth, from spasmodic contraction of muscles. Such cases usually require a surgical operation, consisting in the division of the tendon of the muscle or muscles by which the foot is drawn into the unnatural position.

The variety of club foot where the foot is turned outwards and the person walks on the inner edge may come on after birth, when a child has *weak ankles*. In the natural healthy condition, the weight of the body rests principally on the heel and ball of the foot, the two forming the extremities of what is called the 'plantar arch.'

By this means an elasticity is given to the foot, and consequently to the step or gait, which would be altogether wanting if the 'plantar arch' were not there, or if the parts entering into its structure were joined in one mass of bone, instead of consisting of small bones jointed together accurately, with ligamentous substance. When children are allowed to walk too soon, particularly if fat and heavy, the *astragalus*, or upper bone of the plantar arch, sinks down, causing a lowering of the arch and a flattening of the sole of the foot. High heels tend to the same result. This defect, when slight, is known as WEAK ANKLE; when more decided, it is called FLAT or SPLAY FOOT. In bad cases the bone or top of the arch may descend so much as to render the *inner* side of the foot *convex* where it should be naturally concave. Or in still worse instances, the deformity may increase until it assumes the form of club foot.

*Treatment.*—Children frequently show a tendency to weak ankles, which as they grow older disappears. *No child having such tendency should be encouraged to walk early.* The ankles and feet should be frequently bathed with strong salt and water. Rubbing and properly directed manual extension should be daily practised. Boots should not be worn, the pressure of the top of the boot round the ligaments of the ankle tending to wasting and weakness of the part, instead of proving, as is popularly supposed, a support. A spring, or piece of cork, fitted in the sole of the shoe, so as to press against the flattening of the arch, is sometimes useful, but should not be worn if it causes pain. Low heels and thick soles are necessary. When a person walks, the heel impinges on the ground first. High heels throw the weight of the body on the toes, which is unnatural. If the deformity from weak ankles becomes great, the remedies are peculiar supports constructed by a surgical-instrument maker.

**COLIC.**—This term is commonly given to all severe griping pains in the bowels. It is variously denominated from its different causes and circumstances. When its principal symptoms are sharp and spasmodic pains, it is called *Spasmodic Colic* (or vulgarly 'cramps,' 'spasms,' or 'stomach-ache'); when with the pain there is vomiting, it is called *Bilious Colic*; if flatulency causes the pain, it takes the name of *Flatulent* or *Windy Colic*; when it is caused by indigestible food, it is called *Accidental Colic*; when accompanied by heat and tenderness in the bowels, it is designated *Inflammatory Colic*; when colic is attended with *obstruction* of the bowels and evacuation of fæcal matter by the mouth, it is called *Iliac Passion.* There is also a peculiar kind of colic called 'lead,' or 'painter's' colic.

Colic usually comes on suddenly, often in the night, with spasmodic griping and twisting pain in the bowels, often faintness and nausea, and perhaps vomiting. There is also spasmodic retraction of the muscles about the navel, which part appears drawn inwards. The bowels are constipated at first, and distended with wind. At a later period there is usually strong desire to stool, the passage of which is attended with great relief. Colic, *excepting when inflammatory*, is relieved by pressure on the bowels, the patient frequently rolling about or lying on the belly. Often, if the patient is in bed, or lying on the back, the legs are so bent that the thighs press on the bowels, the legs being retained in such position by the hands grasping the shins. This distinguishes the malady from inflammation of the bowels, in which state pressure is very painful, and the patient lies on the back and remains still, with his legs drawn up (*vide* p. 79). There is ordinarily no feverishness with colic, while inflammation is attended with much fever. *Inflammatory colic* and *iliac passion* or *obstruction of the bowels* are often sequels of the other varieties of colic, which, unrelieved by medicines, may pass into the inflammatory stage or the obstructed condition.

Colic should be further distinguished from a fit of the *gravel*; from the beginning of *dysentery*; from the blind *piles*; from a *stone* passing through the gall-duct; from *cholera*; and from *rupture*. During a fit of the *gravel*, the testicle is often retracted and the leg benumbed, with pain shooting down the inside of the thigh; there is also pain in the loins, and frequent desire to make water. The griping pains felt at the beginning of *dysentery* are not so violent as those of colic, are less 'twisting' or 'wringing' in their character, and are attended with diarrhœa instead of constipation. The pain from *blind piles* is confined to the lower bowel, and there is probably bleeding. The pain from a *stone* in the gall-duct is felt in the pit of the stomach, shooting through to the back. *In cholera*, there is usually, preceding diarrhœa, vomiting and purging of white fluid and stoppage of urine. The symptoms of rupture often at first resemble colic, and *in every case of colic inquiry should be made as to the existence of a rupture*, which appears as a swelling in the groin (*vide* p. 589).

*Treatment.*—The treatment of colic should be conducted after a consideration of the cause. If it appears to be an *accidental* colic, that is, arising from indigestible food, as salted meats, pork, salmon, rich gravies, or 'high' game, an emetic, as Recipe 54, will remove the offending matter, and so relieve the pain. To assist the action of the emetic, the patient should take copious draughts of lukewarm water. After the vomiting, a mild aperient, as Recipe 2, may be taken.

If the colic is of a *bilious* nature, that is, accompanied with faintness, nausea, or violent vomiting of bilious material, with constipation in the first instance, succeeded by desire to go to stool, the malady has probably arisen from a prolonged course of high living. If there is great retching, a mustard-and-water emetic (Recipe 54) will be desirable. Then, unless purging is very severe, the remedies, are, Recipe 1, followed in a couple of hours by Recipe 2. The bilious variety of colic is often connected with, or caused by, a gall-stone passing from the gall-bladder into the bowels (*vide* p. 274); but when this is the case there is not the sudden desire to go to stool as mentioned above.

If the colic is of the *flatulent*, or *windy*, or *spasmodic* variety, arising probably in nervous or delicate persons from unripe fruit, from eating too much vegetable matter (as cabbage or spinach), or from the habit of drinking too much tea, alkaline carminative draughts, as Recipe 38, or 40 drops of sal volatile in an ounce of water, will be desirable. A full dose of tincture of ginger (*vide* p. 14) is a safe and popular remedy. Effervescing draughts of citrate of magnesia (p. 15) may also be given every two hours. If these measures do not succeed, 15 or 20 grains of chloral. The griping pain in the belly often experienced on first going out in the early-morning cold in India is a variety of spasmodic colic, but rarely requires medical treatment.

During any variety of colic, pain in the bowels may be much relieved by pressure with the hands, by hot fomentations, by friction with soap liniment, or by a mustard poultice. Also, in any variety of colic, if pain is very violent, 15 or 20 grains of chloral may be given, in addition to the other measures indicated.

If, *after* an attack of either of the above varieties of colic, pain or uneasiness in the bowels or diarrhœa remains, a dose of 15 grains of chloral will generally afford relief.

[At the commencement of an attack of colic, especially of the bilious variety, if the bowels are obstinately confined, it will be desirable, if possible, to obtain a stronger purgative dose combined with an opiate. This may consist of 5 grains of calomel mixed with 1 grain of extract of opium, to be followed in three hours' time by a draught composed of 1 ounce of sulphate of soda and 30 minims of strong tincture of ginger, in 2 ounces of water. In the flatulent or spasmodic variety, if the medicines as mentioned in the large type fail in affording relief, Recipe 6 if there is acidity, or Recipe 39 if much griping.]

INFLAMMATORY COLIC, AND ILIAC PASSION, OR OBSTRUCTION.—These conditions, as mentioned above, are generally sequelæ of the other varieties. Instead of the patient finding relief from the remedies, and pain being still *relieved* by pressure, the bowels may not have acted copiously, and the belly, *especially on the right side*, may become tender, with some degree of general feverishness. When colic runs on into such conditions, no purgative medicines should be given, and the patient should be treated for *inflammation of the bowels* (*vide* p. 79), or for *obstruction* (*vide* p. 82), as the symptoms indicate.

LEAD, OR PAINTER'S COLIC.—Lead, introduced into the system, excites the symptoms of colic, viz. more or less severe intestinal pain, retraction of the navel, nausea, vomiting, and constipation. Lead in the system also produces a bluish or slate-grey line on the gums, close to the teeth, and at a later period paralysis of the wrists (*vide* p. 344). People whose employment obliges them to use lead are very liable to colic, especially when they neglect the necessary precautions of cleanliness and ventilation—hence the name of the malady, 'painter's colic.' Lead colic may occur from even sleeping in a newly painted or papered room; it may also arise from the introduction of lead into the body with the food or water (*vide* p. 344). Lead colic should be treated in the same manner as advised for the bilious variety, unless remedies as below are available.

[If obtainable, give 2 drachms of Epsom salts, 20 minims of dilute sulphuric acid, and 10 minims of laudanum in 2 ounces of water every three or four hours, until the bowels have been freely moved; give also an injection, Recipe 106. After the first painful symptoms have ceased, iodide of potassium (Recipe 21) should be given. This, uniting with the lead in the blood, forms a soluble *iodide of lead*, which passes away in the urine and other excretions.]

**CONSTIPATION.**—A tendency to confined bowels is natural to many persons. Or it may depend on several causes, the principal of which are liver derangement and deficient action of either the large or small intestines.

*When constipation is natural to the constitution*, it rarely exerts any deleterious influence. Ordinarily the bowels should be moved once daily, but to some this does not naturally occur, and the condition is unattended by unpleasant symptoms. For constipation of this description, medicines, as a rule, are unnecessary, but the manner of diet as explained below may be adopted.

*When constipation occurs from inactive liver*, the symptoms are more or less similar to those noted under congestion and chronic inflammation of the liver, and the treatment should be the same (*vide* p. 318).

*When constipation occurs from deficient action of the small intestines*, there is a sluggish action, the stools being moderate in amount, very dry, and generally, but not always, light in colour; indicating accompanying torpidity of the liver. In most cases there is an uncomfortable feeling or dull pain at the back of the head, while the tongue looks small and is a little red at the tip and edges. The mouth is viscid, or 'sticky,' indicating the condition of defective secretion prevailing in the bowels. There is also loss of spirits and loss of appetite, with probably more or less flatulence, and occasionally slight colicky pains. This form of constipation is more common in unhealthy malarious districts. Purgatives in such cases are not usually required. What is wanted is the presence in the intestines of more liquid. A glass of cold water taken *every* morning on rising is often beneficial. Or, this not succeeding, 2 drachms of sulphate of soda and 2 grains of quinine should be dissolved in a pint of water and taken as a morning draught. Or fruit, such as baked apples or stewed prunes, eaten in the morning, oatmeal porridge for breakfast, smoking after breakfast, brown bread eaten instead of white, the avoidance of pastry, regular exercise, and regular but not hurried visits to the water-closet, will generally be successful. Figs, prunes, and stewed fruit are valuable auxiliaries; but vegetables are objectionable if they produce flatulence. Such measures may be assisted at first by castor-oil or senna, or Recipes 1 and 2, which are good ordinary aperient doses.

*When the large intestines are in fault*, the tongue is furred, the breath fœtid, the complexion sallow, and sometimes jaundiced. There are occasional attacks of colicky pain, and piles are often present, while the stools are dark or mottled, the part first passed being very hard, and the remainder softer, or even liquid. This is particularly the case when the constipation results from accumulation of fæces in the lower gut close to the fundament, known by the stools consisting of round, hard, black masses or balls. Some persons suffering from torpor of the large intestines state their bowels are regular simply because they go to the closet every day, when in reality they suffer from habitual constipation, as they only pass small lumps of hard fæces. Occasionally, also, there may be straining, and the hard lumps may be passed with a little watery discharge, the result of the irritation they cause. This is mistaken for diarrhœa, instead of being recognised as the effect of constipation. This form of constipation is more likely to occur in India than in temperate climates. The bowels, particularly the large intestines, partaking in the general debility and want of tone resulting from lengthened residence in the tropics, become eventually less able to expel their contents, which leads not only to constipation, but also to accumulation of fæcal matter in the gut, and sometimes to the condition described as chronic inflammation of the *cæcum* (*vide* p. 81). For constipation depending on defective action of the large intestines, occasional doses of castor-oil or sulphate of soda (Recipe 2)—sometimes one suiting best, sometimes the other—are among the most desirable medicines. One grain of ipecacuanha taken early in the morning is often very useful in torpor of the intestines. Rubbing and kneading the belly on each side with soap liniment will also frequently promote healthy action. Then a regimen, as noted, for deficient action of the small intestines, should be adopted; while in many cases, instead of repetition of medicine, the periodical use of an enema syringe will prove the better course, especially when there is accumulation in the lower gut, for the expulsion of which medicines are not well adapted.

It should be recollected that the proper stimulus to the periodical action of the bowels is food perfectly digested. Instead, therefore, of constantly resorting to purgative medicines to remove constipation, it is better to accomplish the object by care in not eating hurriedly, so that the food may be well masticated, by some change of diet, and by attention to the teeth if necessary. On the other hand, constipation, unless natural to the constitution, even if requiring medicines, must not be neglected, and the first tendency to it should be guarded against, lest it become habitual. For it is one of the causes of the following and other maladies: anæmia (*vide* p. 46); apoplexy (p. 53); chlorosis (p. 50); colic (p. 131); cramps in the legs (p. 409); discharges from the privates (p. 364); fissure of the anus (p. 272); irritable bladder (p. 73); piles (p. 347); sciatica (p. 378); varicocele (p. 454); varicose veins (p. 456).

[Other medicines useful for occasional constipation occurring to ordinarily strong and healthy people will be found in Recipes 9 and 10. For weakly people, and when there is suspicion of accumulation of fæcal matter in the lower bowel, Recipe 13 or 15 will be more suitable, provided piles are not present. If present, Recipe 12. Torpid bowels may also generally be much benefited by one quarter of a grain of extract of belladonna taken morning and evening. The extract may be made into pills, and the dose may be gradually increased, by a quarter of a grain, every five or six days, up to 1 grain. 'Valoid fluid extract of Cascara sagrada' is a valuable remedy for habitual constipation, especially when associated with piles. Aperient mineral waters are often of service. Of these Friedrichshall and Hunyadi Janos are deservedly in high repute, the latter having the advantage of being almost tasteless. For constipation, especially of females, not apparently due to any prominent cause, the following recipe is advisable. Extract of aloes, half a drachm; extract of nux vomica, 6 grains; extract of hyoscyamus, 1 scruple; powder of ipecacuanha, 1 grain. Divide into 20 pills; 1 to be taken at night.]

Constipation of Children.—Although infants and children are more liable to diarrhœa in India than in Europe, this does not prevent them suffering from constipation. As explained below, constipation is sometimes the cause of diarrhœa. Fever, convulsions, and spasmodic croup may also arise from hardened masses of fæces retained in the bowels; therefore the conditions should never be neglected.

The constipation of infants and children depends on different *causes*, the principal of which are, improper food; sluggish action of the liver; and weakness of the muscular coat of the bowels; the latter usually a consequence of a feeble condition of the general health. Sores at the fundament, perhaps consequent on irritation from thread-worms, cause constipation, the child being afraid to stool in consequence of pain from the sore. One, two, or all these causes may be in operation, and it is by the discovery and appreciation of such causes, and by combating them by change of diet and hygienic measures, rather than by medicines, that the evils arising from constipation of children and infants may be best prevented or cured.

The symptoms of constipation in infants or children

vary. The bowels do not act with regularity, but while in one case there is simple infrequency and hardness of the motions, in another the stools are little balls, scanty, hard, frequently white greenish or mottled in colour, and passed with more or less straining. Sometimes such stools are accompanied by watery greenish discharge, or by white or jelly-like mucus, or are even streaked with blood, the result of the mechanical irritation caused to the lining membrane of the lower bowels by the hard fæcal matter.

When there are simply infrequent and hard motions, the child may be otherwise apparently quite well, or the only indication of ill-health may be fretfulness, uneasy sleep, and irritability of the bladder, causing wetting of the bed. But as the stools assume the appearances last noted other symptoms arise, as flatulence, colicky pains, fœtid breath, indigestion of food, occasionally vomiting, sometimes fever, and possibly in female children discharge from the privates. Infants especially, when constipated, often suffer from indigestion of the food and vomiting, bringing up their milk in lumpy masses, some of which also pass into the intestines undigested, causing irritation, flatulence, and colicky pains.

When constipation is long-continued, alternating with watery discharges as above noted, the irritation of the hardened fæces is apt to establish a more permanent discharge of the kind which may be mistaken for diarrhœa, and treated as diarrhœa in vain, until the real cause is understood and attacked. But as the child becomes more out of health the local irritation excites a true diarrhœa, which succeeds the former constipated condition and requires a different treatment (*vide* pp. 172, 175).

*Treatment.*—As a general rule the constipation of infants and children is best treated by some change of food, or, if the infant is being suckled, by some change in the food and manner of life of the nursing woman. Generally she will require more exercise, and a larger proportion of vegetables in her diet. To afford immediate relief, a dose of castor-oil may be given to the woman, which will usually be followed by some diminution of the infant's costiveness. Or a little cow's or goat's milk may be given. If the child is being fed by hand, a change from cow's to goat's milk, or *vice versá*, may be tried. The mixture of one-third barley-water, or of half a tea-spoonful of fine oatmeal at each meal, sometimes affords relief. The insertion of a pawn stalk into the fundament may be employed for infants; or a piece of soap may be pared to the thickness of a quill, dipped in salad oil, and introduced into the anus. This will frequently be followed by an easy stool. Rubbing the bowels with cod-liver oil or cocoa-nut oil, the friction being principally made from above downwards, is also often efficacious. Injections are sometimes used, but it is well to avoid these means if possible, although they are excellent remedies in cases of great debility with constipation. Warm soapy water is perhaps the best injection, given in the quantities and manner detailed in the Appendix under heading *Injections or Enemas.*

[When change of milk, as advised above, cannot be readily made, or if it does not succeed, peptonised milk may be tried, using Fairchild's peptonising powders. When hand-fed infants, as previously mentioned, suffer from constipation, vomiting of milk in lumpy masses, and flatulence, the milk may be peptonised, Recipe 22 may be used, and lime-water (Recipe 25) will probably be beneficial.]

When constipation appears to depend on an inactive liver (known by want of colour in the stools) or on want of power of the intestines to expel their contents (usually accompanying a generally feeble condition), and it becomes necessary to administer opening medicines to infants and young children, the choice (from the medicine case or from medicines easily procurable; *vide* pp. 15, 23, 26) lies between magnesia, castor-oil, and senna. If there is costiveness with flatulence, fœtid breath, and acidity, citrate of magnesia may be given in doses according to the age of the child (*vide* p. 15). This is a good laxative medicine for a child, having little taste, and it may be rendered more palatable by a small proportion of sugar. If the child is old enough to drink the draught off immediately, the addition of 3 or 4 grains of carbonate of soda increases effervescence, and also efficacy as an antacid. If there is inaction of the liver and white or clay-coloured stools, senna may be used, as mentioned at p. 26. If there is no evident deterioration of health attending the constipation, castor-oil may be used (*vide* p. 23).

The frequent use of purgatives or of the enema syringe is deprecated. The former weaken and disorder the stomach when habitually given; while the latter by persistent use impairs the muscular tone of the rectum or lower gut. The constipation of children should, if possible, be overcome by change of dieting. A little treacle given with the morning and evening meals sometimes answers admirably.

In all cases of constipation in infants and children sores at the orifice of the fundament should be looked for. If present, they should be treated by washing the part with glycerine soap after every motion, then applying with a sponge alum-water (Recipe 100), and afterwards a little simple ointment (Recipe 86). Lastly, when children suffer from alternating constipation and diarrhœa, the possibility of *worms* should be recollected (*vide* p. 482).

[If the child is under two, a tea-spoonful of glycerine every morning will often overcome constipation. When for children of two years of age and upwards the above-mentioned remedies do not prove satisfactory, mineral waters, as Pullna, or Hunyadi Janos water (the latter having the advantage of being almost tasteless) may be tried. Or it may be well to obtain and use Recipe 16, known as 'Gregory's powder.' Or 30 grains of rhubarb powder, 2 scruples of bicarbonate of magnesia, and 2 ounces of peppermint water should be made into a mixture, of which a child two or three years old may take a tea-spoonful every four hours. During the early months of life, especially in children brought up by hand, probably after a previous attack of diarrhœa, constipation as previously described, with hard clay-coloured stools, or mottled green motions, may occur. The stools are passed with pain and screaming, and there is much wind, making the child cry incessantly. A grain of podophyllin should be dissolved in a drachm of brandy, and 1 or 2 drops of the solution should be given to the child twice a day on a lump of white sugar. It will be well to commence with 1 drop, increasing if no effect is produced. Usually under this treatment the motions become natural, the flatulence of the belly disappears, and the child quickly improves.]

**CONSUMPTION** or **PHTHISIS.**—Consumption does not attack Europeans so frequently as in colder climates, and, if not too far advanced, it may be arrested by the warmer climate of the tropics. Consumption consists in the decay of the lungs, arising from the deposit in their texture of a material derived from the blood, which is technically called 'tubercle.' Microscopic organisms, or a form of *bacillus*, consisting of slender rod-shaped living bodies, have been discovered in the diseased product and breath of the consumptive, and it has therefore been advanced that consumption is a localised *tuberculosis* (*vide* p. 88) which may under certain circumstances prove contagious. The first symptom noticed is short dry cough, most troublesome on rising in the morning. The patient is easily fatigued, flushes on slight exertion, and experiences difficulty in ascending heights or stairs. Then expectoration of mucus occurs, and probably spitting of bright-coloured frothy blood. The pulse is also quicker than natural, and there is generally a sensible increase of temperature towards evening. This condition may persist for weeks or months, even sometimes for years. Many persons coming to India in this first stage of consumption are prevented growing worse by the change of climate, but suffer as above either continually or peridiocally—their complaint being often considered by themselves and friends due to weakness or febrile influences.

In the second stage of the disease the cough grows worse, the expectoration more profuse, and becomes of a yellow colour, formed in globular masses which float in water, and are sometimes streaked with blood. *Hectic*, or night fever (*vide* p. 269), occurs, followed by profuse night sweats; and although the appetite may continue good, flesh and strength are lost. There are often now sharp cutting pains in the side and chest, the patient may lose his voice, and diarrhœa may occur. Ultimately the patient dies from exhaustion, or from a large blood-vessel giving way in the lungs, when large quantities of bright-coloured blood are passed by the mouth. This, however, may occur several times without causing death. Until the latest stage of this malady the patient is generally hopeful of recovery, and frequently fails to recognise his danger.

*Treatment.*—More may be done to prevent than to cure this disease. As it is often hereditary, those of consumptive family should be especially careful as to their mode of life. Avoiding injudicious 'coddling,' they should sleep in well-ventilated rooms, should avoid late hours, should habitually live generously, but not richly or intemperately, should shun exposure to cold or damp, and should wear flannel next the skin. When the disease has declared itself, cod-liver oil, and tonics, as iron and quinine, are beneficial. Medicines to allay the cough are also required (Recipe 57). Consumptives should never swallow the expectoration; it should be destroyed if possible by burning, and for this purpose spittoons with movable paper interior may be used. The sharing of a bed, or even a bedroom, with consumptive patients should *not* be sanctioned, and attendants should have as much fresh air as possible. Too much stress cannot be placed on the necessity of parents of consumptive family bringing up their children under strict discipline as regards diet, personal hygiene, and general sanitary conditions of life; for such children are not only liable to consumption as they reach adult age, but are also prone to *Atrophy*, or wasting (*vide* p. 66), and to other ailments.

As medicine, special recommendation is accorded to Fellowes' 'Compound syrup of hypophosphites.' The syrup contains elements essential to the animal organisation—viz. potash, lime, and iron, also magnesia, quinine, strychnine, and phosphorus. The 'Kepler palatable cod-liver oil' is the best. But no cod-liver oil can always be borne by the consumptive's stomach, when the 'Kepler extract of malt' will prove a pleasant and efficient substitute. Special praise has also been given to *altitude* as a curative agent in consumption, the diminished pressure of the air as experienced on mountains having been questionably theorised as an important medical factor. Thus in America, Denver in the Rocky Mountains, and on the Continent, St. Moritz and the Upper Engadine, generally have been recommended for the phthisical. It is, however, only in the early stages that any such change will prove beneficial, and the benefit which unquestionably often results must be credited to the pure dry air, and not to the altitude. The second stage requires a moist equable unstimulating climate, and all patients in the latest stage should remain in the comfort of home. The comparatively equable climate of the Neilgherrie Mountains, especially at Conoor and Kotagiri, also affording any advantage to be derived from altitude, is perhaps as good a climate for the consumptive as can be found. As regards the choice of a climate for the consumptive, the mind as well as the lungs should receive consideration. As a general rule, novelty and employment of the mind are desirable, and a congregation of invalids is depressing, and therefore injurious.

**CONVULSIONS.**—*Vide* FITS, EPILEPSY, HYSTERIA, TETANUS, HYDROPHOBIA, in all of which diseases convulsions are prominent symptoms. Convulsions depend on some cause irritating the nerves of the part, and this irritation may be either at their seat of origin in the brain or spinal cord, as when inflammation occurs in these organs, or when spiculæ, or splints of bone, are driven into them from accident. Or otherwise, the irritation on which the convulsions depend may be at the ends of the nerves, where they divide on the surface of the skin, or on the surface of the bowels, into innumerable filaments. Of this variety of convulsions *tetanus*, or 'lockjaw,' from injuries of the hand; convulsions of lying-in women from irritation in the womb; in children from teething, or from constipation, or worms, are illustrations.

**CONVULSIONS OF CHILDREN.**—Do not usually come on suddenly. There are generally indications that convulsions are threatening, although such signs may not be recognised. Signs of a tendency to convulsions, or, it may be said, a minor degree of convulsions, are turning in of the thumbs towards the palms of the hand, clenching of the fingers, contraction of the toes, startings during sleep, squinting, and twitchings of the face. A slight degree of twitching of the face during sleep has been called by ignorant nurses 'the angel's whisper.' Whenever any of these symptoms are observed the child should be carefully watched, and great attention should be paid to the state of the bowels and teeth, and to the diet.

A few days after birth an infant is apt to suffer from slight convulsive movements, to which nurses give the name of 'inward fits,' or 'nine-day fits.' The baby, after lying as if asleep, rolls its eyes about, or draws them up underneath the lids, perhaps moans gently, breathes a little heavily, has twitchings of the muscles of the hands, and sometimes there is a livid ring round the mouth. This either arises from indigestion, and is a warning that the quality of the food should be looked to (*vide* Chapter V., *Feeding of Children*, or *Index*), or from something wrong with the navel (*vide* Chapter V., *Ulcerated Navel*, or *Index*), which should be investigated. It may be temporarily relieved by gently rubbing the bowels, by giving two drops of aromatic spirits of ammonia (*vide* p. 8), or, if there is also wind and acidity, by using citrate of magnesia (*vide* p. 15). If not relieved the condition will probably pass into decided convulsions.

Children are subject to a nervous affection called *night*

*screaming* or *night terrors.* They wake up suddenly, apparently horribly frightened, and commence screaming violently. While thus screaming, they are generally quite unconscious of what is occurring around them, and cannot recognise, or be comforted by their friends, or they think some object near them is some animal coming to attack them. The screaming may last a few seconds, or it may be continued for an hour or more, and in confirmed cases the sudden waking up and screaming may be repeated several times during the night. There are generally also some of the minor symptoms of convulsions previously noted, and 'night terrors' may terminate in convulsions. It is frequently attributable to dreams and nightmare, or to the cold feeling arising from *wetting the bed* (*vide* p. 460), with which it is often associated. Sometimes the cure of this latter ailment will stop the fits of night-screaming. But generally the cause is something wrong, arising from teething, or from worms, or from the digestive organs, and as a result affecting the nervous system. During the actual fit of screaming, the only thing necessary is to endeavour to soothe and pacify.

The affection designated *spasmodic croup* is also a form of the convulsions of children. It is popularly known as 'child-crowing.' Infants in poor health often wake up in the night with a start, and for some time cannot get their breath—a condition designated by nurses 'a catch in the breath,' but which is in reality a minor degree of spasmodic croup. When fully developed the principal symptom of spasmodic croup is a remarkable *crowing* inspiration, unattended with cough, and coming on suddenly often on first waking from sleep. For a minute or so the child makes ineffectual efforts to draw breath, and struggles violently, but at length the difficulty is overcome and breath is *drawn in* with a loud crowing sound. The difficulty of breathing is during inspiration, and in the intervals between the paroxysms the difficulty ceases, which does not happen in true croup. Of these attacks there may be several during the day or night. In extreme cases the face becomes livid, the whites of the eyes bloodshot, the thumbs are clenched in the hands, the fingers and toes are bent, and the joints of the wrists and ankles are forcibly turned inwards, and very violent attempts are made to breathe. Occasionally death results from suffocation or exhaustion, but the malady is not so dangerous as inflammatory croup (*vide* p. 154). The spasmodic tendency of the parts about the throat sometimes excites a peculiar condition, in which the child is able to swallow solids with ease, but chokes when it tries to drink fluids.

Spasmodic croup depends on spasmodic or convulsive action of the muscles about the upper part of the windpipe. It is distinguished from true croup by the very sudden accession and decline of the fits or paroxysms, and by the perfect freedom of the breathing in the intervals. Also, by the absence of fever or catarrhal symptoms, and generally by the absence of cough. It is usually connected with, and often immediately caused by, the irritation of swollen gums during teething, by glandular enlargements in the neck, and by constipation, or accumulation of fæcal matter in the intestines. It is most common in weakly, scrofulous children who are being brought up by hand. It may occur up to two years of age, but is rare after twelve months.

*Treatment.*—All clothing about the neck should be rapidly loosened, plenty of fresh air should be admitted, and the child should be exposed to the current. The face should be sprinkled with cold water and fanned, while the back should be briskly rubbed. A cloth or sponge, wrung out of hot water, should be suddenly applied to the throat and removed in half a minute, several times, at intervals of five minutes. If the attack has come on after a meal, a finger should be passed into the child's throat to excite vomiting. A stimulant, as a tea-spoonful of wine or of brandy-and-water, may be given with advantage as soon as the child can swallow. If the gums are tender and swollen, they should be lanced immediately. If the fit has come on after a hearty meal, and free vomiting has not been excited by the finger in the throat, an emetic, as a drachm of ipecacuanha wine in a table-spoonful of water, should be given. These measures are usually successful; but if not, as soon as a warm bath can be obtained, the child should be immersed in the water, or its feet may be put in mustard (a tea-spoonful) and warm water (a gallon) if a hot bath is not procurable (*vide Appendix, Baths.*)

But it is during the intervals between the attacks that curative agents are most serviceable, and these must depend on the causes producing the irritation. Bromide of potassium (Recipe 20) should always be used. The condition of the gums and teeth must be constantly investigated (*vide Teething*, p. 429). Constipation or worms must be removed (*vide* pp. 138, 482), and swollen glands in the neck must be treated on surgical principles (*vide Enlarged Glands*, p. 278). If the child is being brought up by hand, a wet nurse should be procured.

*The general convulsions of children* mostly occur in delicate infants about the period of teething, especially when children have been fed with improper food. Convulsions from teething, or from any other cause, happen much more rarely to children nourished on human milk than when fed on other foods. Convulsions may arise from the irritation of worms in the intestines. They may be caused by constipation, and the consequent collection of hard fæcal matter in the bowels, or from a piece of potato-peel swallowed, or even from the flatulence to which such conditions give rise. They may result from the irritation caused by prolonged diarrhœa. They may come on during fever, or from hooping-cough. They have been known to arise from some local irritation, as, for instance, a blister, or from a pin in the clothing pricking the skin. They have followed suckling the child after the mother has given way to a fit of hysterics or passion. They may follow the sudden disappearance of a skin eruption. They may be due to anæmia (*vide* p. 46). *Lastly*, they may be premonitory symptoms of serious maladies, such as epilepsy, or water on the brain, or the prelude to small-pox or scarlet fever.

*Symptoms.*—An attack of general convulsions in a child presents spasmodic contractions of the arms and legs, which are suddenly rendered tense and hard, and are drawn upwards and inwards towards the body; the eyes are also turned up under the lids, the mouth perhaps screwed to one side, while the teeth grate, the lips twitch, and froth appears at the mouth. The head and neck may be drawn backwards, or to one side, and the throat may be affected as in spasmodic croup (*vide* p. 146). Sometimes the convulsions are limited to one side of the body. During the fit the urine and fæces may be discharged involuntarily, and a clammy moisture breaks out over the whole body. The pulse is weak and often irregular, the breathing laboured, and the pupils of the eyes will be found either contracted or dilated, but always insensible to light. This condition may last for a few minutes, or may endure, with intervals of incomplete cessation for hours, the child being more or less insensible during the whole period. At last the child falls asleep or cries loudly, or lies in a kind of stupor, slowly returning to consciousness, or becoming profoundly insensible. In bad attacks it may die from spasmodic closure of the air-passages. In this case the face becomes purple, the head is thrown back, violent efforts are made to breathe, and a crowing noise like that of croup is heard, which gradually becomes fainter as the child ceases to exist.

*Treatment.—In all cases* all clothing about the neck, chest, and head should be rapidly loosened, plenty of fresh air should be admitted, and the face should be fanned, and sprinkled with very cold water, while the back should be briskly rubbed. If there is any throat spasm, a soft cloth, or sponge wrung out of hot water, should be several times suddenly applied to the throat, and removed from it in half a minute, at intervals of five minutes. The next treatment depends considerably on whether there are attempts to vomit, whether the attack succeeded a meal, whether the child can or can not swallow, and whether it had suffered from preceding diarrhœa.

*If there are efforts to vomit,* such efforts should be encouraged, by passing a finger into the throat, or by tickling the throat with a feather. *If there are no efforts to vomit, but the convulsions have come on after a full meal,* and therefore appear due to an overloaded stomach, vomiting should still be excited by the finger or by a feather. If free vomiting does not occur, and *the child can swallow,* weak mustard and water (a quarter the strength of Recipe 54) may be given as an emetic.

*Caution.*—If, as often happens, the child is unable to swallow, no attempt should be made to give medicines, as fluids put into the mouth under such circumstances will not pass into the stomach, but will probably trickle into the windpipe and do mischief. It is true that fluids may be given through the nostrils, but in the absence of medical aid this plan is not recommended.

*After the vomiting,* if the child can swallow,* a stimulant, as a tea-spoonful of wine or brandy-and-water. Then, as it is desirable to open the bowels if *the child can swallow,* and *if the convulsions have not supervened on prolonged diarrhœa,* a purgative, as castor-oil, or sulphate of soda, whichever may be at hand, should be given in doses according to the age of the child (half a tea-spoonful of castor-oil for an infant six months old, and a tea-spoonful at one year old—of sulphate of soda half a drachm at six months old, 1 drachm at a year old, in a little water), to be followed in the course of an hour by an enema composed of, for an infant of six months old, 1 drachm of castor-oil in 1 ounce of soapy water; at one year old, of 2 drachms of castor-oil and 2 ounces of soap water. *If the child cannot swallow,* the enema should be given at once. To unload the bowels is, in the majority of cases, a matter of primary importance, and therefore, if not freely moved, the medicine and enema should be again used after the lapse of two hours.

*If the convulsions have followed diarrhœa* and the child is weak and debilitated, purgatives should *not* be given. *In such cases, if swallowing is possible,* for infants small doses of chlorodyne, according to the age of the child (*vide* p. 12), should be administered every two hours; or, for older children, chloral may be given in a dose of 4 grains for a child two years old, and 2 grains at one year old; the dose to be repeated twice at an interval of two hours.

*In all cases, if the child can swallow,* bromide of potassium (Recipe 20) should be used every two hours, *after* the vomiting is over; or if purgatives are used, *after* the bowels are well open. The first doses of this medicine may be given with the chlorodyne or chloral as above. *But if a child is not able to swallow,* an injection containing 3 grains of chloral and 5 of bromide of potassium in an ounce and a half of water may be given from ten to fifteen months old; half a grain of each and 2 tea-spoonfuls of water being added for every month up to twenty-four.

*If there are no efforts to vomit, and the attack has not*

*come on after a meal*, the irritation causing the convulsions is probably in the intestines and not in the stomach. *In such cases the treatment mentioned above after the vomiting should be pursued* (*vide* asterisk, p. 150).

*In all cases*, if the gums are swollen (*vide* p. 434) they should be lanced immediately; sometimes lancing the gums is followed by cessation of the convulsions. Then, as soon as possible, if the convulsions are not connected with prolonged preceding illness, and if the child is ordinarily robust, it should be put into a hot bath of the temperature of 98° to 100° Fahr., where it should be kept for ten minutes. While in the bath cold water may be applied to the head. If from debility or long illness the child is weak, it may be enveloped in a blanket wrung out of hot water, round which two or three dry blankets should be wrapped. The child should remain thus covered for fifteen minutes, when it should be gradually uncovered and well dried with soft warm towels, being handled with the greatest care and not subjected to sudden jerks. If the child is very weak, it will be advisable to put the feet in warm mustard-and-water (a tea-spoonful of mustard to about one gallon of water) instead of using hot bath or blanket. The child should afterwards be kept perfectly quiet in a darkened room, and all noise, talking, &c., should be avoided. In half an hour or so, if there is return of convulsions, a mustard plaster, or if available the mustard leaf (Recipe 109), protected by muslin, should be put on over the stomach and kept on until the skin is reddened. The child should be kept lying on its left side as much as possible.

[If the above measures do not succeed, and if there is *no heat* of head, *ten drops* of chloroform may be sprinkled on a handkerchief, and the latter held two inches from the child's mouth and nose, so that it may inspire an atmosphere impregnated with chloroform, which will soothe the system and diminish the convulsive tendency. *If the child cannot swallow*, and it appears from previous constipation decidedly necessary to open the bowels, a little croton oil should, if possible, be procured, *half* a drop of which should be mixed with a little sugar, and placed with a feather on the back part of the tongue. *If the child is able to swallow,* and the oil, or sulphate of soda given as mentioned in the large type, do not thoroughly open the bowels, 1 grain of calomel and 2 of rhubarb should be procured for a child one year old, and 2 of calomel and 2 of rhubarb for a child of two years of age.]

*After an attack of convulsions,* unless the seizure has been preceded by prolonged diarrhœa, it is desirable to maintain a free action of the bowels for some days, and for this senna tea may be employed (*vide* p. 26). If the child has been previously flatulent, and the stomach out of order, antacids, as citrate of magnesia (*vide* p. 15), may be given. The existence or otherwise of worms should also be ascertained, and if necessary the treatment appropriate for the expulsion of worms (*vide* p. 482) should be adopted. The teeth should also receive more than ordinary attention for some time after an attack.

Great care should at all times be paid to the diet of children liable to this dangerous affection. One of the most common causes of convulsions is excessive and improper feeding. Convulsions in children following hysterical or other nervous excitement in the wet nurse indicate the desirability of change of nurse; or, if this be impossible, the substitution of animal milk.

**CORNS.**—Are growths from the skin, mostly caused by pressure of the shoe on prominent parts of the feet. If change of boots and attention to the 'fit' do not cure or relieve corns, they may be treated as follows:—Hard corns on the sole of the foot, or on the sides, or on the toes, are best treated by filing with a sharp file having a convex side, until slight pain is experienced, and then applying a plaster of soft leather, having a central hole to receive the corn. By this treatment, and by avoiding pressure from hard or ill-fitting boots, or from rough, creased, or darned stockings, corns in such situations may often be thoroughly cured. Soft corns generally occur between the toes, and are best relieved by keeping the toes separate by a little cotton-wool placed between. A piece cut out from the finger of a kid-glove and put on the toe may be also used. The fit of boots and shoes must be attended to, so that no pressure from ill-made boots or hard leather may be made on the part. By thus preventing the pressure and keeping the parts clean soft corns will usually disappear.

[If the above measures do not succeed, corns may be treated by the application of *liquor arsenicalis* two or three times daily. Stronger applications are *acetic* or *nitric* acid, which should be *lightly* applied by means of a small stick of cedarwood or a small camel's-hair brush. *Only the centre* of the corn should be thus touched, and if a soft corn the toes should be kept asunder for a few minutes, in order that the acid may soak in. Care must be taken that the acid does not touch any part except the corn. Then apply between the toes a small portion of cotton-wool. Repeat every other day until the corn ceases to be inconvenient.]

Corns and Bunions sometimes suppurate from the pressure of the boot, or as the effect of injury. They then require the removal of all pressure, rest, poultices, and afterwards healing ointment (Recipe 86).

**CROUP.**—Croup consists of the formation of a white membranous deposit in the windpipe and air-passages leading to the lungs, which, blocking up these air-tubes, or the small aperture leading from the throat to the windpipe, causes the extreme difficulty of breathing characterising the disease. But milder attacks of a croupy character occur, in which the disease does not proceed so far as to the formation of this deposit. In such cases the symptoms are as afterwards detailed until the coughing up of *mucous fluid is mentioned* (*vide* p. 156), when after expectoration this mild variety of croup generally passes off.

The period between one year of age and five is the time during which children are most susceptible to croup.

After five years of age the tendency to croup gradually declines, while the danger from an attack is less.

The causes of croup are generally admitted to be cold, or exposure to damp, changeable atmosphere. But there is in some children an unexplainable constitutional aptitude or tendency to attacks of the disease, which renders them liable to suffer from an exposure or change of temperature so slight as not to be felt by other children; also, when a child has once had an attack, a recurrence is not unfrequent. Croup has also—doubtless from some unknown atmospheric condition—prevailed epidemically in various localities. As a general rule, low, damp positions are favourable to croup; especially if exposed to north-easterly winds. On the other hand, the changeable temperature of hill stations, especially in the Himalayas, appears to favour croup.

*Symptoms.*—Croup sometimes commences quite suddenly, the child waking in the night with difficulty of breathing. In most instances there is for some days a little feverishness, accompanied by sneezing, watering of the eyes, and dry cough, the child appearing to have only a common cold. The child is probably cross and irritable, and the voice perhaps husky and hoarse. After such premonitory symptoms, or without them, the child suddenly awakes with an appearance of suffocation, and with a hoarse, ringing cough, to which, from its peculiar sound, the term 'brassy' has been applied. The sound of this cough is so peculiar, that once heard it can scarcely be mistaken. It resembles either the crowing of a cock or the bark of a dog, and has a ringing, metallic tone. The breathing is difficult, and the air is *drawn in* with a sound resembling the passage of air through muslin, or through a metallic tube. The cough, as also the difficulty of breathing in a lesser degree, occurs in paroxysms, in the intervals of which the child may have a little restless sleep. At first the cough is dry, but at length *a mucous fluid is brought up*, after which much relief may be experienced and the disease may subside.

If this favourable termination of the attack does not occur, tubes or flakes of a whitish membranous substance appear. The efforts to bring up such material are very great; the countenance is flushed, sometimes almost livid, and the body is covered with perspiration; the hands are clenched, the arms thrown about, the bed-clothes tossed away. The child sometimes sits erect, sometimes lies down, and sometimes the head is rigidly bent backwards. The eyes project, and the whites of the eyes become congested. red, or 'bloodshot.' The pulse is quick and hard, the skin burning, and the thirst great. The little patient frequently carries the hand to the throat, as if to remove some obstruction. In the morning the symptoms somewhat abate, and the child continues better during the day; but this seeming step towards recovery is often deceitful—the return of night being accompanied by a re-accession of suffering. If the case ends favourably, there is gradual amendment, after a considerable amount of *flaky* material has been coughed up. If the disease terminates fatally, the paroxysms of coughing and the difficulty of breathing become more violent and incessant, until from want of strength the cough grows husky, faint, and muffled, when the child dies, partly from exhaustion and partly from suffocation. Often, also, towards the end of the case, one or more convulsive seizures occur, during which the patient may expire. The duration of the malady may be from twenty-four hours to five days.

For the distinction between *croup* and *diphtheria*, see *Diphtheria*, p. 182.

*Treatment.*—On the first appearance of croupy cough or hoarseness, ipecacuanha and paregoric (Recipe 57) should be given, and the patient should be well protected from cold, especially at night. In children subject to croupy attacks, the malady may often be stopped in the first stage by giving, when the child wakes up with hoarse cough, a tea-spoonful of *salad* oil, which, as it is swallowed, lubricates the parts about the entrance of the windpipe; and by lighting several lamps in the room, or otherwise increasing the temperature, often in India so much less by night than by day. For this purpose, when children are subject to croup, several lamps should be put ready, so that they may be lighted immediately. Or, if these means are not available, the child should have some hot tea and be covered up warm.

When undoubted croup is present, an emetic should be at once given. This, for a strong child of two and a half to three years old, should consist of 3 drachms of ipecacuanha wine in two or three ounces of warm water. If the patient is not a strong, robust child, 2 drachms of ipecacuanha wine, with two or three ounces of water, should be given every five minutes till free vomiting occurs. The action of the emetic should be assisted by a warm bath of from 98° to 100° Fahr. in temperature, in which the patient should remain about eight minutes, being then well and quickly dried and wrapped in blankets. If the emetic appears to produce relief, it may be repeated in about one hour, after which ipecacuanha wine in from 5- to 8-drop doses, with a drachm of water, should be given five or six times every hour. If the child is strong and robust, leeches should also be applied over the *upper part of the breast-bone*, in the number of one moderate-sized leech for each year of the child's age. But when the leeches come off the bleeding should be stopped, which can easily be effected by pressure with the finger on the leech-bite against the breast-bone (*vide* p. 512 and *Appendix* No. 117). After the vomiting from the emetics has ceased, if the bowels have not acted freely, a tea-spoonful of castor-oil should be given. Neither opium nor any other narcotic agent should be used to procure sleep, as they would be injurious by preventing expectoration. During the daytime, when symptoms ameliorate, Recipe 57. As blisters or other counter-irritants rarely seem to do good in this disease, their use is not recommended, but a sponge wrung out of hot water and applied to the throat often proves beneficial. In the latter stages of the complaint, stimulants, as wine or brandy-and-water, are indicated. *Throughout the treatment the object is to combat the inflammation, not to weaken the child*; therefore, if possible, the patient should be induced to take strong broth or other nourishing fluids at any period of the disease; and if the child cannot swallow, they should be given as injections; or, if practicable, *digested enemas* (*vide Appendix*) should be used.

The remarks made at pp. 104, 107, under *Bronchitis*, regarding *temperature* of the sick-room and *moistened atmosphere*, are *equally applicable to croup*, and should be *fully attended to*.

When all measures fail, opening the windpipe has sometimes proved successful; but this operation can only be undertaken by a surgeon.

Children subject to any variety of croup require great care as regards their diet, and attention in avoiding catching cold, or ordinary cough, which in those constitutionally predisposed is liable to terminate in an attack of croup.

**COUGH.**—Cough is a symptom of other affections rather than a malady in itself (*vide* p. 37). Cough differs in its character according to the causes. Cough, sometimes attended with expectoration, at others 'dry,' occurs in catarrh and influenza. In consumption, when it is constant, with pain in the upper part of the chest, fever, and wasting of the body. In asthma, with difficulty of breathing coming on in fits, and generally in the night. In inflammation of the lungs, when the cough is followed by expectoration of a rusty colour. In hæmoptysis, when bright-looking blood is coughed up. In pleurisy, when it is attended with stabbing pain in the side. In croup, when it has a brassy sound. In measles, with discharge from the nose, and watering of the eyes. In acute bronchitis, when the cough is accompanied by tenacious expectoration like white of egg. In the teething of children, when it is particularly troublesome at night. Cough may also arise from an elongated uvula, from ear affections, from hysteria, or from stomach and liver derangements. In all these, and in various other maladies, cough is a distinguishing and prominent symptom.

Cough, in the popular acceptation of the term, is, however, mostly the consequence of cold, damp, or draughts, and is usually accompanied with some degree of *bronchitis* (*vide* p. 102). Ordinary cough may be best relieved by measures which promote perspiration. Three or four grains of Dover's powder may be taken twice or thrice a day; or Recipe 56. If the urine is thick, Recipe 57.

[A good cough mixture may be made as follows: Take of honey and treacle, of each 4 ounces; of vinegar 5 ounces; mix and simmer them over a slow fire, then add a dessert-spoonful of ipecacuanha wine, and the same quantity of paregoric. The dose is 2 table-spoonfuls three or four times a day.]

**DELIRIUM.**—Delirium means temporary disorder of the mental faculties, which reveals itself in the language or actions of the patient, and is a symptom of disease rather than a disease itself (*vide* p. 37). It may vary in degree, from slight wandering and incoherence, to complete and thorough derangement of the mind. Frequently the patient has some fixed delusion. Delirium usually tends to be worse at night, or it may only come on at that time. A delirious patient may often be roused so as to become temporarily coherent, or the delirium may be constant. Delirium often occurs after a person has been drinking to excess, when it is generally accompanied by delusions of the mind, by trembling of the hands, and by restlessness and timidity of manner. Delirium also arises from the weakness following continued bleeding, or from almost any cause of great exhaustion, such as bad burns, wounds, or compound fractures. It is also often present during the course of fevers. Of this *febrile delirium* there are two forms—*one* occurring in the early stages of fever, often marked by great excitement, struggling, and displays of strength; the *second* form supervening in the latter stages of fever, when the patient lies prostrate on his bed, utterly helpless, and muttering indistinctly—a condition known technically as *typhoid*. Lastly, delirium is a symptom of inflammation or other disease of the brain, when the delirium is characterised by great fury and violence.

In most instances of delirium the patient will require to be restrained, so as to prevent his getting out of bed or otherwise injuring himself. Persuasion and gentle force, a soothing manner, combined with watchfulness, firmness, and decision, are required from the attendants; for contradiction, and the exercise of authority, always excite opposition from the delirious. As a general rule, delirious people may be sufficiently restrained without mechanical means; but in exceptional cases, or when sufficient help cannot be obtained, the strait-waistcoat may be employed.

*The strait-waistcoat* is made of strong cotton cloth, and should extend from the neck to below the waist. It should have no opening in front, but tie down the back with tapes. The sleeves should be long enough to extend half a foot beyond the hands, and should be closed at the extremities, round which a cord or strong tape is tied. The waistcoat should also be furnished with shoulder-straps. When used, the tapes should be tied down the back, and the cords or tapes attached to the sleeves may be tied to the foot of the bed, if the patient's hands are required by his sides; or to the opposite sides of the bed, if the hands are crossed over the body. Strong tapes or rope, passed through the shoulder-straps, and tied to the bed, effectually secure the patient's body.

**DELIRIUM TREMENS.**—This is the peculiar delirium of the drunkard, and presents certain characteristics differing from any other kind of delirium. It is generally caused by continuous or prolonged drinking, but may follow a single indulgence in excess. Or it may come on after a person, habitually drinking, suddenly ceases doing so. Drunkards are especially liable to this delirium after a severe injury. The patient is incoherent, and fancies he sees all kinds of frightful objects, especially at night; his hands tremble, his eyes wander, his pulse is feeble, his skin moist, he has no appetite, and he cannot sleep. The patient, however, is seldom violent, and may be generally restrained without force or mechanical restraint, although the reverse occasionally happens. But there is cunning with the delirium, and the patient may secrete such articles as razors or knives, so that he requires watching. Often the person exposes himself to injury by endeavouring to effect an escape from his attendants, or from imaginary dangers. In fatal cases the delirium is succeeded by insensibility, in which state the patient dies after a period in which heavy breathing, twitching of the limbs, and involuntary discharge of fæces, with perhaps convulsions, are the most marked symptoms.

The mental delusions in delirium tremens are peculiar. The patient may declare there are snakes under his pillow, or he may be seen listening to the arm of a chair, which he believes to be a hissing serpent; or he may accuse a bystander of a design on his life, or imagine he is besieged by a party of soldiers; or he will pretend to be busy with his daily avocations; or imagine himself possessed of great wealth, which he will either hoard or lavishly distribute.

Delirium tremens must be distinguished from the delirium accompanying inflammation of the brain and its membranes. This is accomplished by a consideration of the history of the case, delirium tremens occurring in persons addicted to drink; inflammation of the brain originating without any evident exciting cause, or after exposure to the sun. In delirium tremens there is an absence of headache, and light is not painful to the eyes, while the reverse obtains in inflammatory delirium. There is in delirium tremens an absence of febrile symptoms and a moist skin, the reverse being the case in affections of the brain. In delirium tremens there is also generally a smell of liquor with the breath. It sometimes, however, happens that delirium tremens occurs in persons who, while drinking hard, have also, from exposure to the sun, or from fever, a congested condition of the brain. The symptoms of delirium tremens may then be somewhat less characteristic than as above set forth. In doubtful cases, in the absence of medical aid, it will be best to treat the case as delirium tremens.

*Treatment.*—In some instances purgative remedies are desirable at the first. These cases are known by the flushed, bloated appearance, the very foul tongue, the bad-smelling breath, and the history of a recent surfeit of eating as well as of drinking; in such cases Recipe 1, followed in two or three hours by repeated doses of Recipe 2, may be given. In other cases the strength must be supported by fluid diet of the most nutritious kind, such as yolk of egg, soups, and the like, which should be given often in small quantities. When there is great depression and feeble pulse, with moist pale tongue and pallid countenance, a small quantity, as one ounce, of wine, or half an ounce of brandy, may be administered with the soup, or in the shape of 'egg-flip.' If the patient continues to take and digest food the danger is diminished, and food adapted to the feeble state of the system, with good nursing, is the *sine quâ non.* The danger all through is from exhaustion, but this cannot be fully combated by its cause, viz. alcoholic stimulants; therefore reliance must be placed principally on nourishing food. The disease, in short, must be treated as one curable, not by withholding stimulants altogether, but by using them in strict subordination to good nursing and careful diet and regimen.

The administration of any narcotic, notwithstanding the apparent indication in the sleeplessness of the patient, requires caution, and should scarcely be given except under medical advice. But when *there is any natural tendency or desire to sleep*, a dose of twenty grains of chloral may be given. It must, however, be recollected that opiates are only safe in delirium tremens when used with the object of aiding or seconding the natural cure of the disease.

If obtainable, *bromidia* may be beneficially used instead of chloral. The dose aud composition of bromidia are given at p. 62.

*Chronic Alcoholism.*—Delirium tremens is not, unfortunately, the only malady to which excessive drinkers are subject. Delirium tremens usually arises from a fit of drinking, or a debauch; but persons who do not thus exceed, yet who are constantly taking fermented drinks (although not in sufficient quantities to produce delirium), are liable to fall into a condition to which the term *Chronic Alcoholism* has been applied. The signs and symptoms are restlessness, sleeplessness, growing indecision of character, with loss of mental and moral power—the latter exhibited by a tendency to tell falsehoods about drink. The features become bloated and flabby, the eyes red and watery, and the whites of the eyes often yellowish. The nose may be red, and there are generally enlarged vessels to be seen ramifying about the nose and cheeks. There is also trembling of the hands. Spirit-drinkers generally become emaciated, but malt-liquor drinkers often grow obese. Then, the digestive organs are always affected, indicated by disgust for food, especially in the morning, by morning nausea or sickness (which the persou probably endeavours to relieve by a secret glass of his favourite drink), by a furred tongue, foul, sour breath, and irregularity of the bowels with fœtid stools. If the constant habit of drinking is not checked, the person probably becomes affected by a special form of liver-disease, known as 'gin-drinker's liver,' or *cirrhosis* (*vide* p. 322); or by chronic disorder of the stomach (*vide* p. 415); or he grows silly, probably from softening of the brain (*vide* p. 87); and perhaps becomes wholly or partially paralysed (*vide* p. 342).

*Chronic Alcoholism* can be cured if the person will abstain from drink; but so great is the 'drink-craving' that the majority thus giving way are unable to avoid taking liquor, and will do so when opportunity presents, notwithstanding any promise to the contrary. When such patients come under medical treatment, they usually do so for the dyspeptic symptoms detailed above, and are not ready to confess to the amount of drink they consume, or to admit that their ailments arise from such a cause. The great points of treatment are to keep the patient altogether from liquor, and to give plenty of food; but as there is a disgust for solid food, it should be given in the shape of milk, beef-tea, soups, meat extracts, and puddings. The morning sickness may be often much relieved by soda-water and milk in equal parts, and drop doses of ipecacuanha wine may be given in a little water every two hours, for the same purpose. *Craving* for drink is best combated by 30-minim doses of tincture of capsicum, or of strong tincture of ginger, in 2 ounces of water, every three hours, or when craving or sinking feelings occur.

[In all cases of the kind, the following may be given with great advantage: Take of bromide of potassium 1 drachm; tincture of capsicum 1½ drachm; aromatic spirits of ammonia 6 drachms; camphor water 6 ounces; 1 ounce three times a day.]

**DIABETES.**—This complaint comes on very insidiously, and is characterised by the passing of large quantities of pale, light-coloured urine, having an apple-like odour, and containing a large amount of sugar. (There is, however, another form of the disease, called *diabetes insipidus*, when very large quantities of urine are passed, but without sugar.) Sugar, when thus voided with urine, may be easily detected by what is known as 'Moore's test.' This consists of boiling in a test-tube held over a spirit-lamp equal parts of the suspected urine and of *liquor potassæ*. If sugar is present, the fluid becomes of a fine deep purple colour. If sugar is not present, no change results. Diabetic urine attracts flies in large numbers, which in some cases has led to suspicion and detection of the disease. The appetite for a long time remains good, and is sometimes voracious, but the skin is always dry, the bowels costive, the gums pale and spongy, there is constant thirst, and the patient wastes away. As this emaciation progresses, the general health suffers, the appetite declines, perspirations occur, there is great debility, the heart becomes weak, and the feet may swell. There is also, in women, frequent intense itching, and sometimes *eczema* (*vide* p. 396), of the private parts, and in men *balanitis* (*vide* p. 282). Persons suffering from *diabetes* are extremely liable to cataract; also to attacks resembling apoplexy (known as diabetic coma), to affections of the lungs (resembling rapid consumption) and to carbuncle, from either of which death may result.

The cause of diabetes depends either on an over-production of sugar, consequent on the liver not acting properly, or, *secondly*, on a diminished destruction of sugar normally produced, consequent on errors in various organs. The result in either case is the same, viz. the entrance of sugar into the circulation and its discharge by the kidneys. Diabetes is very prevalent among well-to-do natives of India who lead indolent lives and consume abundance of butter, rice, sweetmeats, and sugar. Mental strain is also regarded as a predisposing cause. It also appears to be hereditary in some families.

The *treatment* of diabetes is more by appropriate diet than by medicines; but any change of diet made should be gradual and not abrupt. When sugar is being passed, the food should be nutritious, *but free from material containing sugar or starch.*

The articles of food which should *not* be taken are chiefly as follows. *Bread* made from wheats, oats, maize, rice, rye, or barley, or other grain containing starch, and every description of pastry and biscuits made with flour from the same. *Soups.*—All soups in which is flour or other thickening and colouring containing starch or sugar. *Meats.*—Smoked tongues, hams, bacon, and all other cured or smoked meat and fish, if cured with sugar. *Vegetables* containing sugar or starch, such as potatoes, turnips, beetroot, parsnips, carrots, radishes, onions, leeks, ripe fruits of all kinds, cauliflower, peas, sea-kale, the hearts of cabbages, beans of all kinds; dried fruits, such as dates, figs, raisins, currants, grapes, apples, pears, pine-apples, plums. All preparations of ordinary macaroni, vermicelli, semola, arrowroot, tapioca, sago, rice, dried peas, beans, chestnuts, and all farinaceous foods, and all preparations containing sugar. *Drinks.* —All malt liquors, such as beer, stout, porter, cooper, mild and old ales, cider, perry, all sparkling wines, sweet liqueurs, lemonade, ginger beer, fruit syrups, and all aerated waters containing sugar; also milk, unless with permission of medical adviser.

Articles of food which may generally be taken are: *Bread.*—One or more of the several breads, cakes, or biscuits, made from bran, gluten, and almond flour; which, if really prepared as stated without starch, are very beneficial. *Soup.*—Clear soup, mutton and chicken broth, and beef-tea if not thickened with wheaten flour. *Fish.*—All kinds of white fish, fresh, salted, or smoked, oysters and other shell fish. *Meat.*—Beef, mutton, lamb, veal, venison, pork, all kinds of game, bacon, ham, tongue, and other cured meats, if no sugar is used in the curing, cheese, eggs not too much cooked. *Vegetables.*—The green portion of most vegetables, spring cabbages, turnip-tops, spinach, the green tops of asparagus, artichokes, Brussels sprouts, sea-kale, broccoli, the green part of lettuce, cucumber, celery, pickles, olives, nuts, excepting chestnuts, mushrooms. *Pastry.*—None if made with ordinary flour. *Salad.*—Watercress, mustard and cress, endive, celery, salad oil and vinegar. *Drink.*—Claret, dry sherry, dry sauterne, chablis, burgundy, hock, unsweetened gin, whisky, tea, cocoa, skimmed milk, aerated and medicinal waters not containing sugar.

A diet composed principally of skimmed milk, with bran biscuits, has been much recommended by good authority. Diabetic food may be sweetened with saccharin, which allows of a much-needed enrichment of the diet of diabetic patients, inasmuch as they may now enjoy a sweetening flavour in diabetic bread and other nutriment without the introduction of the objectionable elements of sugar (carbo-hydrates) into the system. As medicines, Recipe 75 may be generally taken with advantage; also Recipe 65 in half the dose every night. Cod-liver oil sometimes does good when the emaciation is great and the stomach does not reject the oil.

**DIARRHŒA.**—Originates from numerous causes, and every description is met with in India. *Diarrhœa, premonitory of cholera; diarrhœa, premonitory of dysentery; and diarrhœa accompanying or forming a symptom of other diseases*, are sufficiently treated of under the respective headings. There remain other kinds of diarrhœa, which may be summarised as—(1) *irritative diarrhœa*; (2) *diarrhœa from atmospheric changes, or chill*; (3) *hill diarrhœa*; (4) *infantile diarrhœa.*

*When requiring to distinguish and treat diarrhœa, the first question is, Is it premonitory of cholera?* If there is no cholera in the neighbourhood the idea may generally be safely dismissed. If cholera is in the neighbourhood, immediate treatment, on the assumption that it may be premonitory of cholera, is advisable (*vide* p. 122). The next question is, Is it premonitory of dysentery? This will not be the case if the attack commences as colic (*vide* p. 131), or if it can be attributed to any of the causes mentioned below as exciting *irritative diarrhœa.* Dysentery is more likely to follow diarrhœa arising from atmospheric vicissitudes.

1. Irritative Diarrhœa arises in the majority of instances from *imprudence in diet*, and must be regarded as an effort of nature causing the bowels to throw off offending matter. Such matter is usually indigestible food, unripe foods, badly cooked vegetables, shell fish, inferior tinned provisions, inferior wine or beer, &c. Diarrhœa of the irritative type may arise from a dirty condition of, or from defective tinning of, cooking utensils (*vide* Chapter VI., *Diet*). Brackish water may excite irritative diarrhœa. When persons pass from districts where the water is good into localities where it is brackish, they frequently suffer from diarrhœa, especially if no precautions are taken in the way of boiling and filtering.

The above-mentioned causes of irritative diarrhœa are more or less under the control of the individual, but there are other causes not so much under control. These are *worms* (*vide* p. 482); retained lumps of fæcal matter (*vide* p. 136); indigestion (*vide* p. 203); overflow of bile, or biliousness from congested liver (p. 319).

*Treatment.*—When diarrhœa is excited by any of the causes first mentioned, the purging is nature's remedy to free the bowels of the substances which are irritating them, and often no medical treatment is required.

Diarrhœa from indigestible food may, however, be preceded by an attack of colic, when the treatment for colic must be pursued (*vide* p. 132). Usually irritative diarrhœa is merely accompanied by more or less griping, when a spoonful of castor-oil with 20 drops of chlorodyne will be beneficial. If the purging continue, or if the evacuations are sufficiently copious to cause depression, 30 drops of chlorodyne in half a wine-glass of brandy and a little water may be taken, or Recipe 38 may be used. If there be much griping or nausea, and this is not relieved by the medicine, apply a mustard poultice or a turpentine stupe (Nos. 108, 109) over the bowels. Irritability or sickness of the stomach may be relieved by soda-water, or iced water.

If irritative diarrhœa can be traced to any of the causes *last mentioned*, while pain may be relieved by a dose of chlorodyne, the real treatment must be directed to the cause, whether worms, retained fæcal matter, indigestion or overflow of bile.

2. DIARRHŒA FROM ATMOSPHERIC CHANGES, or CHILL. This often results from sudden changes of temperature, as occur, for instance, at the commencement of an Indian monsoon, or from exposure to damp night air, or from damp clothing or bedding, or even from sitting before an open door or window, or on the first passing out into the cold early-morning air. Diarrhœa, which has been erroneously attributed to malaria, occurs after a person has been actively engaged during the day—perhaps snipe-shooting—in the heat of the sun. He returns home, feels a little feverish, has diarrhœa during the night, and in the morning feels well again. This depends on chill and fatigue, or unaccustomed exercise. On inquiry it will be found there has been exposure, when fatigued, to the evening fall of temperature, or to a dense shade, immediately after the skin has been acted upon by a powerful sun; or the person has been sitting in the wind when perspiring.

Diarrhœa may also arise from an atmosphere impregnated with emanations from foul drains and sewers. When a person is anæmic (*vide* p. 46), he or she is very liable to diarrhœa from such slight atmospheric causes, that a variety of diarrhœa occurring in anæmic subjects has been described as *anæmic diarrhœa.* Also, when persons are subject to mental anxiety and worry, diarrhœa is excited by such slight additional causes that another form has been described as *nervous or mental diarrhœa.* In any climate diarrhœa may be excited, in a weakly predisposed person especially, on exposure to vicissitude of temperature. This is probably more often the case in India, partly owing to the general tendency to bowel complaints in the East, partly to the anæmic or scorbutic taint from which so many suffer, partly owing to the mental strain to which so many Anglo-Indians are exposed, but chiefly owing to changes of temperature so readily inducing chill on a skin rendered excessively sensitive by heat.

*Treatment.*—Diarrhœa resulting from vicissitudes of temperature generally subsides spontaneously unless the person be otherwise in bad health, when it may be the prelude to dysentery. No kind of purgative medicine should be given for this kind of looseness, a dose of chlorodyne, or Recipe 38, being the better measure, with a mustard-leaf over the bowels, quiet, and fluid diet. But prevention is still more desirable, and this may be accomplished by caution in not sitting or sleeping in draughts, especially at the more changeable seasons of the year, by clothing in flannel, by wearing a flannel belt, and by taking a biscuit and a cup of hot tea or coffee before going out in the morning.

3. Hill Diarrhœa.—The prevalence of a peculiar species of diarrhœa at hill stations, and more especially at the Himalayan hill stations, has given rise to the name. But this peculiar diarrhœa, often called 'white diarrhœa,'

or 'sprue,' is not limited to hill stations, but often occurs on the plains, and is one of the worst forms of bowel complaint. The symptoms are peculiar, and consist at first of, often, *painless* diarrhœa, occurring chiefly in the early morning. The stools passed are light, sometimes white in colour, and generally copious and frothy. As the disease advances light stools are also passed in the evening, or soon after meals; but the patient, probably continuing to feel tolerably well, takes little notice of the commencement of the malady. The calls to stool, although unattended by pain, are urgent; but the fæces are passed without straining, faintness, or griping, and are succeeded by a feeling of comfort. The most distressing symptoms are fulness and distension of the bowels by *flatus*, eructations having an odour and taste of rotten egg, and other dyspeptic manifestations. But the stools are sometimes not offensive. The pulse is feeble, the tongue furred in the centre, but the appetite not much impaired. There is also slight sallowness. On inquiry the patient generally confesses to a feeling of uneasiness about the liver, which some describe as 'sense of void.' If this condition be not checked, the person falls into a state of confirmed weakness or *cachexia*. The stools become more numerous, emaciation takes place, the mind becomes weak and fretful, and fever occurs. Then, probably, the stools become dysenteric, containing slime and blood, and the patient dies exhausted.

*Causes.*—It has been attributed to malarious influences and to defective sanitation, and doubtless such conditions predispose to the malady. But the facts that *hill diarrhœa* is most prevalent about the period of the commencing monsoon, and that new arrivals at hill stations are more subject to it than older residents, favour the conclusion that sudden changes of temperature acting on the liver, and preventing the formation of bile, are the chief exciting causes. Persons arriving at hill stations are often attacked with more or less severe diarrhœa soon after ascending into the colder atmosphere of the mountain climate, and this especially if the wearing of warmer clothing has been neglected.

*Treatment.*—Too hot drinks must be interdicted, and the diet restricted to animal broths and farinaceous gruels or puddings, with a little port wine daily. A milk diet often suits well, the milk sometimes agreeing best after boiling (*vide* p. 194). Dover's powder combined with quinine and ipecacuanha (Recipe 17) should be administered every night. But if the ipecacuanha produces sickness, the quinine and Dover's powder may be given *alone.* Chlorodyne and Recipe 38 may be used alternately: the latter compound being not only agreeable, but often especially beneficial. Mustard poultices or leaves should be applied daily, or as often as can be borne, both on the right side over the liver, and also over the bowels. Special care must be taken to keep the bowels warm. But if diarrhœa and emaciation continue, or if the motions become dysenteric, that is, containing blood, immediate change of climate will alone effect a cure.

[Recipe 39 should be used, if obtainable, instead of 38. Other prescriptions for hill diarrhœa are Recipes 40, 47; the first being preferable when there is much acidity of the stomach. The flatulence, having a sulphuretted hydrogen or 'rotten-egg' taste, may be much relieved by a drop of carbolic acid, or of creosote taken on sugar. Should these measures fail after a fair trial of three days, give tincture of cannabis indica, 10 minims; subnitrate of bismuth, 10 grains; compound spirits of chloroform, 20 minims; water, 1 ounce, three times a day. Milk peptonised with Fairchild's peptonising powders should be used if milk as mentioned above does not suit. Valentine's meat juice is also recommended.]

Diarrhœa of any kind occurring in India, if long-continued, requires change of climate, which should be taken before the patient becomes greatly debilitated. A severe chronic diarrhœa requires at least two years in England, even if the person is apparently well soon after arrival, as the disease is very liable to return on re-entering the tropics.

**DIARRHŒA, INFANTILE.**—An infant's bowels should be relieved three or four times daily, and the motions should be of the colour of mustard, and free from fœtor or acid smell. The diarrhœa of children is most commonly caused in the order named, by atmospheric changes, damp and cold; by errors of diet; by undigested food, or accumulation in the bowels of hard fæcal material (*vide* p. 139); by teething; by worms; by tubercular disease of the bowels (*vide Atrophy*, p. 67), or it may come on during hooping-cough. The diarrhœa of children is often accompanied by vomiting, and is always attended with more or less flatulency, and frequently by griping, which is evidenced by the straining cry of the child, and by its legs being spasmodically raised up towards the bowels, when the pain occurs. *When the stools are a natural yellow colour, and there is no fœtor or feverishness,* the diarrhœa is probably caused by an accidental error of diet, or by atmospheric vicissitude, and it may be regarded as of comparatively little importance. *When the stools are yellow but becoming greenish after exposure,* it denotes a large secretion of bile, and there is still little cause for anxiety. *When they are green, or greenish yellow, with sour smell, and containing specks,* or flakes like bread crumbs, or larger masses, of white curdy material (which may be undigested milk, or mucus from the bowels), afterwards becoming green, there is much intestinal irritation and disorder present, and the diet is disagreeing with the child. In such cases curded material may be also vomited. *When the stools are white,* an inactive liver is denoted. *When diarrhœa of a watery character alternates with constipation,* the latter may probably be the primary cause of the mischief (*vide* p. 139). *When diarrhœa comes on suddenly, the stools consisting altogether of greenish-coloured water,* accompanied by much exhaustion, the condition resembles cholera. *When there is slime and streaks of blood,* the malady has passed into dysentery (*vide* p. 195).

In addition to the above phases of diarrhœa, the malady in children in India is very liable to excite an inflammatory condition of the intestines, to which state the term *muco-enteritis* has been applied. This is something more than diarrhœa, and something less than dysentery, although equally dangerous. The symptoms are fever, when the temperature may rise to 104°, thirst, quick pulse, tongue coated white with prominent red spots, skin dry, urine scanty. The stools are semi-fluid, often containing hard lumps, paler than natural, a quantity of whitish mucus, while the bowels are tender, and, if the child is old enough, burning pain is complained of. It is the fever, the white mucus, the tenderness, and the pain which separate the condition from ordinary diarrhœa; and it is the absence of blood in the stools which separates it from dysentery. There is generally much *flatus*. Also nausea, but vomiting is infrequent. In addition to the burning pain, there is griping and straining on passing motions. The child lies with cold feet, hot bowels, pinched face, and shrunken body, often maintaining a short feeble cry, and it is very liable to convulsions, especially if teething. Ultimately, if the termination is unfavourable, the tongue becomes dry, the pulse quicker, and the child dies exhausted. If blood appears in the stools, the probability of a fatal termination is increased.

*Treatment.*—As a rule, diarrhœa in children should not be too suddenly checked, particularly if the child is teething, when it is frequently a salutary effort of nature to relieve the irritation of the system thus excited. If the purging is moderate, the colour of the stools natural, and the motions semi-fluid, it will most usually subside without any medicine. But the diarrhœa of infants and children in India cannot safely be permitted to run on without treatment so long as would be warrantable in a temperate climate. Even the mildest form should not go untreated longer than twenty-four hours, for the rapid exhaustion of the vital powers of a child, caused by continued infantile diarrhœa, is a condition very favourable to the supervention of convulsions and other serious maladies.

The first thing to do is to look to the food, with the view of correcting any error of diet. In the case of infants, diarrhœa is often caused by improper feeding, or by overfeeding, or by some deleterious property of the milk, or by uncleanly feeding-bottles. Infants should not be nursed oftener than every two hours, and as the age advances the periods should be lengthened. If fresh milk is taken into the stomach while some of the last meal still remains, the result is generally either purging or vomiting. When the milk of the nurse is at fault, it will probably be due to improper diet or conduct of the woman, and this may require not only alteration in the food, but also the action of a purgative dose, and perhaps alteration of manner of life. If the milk is scanty or otherwise deteriorated, the nurse should be changed. If the child is hand-fed, the food of the animal from which milk is procured should be looked to (*vide Feeding of Infants,* Chapter V., *or Index*).

When medicines are necessary the best and safest treatment is to give at the onset (but not afterwards) half a tea-spoonful of castor-oil, or, if the child is a year old, a tea-spoonful. This will relieve the bowels of any irritating matter lodged there. If the purging continues, chlorodyne may be given in doses corresponding with the age of the child (*vide* p. 12). If the child is feverish at one time of the day and cool at another, the quinine and Dover's powder

(Recipe 18) may be used. If the breath or stools smell sour, lime-water (Recipe 25) should be used. If there is passage or vomiting of curded material, milk previously boiled should be tried. If the child still passes large, offensive, curdy stools the milk should be stopped and Liebig's raw-meat soup (*vide Addendum*), or, if not attainable, weak chicken broth, should be given for two or three days. Both in the diarrhœa and dysentery of children, especially if being brought up by hand, or who are partially fed by hand, such a change of food is often attended with much benefit whenever the motions show that milk is not being digested. When the milk is resumed it should be well diluted, and a dessert-spoonful of lime-water should be added to each meal. If there are *white* stools the purging will not cease until the liver acts, and podophyllin dissolved in brandy, as detailed at p. 142, may be given. If watery stools alternate with constipation the same treatment should be adopted. *Sudden diarrhœa* with copious, greenish, watery stools and great depression should be treated as cholera (*vide* p. 127). If the stools become slimy and bloody, the child must be treated for dysentery (*vide* p. 195).

If the malady assumes the condition described as *muco-enteritis* (p. 173), and there are any lumps passed in the stools, it will be desirable to give a dose of castor-oil with the view of dislodging irritating material, and which may be repeated next day if lumps are still passed. The bowels should also be well fomented daily. Quinine and Dover's powder (Recipe 18) should also be given. If milk is tolerated it is the best diet, but it is not always well borne. Milk and lime-water sometimes agree when milk alone does not. If sickness follows the milk, or if it passes away curdled, chicken broth, or Liebig's raw-meat soup, should be substituted, being given alternately. Curdled milk is to be distinguished from mucus in the stools by its less slimy and less jelly-like appearance. In this, as in all varieties of diarrhœa, the child should have very small quantities of food, but often. Less than a tea-spoonful every quarter-hour has been kept down when larger quantities were rejected. Children with this disease require stimulants at an early period, and a tea-spoonful of port wine in water may be given two or three times daily after the first day or two.

In all cases of diarrhœa in children flannel round the bowels is advisable. Also in all cases, while using the remedies prescribed, the condition of the gums should be frequently investigated. If the gums are full, red, and swollen at the *commencement* of the attack of diarrhœa, they should be lanced (*vide* p. 434), after which, probably, the succession of remedies noted above will not be required. If, in spite of medicines, the purging continues, and the gums become red and prominent *during* the persistence of the diarrhœa, they should be lanced at the most prominent or swollen part. If the child is discovered to have worms, it should be treated with santonin (*vide* p. 486), but without the oil mentioned at the reference.

[In violent cases, when the above remedies and care in diet do not prove efficacious, Recipe 49 should be procured for simple diarrhœa as first described. If there is acidity of the child's stomach, to be recognised by sour-smelling breath, Recipe 48 should be procured and given night and morning, with Recipe 22 three times a day. If there is much griping pain, the sulphuric acid and laudanum medicine (Recipe 45). When the feeding as recommended does not succeed, Kepler's Extract of Malt and Valentine's meat juice may be tried. And in cases where the breath is very sour, milk peptonised by Fairchild's powders, as it will not afterwards curdle from the acidity of the child's stomach.]

**DIARRHŒA, CHRONIC IN CHILDREN.**—The preceding refers to acute or sudden diarrhœa of infants. But the diarrhœa of children, especially if neglected, often becomes long-continued or *chronic*. Chronic diarrhœa may also arise at a later period from decayed first teeth and gumboils. The child swallows the fœtid discharge from the boils, and is unable to masticate food properly. There are five or six pale putty-like offensive motions daily, occasionally varied by watery discharge, while the child becomes thin, pale, and wastes. The temperature should be taken twice daily (*vide* p. 33). If the temperature is that of health, there is probably nothing serious the matter. If it is persistently above the standard of health, there will be cause for anxiety; and particularly so if this form of diarrhœa has succeeded some other illness, as scarlet fever or measles, when the commencement of tubercular deposit in the glands of the bowels may be feared (*vide Atrophy*, p. 67). The first indication of amendment is the appearance of bile in the motions.

Great attention must be paid to protection from damp and cold, to the ventilation of the sleeping apartment, and to careful regulation of the diet, as detailed at p. 174. If the child is taking other food than milk, or if weaned, potatoes, sweet biscuits, farinaceous foods generally, as arrowroot, sago and rice, also sugars and jams, should be interdicted. Bread and milk, a little fresh meat, green boiled vegetables, and custard, instead of pudding, may be allowed. The gums or teeth should be examined and attended to if necessary.

[Malt food, as Kepler's or Mellin's, should also be given. The great point, however, is to get the liver to act, and for this purpose podophyllin dissolved in brandy should be used (*vide* p. 142).]

**DIPHTHERIA.**—This dangerous complaint is sometimes called *leather throat*, from the appearances which this part presents; it has also been termed *drain throat*, from the malady being found frequently associated with defective drainage and sewage. Diphtheria often prevails in an epidemic manner—that is, it affects several persons in the same house or neighbourhood at the same time; and it then spreads by infection, or by the communication of the disease from one to another, in the manners afterwards indicated. But single cases of diphtheria frequently occur when, so far as can be ascertained, the person affected has not been exposed to infection. But, as the malady is not only communicable by direct contact, but also through the atmosphere, by means, as there is reason to believe, of minute specific microscopical germs rising from the diseased, it can never be said with certainty that infection could not have taken place.

The *causes predisposing* to diphtheria are childhood and youth, fatigue and exhaustion, and probably nervous excitability. But the poison itself is believed to be intimately connected with, if not to arise from, foul drains, sewage, or privies. Hence, in Europe especially, diphtheria is met with in houses having fixed wash-basins, and badly-trapped or ventilated water-closets, in immediate connection with nurseries and bedrooms. Such bad sanitary conditions, if not giving rise to diphtheria, often occasion sore throat, the cause of which is erroneously supposed to be cold; and the measures generally adopted against such presumed cause, by impeding ventilation, and allowing a minimum of fresh air, increase the evil. When diphtheria occurs in a house, if the children are living in good sanitary conditions it falls light; but if the reverse is the case, and especially if the drinking water happens to be contaminated from sewage or drains, the disease spreads with appalling rapidity and mortality.

It has also been shown that outbreaks of diphtheria among human beings have been preceded by the appearance of very similar symptoms among pigeons, fowls, turkeys, pheasants, sheep, pigs, and cats.

Diphtheria has been regarded as allied to scarlet fever in its nature, as these diseases often prevail at the same time or the former follows the latter. But diphtheria is more allied to croup, consisting, like the latter malady (*vide* p. 154), in the formation of a membranous substance in and over the parts about the throat, which are at first seen reddened and swollen, and afterwards covered with a white exudation, often extending to the tongue, palate, gums, to the inside of the cheeks, and to the air-passages. The exact nature of this deposit is not yet determined, although organisms have been detected in it by microscopic examination. However this may be, the *contagious principle* is believed to be associated only, or chiefly, with the peculiar deposit which forms on the throat and other parts; which, coming into accidental contact with a healthy mouth, may take root and spread. Thus the disease has been communicated by kissing, by transferring the feeding-bottle from a sick to a healthy child, and by drinking from the same cup used by the invalid. It has also been communicated to a surgeon who, having opened the windpipe of a patient, sucked the wound to prevent suffocation. It is also believed to have been conveyed from one house to another by a cat. There is also every reason to believe that the contagious principle is also given off in the breath of persons suffering from diphtheria; which may account for the fact of milk kept in the sick-room becoming so tainted by the vitiated air as to convey the disease. The contagious principle is likewise probably contained in the other excretions, as from the nose, or from the bowels. Thus, the disease may spread to any inmates of an infected house; but there is always much more danger in the case of those who are brought into close contact with a patient with diphtheria, who may inhale the breath of the patient, or who are liable to have the morbid products coughed out upon them (*vide* p. 186). It appears from experience that after exposure to infection the malady may come on in thirty-six hours, or be deferred as long as three weeks; but five or six days after exposure is the usual period; it further seems that a person may communicate the disease six weeks after convalescence.

*Symptoms.*—There are two principal varieties of diphtheria: *one*, in which the disease commences as a common sore throat, with some pain on swallowing. *A second*, in which, without any previous sore-throat, the person is suddenly attacked with shiverings and hoarseness, quickly followed by feelings of suffocation and croupy symptoms. *Ordinarily*, the first symptoms are great depression, chilliness, nausea, and occasionally diarrhœa. Then the throat begins to feel stiff, or tender, with some difficulty of swallowing, and probably swelling of the glands about the jaw, but not so much pain as when the affection extends to the nose and air-passages. At first accompanying the sore-throat there is merely redness of the parts; but in a variable time—from a few hours to two or three days—the characteristic exudation makes its appearance, accompanied by badly-smelling breath. This may commence at any spot where the redness has appeared, and generally does so on the tonsils, or on the back of the throat. At first only small whitish specks may be observed, which speedily extend and meet so as to form large patches, or even cover the entire surface. The thickness and colour of this deposit vary considerably in different cases. It is sometimes as soft as cream, at others almost as hard as wash-leather. The colour is usually white, grey, slightly yellow, or brownish, with a rosy-red border. If removed, a raw bleeding surface is left, which quickly becomes again covered with deposit. The exudation may spread over the mouth to the lips; it may penetrate the nose; or it may pass into the windpipe and air-passages, occasioning much increase of pain and difficulty of breathing. It has also been seen on the whites of the eyes, in the ears, and even in the female private parts, and in the lower gut (rectum). The glands about the neck, and especially near the ear, become more swollen and tender, adding much to the distress of the patient, and there is a thin, irritating discharge from the nostrils. When the disease has fully formed there is always hoarse or *husky* cough, great difficulty in swallowing, and fever. If the disease extends into the wind-pipe, known by croupy cough, increased difficulty of breathing, and threatening suffocation, the danger is great. Under such circumstances the only thing which can save or even relieve the patient is the spontaneous separation of some of the false membrane which impedes the respiration. This sometimes takes place, and one or more hollow tubular pieces of membrane several inches long, sometimes branched, may be coughed up. This a favourable sign, although if the disease is very severe, or the patient much weakened, recovery may not occur after it. Whenever the false membrane is spit or coughed out, the breath, previously smelling badly, often becomes horribly fœtid. Growing obstruction of breathing and lividity of face and lips point to a fatal termination. Hæmorrhage or bleeding from the mouth, nose, throat, or air-passages sometimes occurs, and this is a very unfavourable sign; as also are continuous vomiting, the appearance of erysipelas, or of erythema (*vide* pp. 220, 386); or of dark-coloured spots on any part of the body. During the progress of a case of diphtheria, the urine should be examined at least once daily for *albumen* (*vide* p. 101). If no albumen is found it is a favourable sign; and the reverse.

The above is the description of a severe and dangerous case of diphtheria. But sometimes the disease is much milder, and all the signs and symptoms are of less severity. The malady may decline, and the exudation separate, without extending to the mouth or air-passages. This separation may commence after two or three days, or the disease may be prolonged for a fortnight. *Secondly,* diphtheria may be characterised from the very commencement by great depression and debility. In such cases the face and skin generally assume a dirty yellowish tint, and the surface feels hot, although the temperature, as tested by the thermometer (*vide* p. 34) may not be very high. The pulse is frequent, small, weak, and irregular, and the heart's action is feeble. The tongue soon becomes dry and brown, and 'blacks' (*sordes*) form on the teeth; the general condition resembling the later stages of *typhoid* fever (*vide* p. 242). Or, *thirdly*, as previously mentioned, the disease may set in suddenly, the air-passages being first affected, with little or no sore-throat, the attack then very much resembling croup (*vide* p. 154), when it has been called *diphtheritic croup*.

Although diphtheria and croup are undoubtedly allied diseases, there are points of difference. A usual distinction is the formation of the membrane of diphtheria over the tonsils and in front of the windpipe, while in croup the membrane forms inside the windpipe. Diphtheria is contagious, and is therefore the local manifestation of a special organism, while croup is not contagious, being the local results of cold. Diphtheria is infectious, by direct contact of the expectoration of the sick with a healthy mucous surface, or by emanations from an affected person, as is evidenced by the manner in which it often spreads in a family. On the other hand, a child affected with croup lying in a confined room (as so often seen among the poorer classes) does not give it to other children, even although in the same apartment; while under such circumstances diphtheria spreads. Diphtheria often occurs to adults, croup seldom to adults. Diphtheria prevails at all seasons and during all kinds of weather—sometimes as an epidemic, and then often coincident with scarlet fever; but always more or less connected with, or influenced by, the effects of sewage emanations or imperfect drainage. Croup is most frequent during cold moist weather, especially during the prevalence of easterly or north-easterly winds.

Diphtheria is characterised by much swelling of the glands about the jaw, and much pain in swallowing, symptoms not usually accompanying croup. The 'husky' cough of diphtheria is not of the 'brassy' character of that of croup. In diphtheria albumen is generally found in the urine, in croup not. Diphtheria is often attended or followed by paralysis, croup not. Diphtheria may attack other parts, as the nose, mouth, and in females the privates, which croup never does. In one feature there is similarity—viz. the presence near or in the air-passages of the material formed in both diseases, giving rise to very similar symptoms, as regards the sound of voice, breathing, and suffocating paroxysms.

*Diphtheria* in the early stage may be mistaken for *scarlatina*, which often commences with throat affection, but the redness of the throat is not so bright and vivid as that of scarlet fever, while the early occurrence of white deposit on the throat, and the absence of rash on the second day, are distinguishing. (*Vide Scarlatina,* p. 375)

*Treatment.*—The patient should be put in a well-ventilated room free from draughts, and the temperature should be maintained equable, and the air moist, as mentioned under *Bronchitis* (p. 104). Complete quiet and rest should be observed, and, as there is often great prostration, the patient's strength must be stored from the first. Unfortunately there is no drug which can be looked upon as a specific, nor any means by which the disease can be cast off when it has once attacked an individual. But much may be done, even in severe cases, if the disease is recognised sufficiently early. In the first place, if it is found that the room or house is contaminated by defective sewage or drainage, the patient should, if possible, be removed. In the mildest form of diphtheria it is enough to protect the patient from cold; to open the bowels (Recipe 1, 2); to administer some saline, as citrate of magnesia (*vide* p. 15); to allow a good quantity of beef-tea and milk; and to employ such soothing local remedies in the form of fomentation, dry or wet (Recipes 80, 82), to the throat, as may afford most relief; with the very frequent use of alum gargle (Recipe 100), or, if available, *compressed tablets* of chlorate of potash may be sucked. In more severe cases the patient should also inhale the steam from hot water and vinegar three or four times daily, and strong alum solution (alum 3 drachms, water 1 ounce) should be applied to the inside of the throat every six hours, with a piece of stick to which a bit of lint or sponge has been firmly fixed, using fresh lint or sponge on every occasion. The solution should be thoroughly applied with a 'dabbing' motion to all the diseased portion of the throat which can be seen, but not so forcibly as to rub off the deposit, or cause bleeding. Or it may be introduced by means of an ordinary scent atomiser, if such an instrument is at hand. Or four or five grains of powdered alum may be blown into the throat from quills or a glass tube (long, to prevent infection), a method of application sometimes least irksome to the sick person. If the nose is affected, alum solution should be injected, or powdered alum sniffed into the nostrils. If old enough, the patient should also gargle frequently with Recipe 100. As medicine, quinine (Recipe 66) may be given every two hours. In severe cases, although beef-tea, chicken broth, milk diluted with a third part of lime-water (Recipe 25), and eggs may be used, almost *ad libitum*; no solid food should be allowed; and the patient must be fed slowly, as the act of swallowing is always difficult, and sometimes dangerous. In any case, if agreeable to the patient, ice may be given to suck. When diphtheria attacks an infant which is being suckled, the infant should be weaned, as the disease may be communicated to the woman's breasts. Weaning may be practised with the greater confidence, as probably the infant will not be able to continue to take the breast.

In the latter stages of the complaint, or in those cases showing great debility from the first, wine or brandy beaten up with eggs may be freely given, to the extent, for an adult, of a bottle of the first, or eight ounces of the latter, in the twenty-four hours. Good port wine and iced champagne are the most valuable. If a patient cannot or will not swallow, beef-tea, mixed with a little brandy, should be administered as injections; or, if practicable, *digested enemas* should be used (*vide Appendix, Injections*).

[If obtainable, instead of the strong alum solution mentioned above as an application to the inside of the throat, use a strong solution of nitrate of silver. Strength, 10 grains of nitrate of silver to 1 drachm of distilled water. Or, if an atomizer is at hand, use the following Recipe: Liquefied carbolic acid, 30 drops; chlorate of potassium, 3 drachms; glycerine, 3 ounces; distilled water, 5 ounces. Also give every two hours, alternately with the quinine mixture, the following Recipe: Tincture of iron, 2 drachms; chlorate of potassium, 1 drachm; distilled water, 8 ounces. Dose, for an adult, two table-spoonfuls. For children, according to table of proportions at p. 6.]

Diphtheria is a disease requiring skilled professional watching, and particularly so when the air-passages become affected. The question of the propriety of an operation—opening the windpipe or larynx—then presents. As such an operation almost always affords temporary relief and prolongation of life, and as cases do sometimes recover after operation, from an apparently almost hopeless state, it is generally considered advisable to afford the patient the chance. There are, however, conditions, such as extreme debility, or extensive implication of the lower parts of the air-passages, when an operation would not be advisable.

In all cases of illness, when diphtheria is prevalent, it is desirable to examine the throat, as occasionally, when there was no previous suspicion, a spot of diphtheritic deposit will be found. This should immediately be destroyed with strong solution of alum, or, if available, with nitrate of silver, which will very probably prevent the spread of the disease.

As soon as the patient can be moved with safety, change of air from the infected locality is most desirable. Convalescence is often slow, and may be retarded by the presence of *albuminuria* (*vide* p. 100), or by *inflammation of the lungs* (*vide* p. 325), or by *chorea* (*vide* p. 422), or by *paralysis* of different parts (*vide* p. 345). Sudden deaths have occurred after diphtheria, owing, as is supposed, to paralysis of the heart, happening in some yet unexplained manner, as the result of the disease. To guard against such sequelæ, avoidance of chill, generous diet, and good sanitary conditions must be enforced.

*All through the disease the greatest care must be taken to prevent infection, and the rules given in the Appendix under 'Disinfection' (vide also Index) regarding the disinfection of the apartment, of the utensils, of the clothing, of the discharges, and of the hands of attendants, should be scrupulously carried out. Attendants should studiously avoid inhaling the breath of, or the contact of the expectoration of, the patient with their own lips or mouth, as may accidentally occur. This risk may be greatly diminished by the attendants wearing a respirator, composed of a layer of cotton-wool between two folds of muslin: to be burned after use. Rags, which may be immediately burnt, should be used instead of pocket-handkerchiefs or towels. No article of food, especially milk, should be allowed to remain in the sick-chamber, as it may become contaminated, and so convey the disease.*

Experience has shown that the germs of the disease will sometimes cling with remarkable tenacity to a house or apartment in which a patient has suffered, even although every care has been taken to purify and cleanse. Numerous instances have occurred of persons suffering from diphtheria after occupying a room in which a patient had been ill many weeks, and in some cases months, previously. A fortnight at least should be devoted to sanitary measures and ventilation before a room is again occupied.

**DROPSY.**—Dropsy is generally not a disease *per se*, but is a consequence and symptom of other diseases. Dropsy consists of swelling caused by the escape of the watery portion of the blood through the coats of the veins into the surrounding tissues. This is produced by some impediment to the circulation of the blood causing stagnation of that fluid, as, for example, swelling, or in reality dropsy of the leg, may be caused by a tight ligature, as a garter, if allowed to remain sufficiently long. The most usual positions of dropsy are the lower extremities and the belly. The malady is recognised when external by the parts affected 'pitting' on pressure: that is, if pressed upon by the fingers depressions are left which gradually fill up.

Dropsy is generally connected with, and traceable to, one or other of the following conditions: Exposure to cold. Disease of the kidneys. Disease of the heart or lungs. Disease of the liver or spleen. Anæmia. Disorders of the *menses* or 'monthly flow' of females.

Dropsy from Exposure to Cold generally occurs suddenly, after exposure to cold and damp, or from sitting in a draught of cold air while the body is freely perspiring. The action of the skin is suddenly checked, and watery fluid becomes lodged in the loose tissues beneath, forming the condition known as *Anasarca.* Often also the *kidneys* are implicated, and the attack may be the prelude to *Bright's disease. Anasarca* may also occur after scarlet fever, during which malady the action of the skin is impeded. Should sudden general dropsy from cold or from checked perspiration present, the patient should be kept warm and should take Recipe 2, to act on the bowels and produce watery stools; Dover's powder in 5-grain doses three times in the twenty-four hours to act on the skin, and half-drachm doses of sweet spirits of nitre to increase the flow of urine. Warm baths will also be generally advisable. *Dropsy following scarlet fever* should be treated as recommended above, excepting that nitre should *not* be given.

Dropsy from Disease of the Kidneys begins generally in the loose structure of the eyelids and privates, the feet and legs quickly becoming affected.

Dropsy from Disease of the Heart or Lungs commences in the legs and arms, often at the same time, and gradually involves the whole body.

Dropsy from Liver or Spleen Disease first affects the belly, which swells, and may be felt to contain fluid, a condition called *ascites.*

Dropsy from Anæmia is rarely extensive, and does not affect the interior of the body. It is usually confined to the feet, ankles, and eyelids (*vide* p. 49).

Dropsy accompanying Disorders of the Menses is not indicative of dangerous disease, as are most other varieties, and is generally confined to the lower extremities, but may appear also in the hands and face, which become more swollen towards evening (*vide* p. 468).

Dropsy is therefore due in the great majority of instances to some organic internal disease, meaning thereby some disease involving change of structure in the parts implicated, and which sooner or later will prove fatal. The treatment of dropsy must therefore be that of those diseases of which it is a prominent symptom.

**DROPSY, OVARIAN.**—Ovarian dropsy is a different disease from the foregoing. It only occurs in the female sex, and consists in the gradual distension of the parts called the 'ovaries' by fluid. The 'ovaries' being situated on each side, rather above the female groins, the disease presents itself as a tumour or swelling on one or other side in that position. But if both ovaries are affected, the tumour appears central; or, in the later stages of the malady, one tumour extends over the whole of the bowels. The strength and general health of the patient remain long unimpaired, sometimes for years, until the bulk and pressure of the swelling on neighbouring parts bring on difficulty of breathing and swelling of the feet. In some cases there are periodical attacks of pain and tenderness in the tumour, and also cessation of the monthly discharges; but neither of these symptoms is constantly met with. For this malady no medicinal treatment is of any service. Wearing an elastic abdominal belt often affords much relief and support, but the only chance of cure is surgical operation.

**DRUNKEN FITS.**—When a person is in a drunken fit, or, as it is called, 'dead drunk,' there may be doubt as to the cause of the insensibility. Persons suffering from apoplexy have been frequently locked up as drunk, and the distinguishing features are given at p. 56. If a person is insensible from drink the following rules should be followed:—Place the patient on his *right side*, with head slightly raised. Do not allow him to lie on his back or on his face. Remove all constrictions about the neck and the upper part of the chest. Induce vomiting by tickling the throat with a feather. If able to swallow, give lukewarm water to drink. Apply a mustard poultice to the chest, and as soon as the patient begins to recover give some strong coffee. Unless taken in poisonous doses, the person will in a few hours sleep off the effects of the alcohol. But if taken in poisonous quantities, the condition nearly approaches to apoplexy, and the stomach-pump may be required.

**DYSENTERY.**—This disease is most prevalent in India and other tropical climates. A long-continued high temperature predisposes to the disease, which is often excited at the changing period from the hot weather into the damper season of the monsoon. The principal causes of dysentery are a tropical climate; exposure to sudden changes of atmosphere; imprudent change of clothing, particularly of that worn over the bowels; drinking water containing mineral or vegetable impurities; irregularities in diet; famine and want; lying on the damp ground; residence in ill-ventilated, imperfectly-drained, and badly-located habitations; and a scorbutic condition of the system from the want of fresh vegetables. Many also believe that exposure to malaria will excite dysentery. Pregnant women in India are especially liable to dysentery, which generally causes miscarriage.

The first *symptoms* of dysentery are feelings of griping about the navel, often accompanied by nausea. Very frequently this is first felt after incautious exposure to night air, particularly during sleep, and more especially if the wind has been suffered to play on the bowels, even if well covered. Next there are irregular loose discharges from the bowels, which may continue one, two, or three days, forming the *premonitory diarrhœa* of dysentery. Then the irregular griping pains gradually become cutting and shooting, with great heat about the fundament, and frequent straining and purging. Matters now voided consist of liquid fæces streaked or mixed with white mucus and blood. As the disease becomes more severe, shreds or large flakes resembling the washings of raw meat often pass away, and the stools have a peculiarly offensive odour. The desire to stool is generally most urgent during the night; in some instances it is incessant, in others there may be ten or twenty calls in the twenty-four hours. There is frequent desire to make water. The amount of attending fever is variable, in some instances hardly exciting attention, in others evidenced by a flushed face, dry skin, hard quick pulse, and furred tongue. Pressure over the bowel is painful, although the parts are not so tender as when inflammation of the bowels is present. Absence of pain or tenderness of the bowels, and slimy bloody stools unmixed with fæcal matter, indicate that the lowest part of the intestines (the rectum) is chiefly implicated. A cadaverous smell, anxiety of countenance, feeble pulse, hiccough, and involuntary motions pronounce the case hopeless.

In every case of dysentery there is danger of the liver becoming affected, and of liver abscess forming as a secondary consequence of the dysentery. This renders every case more serious, and shows the necessity of prompt, careful, and efficacious remedial measures.

*Treatment.*—In the mildest form of the affection, when griping pains are complained of at intervals, followed or accompanied by the discharge of slightly bloody or slimy stools, fomentations or the turpentine stupe (Recipes 80 and 108), rest in the horizontal posture, and 5 grains of Dover's powder three times a day will frequently effect a cure. The diet should be of the plainest description, consisting of broths and farinaceous gruels without any solid material.

In the more acute forms of dysentery, when the calls to stool are frequent, the pain cutting, the abdomen tender, and the patient feverish, give immediately 40 drops of chlorodyne in a table-spoonful of water; then, if the patient is not a pregnant female, fifteen or twenty minutes afterwards give 30 grains of powdered ipecacuanha in a wine-glassful of water, and then apply a mustard poultice over the pit of the stomach (not the bowels) for twenty minutes. The patient should lie down and remain perfectly quiet, and refrain from drinking, but if thirsty he may suck ice. This treatment will probably cause great nausea and depression; but the after-result is usually free action of the skin, subsidence of griping, and re-appearance of natural stools. Often one dose of ipecacuanha checks the disease. But if it returns, and if vomiting did not occur in a very violent manner from the ipecacuanha, and if the person was not long or greatly depressed, the same medicines should be again given in about eight hours afterwards, and repeated at such intervals during three days, care being taken to allow of a sufficient time between the doses to admit of the patient taking and digesting some fluid nourishment. But the vomiting and depression produced by the large doses of ipecacuanha are sometimes so great that the treatment cannot be continued. In such cases, or when, as sometimes happens, ipecacuanha administered as above fails to prove beneficial, it will be advisable to give 1 grain of ipecacuanha, 5 of Dover's powder, and 3 of quinine every four hours; the quinine being especially required if the patient has been in a malarious district, or if there is accompanying fever of the intermittent or remittent form (*vide* pp. 252, 258). It will also be desirable to use soap-and-water injections twice daily (Recipe 104), in which 30 grains of ipecacuanha powder should be placed, when the medicine is not well borne by the mouth.

*If the patient is a pregnant female*, and especially if also weak, in the absence of medical advice, the treatment by large doses of ipecacuanha is *not* recommended, as vomiting if so excited may bring on miscarriage. The treatment last mentioned is preferable.

In all cases of dysentery the recumbent posture should be insisted upon, and the patient should be instructed to give way as little as possible to the frequent inclinations to stool. In any case it will always be right to apply warm applications to the bowels, as fomentations, hot bran, linseed meal, or rice-flour poultices. The patient should be kept in a well-ventilated apartment. When stools are passed they should be *removed immediately*, and some disinfecting agent should be placed in the pan and also used in the room (*vide Appendix*, No. 126). The food should invariably be of the simplest kind, as good broth or beef-tea (without pepper, which may irritate the bowels), Valentine's meat juice, sago, corn-flour, arrowroot, milk and jellies. If the accompanying fever is slight, a small quantity of port wine and water may be allowed. Soda-water or pure plain water may be given in moderation, but neither drink nor food should be given iced, or even quite cold.

During recovery the appetite often increases before the digestive organs recover their tone; therefore caution must be used, so that not more than a very moderate quantity of food is taken, or a severe relapse may be the consequence.

[If the measures recommended are not successful after four days, pills composed of ipecacuanha, blue pill, and opium (Recipe 24) should be procured, one of which should be given every three hours. The pills should be continued until a metallic taste or slight soreness of the gums is experienced, when they should be stopped, and Dover's powder, quinine, and ipecacuanha, as recommended in the large type, given instead. The unnecessary use of blue pill should, however, be avoided. It is only advised on the failure of other measures as above noted. Laudanum should also be procured, 30 drops of which should be added to each warm-water injection, recommended in the large type. A good medicinal tonic during convalescence is Recipe 69.]

**DYSENTERY, CHRONIC.**—Chronic dysentery may commence as such; that is, a minor degree of dysentery than that described above may occur, and, without assuming any violent form, destroy the health of the patient. But chronic dysentery more frequently results as a sequel of the acute form. It often happens after a severe attack of dysentery that tenderness remains in some parts of the bowels, while the stools are occasionally slimy and bloody, alternating with constipation for a day or so; and there is considerable and increasing debility, with perhaps a tender scorbutic condition of the gums. Under such circumstances, the repeated application of mustard poultices or mustard leaves over the tender part is advisable. The bowels should be regulated by small doses of castor oil, constipation being strictly guarded against. When the bowels are *not* constipated, astringent medicines of various descriptions should be employed. In the absence of the remedies mentioned in the small type below, Recipe 17 may be taken at night, and Recipe 42 three times a day. If the ipecacuanha in Recipe 17 causes too much nausea or sickness, it may be omitted. If there is *alternate* looseness and constipation, it will be better to trust to diet and castor-oil, and not to take astringents; but in any case, both the decoction and syrup of the Indian bael fruit (*vide* p. 22) may always be tried, as the bael possesses both astringent and slightly aperient properties. Or, the bael not proving efficacious, decoction of pomegranate may be used, made with either milk or water (*vide* p. 26). If the patient has been in a locality where fresh vegetables were scarce, he should have lime-juice or pulp of fresh grapes daily, even although no indications of scurvy are apparent. During chronic dysentery it is necessary to examine the gums frequently, and if they are found tender, spongy, swollen, or inclined to bleed, thus showing evidence of a scorbutic taint in the system, lime-juice is still more necessary (*vide Scurvy*, p. 380). This should not be neglected, scurvy with dysentery being a serious complication.

It must be noted that chronic dysentery is frequently associated with *piles*, and in some cases appears to commence from piles. When blood and mucus *follow* a discharge of fæcal matters, the existence of piles is indicated; but it is often difficult to distinguish how much of the distress is to be attributed to the one condition, and how much to the other. If piles are present they must be treated (*vide* p. 347).

In all cases of chronic dysentery a flannel belt should be worn round the bowels, and the feet kept warm by woollen socks. The diet should consist chiefly of soup, broth, rice, sago, arrowroot, or flour and milk well boiled together, seasoned with sugar and spice. Generally a little port wine may also be allowed.

In bad cases a milk diet should be tried. Milk should be taken frequently in small quantities. If quickly swallowed in large quantities it forms a curdled mass in the stomach, difficult of digestion. By taking one and a half ounce of milk every hour during the day and night, one quart would be consumed. At first it is advisable to take one quart, or even less *per diem*, gradually increasing the quantity to two or three quarts in the twenty-four hours. Not, of course, being roused from sleep to take milk, but taking some in the night if awake. But even the small quantity first mentioned should not be swallowed at once, but should be sipped very gradually. Tepid milk usually agrees best, and it is advisable that it should be previously boiled. If milk given alone does not agree, it may be tried mixed with one third of lime-water (Recipe 25); or it may be peptonised. To satisfy the patient a little good bread or sago may also be occasionally given, and exceptionally a little broth, or raw-meat tea. But the less of anything besides milk which is taken the more likely is the treatment to be successful. At first the patient may probably complain of not being able to take or digest the milk, or even of feeling weaker. But, as a rule, if he perseveres he will gradually gain strength and freedom from dysentery.

[Other astringent prescriptions for chronic dysentery are Recipes 46 and 47; the first most useful if scorbutic taint exists. When there is much pain, and numerous motions, the pill as below may be used night and morning. Quinine, three grains; hydrochlorate of morphia, one quarter of a grain; to be well mixed and made into a pill with a little gum arabic.

Many cases of dysentery are, however, little benefited by medicines. If a patient with chronic dysentery is living in a malarious country, then probably no treatment will prove of benefit until he is removed from the influence of such an atmosphere. In such cases a thorough and prolonged change of climate, as to Europe, affords the best chance of recovery. But under such circumstances great care must be taken to escape cold and chill, while imprudence in diet must be strictly avoided. A voyage on the Indian seas, as sometimes recommended, is not likely to benefit a person with confirmed chronic dysentery. When it is recollected that a person transported to Europe may be years before thoroughly recovering, and that he may be subject to aggravation from the slightest imprudence in diet, or from the slightest exposure or fatigue, it is evident that sea voyages in the tropics are not calculated to cure a malady for which rest, quiet, well-ventilated sleeping apartments, good sick-cookery, and freedom from exposure to vicissitudes of temperature, are essential.]

**DYSENTERY IN CHILDREN** may occur suddenly, without any previous warning, or it may be a sequel to diarrhœa (*vide* p. 173). It often happens that an infant has been suffering from diarrhœa for several days, passing green motions, or motions like frog spawn, when a sudden change occurs. The griping increases, there is great straining, and mucus and blood are found in the stools. The diarrhœa has passed into dysentery, and the character of the case is more serious. However commencing, dysentery in children is marked by the same symptoms, as the passing of mucus, slime, and blood, and by the pain and straining characterising the affection in adults. From the commencement some degree of fever generally prevails. *If constipation has preceded the attack*, it will be best to commence the treatment with a small dose of castor-oil; *but if the child has not been previously costive*, no laxative medicine should be given. If constipation has previously prevailed, temporary relief will follow the castor-oil, which is the time to commence the specific treatment. But as children do not usually bear large doses of ipecacuanha well by the mouth, the following treatment is recommended. If the child is not more than six months old, a quarter of a grain of ipecacuanha powder should be given every three or four hours. If the child is more than six months old, 1 grain of ipecacuanha may be given; if more than one year old, 2 grains. At the same time, in severe cases, if the child is more than six months old, 5 grains of ipecacuanha powder; and if more than one year old, 10 grains of the powder, mixed with an ounce of thin *congée*, should be used as an injection. (*For the manner of giving injections, vide Appendix.*) An endeavour should be made to retain the injection by pressure with a napkin for ten minutes or longer, until the child seems quiet and unlikely to void it. If the symptoms persist after two days, Dover's powder should be given night and morning in the proportion of 1 grain for a child above six months old, and 1½ grain for a child above one year old, increasing the dose by a quarter of a grain for each year of age. Warm linseed-meal or bran poultices, or, if available, spongio-piline warmed with hot water, or the india-rubber hot-water bag (*vide Appendix* No. 80), should be frequently applied to the bowels, and during the intervals the bowels should be kept warm by a flannel binder. If the child has much straining, starch injection may be used (Recipe 104). If the teeth are causing irritation, the gums must be lanced; and if worms are present, santonin (*vide* p. 486) may be given, but without any purgative. If the infant is suckling, change of the nurse may perhaps be advisable; or, this not being practicable, or if the infant is being fed by hand, raw-meat soup, or weak chicken broth, may be substituted, as recommended for *diarrhœa* (*vide* p. 175). For older children the food should consist of sago, arrowroot, bread and milk, chicken or mutton broth, and tea. The bael fruit is sometimes beneficial in obstinate cases. The dose of the decoction of bael made as detailed at p. 22 is a teaspoonful for a child one year old; of the syrup of bael made as there mentioned, a little less. When the stools become more natural, 2-, 3-, or 4-minim doses of chlorodyne, according to the age of the child (*vide* p. 12), may be substituted for other medicines, to moderate any remaining looseness. When this ceases 1- or 2-grain doses of quinine will be desirable for some days. Great care should be taken for some time to examine the stools of the child, in order to discover if undigested morsels of food pass; and if so, the diet should be altered.

[The above means not proving successful, Recipes 48 and 49 should be obtained and tried in succession; the first being most useful if there is acidity of the stomach.]

**DYSPEPSIA**, in one or other of its numerous forms, is very common in India, sometimes occurring as a simple dyspepsia unconnected with any other malady; at other times as the result of temporary impediment in the action of the stomach, liver, or bowels; at other times the consequence of permanent disease of these or other organs.

Dyspepsia is, therefore, in various instances a symptom of other maladies, and not the primary disease.

Before dyspepsia can be properly understood it is necessary to have some idea of the progress of digestion and of the organs concerned, and the accompanying woodcut shows the latter.

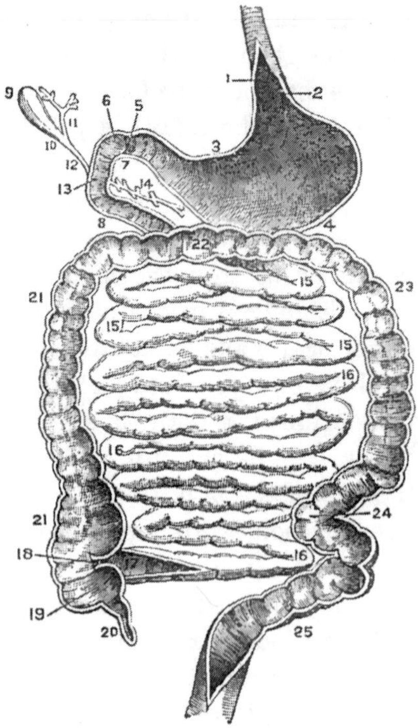


DIAGRAM OF THE DIGESTIVE TUBE

1. The Gullet.
2. The Upper or Cardiac Orifice, or Entrance to the Stomach.
3, 4. The Upper and Lower Borders of the Stomach.
5. The Lower or Pyloric Orifice, or Outlet from the Stomach.
6, 7, 8. The Upper, Middle, and Lower Portions of the Duodenum.
9. Gall Bladder.
10. Bile Duct leading to the Gall Bladder.
11. Bile Duct leading from the Liver.
12. Common Duct, formed by junction of two preceding.
13. Its aperture in the Duodenum.
14. Duct of the Pancreas, opening into the Duodenum close to where the Bile Duct opens.
15, 15, 15. Jejunum } small Intestines.
16, 16, 16. Ileum }
17. Ileum opening into Great Intestine.
18. Ileo-cæcal Valve.
19. Cæcum.
20. Vermiform Appendix.
21, 21. Ascending Colon.
22. Transverse Colon.
23. Descending Colon.
24. Sigmoid Flexure of Colon.
25. Rectum.

The following is a brief *résumé* of the process of digestion :—

Food is masticated by the teeth, and mixed with the saliva, which has the power of converting starch into sugar. The food is then conveyed by swallowing through the gullet into the stomach, where it is brought into contact with the gastric juice. This gastric juice, secreted by the coats of the stomach, is composed of pepsin and acid, and it possesses the power of acting on nitrogenous food, such as flesh, fish, eggs, cheese, butter, wheat, flour, &c. The mass of food is also exposed to a mechanical action by the stomach alternately contracting and expanding. Certain chemical action also takes place. By these means the food is converted into a pulpy mass called *chyme*, which, by the contraction of the stomach, is pressed through its *pyloric* orifice into the next part of the intestinal tube, known as the *duodenum*. Should indigestible food be present, it either causes the stomach to reverse its action, when vomiting ensues, or, overcoming the obstruction the *duodenum* presents to the passage of undigested morsels, it slips into the bowels and becomes a source of future irritation. The *chyme*, while passing through the *duodenum*, now becomes mixed with bile from the liver, and with pancreatic juice from the pancreas, the ducts from both of which organs open into the *duodenum*. The bile has the property of assisting generally in the digestion of food, of preventing fermentative changes, and it also acts as a natural aperient. The pancreatic juice has the property of disposing of fatty matters. After being exposed to the action of the bile and pancreatic juice, the food or *chyme* becomes changed in appearance and characteristics, receiving the name of *chyle*. It now commences its passage through the remaining 24 feet of the intestinal tube. In the small intestines it meets with secretions from the glands they are furnished with, by which the process of digestion is completed. As the process is completed the *chyle* is taken up (or absorbed) by the microscopical mouths of numerous small vessels spread on the surface of the bowels and known as *lacteals*. These converge, forming the *thoracic duct*, which, running in front of the spine, opens into the subclavian vein, where the chyle mingles with the blood. Watery matters, or substances soluble in water, are, however, absorbed directly into the blood by the blood-vessels of the stomach and intestines. Thus while passing through the small intestines the digestion of the food is completed, and all fit for the wants of the body is absorbed from the intestines into the system. In the healthy state no fermentation takes place in either the stomach or small intestines. The food which escapes digestion and absorption, or which is unfit for absorption, together with such items as pieces of bone, husks, woody fibres of vegetables, &c., now passes through the cæcal valve into the large intestines or colon. Here it meets with fæcal matter thrown out by the minute glands of the colon. This excretion is characterised by disagreeable, but not necessarily putrid, odours and gases, and consists of material removed in the renovation of the body. From the colon the fæcal matter passes into the rectum to await expulsion from the body.

DYSPEPSIA is best considered under the heads *Accidental or Temporary*, and *Habitual or Permanent* dyspepsia.

ACCIDENTAL OR TEMPORARY DYSPEPSIA is generally caused by errors in diet, as when some irritating, over-rich or 'high' material is taken. It may occur from eating hurriedly. Also from exposure to chill, from unaccustomed exertion, such as riding in a rough vehicle, from bathing, or from severe mental exertion immediately after a full meal.

*Symptoms.*—Accidental dyspepsia may be of the most trivial character, or more severe. In its milder form it is characterised by sores on the tongue or in the mouth, or by flushing of the face (*vide* p. 274); or by flatulence (*vide* p. 273), or by slight eructations after meals, sometimes tasteless, at others having the taste or odour of the food taken; or by acidity (*vide* p. 45); or by slight headache; and perhaps by a little diarrhœa, when all is well again. There may also be heartburn (*vide* p. 299). But an attack of accidental dyspepsia may be accompanied by giddiness, faintness, nausea, vomiting first of the contents of the stomach, and then of sour, bilious material, with constipation in the first instance, succeeded by desire to stool. Or there may be an attack of colic (*vide* p. 131). Sometimes there is a sudden eruption of nettle-rash (*vide* p. 387). Or accidental dyspepsia, instead of causing any of the symptoms yet noted, may result in sick-headache (*vide* p. 291).

*Treatment.*—The treatment of the symptoms first mentioned, viz., sores of the tongue and mouth, flushings, flatulence, acidity, heartburn, are mentioned under such headings. When there is giddiness, nausea, or vomiting, an emetic of mustard-water (Recipe 54) usually affords relief. When nettle-rash, colic, or sick-headache occurs, the treatment given under those heads should be adopted.

HABITUAL OR PERMANENT DYSPEPSIA results from different causes to those producing *accidental or temporary dyspepsia*, although the causes of the latter will aggravate habitual dyspepsia. Habitual dyspepsia is not, like accidental dyspepsia, the consequence of occasional errors of diet, or of other occasional causes which have been named. Habitual dyspepsia is either the result of constitutional weak digestion, or, more frequently, the result of a continued course of high and improper living, especially if accompanied by sedentary occupations, or by sitting on low chairs, which compresses the bowels, and causes indigestion. Neglect of exercise, stooping when employed, ill-ventilated or crowded sleeping-rooms, or impure atmosphere from any cause, excite indigestion. Overstrain of the mental faculties is a fertile cause of habitual dyspepsia. Idleness, or want of a definite purpose in life, also induces it. Excessive smoking may be the cause. Costiveness is both a cause and a result. Bad teeth, rendering the person unable to masticate his food thoroughly, is a frequent cause. Fœtid secretions from bad teeth or gumboils also interferes with digestion. Tight-lacing, which interferes with the action of the liver, stomach, and bowels, often renders digestion little better than a meaningless term. In females habitual dyspepsia is often an accompaniment of womb affections (*vide* p. 467). Habitual dyspepsia may also arise from worms (*vide* p. 482). Climate also affects dyspeptics, especially when changes occur suddenly. Prolonged residence in a tropical climate causes the digestive organs to participate in the generally anæmic condition of the system induced by heat.

*Symptoms of Habitual Dyspepsia.*—In habitual dyspepsia the stomach, liver, and bowels are the organs chiefly in fault. There are typical cases when the symptoms are plainly referable to one or the other of these organs. But as a general rule they are all implicated, and the symptoms which arise denote defective action of all three.

The stomach secretes an acid fluid called gastric juice (*vide* p. 199), which is the principal agent in that part of digestion which takes place in the stomach. When the coat of the stomach is continually irritated by improper food, this gastric juice may be increased, or diminished, or altered in quality, giving rise to the generation of acids and to acidity, or so-called *acid dyspepsia*. The symptoms of a minor degree of stomach or acid dyspepsia are sufficiently noted under *Acidity* (p. 45). There may also be 'stomach cough,' generally due to an enlarged *uvula* (*vide* p. 444), and vomiting of tough mucus in the early morning. At first there is often a feeling as if the stomach were not large enough for a meal, or as if there were something heavy in it. The nerves of the stomach becoming more sensitive, there is pain of a tearing, dragging, gnawing, or burning character, somewhat temporarily relieved by taking food, for which there is often a craving with thirst. This craving induces people to eat and drink too much, for which they afterwards suffer. There may also be throbbing and tenderness at the pit of the stomach. Shooting pains towards back and shoulders may also be felt, leading persons to imagine the liver diseased. Or pain in the chest, with palpitation and irregular pulse, gives rise to fear of heart disease. The urine often feels hot when passed, becomes thick and cloudy, and deposits red gravel. There is also a loss of nervous or vital power, which leads to diminution of the contractile movements of the stomach necessary for the proper digestion of food. There is also necessarily derangement of the purely chemical processes through which food must pass in the stomach. All these various conditions lead to *slow stomach digestion*, so that the food remaining in the stomach begins to ferment, when eructations having the flavour of rotten egg occur. There is then not only a gnawing pain, somewhat relieved by taking food, but also weight and distension in the stomach some time after taking food, caused by undigested food remaining in the stomach. Then there may be vomiting of this half-digested food, or if not actually vomited it rises into the throat. As a further consequence food finds its way into the intestines without having undergone the full process of stomach digestion. Here it acts as a direct irritant to the intestines, which in their turn resent its presence by altered secretions, and the process of intestinal digestion is not properly performed. Instead of digesting, the food ferments, which causes the formation of various acids and gases, giving rise to much discomfort *after* taking food, to distension of the bowels, to eructations of rotten-egg flavour, to colicky pains, to rumbling and twisting about the navel, and sometimes to irritative diarrhœa (*vide* p. 167). In this form of dyspepsia, diarrhœa is often excited by food, the person having to leave the table for the purpose of nature. Other symptoms are clamminess of the mouth, congested or sore throat, pains in different parts of the body, and weariness. The tongue is red at the tip and edges, with a foul streak in the middle; or if from bad teeth the person eats on one side of the mouth, the foul streak will be more evident on the opposite side. The urine often presents an iridescent film on the surface and deposit sediment.

The stomach and bowels cannot be thus affected without the liver becoming implicated, especially if the original cause is prolonged high and improper living. The bile-duct, which opens into that part of the intestines called the duodenum (*vide* p. 198), partakes of the general irritation and congestion, which passes up the short duct into the liver. The result is alteration in the secretion of bile, which is sometimes deficient and sometimes in excess. As bile is the natural aperient, when it is deficient the bowels become torpid and constipation occurs, while the stools passed are light-coloured. But if bile is secreted in excess, it causes diarrhœa of a bilious character, with griping pain and burning at the fundament; thus adding to the irritative diarrhœa which may be caused, as already mentioned (*vide* p. 203), by partially digested food. Also, as bile exercises an anti-fermentative power, its deficiency leads to increase of fermentation of food, and hence to more *flatus* and colicky pains. Lastly, as bile acts generally in the promotion of digestion, any alteration in its quality or quantity renders the food unfit for absorption from the intestines, and hence to weakness and debility of the person. When the liver is thus implicated there is usually a sallow appearance, due to the retention of the elements of bile in the blood. When dyspepsia of this description becomes very confirmed, the glands at the back of the tongue become enlarged, looking like small warts.

*The symptoms of habitual dyspepsia* occurring in weakly persons differ somewhat, and have been described as *flatulent* or *atonic* dyspepsia. Flatulence, as already noted, is an ordinary symptom of dyspepsia, but it is sometimes the principal symptom, especially in weakly, badly fed females. The subject of flatulent or atonic dyspepsia is usually nervous, often impressed with the existence of some serious malady, and may become hypochondriacal. If a female, she generally complains of pain in the left side. The urine is usually acid, and may deposit dumb-bell crystals (*vide Oxaluria*, p. 341).

Occasional symptoms occur which have not yet been noted. One is 'water-brash' or *pyrosis*, which is frequently seen as an accompaniment of flatulent or atonic dyspepsia. The affection is characterised by a burning sensation at the pit of the stomach, and a sense of constriction, as if the stomach were drawn towards the back, followed by the eructation of a quantity of thin watery fluid, which is frequently tasteless, but sometimes intensely sour, and often described by the patient as being cold. It occurs in paroxysms, which usually come on when the stomach is empty. After the discharge of the fluid the pain lessens and gradually disappears. *Water-brash* seems to be due in a great measure to indigestible food; but there is reason to believe that when it forms a symptom of stomach dyspepsia, it is an effort of nature to dilute and overcome the acidity of that organ.

Other occasional symptoms of dyspepsia are eruptions on the lips (*vide Herpes*, p. 395); inflamed eyelids or stye (p. 222); sudden agonising pain or cramps in the stomach; a trembling sensation commencing at the stomach and passing over the whole body; a feeling that one or several limbs are of an enormous size; 'fidgets,' or an uncontrollable tendency to shake the lower limbs; palpitation of the heart, or attacks resembling *angina pectoris* (p. 298). Dyspepsia is also intimately connected with various other maladies, the principal of which are gout, asthma, constipation, gravel, diabetes.

*Treatment.*—The treatment of dyspepsia is more *dietetic and hygienic* than medicinal. The quantity of food which can be dissolved by the secretions of the stomach and intestines being limited, this quantity cannot be exceeded with impunity, and moderation is therefore the first principle. Persons affected with indigestion should eat slowly. The meals should not succeed too rapidly. The stomach should have time to perform one task before another is imposed on it. Six hours may be mentioned as an appropriate time which should intervene between any two meals. Nothing should be taken between meals. No great or prolonged exertion, either mental or physical, should be undertaken immediately before or after food. The food best suited for dyspeptics is a mixture of well-cooked animal and vegetable food, which is more easily digested than a large proportion of either kind, or than one or the other taken exclusively. Often it is desirable to avoid potatoes, puddings, pastry, sweetmeats, fruit, sugar, and even bread if not toasted. It is well known how readily sugar, and food containing sugar or starch, run into fermentation, and it should never be lost sight of that sugar taken with food or drink furnishes most of the acidity and gases developed. Saccharin may be usefully substituted for sugar, particularly when acid flatulence is present, as saccharin does not contain the objectionable principles of sugar, while it exerts a certain antiputrefactive power. In most cases, dyspeptic persons would do well to avoid all stimulating drinks, although in some instances a little cold weak brandy-and-water, or a glass of sound sherry, or a little ale, may be taken with advantage. Large draughts of tea or other fluids are not advisable for dyspeptics; although in certain instances of what is called 'a fit of indigestion,' when some article taken will not pass through the stomach, and induces nausea and sickness, a draught of water or tea may often relieve the uneasiness. Draughts of very cold or iced water, as so frequently indulged in in India, are prolific causes of dyspeptic derangements, and so is the immoderate use of tobacco. But on all points of eating and drinking a sensible patient will be influenced by his own experience. In most varieties of dyspepsia 'drugging' should be avoided. Care, caution, and self-denial are better for dyspeptics than medicines; and each person should be aware, better than the physician can advise, what particular articles of diet will agree or will not agree with him. No diet table can be given to suit all dyspeptics, the likes, dislikes, and idiosyncracies (*vide* p. 7) of persons being so numerous. The most that can be done is to indicate what articles of food are most digestible as below.

*Animal Food.*—The flesh of young animals, although more tender than that of older animals, is not so easily digested. The flesh of older animals is neither tender nor digestible. Mutton and beef are more digestible than lamb and veal. Mutton is the most digestible flesh of mammals, pork the most indigestible. Ham and bacon are more digestible than pork. Venison, hare, and rabbit are fairly digestible. The liver, kidney, and heart of animals are all indigestible. Tripe, sweetbread, calf's fry, are digestible if not richly cooked. Cheese is indigestible. *The flesh of birds* is more digestible than that of mammals, chicken, fowl, and game being the most digestible; turkey, duck, and goose the least. Eggs lightly boiled are digestible, but not when hard-boiled. *Of fish*, whiting, sole, and pomphres are the most digestible; herring, eel, and mackerel less so; red fish least of all. Shell fish, as lobsters, crabs, prawns, shrimps, mussels, are all indigestible, the oyster being an exception. *Of vegetable food* good bread and plain biscuits, if not too new, are easily digested, and so are dry crisp toast, rusks, and tops and bottoms. Hot buttered articles are indigestible. Cooked vegetables are more digestible than green. Fruits to be digestible must be well ripened and soft naturally, or as the results of cooking. Semolina is more digestible than macaroni or vermicelli. Sago, tapioca, and arrowroot when cooked are readily digested. Asparagus, cauliflower, sea kale, tomatos, and vegetable marrow are digestible, spinach and cabbage less so. Beans, French beans, and peas are not easy to digest unless boiled a long time. Artichokes, turnips, carrots, beet-root, radishes, celery, lettuce, endive, mustard and cress, cucumber, and mushrooms, are all more or less indigestible.

The *hygienic* treatment of dyspepsia consists in preventing the pores of the skin being choked, by the use of soap baths and brushes; in taking exercise short of fatigue, but not before breakfast, especially the early breakfast of Indian life; in avoiding mental strain; in sleeping on a hair mattress with covering only sufficient to ensure proper warmth and to prevent chill; lastly, in change of climate for confirmed dyspeptics.

[With such care in diet and hygiene as indicated above, prominent symptoms may be best relieved as below. Acidity should be treated as given at p. 45. When *heartburn* is the prominent symptom, 10 grains of bicarbonate of soda, or 10 grains of prepared chalk, in a table-spoonful of water, will afford relief. Or 'compressed soda-mint tablets' may be used. There is no better remedy for *flatulence* than peppermint water; or, if flatulence is combined with pain, a tea-spoonful of sal volatile in a wineglass of camphor mixture. If the flatulence is accompanied by a 'rotten-egg' flavour, charcoal biscuits may be eaten, or a drop of creosote or of carbolic acid may be taken on sugar. *Loss of appetite* may be remedied by bitters, such as quinine, or mineral acids, or both combined (Recipes 34 and 60). *For females suffering from dyspepsia with loss of appetite*, debility, and any affection of the womb, 10-grain doses of effervescing citrate of iron three times daily is often beneficial. *Constipation* may be removed by laxatives, as Recipes 12 and 13; or by Carlsbad or Friedrichshall mineral waters, or by the use of brown bread, or occasionally by ripe fruit. Costiveness may also often be prevented by the plentiful employment of salt as an article of diet, and by active exercise. A favourite remedy for costiveness with dyspepsia, at hydropathic establishments, is the use of a cloth wrung out of cold water and applied to the belly. This is called an *abdominal compress*, and is worn under a bandage of mackintosh cloth, to keep the moisture from escaping. It is generally recommended to be used for two or three hours in the earlier part of the day. A tumblerful of cold water drunk at night before going to sleep, and another in the morning on rising, will relieve dyspeptic constipation in some habits; or the sulphate of soda and quinine mentioned at p. 135. When, in tropical residents sojourning in Europe, dyspepsia is attended by both constipation and debility, the mineral waters of Cheltenham, Harrogate, Tunbridge Wells, Spa, and Schwalbach are often beneficial. *In simple dyspepsia*, arising from debility of the stomach, unconnected with other maladies, when a carefully regulated diet does not relieve the sense of oppression following meals, *pepsin* often does much good. Capsicum is especially useful in that dyspepsia of long residents in tropical climates which evidences itself chiefly by a *sense of fulness and distension after meals*, and the following formula may be employed: powdered capsicum, 3 grains; compound rhubarb pill, 5 grains; powdered ipecacuanha, a quarter of a grain. Make into two pills, to be taken an hour before dinner. Recipe 13 is also a good dinner pill, especially if there is tendency to constipation. *Pain, nausea, and vomiting* may be relieved by chloroform, camphor, ether, or ammonia (Recipes 39, 40). Ten or 12 drops of spirits of camphor in an effervescing draught is often an effectual remedy. *Water-brash* usually disappears under a well-regulated diet, aided by mild aperients. Ten or 12 grains of alum, taken in an ounce of water three times daily, is very beneficial. Or compound kino powder in 20-grain doses.]

**EAR, DISEASES OF THE.**—1. ERUPTIONS ON THE SKIN OF THE EAR, OR BEHIND THE EAR.—These 'breakings-out' usually occur to children during teething (*vide* p. 435), and the peculiar form of skin disease thus attacking the ears is generally *eczema* (*vide* p. 396). In such cases, cleanliness must be particularly attended to; otherwise, the skin affection may run into sores. Glycerine soap and water should be used daily, so that all discharge may be gently washed away. Then the treatment should be conducted as given at page 397. But often these affections of the skin about the ears remain more or less prevalent, in spite of any treatment, until the period of teething has passed. Without treatment, and especially without attention to cleanliness, they assume a more prolonged and inveterate form.

2. DEAFNESS.—Deafness occurs in every degree, from mere dulness of perception of sound to absolute insensibility. It may depend on accumulation of wax, or on inflammation and its consequences, on polypus, or on enlarged tonsils, in which cases, if remediable, it can only be treated by the means prescribed for such conditions. In other cases deafness results from some affection of the nerve of the ear, and is called 'nervous deafness.' Such deafness may be caused by blows, falls, violent noises, explosions, or any kind of concussion. Thus deafness may result from rupture of the drum, caused by the sudden compression of the air against the membrane when a person dives into water. Or it may be a sequel of certain diseases believed to leave a poison in the system, as scarlet fever, measles, typhus, malarious fever. It sometimes comes on after great mental excitement, or from taking quinine in large and continuous doses. It may be a consequence of debility, and is then often accompanied by ringing, singing, hissing, or other unnatural noises in the ears. Lastly, it may be connected with disease of the brain.

*Treatment.*—Regard must be paid to the cause of deafness. The most generally useful local means are counter-irritants behind the ears, such as iodine paint or blisters. When deafness arises from enlarged tonsils, it is sometimes necessary to remove them by surgical operation. Deafness from simply nervous debility requires tonics and generous diet.

3. ACCUMULATION OF WAX IN THE EAR.—This often causes more or less deafness. In such cases the wax may

be seen through an ear speculum (a conical tube with bright interior which reflects light into the ear), or often with the naked eye. Sometimes wax in the ear excites a distressing cough, known as 'ear cough.' A drop or two of salad oil or of glycerine should be dropped into the ear at night, to soften the wax, and in the morning it should be *gently* syringed with lukewarm soapy water, which will further soften and expel the wax. A drop of salad oil should then be dropped into the ear, and cotton-wool applied to prevent cold.

*Method of Examining the Ear.*—If an ear speculum is not at hand, take a piece of foolscap 2½ inches square; cut off one corner about half-way to the centre; then roll the paper in the shape of a cone, the cut corner forming the apex, and the paper being rolled only sufficiently tight to allow of the small open end of the cone being introduced into the ear. Then, seating the patient in a chair, pull the ear backwards and upwards with the left hand, and introduce the speculum with the right. This must be done gently, and not more than half an inch of the paper should be introduced. Generally the light of the sun may be thrown into the ear sufficiently for the purpose of examination, by seating the person in the sun's rays for a few moments. Otherwise, light may be reflected into the ear, either from an argand lamp at night, or from the sun by a mirror. If sunlight is used, a plane mirror is required, the concave mirror soon causing great heat.

*Method of Syringing the Ear.*—A bowl should be held by the patient, or by another person, so that the rim is pressed against the skin, close under the lobe of the ear. The operator should then draw the ear upwards and backwards, which tends to straighten the passage. The nozzle of the syringe should be then introduced just within the passage, pressing a little against the upper wall. The syringe should be worked gently, forcible syringing being likely to do harm. Any kind of syringe may be used, but the ear syringe has rings for the two forefingers, so that it may be more easily worked with one hand. A new syringe has been designed, so made that only the necessary length can be introduced into the passage, and which is therefore harmless in the hands of anyone.

*Method of Applying a Poultice.*—One bandage or handkerchief should be passed under the chin and tied on the top of the head, and another should be passed round the head and be tied on the forehead so that the knot may not be inconvenient when lying down. The two should be secured by a pin over the ear. An instrument consisting of two saucer-like receptacles to fit on the ears, and joined by a spring to pass over the head, has been devised for the purpose.

4. EARACHE.—This complaint is in reality neuralgia of the ear. Its causes are those of neuralgia generally, or it occurs from blasts of cold air, or from incautious use of cold water for bathing. But it sometimes arises from a decayed tooth, and in children from cutting the teeth, or from the growth of the second set; or sometimes in adults from the passage of the wisdom teeth. Earache causes very severe pain, shooting over the head and face, increased by opening the mouth and by mastication. It is distinguished from the pain attending inflammation of the ear by the suddenness of its occurrence, by the absence of fever, and by its not being attended with 'throbbing.' Earache in infants is sometimes difficult to distinguish from 'belly-ache.' This may be known by the former being more continuous, without the intervals of freedom occurring when the bowels are affected. Also by the child putting its hand to its ear, and not drawing up its legs, as it would do from bowel-ache. If after giving an infant suitable nourishment, or a drink of water, it still keeps up a continual cry, the cause is most probably earache.

*Treatment.*—The treatment for adults is a purgative dose (Recipes 1 and 2) followed by quinine (Recipe 66), and a small mustard poultice may be applied behind the ear. If the wisdom teeth are appearing the gums may be lanced, and carious teeth should be protected by stopping. If the pain is great, a dose of chloral (Recipe 64) may be taken at night. A bag of hot salt may also be applied to the ear, or it may be fomented with hot poppy-head water (*vide Appendix*, No. 81). A roasted onion enclosed in a muslin bag is a favourite domestic remedy, which should be applied as hot as it can be borne to the ear. In children, in addition to applications as above, if the teeth have not all appeared, the gums may require lancing, and a senna purgative (*vide* p. 26) may also be desirable. Cold applications should be avoided. When earache occurs at regular intervals of hours or days, quinine should be given in doses proportionate to the age of the patient (*vide* p. 19).

Recipe 90 may be obtained for adults and rubbed in behind the ear.

5. INFLAMMATION OF THE EAR.—This may either attack the *external passage* (which leads from the atmosphere to the drum), or, proceeding inwards or commencing within, may attack the *internal part* of the ear (which is on the other side of the drum and contains the small bones and nerves forming the organ of hearing). *Inflammation of the external passage*, or, as it is usually called, the external ear, is attended with smarting, shooting pain, increased by motion or eating. The ear feels hot and dry, and there are shooting pains in the head. After a day or two there is a watery discharge, which in a few hours assumes a yellowish thicker character, when the pain greatly diminishes. Inflammation of the external ear is very frequent in children while teething; but as they are not able to explain the seat of pain, it may be overlooked until discharge presents. When other reasons for feverishness, restlessness, and crying of children are not present, especially if the child refuses to lie on one side, the ear should always be suspected and examined. Inflammation of the external ear often accompanies various skin diseases; it may be a sequel of any weakening illness, it may arise from cold currents of air, from too forcible syringing, or be the result of foreign bodies lodging in the ear. Dust and sand getting into the ear during an Indian dust storm may excite it. Cotton-wool placed in the ear for earache, and allowed to remain without the ear being washed, is a cause. If the inflammation arises from teething, the gums must be lanced. If from foreign

substances in the ear, they must be removed. Other measures are fomenting the ear with hot poppy-water, to relieve the pain (*vide* Recipe 81); using hot linseed-meal poultices during the intervals between the fomentations, or during the night; giving chloral at night to secure sleep; opening the bowels if necessary; and combating fever with citrate of magnesia draughts (*vide* p. 15). When discharge presents, it should be *gently* washed away twice or thrice daily by syringing with warm water, and after the syringing an astringent lotion (Recipe 97), first made slightly warm, may be carefully injected. Afterwards tonics, as quinine and iron, will be advisable (Recipe 70).

*When the inflammation attacks the internal ear*, it is a more serious disorder. The pain is of an acute *throbbing* character, with 'buzzing' in the ears, attended with high fever, and sometimes in children with delirium. Deafness soon occurs, from the pressure of matter forming within, and after the *throbbing* pain has continued for some hours or days, the drum of the ear bursts and matter escapes. When this happens much relief is experienced, but the internal structure of the ear is often destroyed, and permanent deafness is the consequence. Inflammation of the internal ear may present unconnected with any other malady, as the result of cold, or it is sometimes the result of extension of inflammation from the throat, or is a sequel of scarlet fever.

*Treatment.*—If obtainable, leeches should be applied behind the ear, to the number of one moderate-sized leech for each year of the patient's age; purgative medicines should be administered (Recipes 1, 2, for adults, and castor-oil for children); and fomentations of poppy water (Recipe 81), or, if not obtainable, hot water (Recipe 80) should be assiduously applied to the ear; but it will be best not to use a syringe except under medical advice, which, if practicable, should always be obtained.

6. Chronic Inflammation of the Ear.—Should the acute form, as above noted, be neglected, the disease is very liable to result in *chronic* or prolonged inflammation of the external ear. This chronic form, once established, is most obstinate to treatment, and leads to increasing deafness, to polypus, and probably to perforation of the drum of the ear, and destruction of the apparatus of hearing. *Caries*, or decay of the bone in which the ear is situated, may also result, and in some instances it has led to abscess in the brain. There is a persistent discharge, accompanied by dull aching pain, and by a sense of heaviness or pressure, by a variable amount of deafness, and by a feeling often described as like 'a drop of water in the ear,' or by sensations of singing, knocking, or 'surging.' In children the disease is often very insidious in its progress, and may cause great injury before its presence is suspected. Till a discharge appears, the ear may not have been suspected as the seat of any disease, on account of the child's inability to localise its pain, or to mention the deafness; and the child, in consequence of the deafness, may be erroneously regarded as careless or stupid. Instances, indeed, have been known when children thus affected have been punished by, for instance, a 'box on the ear'; the blow directly causing rupture of the drum, already tender from disease. Chronic inflammation of the ear is frequently made worse by even slighter causes, such as the use of an ear-scoop, or exposure to cold or wet. Unless great cleanliness is observed, especially in India, maggots may also form in the ear.

Perforation or rupture of the drum of the ear may be ascertained by asking the patient to blow forcibly while the mouth is shut and the nostrils are firmly pressed together. If the drum is broken, air will pass through the ear, and will be recognised by the patient and heard by the bystander. The flame of a candle held to the ear will be shaken, or even blown out.

The *treatment* of chronic inflammation of the ear consists in perfect cleanliness; daily gently syringing the ear with warm astringent lotion (Recipe 97); and counter-irritants, as a succession of small blisters, or iodine paint, applied behind the ear. The general health should also be attended to, and tonics, as quinine (Recipe 66), will be required. *But, when the disease has gone on to perforation of the drum,* syringing should *not* be employed. Cleanliness, and the protection of the ear by cotton-wool loosely placed in the orifice, is all that may, in the absence of professional advice, be attempted. In all cases the person should avoid exposure to cold or draughts, should be careful in well drying the ear after washing it, should wear a little cotton-wool in the orifice, and should live under the best possible hygienic conditions.

7. POLYPUS OF THE EAR.—This is a fleshy growth in the ear, springing from the lower part of the orifice or near the drum. It generally occurs after a discharge has lasted for some time, or when inflammation of the external ear has assumed the chronic form (*vide* p. 214). A polypus may be vividly red, or slightly red, or almost colourless, looking like a white grape. The consistency of the growth may vary, it sometimes being firm and solid, at others soft and easily bleeding. The presence of a polypus in the ear may be known, if, in addition to more or less deafness and discharge, the characteristic red or less coloured protrusion is seen in passage. The means of cure are extraction by forceps, which must be performed by a surgeon.

**ELEPHANTIASIS.**—Called also 'Barbadoes leg,' and 'Tropical big leg.' Elephantiasis generally affects the leg, and natives are often seen with a swollen leg and foot, which, from a fancied resemblance to an elephant's limb, has acquired the name as above. But elephantiasis may also attack other parts of the body, especially the genitals. It is most common in Western India, but Europeans are rarely affected. In typical cases the disease is ushered in by well-recognised fever, which is known as 'elephantoid fever.' With the fever the leg enlarges, and the glands in the groin are usually swollen. Attacks of fever recur at intervals, attended with additional enlargement of the part affected, the leg sometimes attaining an enormous weight and size; the feet and toes being almost hidden by the increased bulk of the leg. Sometimes there is a gradual enlargement of the leg, without any marked fever. During the progress of the disease small openings appear on the affected part, from which a milky fluid may be emitted. Sometimes the malady, particularly when it affects the privates, commences in this manner. The urine may also be milky (*vide Chyluria*, p. 129). Elephantiasis has been attributed to many causes, such as malaria, new rice, fermented toddy, a fish diet, working in muddy ground, to mosquitoes conveying a peculiar worm or *filaria* into the blood, and to inflammation of the veins and lymphatics. The treatment consists in giving tonics, as quinine, arsenic, and iron in succession (Recipes 69, 71, 75) with iodide of potassium (Recipe 21). But the disease is seldom cured by medicine, although often arrested by change of climate: the Europeans to Europe, the natives to Northern India.

**EPILEPSY.**—Epilepsy is often called 'The Falling Sickness,' or commonly, 'Fits.' Epileptic fits vary in character, severity, and duration. A very minor degree of epilepsy often occurs, which is spoken of as 'blanks,' 'forgets,' 'sensations,' 'absences,' or 'darknesses.' There is a momentary staggering, or peculiar sensation, or transient loss of intelligence; the person stops doing what he was about for a moment, and there may be a spasm or convulsive movement of some one limb. From such slight epileptic tendencies, to the typical seizure described below, there may be infinite modifications.

The symptoms of an epileptic fit are as follows:—After a short *warning*, consisting of perhaps a headache, or pain in the limbs, or spasms of the face or of a limb, or shivering, the patient is seized with loss of consciousness and loss of power, so that if standing he immediately falls to the ground. Or, *secondly*, he may fall without any previous warning. The fit is generally preceded by a loud cry, and consists of strong convulsive movements of the limbs and trunk, with spasms of the muscles of the face and eyes, producing distortions of the countenance. Usually, the first spasm so twists the head round that the sufferer appears to be trying to look over his shoulder. The brows are knit, the eyes fixed and staring, or turned up beneath the lids, so that only the whites can be seen. The eyeballs roll, and the pupils are dilated and insensible to light, but commencing to oscillate towards the close of the paroxysm. The face is at first pale, afterwards becoming red. The skin is cold and clammy. The hands are clenched, and the arms tossed about. The breathing is difficult, or appears arrested, as if the person were unable to breathe. The teeth are gnashed, and foam (often bloody, from the tongue being bitten) issues from the mouth. The fæces and urine are often expelled involuntarily. After the convulsions have continued from one to two, five, ten minutes, or even in exceptionally severe cases several hours, the patient becomes motionless, looks round with a bewildered expression, and generally sinks into a profound sleep. Fits, of a greater or less degree of violence, may occur almost daily, or at intervals of months, or years.

*Causes.*—This disease may be hereditary, may originate during teething, or it may be connected with excessive mental or bodily excitement, or with disease of the brain. In those subject to epilepsy, the malady may be excited by debility, dissipation, fright, passion, worms, plethora, indigestion, and the stoppage of accustomed discharges, as the monthly flow of women, by the irritation caused by stumps of teeth, by a long foreskin, and by bad habits.

*Epilepsy may be distinguished from hysteria* by the total loss of consciousness, by the distortions of the face, by the solitary cry *preceding*, and the deep sleep *succeeding* the fit, none of which signs are characteristic of hysteria. Epilepsy may be distinguished from apoplexy by the *absence* of 'puffing' or *stertorous* breathing, and by the *presence* of the *continuous* convulsions marking epilepsy (*vide* also p. 57).

*Treatment.*—If the stomach is full when *warnings* are felt, a mustard emetic (Recipe 54) will sometimes stop a fit. If the stomach is not full, a draught of cold water. *During the fit*, the patient should be placed on his back with the head slightly raised. Fresh air should be admitted freely and the face should be fanned. The neck and chest should be bared, cravats, stays, and all tight strings or garments about the body being loosed. The patient must be prevented injuring himself by the limbs being firmly held, without any pressure being made on the chest. To do this the attendants should take care not to stand opposite the patient's feet, lest he kick out and cause injury in his struggles; and also, in holding the head, be careful not to allow the fingers to got into his mouth. If sufficient attendants are at hand, the best method for holding him is for one to grasp each leg above the knee and above the ankle, and press them firmly downwards to the ground, and for two others to grasp each a hand and the point of the shoulder, while the fifth holds the head firmly between both hands. To prevent the tongue being bitten, a piece of soft wood or linen pad, too large to slip into the mouth, should be placed between the teeth. Nothing should be given to drink for fear of injuring the mouth. The temples may be bathed with vinegar during the fit, or, if the head is hot, a stream of cold water from the spout of a kettle may be gently poured on the forehead. *After the fit* the patient should be allowed to sleep, but if the patient does not sleep and appears depressed, a stimulant, as a glass of wine, may be allowed.

*In the intervals between the fits*, temperance, exercise, occupation, spare living, and the avoidance of all bad habits should be enjoined. Constipation, worms, stumps of teeth, and too full a condition of system, if present, should be appropriately treated. If the patient is a female the condition of the 'monthly flow' should be inquired into, and medicines given to correct any irregularity of this function. Bromide of potassium (Recipe 19) should always be taken. If the patient is weak and irritable, tonics (Recipe 66) will also be required. The following advice may be safely taken by epileptics. Keep the bowels gently open, the head cool, the feet warm, the mind easy, never wear tight clothing, and avoid intemperance and indigestible articles of diet. The epileptic tendency may sometimes be successfully combated by the use of an exclusively vegetable diet, or by a very considerable reduction of animal food.

*Nitrite of amyl* globules inhaled from a pocket-handkerchief will often stop a fit coming on. *During the intervals between the fits* the following medicines may be used. Iodide of potassium 1 drachm; bromide of potassium 1 drachm; bromide of ammonium half a drachm; carbonate of ammonia 2 scruples; distilled water 8 ounces. Dose—a tea-spoonful before meals, and 2 table-spoonfuls at bed-time in a little water. To be taken until the characteristic effects of iodide and bromide of potassium are produced (*vide* p. 9, and *note* to Recipe 21). This does good in a majority of instances.

EPILEPSY, FEIGNED.—Epilepsy is sometimes feigned, but an impostor does not fall violently, but throws himself down so as to avoid injury.

The eyes are closed, instead of being fixed and staring; the pupils contract on being exposed to light; the tongue is not bitten; the face is red instead of pale; the skin is hot from the necessary exertion; and neither urine nor fæces are voided. Proposing to apply the actual cautery (or red-hot iron), or to shave the head, often frightens the impostor, so that he speedily recovers. Or blowing snuff into the nostrils will change the fit into sneezing.

**ERUPTIONS.**—Eruptions are of different kinds. Those of one class mark various kinds of fevers, which are therefore termed *eruptive fevers,* as typhoid, dengue, typhus, chicken-pox, measles, scarlatina, small-pox. Eruptions also occur without febrile symptoms as skin diseases. Different eruptions are described under the various maladies of which they are a part, or under *Skin Diseases.*

**ERYSIPELAS.**—Erysipelas is often called 'St. Anthony's Fire,' and is a contagious inflammation of a portion of the skin, considered by some to be due to the operations of a microbe. It usually attacks those who are out of health from constitutional debility, or from bad food, from neglect of cleanliness and sanitation, and particularly from exposure to the impure air of hospitals and gaols. Erysipelas is most common on the face, which becomes shining, red, burning, and much swollen, the redness disappearing for a few moments on pressure of the part with the finger. Sometimes the swelling is so great that all distinctive features are quite lost. With the commencement of the redness, or previous to its appearance, there is chilliness or shivering, headache and nausea, followed by vomiting and high fever, with constipated bowels. The redness of the skin now becomes more defined, with severe burning of the part, on which at length small blisters may form, discharging a yellow fluid. *Simple erysipelas* as here described generally runs its course in from ten to fourteen days, the inflammation increasing for four days, after which it declines as the blisters mentioned above form.

*In more severe cases* there is much fever and perhaps delirium, the tissues underneath the skin are also affected, there is intense *throbbing* pain, and matter forms; the resulting abscesses and sinuses (*vide* pp. 39, 44) adding much to the danger, and indefinitely prolonging the disease. If the disease passes inwards to the brain, it may prove rapidly fatal.

Erysipelas frequently attacks wounded parts, or parts which have been subjected to surgical operation, or sometimes vaccinated arms, when the surface of the surrounding skin, or even of the whole limb, becomes red and swollen as above described. When this occurs the discharge from the wound ceases, and if nearly healed it reopens. An unhealed condition of the navel-string renders infants very subject to erysipelas, which spreads from the navel if the child has been exposed to contagion.

*Treatment.*—The part affected should be covered with lint soaked in tepid water, over which oiled silk should be laid. If this does not relieve the stinging pain, salad oil may be tried. A purgative, as sulphate of soda (Recipe 2) or castor-oil, will generally be required at first, after which the strength of the patient must be supported by nourishing diet, by an allowance of brandy or wine, and by the administration of quinine (Recipe 66) every three hours. If blisters form, they should be pricked at the most dependent part for the water to escape. Matter forming will generally require lancing of the skin over the part where it presents. As a general rule, when erysipelas attacks a wound or injured part it should be poulticed.

Of all the predisposing causes of erysipelas, deficient ventilation is the chief; and the greatest care must be taken to admit fresh air, without draughts, into the apartment. Unremitting attention should be paid to the cleanliness of the patient, and everything about him. The bed-linen ought to be frequently changed, and not be allowed to remain when soiled by discharge. The part affected should not be wiped with a sponge but with cotton-wool, which should be immediately burned or buried. The patient's bedroom should be emptied of all but indispensable articles of furniture, and bed-curtains should be taken down. The motions should be at once removed and disinfected. In short the whole of the rules given in the *Appendix* regarding disinfection should be carefully carried out.

Instead of applying lint soaked in tepid water, use carbolic acid lotion if available (*vide Appendix*, No. 119).

[In most cases of erysipelas it will also be desirable to give iron, and Recipe 71 may be procured and given *with* the quinine.]

**EYE AND EYELIDS, DISEASES OF THE.**—AFFECTIONS OF THE EYELIDS. 1. *Stye.*—This term is applied to a small painful boil at the edge of the eyelid. It should be frequently well fomented with hot water, permitted to come to a head, and then pricked with a lancet or needle to let the matter out. If an eyelash grows from the stye, the hair should be plucked out with a pincers. Stye often depends on indigestion, and is indicative of a debilitated condition of system.

2. TINEA, OR OPHTHALMIA TARSI, is a more important affection, consisting of the formation of a number of little styes or pustules at the roots of the eyelashes. They discharge a yellowish brown fluid, which mats the eyelashes together. There is considerable smarting and itching, and often overflow of tears. The malady is most common in children affected by a scrofulous taint. A very similar condition may be caused by the 'crab louse.' If present the insect may probably be perceived on close examination. Or the eggs may be seen attached to the roots of the lashes. If *tinea* becomes chronic, or is

neglected, it may destroy the structure from which the eyelashes grow, so that eyelashes may be more or less wanting. The treatment consists of frequent washing with warm alum wash (Recipe 97) to prevent the accumulation and crusting of discharge. At night simple ointment (Recipe 86) or salad oil should be carefully applied with a camel's-hair brush or feather to the eyelids to prevent them sticking together during sleep. The bowels should be kept open, and tonics (Recipe 66) taken.

[A better ointment, especially if there are lice, is composed of one-third nitrate of mercury ointment and two-thirds simple ointment; and a better tonic medicine is citrate of iron and quinine (Recipe 70). In chronic cases cod-liver oil is advisable.]

3. EPIPHORA.—*Watery eye*, or *overflow of tears*. There is a communication between the eyes and nostrils, by what is known as the *lachrymal sac and duct*, the minute entrances to which may be seen near the *inner* corner of the eyelids. The duct conveys the tears *from* the surface of the eye *to* the interior of the nose, and if this passage becomes blocked watery eye results. The eye fills with water, which collects at the inner angle, and, if not wiped away, falls over the cheek. There is little pain, but the angle of the eye is tender, and the orifice of the duct is reddened, swollen, and closed. If the impediment occurs lower down in the duct, instead of at the orifice, the duct becomes swollen and forms a swelling below the angle of the eye. If the tears are allowed to fall continually down the cheek, the skin becomes irritated, reddened, and eventually excoriated. The causes are various. The stimulus of cold air, or of a bright light after darkness, will produce a temporary constriction of the passage, with a temporary overflow of tears. *Tinea* as described above is a frequent cause. It sometimes arises from the impaired tone and congestion of the parts, consequent on working

with minute objects. In old age the lower lid becomes flabby, and, falling down, exposes the orifice of the duct to cold, which produces congestion, and also by altered position prevents it receiving the tears. A similar result occurs when the eyelid is paralysed. Calcareous concretions sometimes form from the tears in the duct, and so block the passage. Inflammation of the root of the canine tooth, which is close to the duct, may excite inflammation in the duct. It may also arise from injury, and a hair accidentally entering the orifice has been known to cause the affection. If unrelieved, matter often forms in the duct below the corner of the eye, when the duct may burst and be destroyed. Watery eye must be treated with reference to the cause. For a moderate degree of watery eye an astringent lotion (Recipe 97) will be beneficial. The best application for threatening abscess is constant fomentation with hot poppy-water (*vide Appendix, No.* 81). Operative procedure is sometimes required when the passage is blocked.

## Eye, Diseases of the

1. Cataract.—Cataract is a degeneration of the part of the eye called the 'lens.' It most frequently occurs in elderly people, and one or both eyes may be affected. In the healthy eye the *lens* cannot be seen, but when cataract occurs it assumes a white or bluish-white appearance, and may be detected through the pupil or circular central opening of the eye. Cataract may be months or even years forming. It must be distinguished from a white deposit on the front of the eye called 'opacity of the cornea,' and resulting from ophthalmia or ulceration (*vide* p. 233). In cataract vision is impaired, growing progressively worse, and the patient sees best in twilight, or when with his back to the light. Surgical operation is the only cure.

2. Glaucoma.—This term is applied to distension of the eyeball. The symptoms are attacks of dimness of vision, worse one day and better another. The person sees haloes round luminous bodies. There is diminution of the field of vision, as if a cloud obscured some portion. The eyeball feels hard. Pain of a severe bursting kind in the eyeball, above the eye, and at the side of the head, comes on occasionally. Although generally the disease is of slow progress, it may become rapid at any time. Symptoms as enumerated above should therefore lead to obtaining professional advice, and an operation may be required.

3. Iritis.—Iritis is inflammation of the 'iris,' or that part of the internal eye in which the round ring of the pupil is formed, and which gives the various colours of the eye. In this disease, while *the white of the eye is injected, by red vessels running from the middle towards the circumference in generally straight lines,* the cornea or centre of the eye is clear. *Through this* can be seen the 'iris,' which becomes discoloured, reddish if naturally dark, greenish if naturally blue. Afterwards a white deposit takes place, and the pupil may be thereby blocked up. There is intolerance of light, severe stinging pain of the eye and forehead, dull aching in the eye, and feverishness. The causes of iritis may be injuries, over-exertion of the eyes, venereal disease, or perhaps a gouty or rheumatic condition.

*Treatment.*—The eyes should be protected from light by a green shade and darkened room, and fomentation with hot poppy-head water should be frequently applied. If necessary the bowels should be relieved by purgatives (Recipes 1, 2), six or eight leeches should be applied to the temple of the affected eye, and chloral (Recipe 64) may be given at night to relieve pain; if the disease has occurred to a debilitated person, or to one who has suffered from rheumatism or gout, or who is scrofulous, Dover's powder (*vide* p. 12) at night, and quinine (Recipe 66) three times daily.

[The advice of a medical man, or, that impossible, the following remedies, should be obtained immediately. For a patient of fairly good constitution, who is not rheumatic, scrofulous, or debilitated, calomel and opium pills (Recipe 23), which should be given until there is a metallic taste in the mouth, or until the gums are slightly tender. Under the influence of the mercury the deposit will be seen to break up and disappear, leaving the pupil clear. If calomel is given as above, when it is discontinued, iodide of potassium mixture should be commenced (Recipe 21). But if the patient is debilitated or rheumatic, iodide of potassium (Recipe 21) should be substituted for the calomel. In all cases two drops of a solution of atropine (atropine 2 grains, distilled water 1 ounce) should be dropped into the eye twice or thrice daily. This medicine dilates the pupil of the eye, and tends to keep it clear of deposit. If the patient is debilitated from any cause, liberal diet and tonics will be necessary from the first.]

4. Nerve of the Eye, Affections of the.—The nerve of the eye (optic) and its expansion or termination in the eye (retina) are subject to various maladies, which were formerly included under the terms *amblyopia* (meaning indistinct vision), and *amaurosis* (or *gutta serena*, meaning total loss of vision). The ophthalmoscope has enabled surgeons to differentiate the nervous affections of the eye, which are now variously designated, in accordance with the appearances discovered by ophthalmoscopic examination. Nervous affections of the eye are frequently, but not always, associated with some general disease, as syphilis, diabetes, and albuminuria. Constant exposure to bright light, or working with very minute objects, also leads to affections of the optic nerve. Symptoms which may be expected are dimness of vision, distorted vision, sparks or flashes of light, narrowing of the field of vision, perhaps loss of portions of the field as if by a cloud in front, and sometimes night-blindness. Any such symptoms demand early professional advice. In the meantime the eyes should be

rested as much as possible; they should be protected from bright light, and any general malady should be treated.

5. OPHTHALMIA.—This term implies inflammation of the surface of the eye. There are several varieties, marked by a greater or less degree of violence. In mild cases the inflammation may not extend beyond the surface of the white of the eye, which is injected *with red vessels, running in different directions, and not straight from the centre* towards the circumference, as described under *Iritis,* or *Inflammation of the Iris* (*vide* p. 225). There is a smarting feeling as if sand or grit were in the eye. There is intolerance of light, and the eye is watering and weak, and, particularly in children, especially if scrofulous, obstinately kept shut. There is also pain in the forehead, or head generally, and often some feverishness. There is a discharge from the eye, at first clear and thin, but afterwards thicker, and of a white colour. During sleep this discharge collects at the edge of the lids and dries there, gluing together the eyelashes, so that the person finds a difficulty in opening the eyes after sleep without first bathing them with warm water. One or both eyes may be affected. Or one may be affected first, and the other afterwards. It often results from cold, and has been supposed to be caused by a 'flying bug' in the eye, and it may be conveyed from one person to another by common flies. It is infectious, sometimes attacking whole families, and proving the more contagious the more the discharge resembles matter. Therefore, in all cases of ophthalmia the greatest care should be taken that towels, soap, water, &c., are not used in common. The duration of the disease may be a few days or several weeks.

*Treatment.*—Keep the patient in a darkened room with a green shade over the eyes, bathing the eyes frequently with hot water, or with hot milk and water; or, if there is much discharge and the eyelids are painful, swollen, red, and inflamed, fomentation with hot poppy-head water (*vide Appendix, No.* 81) mixed in equal proportions with alum lotion (Recipe 97). Sometimes in slight cases hot applications are not acceptable to the feelings of the patient, in which case Recipe 97 may be used cold. If there is persistent pain, a leech or two may be applied to each temple at the margin of the hair. The edges of the lids should be anointed every night with salad oil or glycerine to prevent sticking; but if they adhere they should not be forced open, but be bathed until they separate. A purgative (Recipes 1 and 2) should also be administered if the bowels are confined. The diet should be light but nourishing.

6. Purulent Ophthalmia is a very severe variety of the disorder, which may result from similar causes, or which may originate from neglect of simple ophthalmia, or from unhygienic conditions, especially overcrowding, or from noxious matter (as the discharge passed in gonorrhœa) being introduced into the eyes, either from using dirty cloths or otherwise. The inflammation is very severe, the whites of the eyes are so swollen that the middle of the eye or cornea is almost hidden, and the pain is very great. Instead of a watery or slightly white discharge, yellow matter is secreted which escapes from the eye in considerable quantities. In some cases the inflammation attacks the deeper parts of the eye, and the organ is destroyed. Purulent ophthalmia often occurs during small-pox. It is highly contagious. Therefore, when the disease occurs, the rules given in the *Appendix* regarding disinfection should be as much as possible carried out. The duration of the malady may be from ten days to two or three weeks; but it often leads to *ulcer of the cornea* (*vide* page 233), or to a rough and irritable condition of the inside of the lids, known as *granular*

*conjunctiva* (p. 230), either of which ailments may prolong the illness for months.

*Treatment.*—The eye should be well fomented every two or three hours with hot poppy-head water (*vide Appendix*, No. 81), and care should be taken that the disease is not communicated by cloths or otherwise, either to the other eye, if sound, or to the eyes of attendants. The face should be kept clean, and the eye or eyes affected should be covered with cotton-wool and a light bandage. The cotton-wool should be frequently removed and burnt. The patient should be kept in a darkened room, and the bowels should be opened, if necessary daily, by Recipes 1 and 2. When the pain and inflammation are great, it will be desirable to apply five or six leeches to each temple; a measure adopted to allay local irritation, not to weaken the patient. The edges of the lids should be smeared nightly with salad oil to prevent them sticking together; and (when the patient is old enough to understand and submit to the procedure) if the discharge hardens under the lids, the nozzle of a glass syringe, charged with tepid milk and water, should be carefully and gently inserted between the eyelid and the eyeball, taking care not to press on the latter, and its contents made to pass quickly over the internal surface of the lids. As the fluid escapes it carries with it any matter which by retention would aggravate the disease. The most useful medicines are quinine (Recipe 66) as a tonic, and chloral (Recipe 64) to allay pain. When the first violence of the inflammation subsides, it will be proper to wash the eyes frequently with warm alum lotion (Recipe 97), some of which should be permitted to fall into the eyes (as described below) several times daily. The subjects of purulent ophthalmia are often of naturally feeble constitution, or are debilitated by prior ill-health, or from other causes. The strength, therefore, should be maintained by good easily digestible food and a little port wine. Thorough ventilation is of the greatest importance, as minute particles of the matter discharged become detached, dry up, and, floating in the atmosphere, are capable of infecting other eyes with which they come into contact. But free ventilation and exposure of such atoms to the oxygen of the atmosphere reduce such danger to a minimum.

[When the remedies as above do not prove satisfactory, blisters should be applied alternately behind the ears and to the temples; and a solution of nitrate of silver, of the strength of 10 grains to an ounce of water, may be obtained, a drop of which should be dropped in the eye from a quill or brush twice daily. It is a painful application, although often very serviceable. It is also sometimes necessary to lance the inflamed eye in order to prevent more serious mischief. The malady is therefore one urgently demanding skilled advice.]

*How to Foment the Eye.*—Place the fluid in a large basin, hold the head over it, dip a piece of lint or soft linen rag in the fluid, and without pressure apply the fluid freely to the eye. This should be continued for several minutes; then lay the patient on his back, open the eye, and squeeze the wet rag over it so as to allow the fluid to run into the eye. This simple method is more satisfactory than the use of glasses or apparatus sold for the purpose.

*How to apply Lotion to the Eye.*—A camel's-hair brush, or a quill cut oval-shaped, may be used. Fill the brush or quill with the lotion, draw down the lower lid, and let the fluid drop into the eye. In order to get the fluid well within the upper lid, move the latter up and down, without pressure on the globe, and the whole surface will be wetted. The brush or quill should be washed in warm water after use.

7. Granular Ophthalmia is often the result of other forms of ophthalmia. It is characterised by the formation of granular bodies on the inner surface of the eyelids, more or less resembling sago grains, which, being rough, irritate the front of the eye. The object is to destroy these granulations by caustics, which can only be attempted by a surgeon. In the meantime, good diet, tonics, and bracing air are desirable.

8. Short Sight.—Short sight most frequently depends on too great convexity of the *cornea* (or front part of the

eye), or of the *lens* (in the interior of the eye), or of both. The rays of light are brought to a focus before they reach the proper part of the eye (*retina*), instead of being concentrated upon it. Short sight often originates in school-children from bad lights and constrained position. An opposite condition of the refractive *media* of the eye gives rise to LONG SIGHT; and as this opposite condition occurs as persons grow old, long sight is most common after forty-five years of age. For similar reasons, *short sight* may improve as people grow older. Short-sighted persons should avoid over-working the eyes, and especially by the examination of minute objects, or by writing in artificial light. Well-adjusted concave pebble glasses should be used; but the weakest power which will serve to assist vision should be chosen. The glasses should only be worn when actually required. Single glasses tend to alter the power of the eyes, and are therefore not to be recommended. For *long sight* convex glasses are required, and they should be so worn that distant objects may be seen over them at pleasure.

There are several other affections of the eye remediable by glasses, the principal being ASTIGMATISM and HYPERMETROPIA. Astigmatism implies an inequality of the refractive media of the eye, the rays of light not coming to a focus at one point. Vertical and horizontal lines drawn on paper are not seen equally distinct at the same distance. Hypermetropia means when neither near nor distant objects are seen distinctly owing to rays of light coming to a focus behind the retina.

9. SPOTS BEFORE THE EYES, OR MUSCÆ VOLITANTES.—Persons of sedentary habits or delicate constitutions, especially if they are in the habit of writing or reading much, or otherwise exercising their sight on minute objects, are liable to suffer from spots before the eyes in the shape of black motes, or grey films, or an appearance of something resembling spiders' webs. In some cases small circles with central spots are apparent. When looked at, these

appearances move slowly downwards. There may also be sparks, or a gradual formation from a point, of an extending 'zigzag' halo of light. Such impediments to vision are more perceived when the sky or some white object is looked at. They often first occur very suddenly, and may be the cause of much uneasiness, as it may be thought they are significant of some serions disease. But as a general rule this is not the case, although sometimes sparks occur as the forerunner of nervous affections (*vide* p. 226). Frequently they are symptomatic of dyspepsia, and spots especially are more apparent or troublesome when the stomach or liver is out of order. They often continue without increasing for many years. They depend, when permanent, on the rupture of a minute vessel in the vascular coat of the eye, probably from overstrain, and the consequent escape and deposit of a minute portion of the colouring-matter of the blood, which, imprisoned in a vessel, still moves with the circulation to a small extent.

*Treatment.*—Any particular employment which may seem to have caused the affection should be discontinued. Tonics, change of air, and rest to the eyes are the main remedies. The state of the digestion should be inquired into, and any error appropriately treated. Care should be taken not to wear tight cravats or collars, and the person affected should not read at night, or when lying down.

If the spots increase, or are very annoying, or if they are accompanied by weakness of sight, blue spectacles may be worn of a lighter or darker shade according to the degree of protection required. Blue spectacles are better than either brown, smoke-coloured, or green. Green spectacles protect the eyes only from red rays; while brown or smoke-coloured glasses intercept all rays equally, thus rendering vision indistinct. But blue glasses intercept only orange rays, which are the most intolerable to a sensitive eye.

10. SQUINTING.—A squint may be either single or double. It depends on want of equilibrium between the muscles which move the eye. It may be present at birth,

or may come on in childhood. It may arise from the irritation of teething, or from worms, or may be a result of the debilitated condition left by fevers. Squinting when a child is out of health is always a matter of anxiety (*vide Convulsions*, p. 145). Sometimes a film or *opacity* on the cornea (*vide* p. 233) leads to squinting. The treatment, therefore, of squinting must depend on the cause, and a surgical operation may be required.

11. ULCERS OF THE CORNEA, or central part of the eye, often result from neglected ophthalmia, from granular lids, and particularly from ophthalmia (sometimes in spite of treatment) occurring in scrofulous children. While the white of the eye presents more or less the injected appearance described as simple ophthalmia (p. 227), one or more red vessels may be seen stretching from the margin towards the centre of the cornea or middle of the eye, in some part of which a small rough-looking or white-coloured spot will be discovered; there is also much intolerance of light and watering of the eyes. In bad cases several of these spots may form, which are, in fact, ulcers of the part. If the case proceeds favourably, the white of the eye loses its injected appearance, the red vessel or vessels on the cornea disappear, and the ulcer heals, often, however, leaving a white spot or film, which may or may not also disappear during the next few weeks or months. When the disease does not progress favourably a large white film is left on the cornea (called *opacity of the cornea*), interfering very much with sight. In still worse instances the cornea is quite converted into a white mass, and the person cannot see at all.

*Treatment.*—A darkened but well-ventilated room must be *insisted* upon, and the eyes should be assiduously fomented with poppy-water (*vide Appendix*, No. 81), until the inflammatory redness of the white of the eye has almost disappeared. Then the essential point will be the improvement of the general health. The diet should be nutritious, and a little wine should be allowed. Quinine should be given, and exercise short of fatigue should be taken in the open air, the eyes being well protected from light and glare.

[During the earlier stages of ulcer of the cornea a solution of atropine (atropine 2 grains, water 1 ounce) should be if possible obtained, and a drop should be dropped into the eye once or twice a day. Blisters should also be obtained and applied, alternately, behind the ears and to the temples. Iodide of potassium (Recipe 21) should be given internally. In the latter stages it may also be advisable for the ulcer to be *very lightly* touched, every second day, with a very fine pencil of nitrate of silver, or caustic point made for the purpose in a glass case. But this is an operation requiring great care and delicacy of touch, and should only be performed by those well aware of the properties of nitrate of silver, and of the appearances rendering its application desirable.]

**FAINTING** or **SYNCOPE** occurs from numerous causes. It may result from loss of blood, or from fright or sudden shock; it may be produced by a blow on the stomach, or by intense pain; or it may be connected in women with irregularities of the 'monthly flow.' It may be caused by a disordered stomach, or may arise from certain diseases of the heart. It may even arise from bad smells or unpleasant sounds. Persons most liable to fainting are females, and young men of nervous temperament. The first symptoms are giddiness, 'swimming' in the head, and pallor. A person in a deep faint is pale, unconscious, with feeble pulse, dilated pupil, relaxation of the limbs, unfrequent, irregular, scarcely perceptible breathing, white lips, and a death-like expression of countenance. The body should be *at once placed in the recumbent position*, the head even being allowed to hang down lower than the body; cold water should be dashed on the face and cold air admitted into the room, or the person should be taken out of doors. The limbs should be well rubbed, and a burnt feather should be held smoking under the nose, which is a better remedy than ammonia. If a feather is not at hand, smelling-salts may be held to the nostrils for half a minute, every two or three minutes; strong salts should not be applied continually, as injury to the nostrils may arise therefrom. In prolonged faints a mustard poultice should be applied over the heart. The subsequent feeling of languor will be relieved by wine in moderate quantities. For the *prevention* of a fainting fit, lying down at full length, without a pillow under the head; or if not able to lie down, the head should be bent forward between the legs. Persons subject to fainting usually require tonics and outdoor exercise, and should avoid constipated bowels.

**FAT, ACCUMULATION OF.**—Both Europeans in India and natives often grow very stout; and sometimes this increase of size occurs rather suddenly, not only giving rise to inconvenience, but sometimes constituting disease. The cause is, probably, too much fat-forming food, and too little exercise at that period of life when the accumulation of a little fatty material is natural. When the fat is equally distributed about the body no immediate disadvantage may be experienced; but when it is accumulated in distinct parts, interfering with the functions of particular organs, its evil influence becomes apparent. The average weight of a healthy adult man in the prime of life, or from twenty-five to thirty-five, five feet in height, is 115 lbs., to which standard 5 lbs. may be added for every inch in height. For females the average is somewhat lower. When persons weigh much above their height, or when their waist girth exceeds their chest girth, they are growing fat, and there is a tendency to impairment of the powers, both of the muscles and of the blood-vessels. The heavier man carries greater bulk, and his heart has to propel into a larger mass of tissue a larger amount of blood. Hence one form of evil, viz. *an* *overworked heart*, resulting from accumulation of fat, and which is characterised by shortness of breath, and sometimes by palpitation. In addition to this, fat may collect about, or in the substance of, the heart, giving rise to the malady known as *fatty degeneration* of that organ. This is marked by aggravated symptoms as above, with probably attacks of giddiness. In elderly people it is often accompanied by a peculiar appearance of the eyes, designated the *arcus senilis*, and known by a narrow opaque or whitish zone presenting near the margin of the *cornea* (or the circle of the eye where it joins the white). Fatty heart is a dangerous malady, as it may lead to dilatation of the organ, and any suspicion of such affection should lead to application for medical advice. In the meantime, persons so affected should avoid *all* kinds of exertion, hurry, or excitement. Another form of evil is fatty degeneration of the blood-vessels of the brain, which may terminate in rupture, and its consequence apoplexy (*vide* p. 55).

When persons are growing fat, the *first great principles of prevention* are *less food and more exercise.* The person who, becoming stout, desires to permanently reduce his flesh *must consume less food and take more exercise.* If he leaves off carbonaceous foods, of which sugar may be taken as the type, he will achieve his purpose the more quickly. There is no royal road *both to become thin and to keep so*. No system of dietary will achieve this. But spare food and physical exercise will do so.

The *second great principle of prevention* is the avoidance of those articles of food which are known, when taken in excess, to produce obesity. Fat of meat, bacon, fat pork, white bread, cheese, butter, thick soups, salmon, stews, preserves, beer, sweet wine, spirits, articles containing much starch, as potatoes, tapioca, rice, arrowroot, sago, and sugar, must be interdicted, or at least taken in moderation. For sugar saccharin may be substituted, as, although possessing more sweetening power than sugar, it is not a food. Brown bread, toast, biscuits, rusks, lean of any kind of meat, fish, fowl, or game, green vegetables, as cauliflower, asparagus, and lettuce, celery, fruit, and light wines, should form the diet. Even if the regimen as above sketched cannot be strictly adhered to, attention to its leading principles will tend to prevent accumulation of fat, and also to lessen the amount present in the system. The change from one diet to another should be made gradually. The sudden withdrawal of accustomed articles of food is unwise, and it is better to lessen gradually the fatty portions of the diet than to go to extremes.

The dietary recommended is a modified form of Bantingism. Many persons placed on the strict system recommended by Banting, while reduced in bulk, feel so weak, dyspeptic, and wretched that they are unable to persevere. They are brought into a state of inanition—a condition unfavourable, especially in any tropical climate, to either physical or mental health and vigour. By such a method they avoid one trouble with partial success, only to fall into another, probably worse. For Bantingism *is no permanent cure, as the tendency to obesity returns immediately the strictness of the system is relaxed.* Similarly with the popular anti-fat cures (*Entfettungskuren*) of Continental health-resorts, also with the preparation known as 'Anti-fat,' which is a fluid extract of the *Fucus vesiculosus*, or 'sea-wrack.'

Other means of growing thin have been advocated. A diet almost exclusively of meat and hot water is one. Lean beefsteak is recommended as the model food, an occasional meal of plain boiled cod-fish, and now and then a few sticks of celery, being the only other articles of diet allowed. About a pint of hot water must be slowly taken three or four times a day between meals, and no other liquid. But a certain mixed diet is requisite for healthy nutrition, and neither fatty, farinaceous, nor albuminoid material can be omitted in any considerable proportion without detriment to health.

Another means proposed for growing thin is by minimising the quantity of liquid consumed. But it is essential there should be constantly passing through the system a sufficient quantity of fluid to hold in solution and wash away the constantly accruing products of bodily waste. For example, uric acid requires not less than 8,000 times its bulk of water at blood heat to hold it in solution, and if it be not so dissolved it rapidly crystallises with more or less disastrous consequences, as in the production of gout, gravel, and other less well-recognised troubles.

A system has been recommended in which the person is encouraged to eat fat, and certain other matters, as salmon and *pâté de foie gras*, &c. This system is based on the principle that fat produces satiety, and thus diminishes the demand for food. But this system, like the previous ones, only produces a temporary effect, and, like all the others, may injure the health if long-continued. *If the result is to be permanent, there must be less food and more exercise.*

**FEET, TENDERNESS OF THE.**—Some persons suffer much from tenderness of the feet, and are unable to wear boots sufficiently thick to protect from jungle, thorns, &c. For the relief of this annoying condition nothing is better than bathing the feet daily in strong salt and water. Tender feet are often found perspiring and *smelling offensively.* Salt and water bathing will also tend to correct this, especially when aided by perfect cleanliness, and clean socks twice daily. Wool socks free from dyes, with divisions for the toes, are made for this complaint. Wool, being a slow conductor of heat, maintains the feet warm and of equable temperature, while it permits the perspiration of the feet to evaporate (*vide* Chapter VI., Clothing). *Cold feet* may be *relieved* by immersing them for two or three minutes every night in cold water, rubbing all the time, and then putting warm socks on.

**FEVER.**—All varieties of fever, from a common cold to the most severe, commence much in the same manner, with lassitude, headache, weakness of mental and physical power, chilliness, and painful sensations in the back and limbs. This is succeeded by heat of skin, quickened pulse, furred tongue, disordered stomach, scanty and high-coloured urine, with great thirst. Such a condition is common in most diseases, and after injuries, also from disordered stomach, and from cold, when the person is said to be 'feverish.' Fever also attends small-pox, scarlatina, measles, chicken-pox, and these maladies are often called the ERUPTIVE FEVERS. Fever, therefore, in many instances must be regarded as a symptom of disease rather than the disease itself (*vide* p. 37).

But fever exists as a disease *per se*, or unconnected with any other malady. And of such fevers there are three divisions: *one class* marked by almost complete *continuance* of the symptoms from the origin to the termination of the attack; such as *Continued Fever*, *Enteric* or *Typhoid Fever*, and *Typhus Fever*.

A *second* class characterised by the more or less temporary or complete *cessation* of symptoms for a variable time, during which the patient may seem in health; such as *Relapsing Fever*, *Intermittent Fever* or *Ague*, *Remittent Fever*, *Masked Malarious Fever*.

A *third* class in which some of the symptoms of several varieties may appear, but not all the symptoms of any kind; such as *undefined climatic fever*, which has also been called *typho-malarial*, *malario-typhoid*, *typho-remittent*, and *hybrid*.

**FEVER, CONTINUED.**—Commences with a chilly sensation, pain in back and head, languor, weakness and loss of appetite, quick pulse, and heat of skin. When a person is thus attacked it is often impossible to foretell into which of the different phases of fever the disease may run. Such symptoms may be caused by exposure to cold and wet, or to the sun, or even by indigestion or over-fatigue. When thus excited it rarely lasts longer than from twenty-four hours to two or three days, and is then often spoken of as *Ephemeral Fever*. When, however, exposure to the sun causes fever, it may develop into a more serious form (*vide* p. 427). Also, the malady may continue by the skin becoming hotter, the pulse quicker, and by disorder of the stomach (evidenced by frequent vomiting and inability to retain food). It is to this condition that the term *gastric fever* is frequently applied (*vide Disorder of the Stomach*,

p. 415). Symptoms as above may also precede acute rheumatism (*vide* p. 367). Sore throat accompanying the fever would point to scarlet fever; headache, vomiting, and pain in the loins to small-pox; sneezing, running at the nose, and cough to measles; very severe headache with shivering and backache to typhus; dull frontal headache to typhoid. If the second day passes without a rash it is neither chicken-pox nor scarlet fever; if the third day passes it is not small-pox; if the fourth day passes it is not measles; if the seventh day passes it is not typhus; if the twelfth day passes it is not typhoid, but may be acute general tuberculosis. In the absence of any symptoms indicating maladies as above, the treatment of simple continued fever consists in perfect quiet, good ventilation, maintaining the bowels moderately open by Recipe 2, in giving citrate of magnesia draughts to allay feverishness, and in treating the accompanying disorder of the stomach as mentioned under that head (*vide* p. 415).

**FEVER, ENTERIC or TYPHOID.**—Typhoid fever is called also *enteric* fever, from its usually affecting the bowels; and it has been termed *pythogenic* fever, meaning fever generated by dirt. It is often, especially in Europe, connected with inefficient conservancy arrangements, such as a water-closet out of order, or escape of sewer-gas into a house. It is also believed to arise from drinking-water contaminated from sewers, and especially from sewers into which the discharges from typhoid-fever patients have been introduced. Thus a pump or well, and a cesspool or sewer, in close proximity, is very likely to give rise to typhoid fever in those drinking such water. Milk also has conveyed the disease, after dilution with contaminated water, or when allowed to stand in proximity to a diseased person. There is also evidence that the contagion may be conveyed by clothings which have been washed in contaminated water. Yet it is not by touch or odour the disease is spread, but by germs (supposed to be microbes or *bacilli*) swallowed with food or otherwise. It is most contagious during the third week. It is more likely to attack young than elderly people; and it is more prevalent during the autumnal months. The period between infection and development of the disease is from ten to twenty days.

*Symptoms.*—The onset of typhoid fever is usually gradual, with feelings of *malaise*, aching in the limbs, headache, loss of appetite, and chilliness. But for some days the sufferer is able to go about thinking there is not much the matter. But sometimes typhoid fever sets in suddenly. Usually the bowels are constipated at first; but often the bowels are *relaxed from the first*, and the person may be supposed to have ordinary diarrhœa. There may also be from the commencement marked symptoms of stomach derangement, as nausea, vomiting, and inability to retain food, which has sometimes led to the disease being called *gastric fever*. At length the pulse, at first feeble, becomes quicker and full, the skin hot and dry, and at about the end of the first week the patient takes to his bed, with the appetite gone, the tongue coated, and the bowels loose. The fever is now found to be slightly *remittent* in type, showing an *exacerbation* or increase in the afternoon, and a slight *remission* or diminution towards morning, although it never varies to the extent of remittent. The urine is scanty and high-coloured, there is increasing restlessness at night, the face is often pale with a pink flush on the cheeks, while the eyes are clear and bright. The diarrhœa continues, and the stools passed are thin and of a yellow colour sometimes resembling pea-soup. If now the hand is pressed on the right side of the patient's bowels, his face will probably express pain, and a gurgling may also be felt and heard under the fingers. About this period also the bowels may become tense and resonant. Between the seventh and twelfth day the peculiar eruption of typhoid fever appears on the chest, abdomen, and back; consisting of a few slightly raised rose-coloured spots, which disappear temporarily on presure under the finger, and fade away in two or three days, being in the meantime succeeded by fresh crops. On the darker skin of the native the eruption of typhoid fever appears very like flea-bites. This characteristic eruption must not be confounded with one of very small watery vesicles, called *sudamina* (*vide* p. 399), and which occurs in most fevers. In favourable cases, and especially in children, after the appearance of the eruption a diminution of the fever takes place. In favourable cases, the patient may improve about the beginning of the third week, when the remissions of the fever become more distinct, the diarrhœa lessens, the tongue cleans, the pains in the limbs cease, the patient sleeps at night, the temperature of the body decreases, and the appetite returns. In more severe cases, about the middle of the second week delirium comes on, at first slight and only noticed at night, afterwards more constant, intense, and noisy. And it should be noted that when the mind is affected the person is apt to reply in the affirmative to every question. As the malady increases what is spoken of as the 'typhoid condition' presents, the tongue becomes drier, red and glazed, and often cracks in various directions, while dry, black crusts, called *sordes*, form on the teeth. The lips also crack and bleed. As the time advances, or during the third week, the patient loses flesh and strength, he lies prostrate, and often unconscious of what is going on around him, and if the case ends fatally he will become quite insensible, his temperature will rise higher, and he will, with trembling hands, pick and 'fumble' at the bed-clothes. A large degree of this picking and trembling is suggestive of much mischief in the intestines. Dilated pupils, bleeding from the nose, blood passed with the stools, urine and stools passed involuntarily, muttering delirium, and convulsions, are all unfavourable symptoms.

The temperature should be frequently tested by the clinical thermometer (*vide* p. 33). If the temperature rises above 105° Fahr. *in the early morning*, or above 107° *at any time*, recovery is rare. In a typical case, during the first week the temperature rises perhaps to 105°; during the second week the daily morning and evening temperatures are identical, a little above 105° in the evening and below 105° in the morning; during the third week the morning temperature is a little lower; during the fourth week there is a gradual fall. A sudden or irregular rise of temperature during typhoid denotes some local complication, probably in the lungs, which are very liable to become congested. A marked fall of temperature not unfrequently precedes dangerous bleeding from the bowels. Sudden variations of the pulse will denote similar complications.

The *duration* of typhoid fever from the commencement of the premonitory symptoms is ordinarily from three to four weeks; but there may be relapses, which happens in about 15 per cent. of cases. The mortality from typhoid fever is one in every six attacked.

*Typhoid fever may be rendered more dangerous* from the accompanying *diarrhœa* being very profuse and exhaustive. There may also be profuse *bleeding* from the bowels. *Perforation of the bowel* may occur between the twenty-fifth and thirty-second day—an accident attended with symptoms of fainting or *collapse*, and always proving fatal. *Inflammation of the bowels* may supervene, or the *spleen* or *liver* may become enlarged. There may be *intense gastric irritation*, marked by incessant vomiting and irritability of the stomach. The *lungs* may become congested, denoted by quick breathing and short hacking cough.

In adults, enteric fever may be mistaken for *typhus*, or for *remittent*, and the distinctions are given at pp. 249, 263. In children, enteric may be mistaken for *water on the brain* and for *disordered stomach* (*vide* Distinctions, p. 418).

*Treatment.*—The patient should be placed in a well-ventilated room without curtains or other impediments to perflation by the air. The light from the windows should be prevented falling on the patient's eyes, and all noises should be stopped. The bed should not be too soft, and an india-rubber sheet should be placed under the patient. If possible there should be two beds for daily change. But the patient should not be allowed to exert himself at all, but should husband all his strength. The greatest cleanliness must be observed, and *all* the rules regarding disinfection given in the *Appendix* (No. 121) should be *carefully attended to.* Bedsores should be guarded against from the very first (*vide* p. 69). Throughout the attack the mouth and teeth should be kept clean. The body should be daily sponged with tepid water, the nurse drying and sponging one part at a time, so as to prevent chill from exposure; this relieves the patient, and tends to remove the unpleasant smell so common during fevers. Headache may be relieved by cutting the hair very short, by ice or cooling lotions. Vomiting and thirst are relieved by sucking ice. Milk, beef-tea, broths, jellies, extract of beef, Liebig's raw-meat soup, Brand's essence, should be the only articles of diet. A milk diet is the best. Given in small quantities, say every hour or two, from two to four pints may be taken in the twenty-four hours. The remarks on milk diet at p. 194 should be followed. Milk may be supplemented by one or two raw eggs *per diem* made into egg-flip, also by the other articles mentioned above; beef-tea not being used if the diarrhœa is excessive. It must, however, be remembered that digestion and absorption are much impaired, and therefore food must not be too much pressed on the patient. No *solid food* should be allowed under six weeks or two months, because in consequence of the ulceration of the bowels occurring, the coats are very thin and liable to burst. Eating an orange or a piece of potato, or drinking an effervescent draught, may cause distension of the bowel and rupture it just when the patient is otherwise doing well; especially during the third and fourth weeks. After the first week, if the pulse is growing in rapidity and losing in strength, port wine and brandy, in the proportion of two ounces of the former or one of the latter every three hours, will be necessary. But in typhoid, *as in all other fevers*, the use of stimulants, and the amount to be given, must be guided by the effects produced. If, after stimulants, the tongue becomes more moist; or if the pulse becomes slower; or if the skin grows more moist, or the delirium less, the stimulants are doing good; if the reverse occurs, they are doing harm. In any case, and at all times, the fever may be moderated by saline cooling draughts, as citrate of magnesia (*vide* p. 15) taken *after effervescence has subsided*, and by cooling applications, as vinegar and water, or Recipe 83, to the head. The diarrhœa need seldom be checked unless the patient is purged more than eight or nine times in the twenty-four hours, and then a starch injection (Recipe 104) may be given, Recipe 68 may be used, and ipecacuanha in two-grain doses may be given night and morning. If this does not succeed, or if there is bleeding from the bowels, a drachm of powdered alum should be added to a pint of boiling milk, which should be then strained. Two ounces of this alum whey may be given after each motion of the bowels. Milk and lime-water in equal parts are also often beneficial. If *the skin is moist, and there is little or no headache*, sleeplessness and delirium may be met by an opiate, as chloral (Recipe 64). But no opiate should be used, except under medical advice, so long as the skin is *hot and dry*. Before giving an opiate it should be ascertained if the patient does or does not sleep, as he will frequently assert he does not do so when sleeping for hours very night. When the patient is unconscious, care must be taken to empty the bladder, as it often happens he is unable to make water. In such cases the catheter will be required (*vide* p. 492).

[From the preceding it will be observed that more is to be done in this disease by care and good nursing than by medicines. Still the following may be recommended. Oil of turpentine, one drachm; white of two unboiled eggs; white sugar, one drachm; distilled water, six ounces. Two table-spoonfuls three times a day. Shake the bottle well before using. Should the diarrhœa become excessive, and not checked by the measures noted, Recipes 43 and 46 may be obtained and tried in succession. The latter recipe (46) is also very serviceable when blood is passed.

During typhoid and other fevers, when the temperature rises above 103°, cold or even iced baths are often used. The patient may be lifted in a sheet, and placed in lukewarm water, which may then be cooled by the addition of cold water to a temperature of 68°, where he should remain from five to seven minutes, after which he should be rapidly dried, and wrapped in dry sheets. Two or three baths should be given daily, and the same water may be used several times. Or the patient may be packed in a wet sheet, which is preferable for children and delicate persons. This treatment is *not* recommended unless under medical supervision; and placing the patient in cold water at first, as sometimes advised, is not recommended at all, as it may induce collapse or internal congestions.

The necessity of medical supervision applies also to the use of *kairin*, *antifibrin*, *antipyrin*, and other drugs which reduce febrile heat, but which also have a tendency to produce nausea, vomiting, and sometimes collapse.]

**FEVER, TYPHUS.**—This disease commences with severe headache, chilliness, loss of appetite, languor, and aching of the limbs. The commencement of the fever is sudden as compared with *enteric* fever, and in two or three days the patient takes to his bed. From the first there is much restlessness and sleepless nights. The head is heavy and confused, with intolerance of light and singing in the ears. When the disease is fully formed, there is a general aspect of a typhus case, which an experienced person will at once recognise. The patient lies on his back, with a dull, stupid expression, the eyes are suffused and watery, and a dusky flush overspreads the face. As the disease advances the eyes are half-shut and the mouth open; the patient lies moaning, and unable to move himself or answer questions; he probably grows deaf; and the lips, mouth, and teeth are dry and covered with black *sordes*. The tongue is covered with black or brown fur, the margins being often pale; and this coat may crack, but the tongue itself does not crack as in *typhoid*. The temperature of the body reaches 104° to 105° Fahr. at the end of the first week, and in favourable cases begins to decline about the fourteenth day. Throughout, the temperature is more sustained than in enteric fever, the morning and evening differences not being so observable. There is also frequently a slight diminution of temperature about the seventh day; and in favourable cases, although the temperature may again rise, it does not rise to the point it attained previously. The pulse ranges during the attack from 110 to 120. On the fourth or fifth day the characteristic rash of typhus appears, probably first on the wrist, then on the bowels and chest. The rash somewhat resembles measles, but soon assumes a darker hue, which has caused it to be termed the 'mulberry rash.' It presents as irregular spots varying in diameter, from three or four lines to a mere speck, being different from the more defined rose-coloured eruption of typhoid; and it must not be mistaken for *sudamina* (*vide* p. 399). Throughout the attack the bowels are constipated, not loose as in enteric fever, and there is often troublesome cough. Unfavourable signs are prostration, muttering delirium, picking at the bed-clothes, bleeding from bowels or nose, blood in the urine, urine and fæces passed involuntarily, starting of the limbs, and insensibility. The average duration of typhus fever is fourteen or fifteen days, when the patient begins to recover, or the bad symptoms as above noted precede a fatal termination, which may not occur until the twentieth day. When recovery takes place the subsidence of the fever is often very marked and rapid, the temperature sometimes falling as much as four degrees in a night. During the progress of typhus there is a peculiar odour from the skin, which has been compared to rotten straw. Deafness, when occurring, is regarded as a favourable symptom. The mortality from typhus fever is one in five of those attacked.

The cause of typhus is considered to be a specific poison emanating from the bodies of persons affected, or which may be generated when human beings are overcrowded in ill-ventilated dwellings. Damp, squalor, filth, and poor diet are also favourable to its development. When typhus fever exists, the disease is communicable, and may be contracted by other persons. It may also be conveyed by contaminated clothing or furniture.

*Treatment.*—As regards ventilation, good nursing, cleanliness, quiet, and disinfection, the remarks under *enteric* are applicable. Similar medicines should also be given for the moderation of the fever. The diet should at first consist of milk and broths; but as there is no injury in the bowels in this disease, so much care under this head is not necessary for so long a period as advised under *enteric* (*vide* p. 245). Brandy or wine will probably be required after the first week. On the cessation of the fever and the approach of convalescence, tonics as quinine and acid (Recipe 67).

The principal distinctions between typhus and enteric fever are shown below :—

| Typhus | Enteric |
| --- | --- |
| Origin connected with overcrowding. | Origin connected with defective conservancy. |
| Occurs at all ages. | Chiefly attacks young people. |
| Onset more rapid than typhoid. | Very gradual and insidious at the onset. |
| Face flushed or dusky, with heavy, stupid expression. | Face pale with pink flush on cheeks, and without the heavy, stupid expression. |
| Eyes suffused and watery. | Eyes bright and clear |
| Degree of fever varies little, if at all. | Fever higher in the evenings, and less in the mornings. |
| Eruption dusky, mulberry-coloured, of irregular form, spots not elevated except at first. The skin appears mottled. | Eruption rose or pink-coloured, regular, defined, spots elevated Skin does not appear mottled. |
| No diarrhœa. | Diarrhœa with yellow stools. |
| No pain of bowels. | Pain of bowels constant. |
| Tongue furred and *fur* cracked. | Tongue furred and *tongue* cracked. |
| Odour like rotten straw. | Not present. |
| Belly soft. | Belly drum-like. |

Cerebro-spinal Fever.—Convulsions, especially of the muscles of the neck, with pain down the spine, may occur during the progress of enteric, of typhus, and of relapsing fever. Sometimes these convulsions are so prominent as to become the leading symptom. This has led to the disease being described as a special fever as above. It should, however, be regarded as a *tetanic* or convulsive phase of the fevers named.

**FEVER, RELAPSING.**—Relapsing fever from the peculiarities of its course, has been called *short fever*, *five-day fever*, and *seven-day fever*, and, from a peculiar condition of the blood noticed below, *spirillum fever*. It is also known as *famine fever*. It is characterised by recurrence at tolerably regular intervals, the succeeding attacks becoming less violent, and the intervals between them more prolonged. Relapsing fever commences with feelings of chilliness, frontal headache, pain in the back and limbs, and prostration of strength. These symptoms may last from one to several hours, when the skin becomes suddenly hot and dry, with increase of headache, of pain of back and limbs, and with thirst. On the second or third day sweating may occur, but without relief to the symptoms. The temperature of the skin ranges from 104° to 108° Fahr., and the pulse from 110 to 120 beats per minute. There is usually no eruption of the skin; but sometimes rose-coloured spots have been observed. Jaundice is often a prominent symptom, sometimes occurring suddenly, sometimes gradually. At first the tongue is moist with yellow fur, then becoming dry and brown in the centre. The bowels are generally constipated, and there is often pain, tenderness, and enlargement of the liver and spleen. Severe shooting pains are felt both in the limbs and in the head, but delirium is rare.

From the fifth to the seventh day there is an abrupt cessation of all the symptoms, generally accompanied by copious perspiration, and occasionally attended with diarrhœa, or bleeding from the nose or bowels. The febrile symptoms are then *absent completely* for a few days, the tongue becomes clean, the appetite returns, and the patient may declare himself well. He may even go about and gain strength, and sometimes there is no second attack. But usually after six or seven days, during which period the pulse is often slower than natural, there is a sudden return of all the symptoms. The relapse lasts from three to five days, when the fever again abruptly declines. Sometimes a second or even a third relapse occurs, but each interval is longer and each attack shorter.

A microbe, which has been named, after the discoverer, *Spirillum Obermeieri*, is often found in the blood and saliva of persons affected with this fever. This worm appears in the form of thin threads, showing corkscrew-like movements. They are usually only found in the blood during the height of the fever, disappearing when the fever declines. It is stated there is no recognisable difference between this spirillum and a worm known as the *Spirillum plicatile*, found in water.

Starvation and destitution are the conditions chiefly tending to produce this disease. But, like other fevers, it is aggravated by overcrowding, want of ventilation, especially as regards the breathing and emanations from the sick, and all other unsanitary conditions. When originated, it is communicable to persons who have not been subjected to want of food, and is therefore contagious. The mortality is about 18 per cent. of those attacked, and the period after exposure to infection till the commencement of an attack is believed to be about eight days.

*Treatment.*—Consists in placing the patient in a well-ventilated room, in promoting cleanliness, and in giving milk and other nourishing diet, such as described in the *paras.* on enteric and typhus fevers. At the commencement of the attack the bowels, if constipated, should be acted upon by a purgative (Recipes 1 and 2). The skin should be daily sponged with tepid water. If there is much prostration with feeble pulse, stimulants will be necessary. During convalescence mineral acids and quinine (Recipe 69) should be given. For some time after the fever ceases the patient requires a generous diet.

**FEVER, INTERMITTENT**, or **AGUE.**—Of Intermittent Fever there are three principal varieties, viz:

The *Quotidian*, or daily ague, coming on every day; usually in the morning. The *Tertian*, or third-day ague, with interval of one clear day; usually coming on about noon. The *Quartan*, or fourth-day ague, leaving an interval of two clear days; usually commencing in the afternoon. Of all varieties, that which returns every day is the most common. But this regularity is not always observed; neither are the cold, hot, and sweating stages, described at page 253, always present as in a typical case. Hence there are *irregular* or *masked* agues, which cannot be classed under any particular form. But in all varieties of ague in well-marked cases the symptoms are similar, and are divisible into the cold, hot, and sweating stages.

*Causes.*—Intermittent and Remittent Fever are both marked by paroxysms of fever followed by decline of the symptoms, although in *Remittent Fever* (*vide* p. 258) the period between the attacks is not so strongly defined by the appearance of returning health. Both fevers are attributed to the poisonous action of MALARIA in the system.

MALARIA has not yet been isolated as a distinct poison. But from various diseases (the chief of which are intermittent and remittent fevers) showing a tendency to *periodicity*, or to renewed force or decline at fixed periods, being found to prevail in certain localities, it has been reasoned that a poisonous emanation arises from the ground, or from something on the ground, to which emanation the term 'malaria' has been applied. Thus, judging from its presumed effects (viz. the prevalence of paroxysmal fever), malaria is mostly produced near the marshy banks of rivers; in the dense jungle usually found at the base of mountain ranges; on lands subjected to periodical inundation or to too profuse irrigation; in dense jungles and ravines; near marshes either of salt or fresh water; in arid, sandy, barren districts with a moist subsoil; and on long-neglected ground freshly excavated or turned up for cultivation. Still, reasoning on observation of the effects produced by malaria, it is supposed to exist in greatest abundance immediately after the monsoons, when the hot September and October sun dries the saturated ground. It has been presumed to be an invisible vapour floating in the atmosphere; but recently the idea has been revived that malaria consists of low vegetable organisms, which have been found by the microscope to exist in the mud of, and in the atmosphere over, certain marshes, which have been named *bacillus malariæ*, and which, introduced into the human system, are said to cause changes in the blood. But so-called malarious diseases have prevailed on all kinds of geological formations, and it is scarcely reasonable to suppose all produce the same kind of vegetable organism. Sufficient malaria having been taken into the system by the lungs, or, as many believe, through the medium of bad drinking-water holding malaria in solution, intermittent or remittent fever is the most usual result; the nature of the disease, and the time when it may appear, being probably determined by the amount of poison received into the system, and by the strength or state of health of the person; the worst variety, or remittent fever, following the largest dose of malaria. On the other hand, the dose of malaria may be so small as to induce no ill effects for weeks, or only to excite the condition presently described as *masked malarious fever*, or even merely simple headache, or *malaise*, or an attack of diarrhœa.

But so frequently do attacks of ague follow cold and chill, that the idea has been advanced, and is gaining ground, that 'chill' alone is sufficient to produce the malady, that there is no such thing as malaria, and that so-called 'malarious influences' are in reality atmospheric or climatic vicissitudes. Unless the *bacillus malariæ* theory is accepted, to which there are fatal objections, malaria is invisible, imponderable, and not recognisable by any chemical test. All that has been taught regarding the characteristics and habitat of malaria has been deduced by inference from *presumed* consequences. *Recognisable* causes of disease may be fairly pitted against hypothetical malaria, as the excitants of so-called malarious disease. Fortunately the means of protection against malaria are the same as the means of protection against other more *recognisable* causes, as cold, damp, and chill.

*Symptoms of Intermittent Fever or Ague.*—Languor, debility, restlessness, yawning, stretching, and a sense of oppression about the stomach. In other instances there is uneasiness or pain in some particular part, as the legs, back, or loins; or there may be burning of the eyes or of the palms of the hands, or beating or other noises in the ears, or simply headache. Often the tongue is coated; there is frequently nausea and sometimes vomiting. Then a chilly sensation is felt all over the body, especially along the spine, the features shrink, the fingers become white and shrivelled, and the skin generally rough. This rough state of the skin is recognised as 'goose skin' or *cutis anserina*, from a more than fancied resemblance to the skin of a plucked goose. This cold feeling may be followed by violent shivering and chattering of the teeth. Sometimes the cold stage, or the shivering attack, comes on without any premonitory symptoms as above referred to. With the shivering, the lips, ears, and nose become bluish in colour, the breathing quick, and the pulse more frequent, while the tongue is white and dry, and severe pains are often felt in the back, loins, and limbs; also nausea and vomiting may be more severe. Towards the end of this cold stage the inner parts appear to burn, while the outer parts freeze. Then, after a very variable time, from a few minutes to several hours, the shiverings and cold sensations gradually become less, and the second or hot stage commences. Flushes of heat are first felt about the neck and face, soon to be followed by the burning heat of the whole body. The face becomes red and flushed, the pulse quicker and strong, the temples throb, and the patient is very restless and irritable. Both during the cold and hot stage there are usually frequent calls to make water, which is passed in increased quantities, but of an irritating or scalding character. At length the sweating stage commences, by moisture first felt on the face and neck, and soon extending to the whole surface. The pulse now lowers to the natural standard, a sense of comfort is experienced, and the patient begins to feel in his usual health, although remaining weak and 'shaky' after the attack. The average duration of a typical attack of ague, such as is here described, is about six hours. But it may terminate much more rapidly, or be very greatly prolonged. Convalescence is marked by scanty, high-coloured, alkaline urine.

The increase of temperature during an attack of ague, as tested by the thermometer (*vide* p. 33), is from the natural standard of 98·4° to 105° or 106° Fahr. The temperature begins to rise several hours *before* the paroxysm sets in, so that, although the patient feels cold, the temperature is really above the normal figure. Also, for some days *after* the disease appears to have departed a periodic increase of temperature may be detected, and so long as this continues the patient is not cured.

Although the above symptoms are always present in a typical case of ague, it often happens, especially after repeated attacks of ague, that the cold stage is not present, or very slightly so, heat of skin coming on without prior shivering. Often the head is affected, and there is, especially during the hot stage, delirium, the patient talking at random, and occasionally failing to recognise his friends. In other instances the stomach is chiefly affected, and there is continued vomiting, neither medicine nor food being retained. And the case may be complicated by affections of internal organs, particularly of the spleen and liver, which will be evidenced by pain or uneasiness in the parts. Certain other maladies, viz. browache, palpitation of the heart, diarrhœa, nose-bleeding, headache, noises in the ears, and troublesome cough, may alternate with ague (*i.e.* may appear instead of the expected ague on every other day).

*Treatment.*—The great object is to shorten the cold and hot stages. The patient should be put to bed, covered with blankets, and have hot bricks or hot-water bottles put to the feet. He should drink freely of hot tea or *congee*, or cold water if more agreeable. A pan containing hot ashes placed under the bed is a useful means of promoting warmth. Emetics are sometimes desirable in the first stage of ague. When there is nausea and inclination to vomit, and when the attack has come on shortly after a meal, a mustard-and-water emetic (Recipe 54) may be given with advantage. But the practice of administering either purgatives or emetics in every case is objectionable. Their operation disturbs and inconveniences the patient, and may expose him to cold at the critical periods of the passage of one stage into another.

*In the second, or hot stage*, the patient should be encouraged to drink freely of cold water (which is one of the best means of promoting perspiration), the body may be sponged with tepid water, or vinegar and water, and cold lotion (Recipe 83) may be applied to the head. Small doses of citrate of magnesia (*vide* p. 15) may also be given, which will tend to promote perspiration and to allay the irritability of the stomach.

*When the patient begins to perspire*, if not profusely, the perspiration should be encouraged by still keeping the body well covered, and by giving tea, or, if preferred, cold water. If weakness is complained of, a little wine or brandy-and-water will be desirable, and he should not sit up for some time, lest fainting may occur. Great care should be taken that the patient does not get chilled when he changes his clothes after perspiration, and he should be carefully rubbed dry with warm towels.

It is during the intervals between the paroxysms that *curative* treatment must be employed. If the bowels are not in good order, if the tongue is furred and the liver inactive, a purgative, as Recipes 1 and 2, should be taken. Then quinine should be administered, either with sherry wine, as Recipe 66, or by itself in water and lime-juice to the extent of 5, 6, 8, or even 10 grains every three hours during the intermission, or until singing of the ears, or noises in the head, or perhaps partial deafness, occurs as an effect of the quinine, when it should be at once stopped. Quinine proves most efficacious when given at the shortest possible interval after the paroxysm, and if the bowels are open the first dose should be given during the sweating stage. Except under medical advice it is not right to give quinine until the fever has abated and perspiration commenced. If this treatment is adopted the next paroxysm may be either altogether stopped or checked in violence. Those subject to ague, and who are well aware of the premonitory symptoms they usually experience, often prevent an attack by an early recourse to quinine, and by attention to the state of the bowels. In some constitutions, or in malarious districts, it may be necessary to give more quinine than the quantities mentioned. 'Experienced hands in ague do not think of measuring or weighing the dose [of quinine] at all, but unhesitatingly take from their bottle, always with them, a flat tea-spoonful of quinine powder, which probably contains about twenty grains.' A generous but easily digestible diet is desirable for those suffering from recurring ague, or when living in a malarious locality. The most likely time for a relapse is a lunar month from the date of the first attack, and preparatory to this, the system should be again brought under the influence of quinine. When ague recurs a change of locality and climate should, if possible, be obtained.

When, during intermittent, the liver, spleen, or lungs become affected, the treatment must be that detailed for such ailments in combination with the quinine treatment for the cure of the ague. Intermittent fever, not being usually attended with any serious immediate consequences, often meets with little attention, particularly in children. But successive attacks will assuredly lead to blood deterioration, anæmia, and enlarged spleen.

[Quinine is not always successful, and when this occurs the fever may probably be re-excited by some disordered condition of the liver and bowels. In such cases it will be desirable to give a laxative, as 5 grains of blue pill every night, and the draught, Recipe 2, every morning, until the motions are of the natural colour; also to alkalise the blood by effervescing draughts (Recipe 36). After two days of such treatment quinine may again be used with greater probability of success.

There are numerous other remedies reputed effective in ague. Thus the 'cinchona febrifuge' (*vide* p. 20) may be successfully substituted for quinine in many cases of fever. Arsenic is the next best approved antiperiodic; and quinine failing, or in cases where quinine cannot be taken in consequence of some peculiar constitutional idiosyncrasy (*vide* p. 18), Recipe 75 may be administered.

In cases of obstinate recurrent intermittent fever it will be desirable to try 'Warburg's Tincture.' This is composed of various aromatic substances digested in spirit with aloes, chalk, and camphor. The following are the directions for the use of this medicine:—Prior to the administering of the tincture it is necessary that constipation of the bowels, if present, be removed by a dose of castor-oil or other form of aperient. For an adult one-half of the quantity contained in the phial should be given unmixed and undiluted, a little before or at the first appearance of the next returning paroxysm of an intermittent fever; the other half, also unmixed and undiluted, after a lapse of three hours. During the interval between the first and second doses, and also for a full hour after the second dose, the patient must abstain entirely from food and drink. Immediately after taking the dose the patient should retire to bed. The perspiration induced by the tincture should be promoted.]

**FEVER, INTERMITTENT, or AGUE OF CHILDREN.**—When a child who immediately before was in its usual health declines its food, yawns, and lolls about, and yet does not complain of feeling ill, an attack of ague may be suspected. If the hands and feet feel cold, while the bodily heat, as tested by the thermometer, is above the natural standard (*vide* p. 33), there is almost certain additional evidence. The suddenness of the attack is usually sufficient to distinguish it from other fevers, and the symptoms do not differ from those in adults. Very similar symptoms sometimes arise from large abscesses, or diseased joints, which points should be inquired into. When ague occurs to children, it has always a great tendency to assume the *remittent* type. Instead of seeming apparently well, children are feverish, restless, and poorly all through the intermission. Occasionally, when pregnant women suffer from ague, the malady attacks the infant in the womb on alternate days, when the shivering of the unborn child is plainly felt by the woman. The treatment of intermittent fever in children must be conducted on the same principles as advised for adults, quinine and other medicines being given in accordance with the age of the patient (*vide* p. 6).

**FEVER, REMITTENT.**—Remittent has been called *Jungle Fever, Teraí Fever, Bengal Fever,* &c., from the locality in which it originated; but all these so-called local fevers are essentially the same. Although remittent fever is usually described as a distinct disease, it is really an exaggerated intermittent. It often commences as an intermittent fever (*vide* p. 251), the *intermissions* becoming less marked until *after a few days* they become *remissions* —that is, the period of apparent health between the paroxysms does not present, the fever only slightly declining or remitting. The symptoms of a remittent fever are those of ague without either any distinct intermission or any distinct cold stage. When the remittent phase of the fever is early declared, the commencement of the attack is still as noted of intermittent fever (*vide* p. 253). But instead of the hot fit subsiding in two or three hours, it continues longer, frequently for eight hours, and is characterised by the pulse becoming quicker, by heavy breathing, with great restlessness and heat of surface; the temperature, as shown by the clinical thermometer, being often, as early as the evening of the second day, as high as 106° Fahr., and the pulse varying from 100 to 120. The countenance is flushed, and the eyes 'bloodshot.' There is generally incoherence or delirium, and often yellowness of the whole body, which come on suddenly, or, more commonly, gradually. There is also sometimes great irritability of stomach, hiccup, and obstinate vomiting, of greenish yellow or brown material, and sometimes of black. After a variable time, usually about six hours, but sometimes not till twelve hours have passed, the *remission* occurs, which is more or less complete, according to the severity of the disease. This is characterised by perspiration, reduced temperature, softer pulse, and sometimes refreshing sleep. But often the *remission* of the symptoms is very slight, and the condition marking the second stage recurs, perhaps without any prior feeling of cold. As a general rule, the *remission* occurs in the early morning, lasting till noon. In severe cases it may be difficult to distinguish the remission, but it should always be watched for. *The continuance of the symptoms, without any prolonged or very decided interval of freedom from fever, constitutes the distinction between an Intermittent and a Remittent.* Also, the occurrence of a *remission*, although slight, is one of the features by which *Remittent* is distinguished from *Typhoid.*

The duration of a single paroxysm of remittent fever may be stated to average about twenty-four hours, but recurring paroxysms (unless cut short by medical treatment) generally tend to become of longer duration than the first. The duration of the disease by such recurring paroxysms is usually from five to seven, nine, or eleven days, but it may last much longer. The days mentioned have been regarded as critical when either a favourable termination or the reverse results. Favourable symptoms are distinct remissions, lowering of temperature and pulse, subsidence of gastric irritability, and copious perspiration. Unfavourable signs are increasing weakness, the passage of blood by stool, blood in the urine, cold sweat, delirium, insensibility; in short, the state described at page 242 as the *typhoid condition*.

During Remittent, affections of internal organs are very likely to present. The occurrence of great irritability of stomach and obstinate vomiting, especially during the hot stage, has already been enumerated among the ordinary symptoms. *This gastric disturbance is sometimes the most prominent and urgent symptom*, every article of food or medicine being rejected. Thus, persons with remittent fever, accompanied by disorder of the stomach, have often been erroneously regarded as suffering from *gastric fever*, the stomach derangement being really caused by the fever present (*vide Disorder of the Stomach*, p. 415). From the effect on the brain, particularly during the remission, sudden fainting may take place, probably after the patient has been imprudently raised into an erect posture, which should therefore be *carefully avoided*. There may be irritation, or even inflammation of the brain or its investing membranes, characterised by great heat of scalp, delirium, and injection or redness of the whites of the eyes, which condition may gradually pass into complete insensibility or stupor. Bronchitis or inflammation of the lungs may occur, when symptoms may present as detailed under the headings of these maladies. Sometimes, during the progress of remittent fever, chest affections arise very insidiously; the symptoms, masked by the fever, not being prominent; and therefore, unless attention is directed to this probability, much mischief may occur before the complication is recognised. Chest affections, it may be noted, are very liable to supervene on remittent fever, occurring to natives, especially in the cold season, of the northern districts of India (*vide* p. 103). Congestion or inflammation of the liver or kidneys may occur, known by pains and other signs distinctive of these maladies (*vide* pp. 318, 314). The spleen may be chiefly implicated (*vide Spleen Disease*, p. 412). Remittent fever and delirium tremens are not unfrequently combined (*vide* p. 161). Diarrhœa may prevail. Dysentery may come on. The attack may be marked by great debility, and tendency to the *typhoid condition* (*vide* p. 242), from the first.

*Treatment.*—In ordinary cases, when no affection of internal organs is evident, a purgative, as Recipe 1, followed after three hours by Recipe 2, should be given daily, until the stools are of a healthy yellow colour and free from all lumpy material. Citrate of magnesia draughts (*vide* p. 15) should also be given two or three times daily. Headache may be relieved by a few leeches to the temples or behind the ears, or, if not so severe, by cold lotions (Recipe 83). Immediately on the first sign of remission, or when moisture of the skin presents, 15 grains of quinine with, if available, half a tea-spoonful of lemon-juice should be given, dissolved in 2 ounces of water. Quinine in 6-grain doses should be administered afterwards every three hours until recurrence of heat and dryness of the skin, when the quinine should be stopped; or until two days have been passed without fever, when the quantity of quinine should be gradually reduced, the more rapidly if singing or noise in the ears or deafness occurs. If the fever returns after the first remission, and after the first doses of quinine have been taken, citrate of magnesia draughts, and laxatives if required, should be again given, quinine being a second, or third, or fourth time resorted to, on return of moisture of the skin and diminution of febrile symptoms. Some practitioners do not wait for the remission of the fever to give quinine, as here recommended. But this plan should only be followed under medical supervision. In the absence of such superintendence, the safer plan will be to wait for abatement of febrile symptoms before administering quinine, as the medicine is powerless to arrest a paroxysm after it has commenced. If, in consequence of the gastric irritability, quinine cannot be retained on the stomach, it should be given in 20-grain doses, in an injection of beef-tea. Vomiting may be sometimes relieved by sucking ice. Quarter-grain doses of ipecacuanha given every two hours may also be tried for the same purpose. Mustard poultices may also be applied over the stomach.

In cases where either the bowels, chest, liver, or spleen is affected, the same plan must be pursued for the cure of the fever. But *when the symptoms point to affection of the brain* quinine should *not* be given, excepting under medical advice. Affections of various organs supervening during remittent fever must be further treated generally as mentioned under the different headings.

During the whole progress of the malady good nourishing diet, in the shape of animal broths or jellies, and farinaceous puddings and gruels, should be given. If great debility occurs, or if fainting feelings are experienced, or if the tongue becomes dry and brown, with weak quick pulse, perhaps also accompanied by muttering delirium, stimulants at regular intervals will be urgently demanded, and which should be given in the quantities, but *subject to the same rules* as mentioned at p. 245 under the treatment of *enteric.* When great debility occurs the patient should not be permitted to sit up, or even to raise himself in bed.

[When from irritability of the stomach quinine is not retained, 12 drops of *strong* nitric acid in an ounce of water should be given instead, until the sickness of stomach subsides. Or quinine may in such cases be injected beneath the skin; but this operation requires a peculiar instrument and special skill. For severe vomiting a pad of lint soaked with chloroform, laid on the pit of the stomach, and covered with oil-silk, is also often beneficial. When the purgative medicines recommended do not produce healthy stools, a mercurial dose, as Recipe 8, should be given. These means failing, 'Warburg's Tincture' may be tried (*vide* p. 257), or the cold bath, or packing (*vide* p. 246), may be desirable.]

Enteric fever being the disease with which remittent fever is most usually confused, the chief distinctive points are given below:—

| Enteric | Remittent |
|---|---|
| Onset gradual. | Onset sudden. |
| Shivering little marked. | Shivering more marked. |
| Temperature does not rise at first for some days. | Early rise of temperature, often on first day. |
| Origin connected with defective conservancy. | Origin connected with exposure to malaria. |
| Usually diarrhœa from the first, with yellow stools. | Constipation at first, or dark bilious stools. |
| Tenderness and pain of bowels. | None. |
| Eruption of rose or pink-coloured spots. | None. |
| No decided remission of fever. | Daily remissions, generally occurring in the early morning. |
| Jaundice, or yellowness of the skin, very seldom occurs. | Often occurs. |
| Gastric symptoms, as nausea, hiccup, and vomiting, occasional. | Gastric symptoms nearly always present. |

**FEVER, REMITTENT, OF INFANTS.**—Infants and children are very subject to fever of the remitting description, although not always arising from so-called malaria. The main symptoms are much the same as those described above, but a shivering fit is very seldom noticed, although the hands and feet feel cold. As in the adult, the malady is marked by *incomplete* cessation of the febrile state. This incomplete cessation of the fever is generally most marked in the early morning, while the aggravation of the symptoms is most developed towards the evening and in the early part of the night. The decline or *remission* is generally attended with some degree of perspiration, but not always. In remittent fever of children there is always a tendency to wandering of the mind, or to convulsions, and delirium or stupor often occurs, the latter accompanied by much restlessness, and probably moaning. Remittent fever in children may occur from a number of causes, of which malaria, the irritation of teething, worms, improper diet, and collection of fæcal matter in the bowels, prolonged diarrhœa, large abscesses, affections of bones and joints, lung affections, and disordered stomach are the chief. In perhaps the majority of cases of remittent fever occurring to children the malady is *not* caused by malaria, but arises from one of the other reasons named. Remittent in children can therefore only be correctly treated by first ascertaining the cause, and then using the remedies recommended for such a condition. When there is no other cause evident, and the attack appears to arise from malarious influences, the bowels, if confined, should be opened by castor-oil, citrate of magnesia (*vide* p. 15) should be given during the paroxysm, at the first decline or remission; or when perspiration appears, quinine in doses according to the age of the child (*vide* pp. 6, 19).

**UNDEFINED CLIMATIC FEVER.**—Called also *malario-typhoid, typho-malarial, typho-remittent, hybrid.* A considerable proportion, if not the great majority, of the fevers of tropical countries are a mixture of several phases based on a few prominent symptoms common to all.

*Undefined climatic fever* commences, like all other fevers, with an indefinite period of languor, lassitude, and chilliness, or sometimes shivering, with more or less headache, succeeded by a gradual, but sometimes by a sudden, rise of temperature. From the time when the temperature rises to 101° or 102° till the date of death or recovery is ordinarily from a fortnight to three weeks, occasionally shorter, but often much longer, extending even to 120 days. During this time there are always morning and evening variations, the range of temperature being sometimes as much as 9°. There are also frequent but variable *remissions*, and often amelioration about every ninth day, when the appetite may return, and the inexperienced be led to believe there is little the matter. Occasionally, also, there is complete abrupt cessation of the fever. Thus, while in the *temperature changes* the fever somewhat resembles *remittent*; in the *duration* of the fever it more resembles *enteric*; while in the *tendency to periodical amelioration* and occasional *abrupt cessation* it simulates *relapsing*. Spots or eruptions may or may not be observed; sometimes the rose spots of enteric, at others the darker spots of typhus, sometimes none. Diarrhœa, light or dark, may or may not occur, while the tenderness, gurgling, and resonance of the bowels marking enteric (*vide* p. 241) are equally uncertain. About the middle of the second week there is generally delirium. During the whole attack debility is strongly marked. The spleen is generally enlarged, often also the liver, and not unfrequently there is sallowness of the skin, or even jaundice. Thus *undefined climatic fever* may sometimes most resemble remittent; at others, enteric, typhus, or relapsing; still not be distinguishable as either, but yet the blurred image, of all. Any complications or sequelæ which occur during or after any other phase of fever may present during or after *undefined climatic fever.*[1]

*Treatment.*—In mixed cases the best treatment is to give quinine as recommended under *remittent*, and otherwise to treat the patient as advised under *enteric.* If the fever is enteric the quinine will do no harm, and is indeed recommended by high authorities for its power of reducing the temperature; while if the fever is *remittent*, the general treatment advised for *enteric* will be applicable.

**FEVER, MASKED MALARIOUS.**—It consists of very slight febrile excitement, which may be *intermittent* or *remittent.* It is often present in delicate females, and is frequently found associated with a scorbutic state of the system. It is common in the autumnal and winter season among the inhabitants of notoriously malarious districts. The individual affected complains chiefly of heat, dryness, and burning in the palms of the hands, less frequently in the soles of the feet, and he may be annoyed by occasional periodic beating or singing in the ear. There is more or less general uneasiness, perhaps slight headache, and depression of spirits, but no decided pain anywhere. The pulse is not excited; the skin, excepting in the palms, does not feel warm to the touch; but the clinical thermometer will show that the temperature is higher than natural. The appetite probably remains good, but the sleep is restless. The burning of the palms may be

[1] It has been sought to explain the undefined or hybrid fevers met with in the tropics by regarding them as *enteric* modified by *malarial poison*, or as *malarious* modified by *enteric* poison. With this view the author does not agree. He holds there is one disease, *Fever*, of which fevers described as distinct diseases are simply phases or modifications; the particular phase depending on the temperament, constitution, and surroundings of the individual. This is not the place for a discussion on the subject, which will be found in the author's 'Manual of the Diseases of India,' second edition, article 'Fever.'

persistent, with slight remissions, when the parts become a little moist; or there may be distinct intermissions. This condition may prevail for months or even years, and is oftentimes so slight as scarcely to attract much attention. But in other instances it constitutes a perpetual source of discomfort. Persons so affected are not especially prone to attacks of fully developed fever. They appear often to escape the latter by the morbific influence expending itself in the constant induction of the masked form. But they generally become *anæmic* (*vide* p. 46). To this condition the term *malaria cachexia* is often applied.

*Treatment.*—Quinine (Recipe 66) or other tonics, and attention to the general health. A liberal diet and a moderate amount of wine or beer, with coffee at least once a day. So-called *malarious cachexia* is often benefited by lemon-juice. A fresh unpeeled lemon should be cut into thin slices and put in a pint of water, which should be boiled down to two-thirds of a pint in an earthenware jar. The liquid should be allowed to stand all night, and should be strained and taken in the morning. Change of climate is the certain remedy.

[The other tonics referred to above are iron and arsenic (Recipes 70, 75, 76). A condition resembling masked fever sometimes arises from saturation of the system with quinine or arsenic, given for the cure of fevers. The blood is poisoned by these agents; which, although necessary to cure fevers, are known to be capable of exciting a febrile condition. If it should appear that a continued use of quinine or arsenic has induced a febrile state, mild purgative and diuretic medicines should be administered (Recipes 9, 2, and 50), with the view of eliminating such excitants from the system. If the patient is not too debilitated, the Turkish bath may also be used (*vide Appendix, Baths*).]

FEVER, YELLOW, is an infectious fever which usually confers protection against a second attack. It ordinarily commences suddenly with shivering, followed by fever. There is constipation, much headache, troublesome vomiting, tenderness at the pit of the stomach, redness of the eyes, and pain in the back and limbs. On the third or fourth day the symptoms subside, and the person may recover. But most frequently the stomach tenderness returns and black vomit sets in, *i.e.* the vomit contains blood, the stools being dark from the same cause. Jaundice also occurs, and the patient sinks into the typhoid condition (*vide* p. 242). It is stated that, although common in other hot climates, yellow fever does not occur in India, which may be doubted, as black vomit sometimes appears in cases called remittent. *Treatment* consists in supporting the strength by light liquid nutritious food and stimulants, which, if not retained on the stomach, should be given as injections. Liquefied carbolic acid in four-minim doses every three hours as a medicine.

**FEVER, DENGUE.**—Usually the first symptoms of dengue fever are headache, restlessness, chilliness, debility, pains in the back, limbs, joints, and eyeballs of a very severe character, with more or less feverishness, and often irritability of the stomach. But dengue sometimes commences with a sudden pain in some joint, and without symptoms as enumerated above. Shortly afterwards, generally within twelve hours from the first feelings of uneasiness, an eruption of a red or scarlet character appears on the face, chest, palms, and elsewhere, lasting about forty-eight hours. During the fever the temperature rises to 103° or 104°, while the pulse ranges to 120 beats in the minute. But this rise of the heat of the body and the increased frequency of the pulse only last during the limited first febrile state, and the condition is not ordinarily indicative of danger. As the rash disappears the fever lessens, and for two or three days there is generally an almost complete cessation of pains and fever. Then, with an accession of fever, a second eruption, more resembling that of measles, occurs, probably first seen on the palms of the hands. This may be so slight as to escape notice, or it may last a few hours or persist for two days. Sometimes this second rash resembles 'nettle rash' rather than measles, and there is often intense itching, and sometimes scurfiness of the skin as in measles. This second fever and second eruption often leave the patient much weakened and depressed, with rheumatic soreness, stiffness, and pains in the joints, and perhaps enlargement of the glands of the neck or groin. A third attack may also occur. Dengue fever prevails epidemically, and is contagious. It attacks both adults and children—even infants—when the startings occasioned by the pain may be mistaken for convulsions. But the after pains, so distressing in grown-up people, seldom cause much trouble to infants and young children, who recover with rapidity. Dengue fever, from the accompanying eruption, has also been called 'red fever,' also 'scarlet rheumatism.'

*Treatment.*—Attention should be directed to the state of the bowels, and constipation, if present, should be relieved by Recipe 1, followed by Recipe 2. If there is much fever small doses of citrate of magnesia (*vide* p. 15) should be given; if there are sleeplessness and great pain in the limbs, but the head is *not* complained of, 10 or 12 grains of Dover's powder, or 20 grains of chloral, may be given at night. If there are periodical returns of pain or feverishness, quinine, as Recipe 66. Warm baths in which a couple of pounds of common washing-soda has been dissolved are also useful. For children little treatment is required. A senna purgative (*vide* p. 26) and cooling draughts of citrate of magnesia will be advisable, and if the child is teething the gums should be lanced if hot and swollen.

[Tincture of belladonna in 10-minim doses often relieves the pain and mitigates the fever. This may be given three times a day in water. Or colchicum mixture (Recipe 52) may be tried if belladonna is not efficacious.]

**FEVER, HECTIC.**—Hectic fever is a consequence of profuse or of long-continued discharge from an abscess (*vide Abscess*, p. 41), or from the lungs, as in consumption (*vide* p. 142), or from *diseased joints* (*vide* p. 311). Hectic fever does not declare itself as long as the matter is pent up; but after matter begins to flow hectic fever may be expected. The fever always commences towards evening, and declines in the early morning. Often the commencement of the attack is marked by shivering or sensations of cold. Then the skin becomes hot and dry, while the eyes look brilliant, the cheeks flushed, and the pulse rises to 120 beats in the minute. The urine passed is turbid and offensive; the bowels are usually costive at first, but after repeated attacks diarrhœa generally prevails; the tongue presents a white fur in the centre, while the tip and edges are clean and red (*vide* p. 36). There is often considerable headache, restlessness, and a complaint of burning heat felt in the interior of the body. After a variable time, generally in the early morning, the skin becomes moist, and the fever terminates in profuse sweating, often attended by great exhaustion. During the day the patient remains free from fever. The appetite often remains good, and is sometimes excessive. But periodical recurrences of hectic are always attended with failing strength and increasing emaciation; consequences both of the fever and its termination in profuse perspiration, and of the discharge of matter causing the fever. As a rule, a hectic patient is easily depressed and easily excited; his mind is buoyant and hopeful, and as soon as relieved from present distress he is sanguine of recovery. Hectic fever may continue for weeks or months, or as long as the exciting cause—the discharge of matter—persists. After a variable period diarrhœa occurs, and this is an unfavourable sign, as it adds much to debility.

*Treatment.*—This consists of a liberal diet, meat, chicken, game, broth, soups, jellies, being given to as free an extent as the digestion of the patient will allow. A small quantity of port wine will also be advisable, but it should not be used towards evening, as it may add to the febrile excitement. The best time for the stimulant will be at the period of exhaustion consequent on the termination of the fever in the characteristic debilitating perspiration. Broths, soups, and jellies may also be *offered* at this time, but should not be forced on the patient, whose appetite will probably return later in the day. As medicine, cod-liver oil, iron, and quinine, either in combination or alone, will probably be required. If a wound exists, matter should be prevented 'bagging,' or collecting in sinuses or fistulæ, by suitable dressings (*vide* pp. 43, 44). If the strength permit, carriage exercise, or even walking exercise short of fatigue, may be taken with advantage. But the most important point is placing the patient under good general sanitary and individual hygienic conditions, avoiding all late hours and excitements; plenty of fresh air, especially in the sleeping-room, coupled with avoidance of chill.

[Perspiration may be usually lessened by acid mixture (Recipe 43) taken every two hours on the accession of the fever. Diarrhœa may be combated by Recipe 46, or, if this does not succeed, Recipe 47.]

**FISTULA.**—This term is applied to any sore which burrows under the skin. A deep-seated abscess, having only a small opening through which the discharge passes, comes under the denomination *Fistula*, and, if extensive, is a condition with which *hectic fever* (*vide* p. 269) is often associated. Fistula may occur in almost any part of the body, but the term is more popularly used with reference to fistula near the *anus*. This, technically termed *fistula in ano*, results from the formation of abscess. The cause of abscess near the anus is sometimes obscure. External injury, or internal injury, as from a swallowed fish-bone sticking in the gut, may excite abscess. When matter forms near the anus it is characterised by throbbing pain and fever, and the parts should be fomented and treated as advised for *abscess* (*vide* p. 41). As matter forms a swelling becomes apparent, and it usually points close to the orifice of the anus, and should be opened *early* with a lancet (*vide Abscess*, p. 44). Then the abscess may gradually cease discharging matter and heal, or otherwise a fistula remains which usually communicates internally with the gut. The treatment of nearly all kinds of fistula requires surgical operation.

**FISSURE or ULCER OF THE ANUS.**—This consists of a crack or ulcer of variable extent, situated at the junction of the skin with the gut, and extending inwards. The causes are habitual constipation, and the passage of large hard stools. Scratching the part in consequence of some local irritation sometimes originates fissure. It is very frequently associated with piles. The chief symptom is pain on going to stool, of a very acute character, often continuing for hours. Often the fæces are streaked with blood; and if the fissure is deep and large, there may be bleeding each time the bowel acts. There is also usually frequent spasm of the muscle round the orifice of the anus, accompanied by intense pain. The spasmodic pressure thus exerted by the muscle gives the stools a flattened or ribbon-like appearance. It may cause irritability of the bladder, and in females symptoms referable to the womb. When such symptoms present, fissure or ulcer may be suspected; but the fact cannot be ascertained without examination. The treatment requires laxatives (Recipe 2) to soften the fæces and prevent straining at stool. Or injections of warm water may be administered for the same purpose. The parts should be kept very clean with soap and water, and be bathed several times daily with alum wash (Recipe 100). But when the fissure is deep or large, a somewhat painful although slight surgical operation will be required.

Instead of alum wash, if available, use carbolic acid lotion (*Appendix*, No. 119). Caustic (nitrate of silver) is the best local application; and in simple cases, if applied to the bottom of the fissure, previously well washed, often effects a cure.

**FITS.**—The term 'fit' is commonly used to signify almost any sudden attack; especially such as Apoplectic, Epileptic, Hysterical, and Fainting. These are treated of in the order named at pp. 53, 216, 234.

**FLATULENCE.**—Flatulence is an accumulation of gas in, and its discharge from, the stomach and bowels. The gas formed is generally sulphuretted hydrogen (*vide* p. 203); but in hysterical females it is inodorous and chiefly carbonic acid. Flatulence causes rumblings, colicky pains, nauseous eructations, vomiting, and palpitation of the heart. Care in diet, and abstaining from those articles of food after which flatulence occurs, is more satisfactory than medicines. Thus sugar, pastry, rice, sago, and arrowroot are not well digested by those subject to flatulence. Flatulence, however, can only be radically cured by considering it and by treating it as a symptom of dyspepsia (*vide* p. 197) or of hysteria (*vide* p. 305).

**FLATULENCE OF INFANTS.**—Flatulence or 'wind' in the stomach of infants usually results either from food being unsuited to the child, in which case it should be changed; omitting sugar, increasing the quantity of water and adding salt, is often successful. Or flatulence may arise from the child taking food too quickly, or in too large quantities, which should be guarded against. It is frequently the cause of great suffering to the child, from the pain it occasions in the bowels. Infants thus affected scream violently, often stopping for a few moments suddenly, as though straining, and their legs are drawn up towards the bowels. The best means of relief is rubbing the child's belly gently with the palm of the hand, and a few grains of citrate of magnesia (*vide* p. 15) may be given. If this does not stop the pain in the course of ten minutes, a drop or two of chlorodyne (*vide* p. 12) in a little water.

[A much better remedy, however, is the magnesia and aniseed mixture (Recipe 22), which should be procured from the chemist.]

**FLUSHING OF THE FACE** is a symptom of dyspepsia often met with, without much other disturbance of the health, and generally occurring after meals. It frequently occurs to women about the 'change of life.' If any article of food is followed by flushing, it should be avoided, and little or no wine or other fermented drinks should be used. The bowels should be maintained moderately open, and plenty of exercise should be taken.

[In some instances 10 drops of dilute sulphuric acid in water three times a day is very serviceable. For the flushing of females at the 'change of life,' if attended with mental depression, bromide of potassium (Recipe 19) may be used; if attended with hysterical symptoms, weight in the head, and perspirations, tincture of nux vomica may be taken in 2-drop doses, in a dessert-spoonful of water two or three times a day. For flushings with 'hot and cold perspirations,' nervousness, throbbing at the temples, and 'fluttering' at the heart, valerianate of zinc 2 grains, extract of gentian 3 grains, made into a pill, may be taken three times a day.]

**FUNGUS FOOT DISEASE** is most common in Western India. It principally attacks natives, and is supposed to arise from the entrance beneath the skin of a vegetable spore or germ. It is generally seen in the feet, but may occur in other parts. Its first sign is swelling under the skin, in which may be seen a bluish or black appearance. After a variable time the skin bursts, and an open sore results, discharging a black substance with matter. The removal of the diseased part by surgical operation is the only means of cure.

**GALL-STONES.**—Gall-stones are small substances which form by the deposit in the gall-bladder, of certain elements of the bile, present in too great redundancy. Their formation is much favoured by sedentary habits, want of exercise, and too much animal food. Mental worry also predisposes to gall-stones. Women are more liable to the complaint than men. So long as the stone remains in the gall-bladder it is not productive of inconvenience, and often its presence is unsuspected. But the flow of bile sometimes carries a stone into the short duct or tube leading from the gall-bladder into the intestines. This often occurs after a full meal, or after some muscular effort. A small stone may pass through the tube without causing any, or only slight, pain. A larger stone causes sudden attacks of shivering, followed by excruciating pain, immediately to the right of the pit of the stomach, shooting to the back, with vomiting, first of the contents of the stomach, and then of sour bile. There is occasionally sudden jaundice, when the stone, exactly fitting the tube, blocks the passage altogether. If a small stone remains impacted in the duct the flow of bile is prevented, but not altogether stopped, and jaundice comes on more slowly. From the pain mentioned above there are intervals of comparative ease, and pressure will, to a certain extent, relieve it, the person throwing himself about the bed, or pressing his thighs on the belly to get relief from change of posture. This distinguishes the malady from inflammation, when pressure and motion are painful. In exceptional cases an impacted gall-stone may excite inflammation of the parts. And a gall-stone may sometimes become the cause of obstruction of the bowels (*vide* pp. 81, 82).

The passage of *gall*-stone may be mistaken for the passage of *gravel* stone from the kidneys, especially if the right kidney is affected. The distinctions are as follows :—

| Gravel Stone | Gall-Stone |
|---|---|
| Pain in loins, usually on one side. | Not. |
| Pain shooting from loins down groin and thighs. | Pain to right of pit of stomach shooting to the back. |

| Gravel Stone | Gall-Stone |
|---|---|
| On either side. | Pain most on right side. |
| Numbness of thigh or leg. | Not. |
| Testicles drawn up. | Not. |
| Frequent desire to make water. | Not. |
| Making water may be painful. | Not. |
| Water scanty, high-coloured, or bloody. | Not altered. |
| Not so frequent. | Shivering usual. |
| Vomiting usual. | Vomiting usual. |
| Previous history of gravel. | Previous history of gall-stone. |
| Most common in men. | Most common in women. |

*Treatment.*—If possible a hot bath, or otherwise the painful part should be fomented with very hot water. At the same time the part may be gently shampooed or kneaded. If the attack comes on after a full meal, an emetic (Recipe 54). If not after a full meal, a tumbler of hot water in which a tea-spoonful of carbonate of soda has been dissolved. Chloral to the extent of fifteen grains every three hours for three doses. If much sickness exists, the chloral should be given as an enema. If the bowels are costive, Recipes 1 and 2 should be administered as a purgative. During the attack the patient should try and walk about. At the end of an attack the fæces passed should be examined for gall-stones, by washing the stools through muslin or through a sieve. Gall-stones are brown or greenish-yellow in colour, are round or oval, or where several have been in the gall-bladder rubbing together, they may present flattened facets. They vary in size, from that of a millet-seed to that of a peppercorn. In exceptional cases they may be as large as a walnut. It is always desirable to ascertain whether gall-stones have or have not been passed, because if a single stone comes away *smooth and round*, it may be assumed there are none left behind, and that the trouble is over. Persons subject to gall-stones should always keep the bowels well open, for which Carlsbad salts or Hunyadi Janos water are recommended. Very plain living, abstinence from fatty substances, no spirits or beer, and a fair amount of exercise are the other means of prevention.

Various preventive measures have been recommended, viz. olive oil from four to eight ounces every day; sixty minims of liquor potassæ in a glass of beer three times a day; from ten to twenty drops of a mixture of three parts of sulphuric ether and two of oil of turpentine, to be taken in capsules thrice daily; phosphate of soda sixty grains twice or three times a day. Whichever of the above is chosen must be continued for some weeks. But none of them are advised excepting the phosphate of soda, which may be obtained in the effervescing form, the most pleasant method of taking this aperient; dose, from one to three drachms. Occasionally a gall-stone may be felt and pressed out of the gall-bladder, but this should not be attempted except by a medical man.

**GASTRIC DISEASES.**—Gastric diseases are stomach complaints. The term *Gastric Fever*, in common use, conveys an erroneous idea of a fever of a special type, the fact being that it is one or other of the varieties of fever accompanied, as mentioned to be the case (*vide* p. 239, 241, 255, 260), with great irritation of the stomach, pain, and obstinate vomiting (*vide Disorder of the Stomach*, p. 415).

**GIDDINESS or VERTIGO.**—This sensation is often described as 'dizziness,' or 'swimmings,' not amounting to actual fainting. Objects around appear to be moving in different directions. There is a sense of dimness or darkness, and perhaps sounds of bells or drums in the ears. There is loss of power to balance the body, with more or less mental confusion. It varies much in intensity, and may be frequent or occasional. In many cases it is only felt on movement, as on rising quickly, or in certain positions, as when the head is hanging down. Giddiness may occur as a symptom of simple weakness or debility, or as premonitory to a fainting fit. Or it may be connected with disordered stomach, or indigestion, or gout. It may arise from excesses of various kinds, from tobacco, and from too much mental work. It often occurs to females at the 'change of life.' In other instances it may be premonitory of epilepsy or apoplexy, or be consequent on diseased heart. Giddiness must therefore be regarded as a symptom of disease rather than as a disease itself (*vide* p. 37), and the conditions causing it must be discovered and treated. For temporary relief sal volatile (*vide* p. 8).

**GLANDS, ENLARGED.**—There is a system of minute vessels throughout the body termed *absorbents*, and on their course are little bodies termed *glands*. In health these glands are scarcely perceptible, but when enlarged they attract notice. The glands most liable to enlargement are as below.

ENLARGEMENT OF THE GLANDS OF THE NECK.—This occurs in young persons, especially if of scrofulous habit, and is often absurdly spoken of as the 'glands of the ears down.' The glands may enlarge, remain swollen for days, or even weeks, and then subside. But they sometimes inflame, gather and form matter, and cause an ugly sore, which leaves a disfiguring scar. When the swelling is not painful and *before throbbing* indicates the formation of matter, cold lotion (Recipe 83) should be assiduously applied. If this does not *stay* the gathering, it should be *hastened* by poulticing, and when the matter points, the abscess should be opened with a sharp lancet, the puncture being made longitudinally, or in a line with the folds of the skin of the neck, by which a remarkable scar will be avoided. After matter has ceased to flow the part should be dressed as an ordinary ulcer. Quinine and nourishing diet should be given. If possible a surgeon should be consulted early before the glands inflame as to the propriety of removing them by operation.

[If the enlargements are not tender, and there is no throbbing pain, iodine paint should be applied daily (*vide Appendix*, No. 111). Cod-liver oil should also be given. If the patient is pale and feeble, citrate of iron and quinine (Recipe 70). Previous to the formation of matter, sulphide of calcium is recommended. Take of sulphide of calcium 2 grains, sugar of milk 40 grains, to make 20 small pills or powders. For a child three years old, one every four hours, dissolved in water; at six years old, two powders.]

THE GLANDS OF THE ARMPIT may enlarge from similar cause, or from injury to the hand, or from cancer of the breast.

THE GLANDS OF THE GROIN may swell and gather from similar causes, or from venereal disease, forming bubo (p. 109).

The treatment of the two latter descriptions of enlarged glands is the same locally as when the glands of the neck are affected. But general treatment must depend upon the diseases causing the enlargement.

ENLARGEMENT OF THE GLANDS OF THE BOWELS is referred to at p. 67.

Lastly, swelling of the *glands behind the jaw* not unfrequently occurs, forming *mumps* (*vide* p. 338).

**GOÎTRE, or DERBYSHIRE NECK.**—This consists in enlargement of the thyroid gland, which is a gland situated in the front of the neck. It sometimes attains a great size, causing, by pressing on the windpipe and blood-vessels of the part, difficulty of breathing, difficulty of swallowing, headache, and prominence of the eyes, change in the pitch of voice, which becomes reduced, and sometimes diminished muscular power on one or both sides of the body. A severe form of the disease is called *exophthalmic goître*, or 'Grave's disease,' in which prominence of the eyes is a very marked symptom. Goître is frequently associated with idiocy, and a condition called *cretinism*, in which there is imperfect development and deformity, especially of the head. Both forms of goître are most common in females. It occurs principally in hilly districts, and particularly where lime is contained in the water. It has therefore been thought due to the latter cause, and removal to another locality is a better remedy than any medicine.

[The best application is biniodide of mercury ointment (Recipe 94), which should be rubbed on the part daily, the patient sitting in the sun or before a large fire; iodide of potassium (Recipe 21) internally.]

A condition termed MYXŒDEMA sometimes occurs in connection with affections of the thyroid gland. Myxœdema results more in connection with atrophy or shrivelling of the gland than with enlargement. It is characterised by swelling of the skin, especially of the face, which appears enlarged, and of the hands, which lose shapeliness. The skin looks waxy, dry, and rough. But the skin does not pit on pressure with the finger as in dropsy (*vide* p. 186), the cause of the swelling not being water but a gelatinous deposit. A similar deposit takes place in internal organs. Irritability of temper, slowness of speech, loss of memory, are other results. The malady principally occurs to adult females. Tonics, as quinine, iron, and arsenic, and medicated baths, are desirable. Preparations of the thyroid glands of sheep have been advised as curative.

**GONORRHŒA.**—Gonorrhœa arises from contagion. It may occur in either the male or female. It commences, usually on the third day after exposure, with itching and redness of the urinary passage, accompanied by a thin whitish discharge. In two or three days there is swelling of the private parts, severe scalding pain in making water, and a copious discharge of thick yellowish-coloured matter. The groins, thighs, and testicles ache and are tender, and there is often, particularly during the night, partial hardness of the penis, known as *chordee.* The duration of gonorrhœa is from ten to twenty days.

But gonorrhœa frequently causes one or other of the affections enumerated below. The inflammation may extend to the *testicle* (*vide* p. 438). The *bladder* may become inflamed (*vide* p. 70). *Bubo* may form (*vide* p. 109). *Phymosis* or *paraphymosis* may be excited (*vide* p. 346). Inflammation of the end of the penis, called *balanitis,* may occur (*vide* p. 282). *Gonorrhœal rheumatism* is another sequel (*vide* p. 282). Gonorrhœal *warts* may grow (*vide* p. 282). *Retention of urine* may result (*vide* p. 420).

*Ophthalmia* may result (*vide* p. 228). *Lastly, gleet* may remain, and ultimately cause *stricture* (*vide* pp. 282, 419).

*Treatment.*—If the disease cannot be treated at the onset, as mentioned in small type, the bowels should be kept freely open by sulphate of soda (Recipe 2), and citrate of magnesia draughts (*vide* p. 15) should be given. Pain may be relieved by fomentations, or hot hip-baths, by chloral, or by chlorodyne. If chordee occurs, the part should be immersed in cold water, and thirty drops of spirit of camphor (*vide* p. 24) may be taken in water. In all cases rest, in bed if possible; the person should drink plenty of barley water or potash water; the diet must be low, fermented liquors, spiced dishes, and coffee being avoided; and the part should be well supported and not allowed to hang down.

[If gonorrhœa in the male be detected at the first, when only a little itching or watery discharge is present, it may be often cut short by injecting, once every four hours, a solution of nitrate of silver of the strength of 2 grains to 8 ounces of water. (For method of injection, *vide Appendix*, Injections.) This should be repeated six or eight times, desisting sooner if the discharge is in the least bloody, or if any pain is excited. The patient should take an aperient, as Recipes 1 and 2. After the aperient he should take 1 drop of tincture of nux vomica every hour, in a tea-spoonful of water. He should also lie down as much as possible, and the private part should be enveloped in a rag kept wet with a lotion (Recipe 84).

As soon as the patient is free from febrile symptoms, he should take copaiba prepared in a capsule, which may be swallowed like a pill, and the nauseous taste thus avoided. But in some persons copaiba induces an eruption like 'nettle-rash.' If so, the following mixture may be substituted. Infusion of cubebs (made by infusing 1½ ounce of bruised cubebs in 12 ounces of water) 12 ounces; iodide of potassium 1¼ drachm. Dose—2 table-spoonfuls three times a day. A sulphate of zinc injection, as Recipe 98, should be used twice daily.]

*Gonorrhœa in the female* is marked by the same symptoms as in the male. There is heat, pain, and swelling of the parts, pain in making water, and in walking. For females, internal remedies are useless. For the first few days warm poppy-water (*vide Appendix*, No. 81) should be used daily, with a female syringe, as an injection; and afterwards alum injection (Recipe 100) should be made tepid, and injected frequently and freely.

The treatment of the affections mentioned as sometimes resulting from gonorrhœa is as below:—

When the *testicle* becomes affected, injections, if being used, should be discontinued; and the treatment indicated at p. 438 should be adopted. When the *bladder* is inflamed the treatment should be that mentioned for inflammation of the bladder (p. 70), and injections, if being used, should be discontinued. The treatment of *bubo, phymosis,* and *paraphymosis* is given at pp. 109 and 346. *Balanitis* means an eruption of, and discharge from, the end of the penis, accompanied with much pain and swelling, for which frequent bathing and washing with warm water and soap, and afterwards alum wash (Recipe 97), is the best treatment. *Gonorrhœal rheumatism* presents the same symptoms as acute rheumatism (*vide* p. 367), and is to be similarly treated. *Gonorrhœal warts* arise from the irritation caused by the discharge, aided by uncleanliness. Warts should be washed twice daily with salt and water, and then sprinkled with *calomel*, which generally cures without pain; but warts may require to be cut off by a surgeon. The treatment of retention of urine is indicated at p. 421, of ophthalmia at p. 228. *Gleet* signifies a watery discharge, accompanied by scalding. It is often tedious, requiring lengthened treatment and very temperate living. The daily use of a sulphate of zinc injection (Recipe 98) and attention to the general health, with iron and quinine, will generally prove successful. *Stricture* may arise from neglected gleet, when the discharge will not cease until the stricture is treated (*vide* p. 420).

**GOUT.**—Gout is a very painful affection arising from *lithic acid* being generated in the blood and deposited in the parts. Lithic acid may be formed as the result of prolonged excess, or indiscretions in diet causing defective action of the liver or kidneys; or it may be a consequence, in persons hereditarily predisposed to gout, of failure of action of the liver and kidneys, even without evident indiscretion in diet. In some characteristics gout resembles rheumatism. But gout first attacks the smaller joints, as the toes and fingers; rheumatism the larger joints. Gout generally attacks the indolent and those feeding luxuriously; rheumatism, the ill-clothed and ill-fed poor. Gout is a disease of advanced life; rheumatism often attacks the young. But gout may be combined with rheumatism, when it is known as rheumatic gout.

An attack, or, as popularly termed, 'a fit of gout,' is usually preceded by irritability of temper, feverishness, headache, and symptoms indicating indigestion. Gout most frequently comes on during the night. There is acute grinding pain in the part, most usually the great toe, abating towards morning, but leaving the toe red and swollen, tender and shining. There is also acid perspiration; the patient's temper is increasingly irritable; and the urine, at first scanty, high-coloured, and clear, afterwards becomes more copious, and deposits a sediment resembling pink sand or pounded brickdust. For several nights the pain may return, although it is usually lessened as the swelling increases. As the pain and swelling subside the skin of the part peels off in flakes. The disease then disappears, perhaps not returning for months. Repeated attacks may lead to ulcers and *chalk-stones*. Gout may occur in the fingers with similar results. The nails of gouty persons become hard, brittle, and marked with lines. In rarer cases it may suddenly leave the toe and attack the stomach, which will be known by sudden and excruciating pain at the pit of the stomach, with flatulence, faintness, nausea, and feeble irregular pulse. Gout may also attack other internal organs, causing giddiness, bronchitis, asthma, and affections of the skin, eye, ear, heart, and brain. This is due to the deposition of lithic acid in the parts affected; but such conditions can only be diagnosed or treated by medical skill.

*Treatment.*—On the approach of the attack, or 'fit,' the bowels, if confined, should be moved by Recipes 1 and 2, and in the absence of *colchicum*, mentioned in the small type below, sulphate of soda should be given in 2-drachm doses three times a day. But the medicine must not be allowed to depress the patient, and should be reduced in quantity if it acts too much on the bowels. The local treatment consists in wrapping the inflamed part in cotton wool, previously steeped in a strong hot solution (4 drachms to 1 ounce of water) of carbonate of soda, and then keeping the limb well raised from the ground, and as still as possible. In all cases warmth is the great thing, cold having a tendency to drive the gout to some internal organ. Rest must be absolute, and the diet must consist only of milk, arrowroot, and the like. Toast water, Vichy water, or seltzer water may be taken freely. If there is need for a stimulant, Scotch whisky or gin may be used in small quantities, but for a time stimulants are better avoided.

*After the fit* the diet should be mainly vegetable. Fish is better than flesh, and chicken than beef or mutton. Sweets and articles containing sugar must be altogether avoided. As a rule fermented liquors should not be taken, although in some instances a little claret, chablis, hock, or gin-and-water does no injury. Regular exercise and attention to the bowels, so as to prevent costiveness, are also enjoined. If the attack cannot be traced to high living or indiscretion in diet, the kidneys or liver, or both, will probably be in fault, and the urine will be clear and pale, or the stools light and constipated. In such conditions citrate of magnesia (*vide* p. 15) and Recipe 1 will be useful.

*If the stomach is attacked,* brandy-and-water must be given, and mustard poultices should be applied to the feet, with the view of restoring the external inflammation.

[Those liable to gout should obtain colchicum wine and colchicum and potash mixture (Recipe 52). On the approach of a fit of gout, 30 minims of colchicum wine should be taken in a couple of ounces of water and afterwards the colchicum and potash mixture (Recipe 52) every four hours until the pain ceases, or until depression or nausea results. Usually this will stop the attack in twenty-four hours, after which in any case the treatment should not be continued without an intermission of a day. Also, if there is any affection of the heart, the colchicum treatment should not be pursued, except under medical supervision. Cotton-wool on which half a drachm of chloroform has been scattered is a better local application than the carbonate of soda mentioned in the large type. If this does not succeed, a lotion composed of acetate of lead 1 drachm, acetate of morphia 3 grains, water 8 ounces, should be obtained and applied *warm.* It should be recollected that it is *poisonous.* When after an attack of gout there are dyspeptic symptoms, Recipe 13, as a dinner pill. The following prescription may be also taken with advantage: Citrate of lithia 80 grains, citric acid 3 drachms, syrup of orange peel 3 drachms, distilled water 16 ounces, to be made into a mixture. Bicarbonate of soda 3 drachms, distilled water 16 ounces. Two ounces of each mixture to be taken *together* while effervescing. As preventive of gout the use of the waters of the places mentioned below may be advised: Aix-les-Bains, Bath, Buxton, Cheltenham, Contrexéville, Harrogate, Leamington, Wiesbaden, Vichy, Carlsbad, Kissingen, Aix-la-Chapelle.]

**GRANULATIONS** are little red portions of flesh which grow in and fill up wounds. When more than ordinarily luxuriant they are commonly called 'Proud Flesh.' Granulations are the consequence of the natural healing process. When they are high, pale, and spongy, they require touching with alum, or sprinkling with powdered loaf-sugar, which reduces their growth and allows the wound from which they spring to heal.

**GRAVEL.**—Gravel signifies a deposit in the urine. There are two principal kinds, viz. *red* and *white* gravel.

*Red Gravel* is composed of *uric* or *lithic* acid, or of other salts termed *urates* (the principal being *urate of ammonia* or *soda*) more or less mixed with the colouring-matter of the urine. Sometimes, from variation of the latter, such deposits are rather pink than red. The urine of persons passing red or pink gravel is clear, acid, of dark golden colour, and often less abundant than the urine of health. After it has cooled the red or pink deposit appears as a sediment. Persons noticing such deposits in the urine after it has stood are apt to believe they may aggregate and form a stone. If voided with the urine, or if the deposit occurs before the urine has completely cooled, there is such risk. But not if the sediment disappears by heating the urine in a test-tube, or silver spoon, to the temperature of the interior of the body, about 100° Fahr.

*White or Yellowish Gravel* consists chiefly of crystalline salts formed from the urine, the principal being *phosphate of lime,* or *ammonio-magnesian phosphate of lime.* This kind of gravel is of more grave significance than the presence of red or pink gravel. The white or yellowish gravel is formed from the urine *before* it passes from the body, and the urine is therefore *turbid when passed*, and if heated does not become clear like urine containing urates.

The passage of *red* or *pink* gravel is connected with a variety of conditions. Tawny or reddish sediments arise from a common cold, and are frequently associated with heartburn, acidity of the stomach, and other symptoms of indigestion or disordered liver, consequent on too rich diet. The pinker varieties are generally associated with acute rheumatism or gout, often following or alternating with attacks of the latter malady. Sometimes passing red gravel causes dull pain in the loins, and repeated calls to make water, but frequently there are no symptoms referable to the urinary organs; but of *malaise*, headache, and depression.

When *yellow gravel* is passed there are shooting pains in the loins, running towards the groin and thigh, often numbness of the leg, with desire to make water, and pain at time of doing so. In the male the testicles are usually spasmodically drawn up. These symptoms are accompanied by feverishness, constituting what is popularly termed 'a fit of the gravel.' In some instances, without warning, the patient is seized with a most acute pain in the back and loins, accompanied by violent sickness and vomiting. There is frequent tendency to pass urine, which is scanty, high-coloured, or bloody. At length, during a violent retching, the patient experiences a sudden sensation as if he were stabbed, and from that time his acute pain gradually ceases. When these symptoms happen to a person passing white gravel, a small gravel-stone, formed in the kidneys, has passed through the ureter (a small tube connecting the kidney and the bladder) into the bladder, where it may remain, increase in size, and become stone in the bladder, or from which, if small enough, it may pass out with the urine. (For the distinctions between passage of gravel and gall-stones, *vide* p. 275.) But if a gravel-stone is too large to pass from the kidney to the bladder, it may remain in the kidney and excite inflammation or abscess (*vide* p. 314).

*Treatment.*—When a 'fit of the gravel' occurs, the great desideratum is the relief of pain. The patient should be placed in a hot bath and be given 25 grains of chloral, which may be repeated in six or eight hours if the pain continues or returns. Fomentation (*vide Appendix*, No. 80) may be used over the loins; and the bowels, if confined, should be opened by a purgative (Recipe 2). The patient should also drink plentifully of barley water, or linseed water, or weak tea.

[When the *red* variety is present, a diet chiefly vegetable, and in some cases strictly so, should be adopted. Sugar, tea, coffee, pastry, butter, cream, should be avoided. Alkaline medicines (Recipe 35) should be given so long as the urine remains, as it generally is in such cases, of an acid character. This may be ascertained by testing the urine daily with *litmus* paper sold for such purpose. Acid urine turns blue litmus paper red; alkaline urine turns red litmus blue. Aperients, such as Recipes 1 and 2, should be taken every other night and morning. Alkaline aerated waters, as Vichy or seltzer, are often very beneficial.

The time when the urine is most acid, and alkalies are most required, is about three hours after the principal meals. An alkali and an aperient may be then combined with a bitter tonic as follows. Take of bicarbonate of soda 10 grains, sulphate of soda 2 drachms, infusion of orange peel 3 table-spoonfuls, for a draught to be taken a couple of hours after eating. When indigestion, red gravel, and costiveness are combined, this will be found very useful, and the salts may be increased or diminished according to circumstances.

In cases of white or yellow gravel the urine is faintly acid or alkaline, and acids are the best medicines. *Dilute* nitric acid may be given in doses of 20 minims in water. Tonics, as quinine, will also probably be required. When yellow gravel is deposited, a more generous diet may be allowed than when red gravel appears, and a moderate quantity of wine will usually be proper. Meat, soup, milk, eggs, good bread, sound sherry, or bitter ale, are the articles to be preferred. Sugar, pastry, sago, arrowroot, and bad wine are to be avoided. Fresh vegetables, as cabbage, lettuce, mustard and cress, may generally be taken with advantage, but not rhubarb.

In all cases of gravel, and especially when *lithic acid* is passed, the amount of water drunk should be increased. A tumbler of hot water should be *sipped* in the morning, middle day, and in the evening. Too long time should not elapse between meals, as eating lessens the acidity of the urine; and persons should not lay too long in bed, as urine then lingers in the kidneys and bladder, and is more likely to deposit. Warm baths, friction with rough towels, flannel clothing, and exercise short of fatigue are desirable.]

**GUINEA WORM.**—The usual positions in which it appears are the lower extremities, but it may present in almost any part of the body. Attention is generally first attracted by the feeling of a thin cord beneath the skin, or otherwise by the formation of the characteristic blister always attending the presentation of the end of the worm on the surface of the skin. The blister so forming assumes the size of half a pigeon's egg, and is frequently accompanied by itching of the body, or by an eruption like 'nettle-rash.' When the blister breaks or is opened, it is found to contain a glairy whitish fluid, in which the end of the worm may be found, thin and fragile as a hair.

A full-grown guinea worm may be three feet long. It is slender, about the thickness of packthread except at the extremity, where it is attenuated to the calibre of a hair. It is opaque, of a milk-white colour. On each side there is a longitudinal line, and when examined with the microscope it is seen to be marked with numerous transverse *striæ* or stripes. The interior of the worm contains a vast number of young worms rolled up in coils. The young or ova of the guinea worm are believed to exist in the water of dirty tanks and wells, and they probably enter the system in two ways. They may penetrate through the perspiratory ducts, of which there are some 3,500 in every square inch of skin, or they may be taken into the stomach with drinking-water, making their way thence into various parts of the body. However the ovum or young worm is introduced, it slowly grows until it attains several feet in length, giving probably, during this period, little or no indication of its presence. The period which elapses from the reception of the embryo into the system till the appearance of the worm is from three to six months.

*Treatment.*—The end of the worm as it presents in the blister should be caught by, and coiled round, a roughened feather stem. Then, by very delicate management, a little may be extracted daily, by gradually winding the worm round the quill. But care must be taken lest the worm break, or lest the part of the worm round the quill becoming dry breaks, even without the application of force. An alum lotion (Recipe 100), applied with lint over the part, both softens and strengthens the worm, and so tends to prevent breakage. Extraction should only be attempted once in twenty-four hours, when perhaps an inch, and perhaps a foot, may be gained. The force applied should not be great, and the pulling should be delicately and yieldingly managed. During the invervals between extraction the quill should be secured to the adjacent part

U

by strips of sticking-plaster. Slight friction with oil along the line of the worm tends to loosen it. Also a stream of water over the part will often assist extraction. If the worm breaks, abscess and fever are the general results. The part must then be poulticed, and any matter forming liberated by means of the lancet; and if the broken end of the worm can again be seized, it should be extracted gradually, as before. Otherwise it comes away piecemeal, with matter forming in various parts of its course, entailing an oftentimes long, tedious, sometimes dangerous illness.

If the worm can be felt lying beneath the skin for a considerable distance, and there is therefore reason to believe its situation is altogether superficial, it may be cut down upon, a ligature passed beneath it, and the worm may be gradually extracted. But this should not be attempted without skilled advice.

**GUMBOIL** is a small abscess, generally commencing in the socket of a carious tooth, and bursting through the gum; or, if neglected, through the cheek. There is great tenderness of the tooth, especially on pressure, severe throbbing and aching pain, and a feverish condition of the body.

*Treatment.*—Fomentations are useful at first; but as soon as matter can be detected it should be liberated by a prick with a lancet. If the tooth causing the gumboil is much decayed, or there is only a fang, it should be removed; otherwise there will be a succession of gumboils.

**HAIR.**—1. Loosening and Falling off of the.—In young persons this may occur from natural weakness of constitution; or it frequently happens after fevers, or to women who have suffered much during childbirth. First, the ends of the hair over the whole head should be snipped off. Then the long hair should be carefully separated, and the weak short hair snipped once every nine days. The head should be well washed with solution of 'areca nut' every morning, and then rubbed with a rough towel sufficiently to cause heat and redness of the scalp. The use of the brush should be frequent, and it should be so employed as to cause warmth to the scalp. The above measures are more applicable for women desiring long luxuriant hair than for men. The hair of men will be best preserved strong and thick in India by keeping it cut short, and by cleanliness and the use of the brush. *Scurf* or *dandriff* is to be got rid of and prevented by similar means.

[When this does not do good, the following will be found to be an excellent application:—Take of olive oil 2 ounces, bicarbonate of potash a quarter of an ounce, solution of ammonia a quarter of an ounce, tincture of cantharides 2 drachms; mix well. To be applied by rubbing on the surface of the scalp and at the roots of the hair, after washing with cold water. It should produce a glow. An excellent hair-lotion for after-use is—2 ounces of eau de Cologne, 2 drachms of tincture of cantharides, 10 drops of oil of rosemary, and 10 drops of oil of lavender.]

2. Falling off of the Hair in Patches.—If the patches are circular, and pimples are seen on the denuded part, or at the roots of the hair round it, or if hairs are seen broken, or running in an unnatural direction, ringworm is present (*vide* p. 389). When no pimples are seen, and the skin of the denuded portion is quite white, it is the affection known as *Alopecia*, and for this a strong solution of borax of soda applied daily will be the best means of cure.

**HEADACHE.**—Headache is a symptom of disease rather than a disease itself (*vide* p. 37.) The principal kinds of headache (which may be distinct, but are often combined) are as follows:—

1. Dyspeptic Headache may arise from stomach, bowel, or liver derangement. When the stomach is most in fault, the pain is of a bursting or throbbing character in the forehead, and may be attended with nausea. Pain

without nausea occurs to stronger persons who have exceeded in eating or drinking. The pain sometimes ceases suddenly with a 'click' felt at the pit of the stomach, and which signifies the escape of some indigestible article of food from the stomach into the next part of the intestines (*vide* p. 198). Such headaches may sometimes be relieved by a draught of soda-water, or by a dessert-spoonful of citrate of magnesia in water. If they commence shortly after a meal, a mustard-and-water emetic will often afford effective relief. When the liver or bowels are most in fault, there is tightness across the head, and the pain is of a stupefying character. In such cases the bowels should be moved, and Recipes 1 and 2 may be used.

2. Nervous Headache.—This is common in delicate persons leading a sedentary life, and in nervous females about the monthly period. Those subject to this headache are usually pale, feeble, and easily flushed or excited, and the headache is often brought on by mental or emotional excitement. The pain may be confined to one spot, or it may be general, especially over the front part of the head. It is sometimes preceded by, or attended by, a peculiar defect of vision, consisting of the appearance of a small hazy spot, which gradually extends into a zigzag halo of light. Nervous headache occurring to women at the monthly periods is frequently spoken of as *megrims*. Hysterical girls are often subject to attacks of nervous pain in one particular spot, which has been likened to driving a nail into the head, and hence the Latin name *clavus* has been given to it. Stumps or bad teeth often localise nervous pain in the jaws. Those liable to nervous headache usually feel chilly, listless, and depressed before an attack. They often wake in the morning with a slight degree of pain, which disappears in a short time. Or they may awake suffering severely, unable to swallow food, and probably feeling sick. The head throbs, and movement

is painful; the face is pale, the pupils contracted, and there is often a dark appearance under the eyes. The head feels hot, and the application of cold is generally refreshing. The patient begs to be left alone and to be quiet.

Nervous headache may arise without evident stomach or liver derangement, but such conditions are often present when nausea, retching, and vomiting, may occur, which does not give relief. Persons who suffer from it, if not erring in quantity of food, do so as regards quality. Many abstaining from alcoholic stimulants drink tea or coffee in excess, and thus irritate the nervous system. Others, intent on business or pleasure, neglect taking food at the proper periodical hours; some, forgetful that motion is one of the laws of existence, remain in close apartments without exercise; and some inflict injury on their nervous systems by the immoderate use of tobacco. Relief at the time is to be best obtained by repose, sleep, and sal volatile. To escape nervous headaches the habits must be altered. The immoderate tea or coffee drinker must take milk-and-water; the devotee to pleasure or business must relax; the indolent or sedentary must adopt regular hours and exercise; the tobacco-smoker must abandon the practice, or at least lessen his consumption; lastly, plain wholesome food must be substituted for made dishes and pastry. When headache of this character occurs to females about the monthly period, bromide of potassium (Recipe 19) may be taken.

3. TIC-DOULOUREUX is an affection of the nerve (*trifacial*) which, proceeding from the brain, divides on each side into three branches. The upper branch (*supra-orbital*) perforates the bone above the eyebrows; the middle branch perforates the cheek-bones below the eyes; the lower branch perforates the middle of each side of the lower jaw. All then divide into numerous filaments,

which are distributed to adjacent parts. The upper branch is the division most usually affected by tic, hence the term BROW-AGUE, or BROW-ACHE. But sometimes the pain is localised in the eye itself, and it is then often spoken of as *migraine of the eye*. When the middle branch of the nerve is affected, the pain may be localised in the upper jaw or teeth, especially if the latter are decayed. When the lower branch of the nerve is affected, the pain may be localised in the lower jaw, the teeth, or in half the tongue. Occasionally, when the whole three divisions of the nerve are implicated, exactly half the face, or even half the head, is painful, and the term *hemicrania* is applied. Tic-douloureux has also been termed 'sun-pain,' as sometimes it only continues as long as the sun is above the horizon. As it usually occurs at intervals, it has been called *intermittent headache.* Lastly, it may be included in the general term *neuralgia*, or *facial neuralgia* (*vide* p. 341). The description and treatment of *brow-ache*, which is the most frequent phase of facial neuralgia, is applicable, *cæteris paribus*, to the other varieties.

BROW-AGUE or BROW-ACHE is always most prevalent in so-called malarious localities, and sometimes takes the place of a paroxysm of ague; that is, a person may have ague one day and brow-ache the next. It occurs at regular intervals, as daily, or every second day, and is confined to the course of the *supra-orbital* nerve, commencing from near the middle of the eyebrow, and passing outwards across the forehead. It may be preceded by or attended with twitching or drooping of the eyelid. The pain is very intense, and increases in paroxysms, causing the eyes to water and the nose to discharge, and rendering the sufferer unfit to attend to any business. Sometimes there is a visible red line in the track of the nerve. It may persist during the whole day, but ordinarily subsides in the course of two or three hours. In those subject to it it may be excited by dyspeptic derangements. Any cause, in fact, which produces a strong impression on the nervous system of those who are disposed to it will bring on an attack. Exposure to heat, and fatigue, working late at night, chill and cold, damp, dinner parties, loss of usual rest, will frequently re-excite the malady. When women have been subjected to weakening influences, such as frequent child-bearing, prolonged suckling, or profuse menstruation, there are additional reasons rendering the system more liable to brow-ague.

*Treatment.*—In India first attacks are generally of malarious origin, and may be cured by 5- or 6-grain doses of quinine every three hours, preceded, if necessary, by Recipes 1 and 2, to open the bowels. 1 grain of quinine mixed with 3 of starch, used as a snuff, will often afford relief. Decided relief is to be obtained sometimes by pressure with the finger over the most painful part; sometimes by a tight wet bandage round the head; by quiet, and by a darkened room. Holding the arms above the head occasionally gives ease. Hot tea or coffee will also often soothe the nervous system and give relief; or, in some cases, a glass of wine or a dose of sal volatile. Medicines at the time of pain do not, as a general rule, do much good. A small mustard poultice may be placed on the temple or forehead. Equal parts of chloral and camphor, mixed together, form a syrupy liquid, which, rubbed on the parts, generally affords much ease. Sometimes hot fomentations give most relief, but in the majority of cases more ease is experienced from cold or ice. Repeated attacks will be generally due to a combination of the effects of malarious or debilitating influences, and stomach or liver derangements, and therefore, existing indigestion and dyspepsia must be first treated, after which tonics, as quinine (Recipe 66), may be used. When the malady occurs to females, attention to any irregularity of the monthly flow is demanded (*vide* p. 467). Bad teeth should also be attended to.

[If quinine does not stop the attacks, iron should be tried (Recipe 71), and this not proving successful, arsenic (Recipe 75). But each tonic should have a fair trial of at least a fortnight's duration. Antipyrine, given in 10- to 15-grain doses in two or three ounces of water, thrice daily, often affords immediate and marked relief, but should not be continued more than two days. Local applications are Recipes 89, 90, 91, the latter being perhaps the most generally successful. Chloroform applied to the part on a piece of lint, and covered with a watch-glass to prevent evaporation, is often beneficial. Cocaine injected beneath the skin is probably the most successful.]

4. BRAIN HEADACHE.—Different from the above varieties is headache occurring in older persons, and caused by what is popularly known as a 'flow of blood to the head.' It often presents as 'warnings' (*vide* p. 53) of more serious disorders, as apoplexy or sunstroke; or from the stoppage of accustomed discharges, as from piles; in women not unfrequently occurring in consequence of the 'change of life.' In such cases the habit of body is usually full and plethoric, the complexion florid, and giddiness is apt to come on in stooping. In severe cases the pain is throbbing, with redness of the eyes and flushing of the face, a feeling of tightness across the head, a fulness or whizzing behind the ears, and often thirst and feverishness.

*Treatment.*—If the pain is slight, purgatives (Recipes 1 and 2), no stimulants, restricted diet, rest from brain-work, and care against exposure to the sun, with moderate exercise. When severe, with feverishness, rest in a sitting posture, quiet, cold lotions to the head (Recipe 83), cutting the hair short, and eight or ten leeches behind the ears.

5. RHEUMATIC OR GOUTY HEADACHE.—Headache may be due to rheumatism or gout of the muscles of the scalp. The pain will be felt to be *outside* the head in the scalp, becoming worse on wrinkling the forehead; there will be

pain in other parts, and probably red deposit in the urine. *Treatment* by alkalies and colchicum, as advised for *Rheumatism and Gout* (p. 282).

**HEART, DISEASES OF.**—To distinguish the diseases of this organ requires a high degree of medical skill, and accurate knowledge of the anatomy of the organ, a correct ear to judge of the sounds of the heart, and much practice. When the heart is affected there are alterations of the sounds only to be appreciated by the educated ear of a medical man. But in addition to alteration of sounds, there are other symptoms indicative of heart disease. Intermittent pulse, palpitations, fainty feelings, a sense of weight and oppression, shortness of breath, livid face, cold extremities, pain in the left arm, and swelling of the legs all more or less accompany heart disease. But some of these symptoms also accompany indigestion, so that without a knowledge of the healthy and diseased sounds of the heart a proper conclusion regarding the true significance of such symptoms cannot be arrived at. If, however, pain or uneasiness in the left breast is accompanied (without any evident cause) by pain in the left arm, or by other signs as enumerated above, and if dropsy or swelling of the legs occurs, unless the patient be a young woman with disordered menstruation, some serious malady may be suspected. When such is the case the following rules may be always adopted:—1. *The work of the heart should be lessened* by resting a good deal in the recumbent posture, by avoiding stimulants and sudden changes of temperature. 2. *Regularity of the heart's action should be ensured* by avoiding mental excitement, by avoiding sudden muscular exertion (as rapid walking, lifting heavy weights, &c.), by not partaking of a large distending meal, by not drinking large draughts of cold fluid, by guarding against indigestion and constipation.

HEART, PALPITATION OF THE.—This, being a very

common symptom, requires special notice. The term denotes a sudden and irregular action of the heart, often accompanied by sensations of distress and faintness. In the majority of cases this does not signify serious disorder, but is caused by indigestion, flatulence, or tobacco. It often accompanies anæmia, hysteria, and amenorrhœa (*vide* pp. 46, 305, 468), and is common during pregnancy. Palpitation arising from disease of the heart itself and palpitation depending on other causes may be distinguished as below.

| *Palpitation depending on Disease of the Heart* | *Palpitation arising from other Causes* |
|---|---|
| Most common in men. | Most common in women. |
| Comes on gradually. | Comes on suddenly. |
| Constant, though more marked at one time than another. | Occurs at intervals of perfect freedom. |
| Frequently accompanied by pain in the left shoulder. | Frequently accompanied by pain in the side. |
| Lips and cheeks often livid, and countenance florid. | Countenance pale. |
| Most common after forty-five. | Most common in young persons. |
| Often not much complained of by the patient. | Usually very much complained of. |
| Sounds of the heart altered. | Sounds of the heart healthy. |

To relieve palpitation give a tea-spoonful of sal volatile in a glass of water, or a little wine; attend to the state of the digestion; use remedies for constipation if prevailing, and forbid tobacco and strong tea or coffee.

HEART, SPASMS OF THE, also called *Angina Pectoris*, and *Suffocative Breast Pang*.—Occurs chiefly in advanced life. It is a temporary stoppage of the heart, and is attended with *intense* pain of a shooting, tearing character, extreme difficulty in drawing the breath, great anxiety, and sense of impending death. The attack ordinarily passes off in a minute or two. It leaves the patient tolerably well, but weakened. The first paroxysm usually occurs when the patient is walking uphill, or after a heavy meal, especially if taken at night. The attack is very likely to recur, but at no fixed interval, months or years sometimes elapsing. It is rarely that the earlier attacks of breast-pang terminate fatally; but as the spasms depend on organic change in the heart or its arteries, *angina pectoris* is a most serious malady.

*Treatment.*—During the attack, a stimulant, as wine or brandy, is required immediately, and afterwards remedies to relieve any attendant dyspepsia. The great point is to ward off future attacks, and this is only accomplished by the greatest care in diet, and by refraining from all exertion which accelerates the breathing. A person subject to this disease should carry an ounce of brandy, or a tea-spoonful of sal volatile in a little water, on his person, which should be taken immediately on an attack.

[The best remedy is *nitrite of amyl*, which is a pale straw-coloured liquid having an odour something like pineapple. Five or six drops should be sprinkled on the pocket handkerchief, which should be held to the nose and mouth, so that the vapour may be inhaled. Or it may be obtained in glass capsules, each containing enough for a single inhalation, to be carried in the pocket.]

**HEARTBURN.**—This term is applied to a feeling of heat in the chest and throat, often accompanied by hot or cold acid eructation of watery matter (*vide Water Brash*, p. 204). This malady has nothing to do with the heart, but is a symptom of indigestion, and should be treated as dyspepsia (*vide* p. 207).

**HICCOUGH.**—Consists of sudden, short, convulsive, spasmodic *inspirations*, attended by a peculiar sound produced in the *larynx* or upper part of the windpipe, and immediately followed by *expiration*. These convulsive inspirations often occur in paroxysms, and may succeed each other at intervals of a few seconds. The paroxysm may last only a few minutes, or may extend to hours or days. Hiccough in most instances arises from indigestion, or from food being hastily swallowed. But it is sometimes present as a symptom during the progress of diseases of the liver and stomach, and it may come on after cholera. When depending on indigestion it may be generally relieved by taking a few grains of bicarbonate of soda and ginger, or by a little brandy-and-water. Sometimes in the case of indigestible food lodged in the stomach vomiting is required to produce relief, and a mustard emetic may be given. Spirits of camphor, chlorodyne, and sal volatile are also good remedies. Swallowing a piece of ice will sometimes give relief. When the attack is slight it may often be stopped by making a very full inspiration, and then holding the breath as long as possible. Strong pressure, as a belt tightly drawn round the body, over a pad on the pit of the stomach, will sometimes stop hiccough. Or pressing firmly near the end of the collarbones next the throat with the thumb may be successful.

**HOUSEMAID'S KNEE.**—This term is applied to inflammation of the 'bursa,' or little water-bag situated over the knee-cap. The *front* of the knee-joint is swollen and tender, with a feeling of 'crackling' if touched, and there is considerable pain. It results from injury or from constantly kneeling; hence the term 'housemaid's knee.' The swelling should be leeched, warm fomentations should be applied, and perfect rest enjoined. After recovery a bandage should be worn for some weeks.

**HYDROPHOBIA.**—The saliva from the mouth of a rabid animal, as a dog, jackal, wolf, or cat, is the poisonous agent causing this disease. A very slight wound, either from teeth or claws, if saliva be on the latter, is sufficient to introduce the poison into the system. After a bite from a mad dog hydrophobia may come on after some weeks, or it may be delayed months, or even, in exceptional cases, years; but it is rare after the fortieth day. It does not follow that everyone bitten by a mad dog must suffer from hydrophobia. The saliva may be wiped off by clothing, through which the animal's fang passes; or the person may escape without any assignable reason. Only one in twenty of those bitten by mad dogs suffer.

*Symptoms.*—In most cases there is slight irritation at or near the scar of the wound, and there may be vague feelings of uneasiness, melancholy, gloom, with irritability of temper, frightful dreams, or shivering. Sometimes there is twitching of the muscles of the face, also in many cases fear and dismay lest hydrophobia should occur. After a few hours or days the patient complains of stiffness of the neck and difficulty of breathing, which suddenly pass into suffocative spasm, most probably on some occasion when the patient attempts to drink. These spasms recur at variable intervals of minutes or hours, and eventually extend from the throat and chest to the muscles of the whole body, which are convulsed. The face is turgid, the eyeballs protruding, the patient foams at the mouth, and claws at the throat as if to remove some obstruction. These general spasmodic seizures are succeeded by intervals of ease and relaxation. Between the spasms saliva which cannot be swallowed collects about the mouth, causing perpetual hawking and spitting. At first these spasmodic attacks are excited only by attempts to swallow fluid; afterwards the sounds or sight of fluids, suggestions to swallow anything, movements or looks of bystanders, draughts of air, rays of light, the sight of anything white, or of a dog, may excite spasms. As the throat spasm spreads to wide convulsions, so the mental distress may proceed to frenzy, causing the patient to rush wildly about, in a state of maniacal fury. It is popularly supposed the patient barks like a dog, for which the hawking has been mistaken; and that he tries to bite his attendants, for which the spasmodic movements of the jaws have been mistaken. The ordinary duration of hydrophobia is from one to four days, after which the person dies exhausted, or suffocated from spasm of the throat. Hydrophobia may be mistaken for tetanus, and the distinctions are given at p. 440.

In some cases, at the commencement, or before the beginning of the disease, the presence of a vesicular eruption under the tongue has been noted. This has been thought distinctive of hydrophobia, as other eruptions are of other diseases. This should be looked for daily. It should also be looked for in persons who have been bitten by a mad dog, as it has occurred as early as the third day after the injury, long before any other symptoms.

There is an affection, arising from nervous influence, or fear, after an injury by an animal which is *not* mad. This is called *spurious* or *false hydrophobia*, but the symptoms are very similar to those of the real disease. Instances of reputed recovery from hydrophobia are usually from this false form of the malady, which may be regarded as present when it can be proved that the sufferer has *not* been injured by a rabid animal.

*Treatment.*—Recovery is rare. Bromide of potassium (Recipe 19) should be given every hour, and ten grains of chloral every four hours. Thirst may be alleviated by ice, and mustard poultices should be applied to the upper part of the chest. A darkened room, protection from draughts, quiet, and nourishment if it can be taken, are important. Sometimes the patient can swallow nourishment if he shuts his eyes. If the eruption under the tongue is found, all the vesicles should be pricked.

*Symptoms of Rabies or Canine Madness.*—The dog affected is at first restless and irritable and hides in corners, while food is refused. The look is suspicious and 'sneaking,' the tail drooping, and there is often redness or watering of the eyes. Sometimes the animal wanders about looking for bits of paper or pieces of straw, which it seizes and eats. It is also fond of rubbing the nose on cold objects. The bark becomes changed and hoarse, the hair set or 'staring,' and the dog snarls and snaps at children and others with whom he was previously on the best of terms. In a short time saliva begins to flow from his mouth, and the throat becomes inflamed, but there is no dread of fluid, as in the human subject, the dog lapping water during the whole illness, which, however, is often not swallowed, but flows out of the mouth.

*Treatment of the Bite of a Rabid Animal.*—The poison remains dormant near the wound until hydrophobia is excited, and does not, like snake poison, enter the system immediately. When the arm or leg is bitten, a pocket handkerchief or piece of string should be tied tightly round the limb above the bite. The person should then forcibly suck the wound; or, if from position he is unable to do so, some friend may perhaps perform the office. No danger is incurred, provided there is no wound on the lips or mouth of the person sucking. As soon as possible the bitten part should be cut out if surgical aid is obtainable, and water-dressing applied. If not done at the time it should be effected days or even weeks afterwards, *should the person appear fearful of hydrophobia.* If position forbids cutting the part out, several punctures should be made near, and bleeding should be encouraged, as recommended for snake bite, p. 608. But when the patient is not seen until the wound is healing, it will be better, in the *absence of fear*, and in the absence of symptoms, to leave it alone. In all cases everything should be done to reassure the patient, and he should be made to understand that all has been done which can be effected.

If after a bite from a mad dog the person will not submit to the knife, or if a sharp knife is not at hand, nitrate of silver may be thoroughly applied; or, if not available, strong nitric acid or sulphuric acid, or caustic potash, or boiling oil, may be applied to the wounds. One or two drops of either of the agents named should be dropped into the wound, taking care that the fluid used does not run over the surrounding skin. Or the *actual cautery* may be used. This means a red-hot iron, such as a thick iron wire, introduced for a few moments into the wound. The pain of the actual cautery is not nearly so acute as is supposed, especially if the iron is very hot, and if it is pressed firmly against the part. Filling the wound with gunpowder, and flashing the gunpowder, is also a ready method of destroying the virus which may have been introduced.

*Hydrophobia, Prevention of.*—M. Pasteur has proved that inoculation renders dogs proof against rabies, and similar success has been recorded after inoculation of the human subject. But this cannot be regarded as an established method of either prevention or cure. It does not follow that a person bitten will get hydrophobia, and before prevention is asserted it must be proved that the person would have had hydrophobia, or success must be invariable, which is not the case, deaths having occurred from hydrophobia after inoculation. Moreover, there is reason to believe that inoculation excites other anomalous affections, especially *paralytic hydrophobia*. Another method of prevention is M. Buisson's daily vapour bath at a high temperature for seven consecutive days, by which it is asserted the poison is taken out of the body in profuse perspiration. Neither of these methods is recommended.

**HYPOCHONDRIASIS.**—This condition, popularly known as *hypped*, or *the vapours*, may be regarded as the correlative in the male sex to hysteria in the female. It may arise from too good living and too little exercise, combined with absence of mental occupation. Or it may originate from overworking the brain, or from worms. The person fancies himself the subject of various bodily ills, and does not believe if told there is little the matter with him. Very frequently there is some functional disorder of the liver, or indigestion, present, which laxative medicines and exercise in the open air will soon carry off. Next to slight dyspeptic symptoms, the most common complaints of the hypochondriac are of neuralgic pains of a burning character, but not the throbbing, excruciating aching of true neuralgia (*vide* p. 341). For the proper *treatment* of this malady the cause must be sought. The person suffering from the effects of severe or long-continued mental labour will require relaxation and bodily exercise; the man having nothing to do will require some employment. Medicines are not of much use. When a person is really 'hypped,' there is only one decisive remedy—namely, change of air and scene. A very short time will often work wonders, and it is in such cases that the ability to take three months' leave for the trip to England is invaluable. It often happens that 'home-sickness,' or longing for home, known as *nostalgia*, is a prominent idea in the mind of the hypochondriac. And this is especially the case with natives of one part of the Eastern Empire serving in another, and who are often the subjects of the hypochondriacal condition. It would appear as if this longing for home were nature's method of pointing out the path of cure.

**HYSTERIA.**—A deranged state of the nervous system of females, especially those in easy circumstances and of sedentary habits. Hysteria manifests itself in two ways: *first*, by a long train of nervous symptoms; *secondly*, by attacks of convulsive fits, commonly called 'hysterics.' A person may suffer from the nervous symptoms presently named, and from occasional hysterical fits; or she may suffer from occasional hysterical fits, the intervals between such fits being more or less free from nervous symptoms.

The principal nervous symptoms are flushings, flatulency, hiccup, palpitations, difficulty of breathing, choking sensations, a feeling as of a ball in the throat, and loss of voice. Pains in various parts of the body are also very common. One called *clavus* is described as like a nail being driven into the head (*vide* p. 292). The left side, the nipples, the joints, are also often affected. Nearly every ailment may be simulated by hysteria, and the patient will plaintively detail symptoms very similar to those of real disease. Thus it may be supposed that an hysterical female is suffering from inflammation of the bowels, or of the womb, or of the throat, when there is nothing of the kind the matter. Stiffness, or. even paralysis of a joint, affections of the spine, retention of urine, structure of the gullet, are well-known hysterical complaints. But all pains described by hysterical females are *terrible*, and not in accordance with those of the real disease. The skin is touched, and the patient screams; but on pressing firmly there is no increase of pain, which would be the case were inflammation and real disease present. The face is not worn, and expresses no suffering. There is a peculiar expression, and a drooping of the eyelids, very characteristic of hysterical persons, and questions are answered abruptly. The temperature of the body, as shown by the thermometer, is not increased, whieh would be the case if inflammatory disease were present. *Lastly*, there is the history of the hysterical tendency, as evidenced by the minor symptoms first mentioned; so that there is rarely any difficulty in arriving at a correct conclusion, whether a malady presenting in an hysterical person is real or the reverse. As a rule, the disorder is, in the mind of the patient, firmly believed to exist; and there is no doubt that the pains complained of are real (although nervous pains), and aetually felt by the patient. But in some instances hysterical persons are fond of making diseases, and will stick pins or needles into the flesh, or swallow them for that purpose. They will sometimes refuse food, unless they ean obtain it surreptitiously; or they will secrete and swallow blood or other fluid, so that they may afterwards vomit it up, as if from disease. Frequently, in cases of hysteria, the monthly functions are irregular: or there may be worms.

Similarly, *hysteric convulsions*, or the *hysteric fit*, is very different from other convulsive affections. It is preceded by sobbing, yawning, hiccup, feeling of a ball rising in the throat, or sensations of choking. There is no insensibility, and the countenance is natural. The patient, if she falls, does not do so heedlessly, but in some comfortable place, and avoids injuring herself. There are convulsive movements of the limbs, which are, however, still partly under the control of the will, and there is often alternate crying and laughing. After the fit there is frequently a copious discharge of light-coloured urine. For distinction from epilepsy, with which it is most likely to be confused, *vide* p. 218.

*Treatment.*—During the paroxysm the dress should be loosened, plenty of fresh air should be allowed, a fan should be used, and cold water, vinegar, or eau de Cologne may be sprinkled on the face, smelling-salts, or the smoke from burnt feathers applied to the nostrils, and the extremities should be well rubbed. If the patient can swallow, a tea-spoonful of sal volatile in a wineglass of water may be administered. If the person is young, strong, and healthy, the mouth and nostrils may be compressed or closed, until efforts to breathe become powerful and then suddenly let go, which often terminates the fit. In prolonged cases cold water may be poured from the spout of a kettle on the head. Hysterical persons should not, however, be treated roughly; for it does not follow that because a person is hysterical she may not have some other disease. On the other hand, sympathy is misplaced, and will usually make an hysterical person worse. Although hysterical patients cannot altogether avoid their attacks, they can to a certain extent guard themselves against the seizures; and this, they should be made to understand, they are expected to do. In the intervals between the fits, good food, good air, exercise, employment for the mind, attention to the bowels, and cold bathing are necessary. If the monthly flow is deficient or irregular, attention must be directed to this condition (*vide Amenorrhœa*, p. 468).

In cases in which hysteric paroxysms are prolonged or associated with unusual symptoms, there may be some affection of the urine requiring skilled advice. A form of nervous disturbance much resembling hysteria, but of very serious import, sometimes attends Bright's disease.

**HYDROCELE** signifies a collection of water in the cavity or bag enveloping the testicle, which comes on gradually. It begins from the bottom of the purse, and forms a pear-shaped swelling, smooth on its surface, soft to the feel, free from pain and tenderness, but causing uneasiness from its weight. It may originate from injuries, it may occur without assignable cause, and it may be congenital. It may be mistaken for *rupture* or *varicocele*, and the distinctions are given at p. 593. The only cure is a surgical operation known as 'tapping and injection.'

**INFLAMMATION.**—Inflammation manifests itself in increased vascularity and sensibility of the part attacked, which may be any part of the body. Inflammation of internal organs is the most dangerous. It produces heat, swelling, and redness from engorgement of blood, attended by pain, increased on pressure. If extensive, the whole system sympathises with the local mischief, and there is fever, quick pulse, generally constipation, and high-coloured urine. Unless cut short at first, inflammation goes on till an effusion of liquids takes place in the inflamed part, and what are called *lymph* and *serum* escape from the blood. These matters quickly become *pus* (or matter), and the result is an *abscess*. The symptoms and treatment of *external* inflammations are those of acute inflammatory abscess (*vide* p. 39). *Internal* inflammations are treated of under the headings of the different organs (*vide* also p. 587, *Defensive Inflammation*).

*Inflammation* often leads to *mortification* or *sloughing* (*vide* p. 337), or may cause an ulcer or open sore.

**INFLUENZA.**—This is a severe epidemic *catarrh*, spreading usually from the north-west towards the south-east, over large tracts of country. The causes of influenza are not understood; but it has been theorised to depend on a specific poison or microbe. As it occurs in greater force periodically, or at intervals of years, and at any season of the year, it is argued that it is not, like an ordinary cold or catarrh, caused by chill, or sudden vicissitudes of temperature, and therefore must *not* be confounded with ordinary catarrhal attacks, which occur most frequently at the colder or changeable seasons. Nevertheless there is no doubt that cold and chill, if not actually causing influenza, place the person in that condition most favourable to the initiation of the malady. A weak state of health, overcrowding, and insalubrious surroundings of all kinds are predisposing causes. Although influenza occurs in greater force periodically, influenza is always present, being in these respects like various other maladies. There are no broad distinctions between a bad cold and an ordinary attack of influenza. There is little doubt that all bad colds, characterised by other symptoms than running and stuffing of the nose (being in reality inflammation of the membrane of the nose) are influenza, although not usually called so. The public have long appreciated this, as is evident from the term in common use, 'an influenza cold.' The symptoms of influenza are, *first*, those of a very bad cold or *catarrh* (*vide* p. 113), to which are added a sudden, early, and extraordinary subdual of the strength, great depression of spirits, restlessness, and anxiety. There is usually cough, and there is always danger of bronchitis or inflammation of the lungs, or of rheumatism supervening. Often the pit of the stomach is tender, the digestive organs are disturbed, the tongue is white, the appetite and taste are lost, and there may be nausea and vomiting. Pains in the limbs and body are also present. The skin, at first hot, afterwards grows moist, and perspires profusely, exhaling a musty odour. The very young and the very old bear influenza less favourably, owing to the great debility it occasions, and the liability to chest affections. The duration of the disease may be from four or five to ten or twelve days. But convalescence is often protracted, and is then characterised by debility, or troublesome cough, or neuralgic pains, or loss of taste, or various other nervous affections.

*Treatment.*—The patient should be placed in a cool, well-ventilated room, but free from draughts. If the bowels are confined, Recipes 1 and 2 may be given. Then, citrate of magnesia (*vide* p. 15) to subdue feverishness, and Recipe 57 to meet cough or bronchial irritation. After the first day or two the diet should be nourishing and liberal; elderly persons also requiring a moderate amount of stimulants, which may be port wine or brandy. As soon as feverishness begins to subside quinine (Recipe 66). If bronchitis, inflammation of the lungs, or rheumatism occur, the treatment for those affections should be pursued.

**JAUNDICE.**—In this disease the skin becomes greenish or yellow, which has led to the malady being spoken of as *green* or *yellow jaundice*, as if there were two distinct kinds. The difference of colour depends on the amount of bile contained in the blood, and does not signify a different affection. The whites of the eyes assume a similar greenish or yellow tint; vision is often affected, everything appearing yellow; the bowels are confined, the fæces are white or clay-coloured, but the urine is of a deep yellow; the skin generally itches, and there is a bitter taste in the mouth, with coated tongue, and nausea, especially in the mornings. The cause of all these appearances is bile in the blood. From some one of various causes bile escapes into the blood, and is partly passed away by the kidneys through the urine. The jaundiced condition may be either *permanent* or *temporary*.

*Temporary jaundice* may be the result of congestion of the liver (*vide* p. 318). Or it may arise from a gall-stone in the bile-duct preventing the passage of bile (*vide* p. 275). It also occurs during certain kinds of fevers. But usually temporary jaundice depends on congestion about the bile-ducts, and Recipes 1 and 2 may be taken every night and morning; while a mustard poultice should be applied daily, or as often as can be borne, over the liver. The food should be light and nutritious, and stimulants should be avoided.

[It will be advisable for the patient to procure Recipe 9, to be taken at night, and Recipe 6 for the morning; to be repeated every or every other day, according to the effect produced. Recipe 32 should also be taken by a weakly person, or if dyspepsia is present; and Recipe 33 by a stronger person, when there is no dyspepsia, three times daily. When constipation exists, a course of Carlsbad salts may be used.]

*Permanent jaundice* depends on some serious or organic disease of the liver or other internal organ, and the disease thus producing the jaundice generally ends fatally.

A form of jaundice sometimes occurs, accompanied by atrophy or shrinking of the liver, which from its rapid course and frequent fatal termination has been termed *malignant*.

**JOINTS, INFLAMMATION OF.**—Occurs as a consequence of injuries, rheumatism, gout, and scrofula. The joint affected becomes swollen, tender, and painful, and if large, as the knee, there is also much feverishness. Leeches, fomentations, and rest are the appropriate *local* remedies, any existing constitutional disease being also treated. If stiffness remains after the acute stage, liniments and bandages should be used.

*Affections of the hip and knee-joints* are sufficiently common and important to demand separate description.

JOINT, HIP-, DISEASE OF THE.—Usually occurs to children who have inherited a scrofulous taint. It frequently arises without any assignable exciting cause, but is often attributed to slight accidents. The earlier symptoms are trifling, and therefore often remain undetected, or unattended to. If, after a slight injury, a child complains of pain in the hip, or *in the knee*; if the child limps when tired, or if it drags one leg, a suspicion of incipient hip-joint disease should be aroused. The limb should be carefully measured, both when the child is standing up and when lying flat on the back. If one leg appears *slightly* longer than the other, the suspicion of hip-joint disease of the limb, thus *apparently* lengthened, is materially confirmed. For, in order to take the weight of the body off the affected joint, when the child stands he bears upon the sound limb, throws out the sound hip, and *lowers* that of the opposite side. If, when the child lies on the back, the lengthening of the limb is still evident, it depends on effusion of fluid within the joint, which mechanically presses down the limb, rendering the existence of disease beyond doubt. Even if this lengthening cannot be detected, a suspicion of hip-disease may be usually confirmed by the following tests. If the projecting bone of the hip-joint is smartly tapped, or if the heel of the foot is struck, when the child is lying down and the leg is straight, pain, more or less acute, will be felt in the affected hip-joint. As the disease progresses the child becomes less able to walk, the lameness increases, and at last he is unable to stand. The buttock becomes flattened from wasting of the muscles, and the joint grows tender; while movement of the limb is very painful. Instead of the limb being *lengthened*, it now becomes gradually *shortened*; the knee of the affected limb becomes directed over the opposite thigh, the foot is turned inwards, chronic abscesses form (*vide* p. 41), and hectic fever (*vide* p. 269) prevails.

*Treatment.*—The most important point is perfect and early rest of the affected limb. On *suspicion* of hip-disease the child should be kept on the bed; and if there is *certainty* of disease, motion of the limb should be prevented by the use of a long well-padded splint, as figured at p. 571 for fracture of the thigh. The bowels should be kept open, and feverishness subdued by magnesia (*vide* p. 15). Quinine (Recipe 66) will be generally advisable. When the joint becomes tender, fomentations will be required; and if matter forms, it must be evacuated by puncture with a lancet. But the disease requires treatment by a skilled surgeon. Here it will suffice to mention the great importance of good hygienic conditions.

JOINT, KNEE-, DISEASE OF THE.—This mostly occurs in scrofulous children, and has obtained the name of *white swelling*, because, although the joint may be considerably enlarged, and the parts inside much diseased, the skin retains a white colour, and gives little indication of the inflammation underneath. It is generally attributed to some injury, but the malady is constitutional, and the injury can only be regarded as the determining cause of a constitutional taint showing itself in a particular part of the body. In white swelling the pain and enlargement are at first trifling, causing merely stiffness of the joint, and uneasiness only when moving or attempting to use it; so that the disease often makes considerable progress before it is recognised. Afterwards the pain is greater, and generally worse at night. The malady, if not checked, usually terminates in abscess, and in disease of the bones of the joint. Stiffness, swelling, or tenderness of the knee or hip joints, or 'limping,' occurring to children, should lead to application for medical advice. In the meantime it should be recollected that a diseased joint requires absolute rest, although fresh air should be afforded to the patient. The diet should be light but nourishing.

**JOINTS, HYSTERICAL.**—Certain symptoms of joint disease often present in hysterical females (*vide* p. 305), such as pain, tenderness, stiffness, and difficulty of motion. But the hysterical joint is neither swollen, hot, nor red. Tenderness on pressure is as great when the pressure is slight as when it is severe. If the hip is affected there is no pain in the knee so often attending hip-joint disease (*vide* p. 312), and striking the sole of the foot will not produce pain (*vide* p. 312). If the knee is affected pain is usually felt just below the knee-cap, and not generally throughout the joint. Usually persons so suffering have been subject to hysterical fits. The joint may be rubbed with soap liniment and the person treated for hysteria (*vide* p. 307).

KNOCK-KNEE.—Knock-knee comes on about the age children begin to walk. It is also found in growing boys and girls who stand too much, or who carry heavy weights, especially if of delicate constitution. Usually one knee is more affected than its fellow. There is sensation of weakness and aching pain. It is often due to mechanical yielding of the parts concerned. But it may also be associated with rickets (*vide* p. 371). The weakened ligaments must have time and rest given them to contract and grow strong. Exercise should be abridged, and supports of the lightest description should be procured. Diet must be nutritious.

**KIDNEYS, INFLAMMATION OF THE, or NEPHRITIS.**—This is known by the pain in the loins, usually on one side, but on both if both kidneys are affected. The pain strikes downwards towards the groin, and in males the testicle is often drawn up by spasmodic action of the muscles. The pain is of a dull, diffused, deep-seated character, increased by firm pressure, by coughing, or sneezing. It is also increased by straightening the leg of the affected side, and the patient lies on his back, or perhaps on the affected side, with his leg or legs drawn up. There is also often numbness in the inner part of the thigh. The urine is scanty, and voided painfully at short intervals; it frequently contains *albumen* (*vide* p. 101), and often becomes bloody. There is usually considerable feverishness, and the bowels are mostly confined. The causes of inflammation of the kidney are cold, external injury, long-continued and violent exercise of the muscles of the back, as in riding; gravel; diseases of the bladder and urinary passages, and scarlet fever. Inflammation of the kidney often lays the foundation of 'Bright's disease' (p. 100), or of abscess. For distinction from lumbago, with which it may be confounded, *vide* p. 324.

*Treatment.*—The bowels should be opened by Recipes 1 and 2; medicines encouraging perspiration should be given, as citrate of magnesia (*vide* p. 15), and the patient should drink freely of barley water, rice water, or linseed tea. A hot hip-bath should be given daily, and pain at night may be alleviated by Dover's powder or chloral. Perfect rest should be enjoined, and the diet should consist of nourishing broths and gruels.

**LARYNX, INFLAMMATION OF THE.**—The larynx is the upper portion of the windpipe, containing the parts forming the organ of voice. Inflammation of this part often commences with sore-throat or catarrh. It may be brought on by cold or by too great exertion of the voice; or it may be connected with consumption, or be a consequence of venereal. It may occur to so slight an extent as to produce *hoarseness*, or it may go on to total loss of voice, and ultimately cause suffocation. It may be *acute*, terminating, often fatally, in a few hours; or it may be *chronic*, lasting weeks or months. When inflammation of the larynx is acute and severe, it is a dangerous disease. There are fever, pain, and tightness about the throat, husky croaking voice, cough of the clanging croupy character, thick tenacious expectoration, difficult breathing, long-drawn hissing inspiration, inability to swallow easily, sleeplessness, attacks of suffocative spasm, urgent fears of suffocation, and towards the end gasping for breath and convulsions. The throat may be seen red and swollen within, and on pressing the tongue downwards the upper part of the larynx or 'epiglottis' may be seen erect and inflamed (*vide* p. 548). The small aperture into the windpipe is, from the swelling of the parts, more or less closed, thus preventing the entrance of air. Laryngitis may be confounded with croup or diphtheria, the distinction being the absence of the false membrane and deposit described in those diseases (*vide* pp. 154, 177).

*Treatment.*—When the malady presents as simple *hoarseness*, or loss of voice, occurring, perhaps, chiefly in the morning, avoidance of cold, especially at night, flannel round the throat, or a mustard poultice, the feet in mustard-and-water at night, and an expectorant mixture (Recipe 57) may be sufficient. But when the disease is severe very active measures are required. Leeches should be applied to the *upper part of the chest*—one for each year of the patient's age to the number of thirty. The steam from hot water should be frequently inhaled, and hot moist sponges should be applied to the throat. Dover's powder should be given in 5-grain doses three times a day, and if necessary the bowels should be moved by Recipes 1 and 2. The patient is to be kept from talking, in a warm room free from draughts, the temperature of which should be maintained as equable as possible, and not be allowed to sink below 80° Fahrenheit. The air should be rendered moist by steam from a kettle of boiling water (*vide* p. 104).

The diet must consist of fluids, as strong soups and broths, and no stimulants should be allowed. The operation of opening the windpipe may be required.

[As soon as possible calomel and opium (Recipe 23) should be obtained and given instead of the Dover's powder mentioned above. The calomel should be continued until there is a metallic taste in the mouth, or slight soreness of the gums. If the patient is a strong, robust person, it will also be advisable to give the tartar emetic mixture (Recipe 59).]

Chronic Laryngitis is often associated with scrofula, venereal, or cancer. The disease generally passes from bad to worse, and surgical operations may be required. But, in spite of all that can be done, the result is either sudden death from suffocative spasm, or lingering death from extension of the disease.

**LEPROSY.**—Leprosy appears in *three* forms. *First*, as circular spots, or blotches of irregular size and coppery hue, on any part of the body, which afterwards assume a whiter appearance, becoming dry, hard, horny, and glistening. *Secondly*, as loss of sensation in the fingers or toes, or of some part of the face or body. *Thirdly*, as a gradual growth of solid prominences or tubercles, varying in size from that of a pin's head to a walnut, causing the part to assume a curiously nodulated appearance. Ultimately the parts, however affected, ulcerate, the ulcers gradually eating away the flesh and bones, so that the fingers and toes are lost. It is hereditary, but may be communicated by contact of a sore or abrasion of the skin with leprous discharge. There is no cure for the disease, but its progress may be delayed by good diet, fresh air, and tonics.

The best tonic is arsenic (Recipe 75). Gurjon oil is also much recommended. The dose of oil is 2 drachms twice daily, with an equal quantity of lime-water. One part of oil with three of lime-water must also be rubbed into the body and limbs for two hours twice a day.

**LIVER, DISEASES OF THE.**—The liver is the largest organ in the body, and is situated in the right side, stretching across to the left.

The liver commences in a line immediately below the nipple, while its lower border comes down as low as the margin of the ribs. Its size varies a good deal in health, and in women who wear tight stays it may come down an inch or two lower. Its function is the secretion of bile, a fluid by which is effected the conversion of the food prepared by the stomach into material or 'chyle' required for the nourishment of the body. It also prepares materials which are destined to maintain animal heat by the slow combustion which a portion of the blood undergoes in the lungs. A third purpose of the liver is to remove effete or useless matter from the blood, *i.e.* to purify that fluid; and this effete matter is the main agent in the formation of the contents of the bowels into a suitable condition and consistence for their removal without injury. It thus acts as a natural aperient. Whenever the liver is disturbed or disordered, there cannot be health. Next to the stomach it is the part of the body most directly influenced by food or drinkables.

1. Congestion of the Liver.—This term implies a distension of some part, or of the whole, of the organ. Or sometimes the gall-bladder and gall-ducts only are implicated. The causes are overcrowding; a sedentary life; too much sleep, especially in the daytime; excessive eating and drinking; rich and hotly seasoned food; stimulating liquors, especially those containing much sugar; the sudden cessation of accustomed discharges from piles; repeated cold stages of intermittent or remittent fever, during which the blood is driven forcibly into internal organs, which thereby become distended. But the principal cause of congestion, inflammation, and abscess of the liver in the East is climatic. The liver is excited by more secretory work falling on it than in temperate climates, some of the effete material which would in temperate regions pass away by the lungs being removed from the system by an increased flow of bile. From solar exposure, heat, and consequent perspiration, the skin is rendered irritable and weakened, and is therefore more susceptible to

changes of temperature, which, both seasonal and daily, are rapid and great. Hence, the surface of the body being easily chilled, the internal organs, especially the liver in its excited condition, suffer much in the same manner as in the cold stages of fever (*vide* pp. 253, 676).

The *symptoms* are coated tongue, bad taste in the morning, depression of spirits, defective appetite, headache, bowels acting irregularly, stools dark, or sometimes light in colour, occasionally bilious diarrhœa, but often constipation, nausea, a sense of weight and fulness in the right side, and pain or uneasiness in the tip of the right shoulder, or in the shoulder-blade. Similar symptoms are sometimes spoken of as *torpor of the liver.* When such symptoms exist in a minor degree the person is regarded as *bilious.* Biliousness may, however, be evidenced by dyspeptic headache (*vide* p. 291), or by bilious colic (*vide* p. 131), or by irritative bilious diarrhœa (p. 167).

*Treatment.*—Recipes 1 and 2 should be taken, with care and abstinence in diet. Mustard leaves should be applied over the liver, and moderate exercise short of fatigue should be taken. Horse exercise is advisable.

[If the above treatment is not successful, it will be desirable for the person to take several mercurial purges, as Recipe 8, followed by Recipe 6. In two or three days after the bowels have been frequently opened Recipe 7 will be useful. Iodine paint may also be applied daily over the liver, until the skin becomes tender (*vide Appendix*, No. 111). In chronic cases, Recipe 33 if there is tendency to jaundice, and Recipe 34 if there is no tendency to jaundice. The nitro-muriatic bath should also be used (Recipe 114). The use of Friedrichshall, or Hunyadi Janos, or Carlsbad mineral waters will also be beneficial. For *biliousness*, euonymin 1 grain; compound extract of colocynth 1 grain; extract of hyoscyamus half a grain, made into a pill: one or two to be taken at night.]

2. Liver, Inflammation of the.—The causes of inflammation of the liver are similar to those of congestion, especially chill. Congestion, if not checked, will often

terminate in inflammation. It is also sometimes connected with dysentery, appearing then to arise from absorption of dysenteric material, secreted in the intestines, by the veins passing between the latter parts and the liver.

The *symptoms* of inflammation of the liver are pain in the *right* side, increased by pressure under the ribs, by a long breath, by coughing, by lying on the *left* side. There is also pain in the shoulder, and often a dragging sensation at the pit of the stomach. The whites of the eyes may turn yellow, the urine is highly coloured, there is nausea or vomiting, there may be either costiveness or diarrhœa, and the stools may be dark or light in colour. The disease is generally marked by febrile symptoms, but in some cases there is little fever. Sometimes it may be distinctly made out that the liver is enlarged, but often this is not the case.

When the pain is very acute, with much fever, the covering of the liver will be chiefly involved in the inflammation. If the bladder is irritable, and the pain more towards the loins, the under part of the liver is most affected. When vomiting is a prominent symptom, with perhaps hiccup, and pain at the pit of the stomach, that part of the liver nearest the former organ is most implicated. When difficulty of breathing, inability to draw a long breath, and cough are prominent symptoms, that part of the liver supporting the right lung, and probably the lung itself, are implicated.

*Treatment.*—In the absence of medical advice, administer a purgative, as Recipe 1, followed by a saline draught (Recipe 2) four hours afterwards. If the bowels are costive, and *there is no dysenteric complication*, these medicines should be repeated every or every other day, so that a continued free action may be secured. *But if there is dysentery*, castor-oil should be given, and after the bowels have been once thoroughly cleansed, ipecacuanha and Dover's powder (Recipe 17) night and morning. Effervescing solutions of citrate of magnesia (*vide* p. 15) may be taken with benefit, as they allay thirst and sickness. Mustard poultices should be applied daily, or as often as can be borne, over the liver. Milk, broth, beef-tea, toast, and biscuits may be taken, but no stimulants should be given.

[For inflammation of the liver *without accompanying dysenteric symptoms, occurring in a moderately healthy and robust person*, it will be desirable, when the materials are available at the onset, to adopt the tartar emetic treatment, as soon as the bowels have been once thoroughly moved by the means indicated above. Two grains of tartar emetic are to be thoroughly mixed in a mortar with 2 drachms of nitrate of potash, and the mass divided into eight powders, one of which should be given in 2 ounces of water every hour until local pain and tenderness subside. If the tartar emetic produces distress by exciting nausea or vomiting, or too much purging, or great depression, the proportion should be reduced to 1 grain in the eight powders. *For less robust persons*, 20 grains of chloride of ammonium should be given three times daily in water. If, after the subsidence of the acute symptoms pain or tenderness continue, a blister should be applied, and podophyllin with nitric acid (Recipes 7 and 12) should be given, the latter being most useful if the skin is dry and the bowels constipated.]

3. CHRONIC INFLAMMATION OF THE LIVER.—This may be a sequel of the acute form, or it may arise from repeated attacks of congestion, or it may come on so gradually that it is often long unattended to. The first symptoms are sensation of weight in the right side, or feeling as if a lump were there, occasional pains of a shooting character, with loss of appetite, flatulence, and other dyspeptic symptoms. These symptoms are very similar to those of congestion, but instead of disappearing, as temporary congestion does, they become permanent. Then the liver *in one form of the malady* becomes enlarged, and may be felt below the ribs. From the pressure of the enlarged liver upwards, there is also cough, difficulty of taking a long breath, and pain in one or both shoulders.

*But in another form* known as *cirrhosis* (*vide* p. 163) brought on usually by spirituous liquors, the liver becomes *atrophied* or smaller than natural. In both forms the countenance becomes sallow, the skin dry, the patient desponding and debilitated. The stools, which may be loose or the reverse, are generally clay-coloured, while the urine is often high-coloured from bile. Sometimes the person becomes jaundiced. Discharge of blood from the bowels and bleeding from the nose are also liable to occur.

*Treatment.*—Saline aperients in the morning, as Recipe 2, and care in diet, with avoidance of stimulants, are the means of relief. But if the disease persists, as it probably will, change to a temperate climate must be taken.

[Nitro-muriatic acid (Recipe 34), taraxacum and acid (Recipe 33), podophyllin (Recipes 7 and 12), iodide of potassium (Recipe 21), all prove useful; sometimes one prescription, sometimes another, agreeing best, and they may be tried in the order named. The nitro-muriatic bath (Recipe 114) should also be used.]

4. Abscess of the Liver.—Abscess of the liver originates as below:

(1) *Suddenly, during an attack of congestion or acute inflammation.*—If during such conditions shivering occurs, followed by cold sweats, obstinately furred tongue, scanty and high-coloured urine, depositing much sediment, fever increased at night, and diarrhœa, there will be every reason to fear formation of abscess.

(2) *Gradually, or during chronic inflammation.*—The most frequent manner, however, in which abscess manifests itself is after the prominent symptoms of acute inflammation have been relieved. The patient does not recover health, remains weak and languid, and after a variable period experiences occasional chills, with feverishness towards evening. This soon assumes a hectic character, and is accompanied by a tongue furred in the centre, red

at tip and edges. Weight and uneasiness are experienced in the right side, and the palms of the hands are dry.

(3) *Insidiously, or without previous inflammation.*—But liver abscess sometimes occurs without any previous decided symptoms, or there may be simply loss of flesh, or a vague sense of uneasiness or obtuse dull pain, or feeling of weight in the side, with perhaps slight cough. These anomalous feelings are signs often scarcely appreciable; or, if observed, are considered too trivial to induce application for medical advice. Often it is not until shivering and cold sweats, with swelling of the liver, appear, that the serious nature of the disease is recognised.

(4) *During the progress of dysentery.*—If the languor, the emaciation, and evening fever are greater than can be accounted for by the violence of the dysentery, if the tongue becomes furred in the centre and red at the tip and edges, and if there is uneasiness and weight in the side, there will be little doubt that abscess has occurred. A fit of shivering in addition would render the matter certain.

When abscess forms it may appear as a swelling in the side or near the pit of the stomach, when it is said to 'point' externally; or it may burst into the stomach and be emptied by vomiting; or into the bowels, and the matter may pass away with the stools; or into the lungs, when the contents may be coughed up; or otherwise into the cavities of the chest and bowels, from which there is no escape.

If the abscess points externally, in the absence of medical aid, the skin must be allowed to become red, when it may be opened with a lancet and poultices applied. Then the abscess, if not large, may discharge its contents, contract, heal, and the patient recover. In other instances, little can be done except supporting the strength of the patient by good diet, and relieving pain by chloral.

5. Hepatalgia, or Neuralgia of the Liver.—The symptoms are slight uneasiness or sense of weight in the side—so slight as to be forgotten when the person is occupied. There is also uneasiness in the shoulder, which feels tired. These symptoms may be absent for days, returning from exposure to cold, or without any probable cause. Sometimes twitches are felt in the side, which the patient may state to be tender. But examination does not confirm this, or detect anything unnatural. The mind dwells on this uneasiness, and the individual dreads some serious disease appearing. There is also languor, want of resolution, and despondency. But the appetite and digestion are good, and the patient sleeps well. These symptoms may recur for years, and may at first be regarded with suspicion, as indicative of insidious abscess. When, however, months elapse during which the individual enjoys good health, and probably gains flesh, the neuralgic character of the affection becomes, even to the patient himself, undoubted.

*Treatment.*—A mustard poultice will relieve the pain temporarily, and tonics, as quinine (Recipe 66), will probably prove beneficial. But occupation of the mind and moderate exercise are the best remedies.

[In some instances it may be desirable to apply a blister over the liver, when the pain is more than ordinarily complained of. Solution of arsenic (Recipe 75), taken daily for some weeks, is the best tonic.]

**LUMBAGO.**—This term implies severe pain and tenderness of the muscles of the loins, aggravated by motion, often preventing the patient from walking, and frequently occurring suddenly. It is a variety of rheumatism. It generally arises from cold. It is distinguished from disease of the kidneys, in which pain occurs in the loins (*vide* p. 314) by being aggravated by motion, by the absence of frequent desire to make water, and from there being no *albumen* (*vide* p. 101) nor blood in the urine.

*Treatment.*—When, at the commencement of the attack, the bowels are costive and the urine scanty and high-coloured, becoming turbid on cooling, Recipes 1 and 2 may be taken, with 8 grains of nitrate of potash (*vide* p. 26), three times a day. But when the bowels are regular and the urine light-coloured and abundant, hot local applications are the best remedies. Mustard poultices may be applied, or the back may be well rubbed with hot 'grass oil.' Powdered sulphur wrapped up in a flannel belt, and worn habitually, is praised as a local remedy. Ironing the back with a hot flat iron, a piece of brown paper intervening, is often beneficial. When the pain is very distressing at night, Dover's powder or chloral may be used.

[A better medicine, when the urine is thick and high-coloured, is colchicum with alkalies (Recipe 30). If the patient is feverish, Recipe 52. As external applications, turpentine and salad oil in equal parts; a belladonna plaster; ammonia and oil in the proportion of one-third ammonia; iodine paint; chloroform and opium liniment (Recipes 89, 90), are all sometimes useful. Galvanism, or Faradisation, or wearing a Pulvermacher's galvanic chain may also be tried. In severe cases a surgeon would probably use acupuncture needles, or inject morphia.]

**LUNGS, INFLAMMATION OF THE.**—This disease, technically known as *Pneumonia*, is ordinarily the result of cold. The disease usually commences as a severe cold, with chills and flushes of heat. Or it may begin as an attack of bronchitis (*vide* p. 102). There is a short dry cough, afterwards attended with a thin, frothy, very tenacious expectoration, which at a later period becomes *rusty*-coloured, or streaked with blood. This coloured expectoration is, in adults, the great distinguishing characteristic between *bronchitis* or inflammation of the tubes leading to the lungs, and the still more dangerous *pneumonia*, or inflammation of the substance of the lungs. There is no acute pain attending this disease, unless it is also, as often happens, combined with some degree of *pleurisy* or inflammation of the covering of the lungs, when there will be a 'stitch,' or stabbing pain in the side, or under the nipple, more or less acute as the covering of the lungs is affected in a lesser or greater degree (*vide Pleurisy*, p. 352). But whether there is this acute pain, denoting the pleura to be affected or not, there is always a deep-seated, dull aching in the chest, and the respiration is frequent and short, rising from fourteen or sixteen (the number of respirations in the recumbent posture during health) to forty or upwards; while the temperature of the body rises to 104° or 105° Fahr. (*vide* p. 33). In favourable cases the disease may decline on the fifth or sixth day, or it may be protracted to a fortnight. As a rule, if the mean of the bodily temperature, taken several times daily, is not above 104° Fahr.; if the pulse does not rise above 120 beats in the minute; and if the respiration does not rise above 35 in the same period, the patient, if otherwise healthy, will begin to get well in eight or ten days. In unfavourable cases, on the fourth or fifth day the breathing becomes more frequent and difficult, the pulse quicker, the skin hotter, and delirium, followed by stupor, ensues.

There are certain physical signs to be discovered by listening to the breathing. The parts generally affected are the lower halves of the lungs, and by listening below the shoulder-blades at the commencement of the disease, a peculiar creaking noise will be heard, very similar to that produced by strongly rubbing the hair near the ears between the finger and thumb. This is caused by the passage of air through the sticky glutinous fluid secreted in the lungs. In the more advanced stages of the malady, the lungs, where chiefly affected, may become hardened, and therefore when the chest or lower part of the back beneath the blade-bones is tapped with the fingers, a more or less dull sound results instead of the resonant sound of health.

Inflammation of the lungs, instead of presenting all the characteristic symptoms noted, sometimes comes on very insidiously. This is especially the case with natives of India, with children, and with old people. Also during the progress of fevers. Natives of India thus suffering frequently die from affection of the lungs, without having shown any prominent symptoms.

*Treatment.*—The patient should remain in bed, and the atmosphere of the room should be maintained equable, free from draughts, and moist from the steam of boiling water (*vide* p. 104). The great thing is to avoid variations of temperature and chills. The patient should not be allowed to talk much, and movement, which often causes great distress by accelerating the breathing, should as much as possible be avoided. A large hot linseed-meal poultice, or spongio-piline moist with hot water, should be applied to the chest. After the linseed poultice, which may be repeated daily, cotton-wool should be applied. As medicine, ipecacuanha wine and paregoric (Recipe 57) should be given every three hours. The diet should be light and nutritious, as milk, light pudding, eggs, beef-tea, broth, and jelly. For previously strong and healthy persons stimulants will seldom be required, provided the case progresses favourably; but if signs of exhaustion occur, brandy should be given freely. A rapid pulse, amounting to 120 beats in the minute, respirations above 35 in the minute, or delirium, are indications that stimulants are necessary. In weakly or elderly people it will sometimes be desirable to treat the case altogether with stimulants from the first, adding 15 minims of aromatic spirits of ammonia to each dose of paregoric mixture. Similarly, when inflammation of the lungs occurs in very old people, a stimulating plan should be adopted.

[If the patient is strong, robust, and young, it will be more advisable to give tartar emetic mixture (Recipe 59). The tartar emetic mixture diminishes the force of the circulation, and also acts on the skin, promoting perspiration, and thus lessens the difficulty of breathing.]

INFLAMMATION OF THE LUNGS, OR PNEUMONIA, OCCURRING IN CHILDREN, demands special notice. *Pneumonia* in children occasionally comes on very insidiously, and may be overlooked. This is most likely to be the case when the lungs become affected during the progress of various diseases, as measles, teething, atrophy, fevers, and bowel complaints. When inflammation of the lungs in children arises from cold, as it often does, and is not a consequence of, or connected with, and masked by, some other malady, the symptoms are better marked. When the disease is commencing, there is feverishness, headache, sometimes vomiting, and talking in the sleep, and a dull heavy expression, soon followed by hard dry cough, parched lips, flushed countenance, furred tongue, hot skin, high-coloured urine, and short, panting, oppressed breathing, the nostrils dilating with each inspiration. The breathing is also chiefly performed by the muscles over the bowels, which may be observed moving more than occurs in a state of health. The mouth is instinctively kept open so that more air may enter, and this tends to make it hot and dry. Usually there is crying only during the spells of coughing, at other times a moan. The number of respirations may rise from 30 to 50 per minute; the pulse to 150, or even higher, and the temperature to 105° or more. This condition in children is very likely to be mistaken for simple bronchitis, and the more grave nature of the case may not be understood, especially as children rarely expectorate, and the distinctive sign, previously mentioned, of rusty-coloured discharge is generally absent. The following contrast of the symptoms of pneumonia and bronchitis is added:—

| *Bronchitis, or Inflammation of the Air-tubes leading to the Lungs* | *Pneumonia, or Inflammation of the Lungs* |
|---|---|
| Skin warm and moist. | Skin hot and dry. |
| Mouth warm and moist. | Mouth hot and dry. |
| Breathing hurried, with wheezing. | Breathing short and panting, unaccompanied by wheezing, although a slight crackling sound may be heard. |
| Cough loud, noisy, and loose. | Cough hard, short, feeble, and dry. |
| Expectoration, if coughed out, white and glairy. | Expectoration, if coughed out, rusty and frothy. |
| Child cross and fretful. | Child dull and heavy. |

The fever, headache, vomiting, and talking in the sleep, which occur in children, may be mistaken for affection of the stomach or head. But in chest maladies the vomiting does not continue so long as in stomach and head affections. The early cessation of vomiting, the quickened breathing and the cough, are usually sufficiently distinctive.

*Treatment.*—If confined, the bowels should be loosened by castor-oil or senna tea, after which Recipe 57 should be given in doses according to age. If necessary the gums should be lanced (*vide* p. 434). Hot poultices should be applied over the chest (*vide Bronchitis*, p. 108). All through the illness the patient should be encouraged to take broths, jelly, milk, or other digestible fluid food. If after two or three days the child is low and feeble, small quantities of wine-and-water may be allowed, for the disease is one rapidly producing exhaustion, which should be early guarded against. The atmosphere of the chamber should be maintained moist, and at an equable temperature, in India about 80° Fahr., if possible both day and night. But whatever the temperature may be, it should be *equable, and the colder atmosphere of the night should be guarded against,* a very slight fall of temperature aggravating the malady.

**LUNGS, EMPHYSEMA OF THE.**—This is the same disease which in horses is called 'broken wind.' The lungs are composed of a vast number of air cells. Emphysema signifies the dilatation of these air cells, and their eventual rupture into each other. Emphysema occurs in connection with, and may be the cause of, such maladies (as chronic bronchitis and asthma) as are attended by violent or prolonged cough. On the other hand, emphysema may be caused by such maladies. The straining consequent on whooping-cough may lay the foundation of future emphysema. It may originate from violent athletic exercises, which necessitate holding the breath long. It may also be induced by playing on wind instruments. But in the majority of cases there is hereditary predisposition, or probably some imperfection of lung structure, perhaps arising from a gouty condition, or from deposit of fat. When emphysema occurs the lung tissue loses elasticity, and acts slowly, the air not being properly expelled. The consequence is difficulty of breathing, especially on exertion, and cough with expectoration of a thin character. There is no acute pain, but a feeling of oppression in the chest, and there are often asthmatic attacks. As the disease grows worse the countenance may become dusky, especially the lips; and the nostrils dilate widely when the breath is drawn in, which is done shortly and quickly, followed by prolonged and wheezing expulsion of the breath. There is frequently some swelling of the feet and ankles of a dropsical nature, and in bad cases the voice becomes feeble, the body wastes, and more decided dropsy may ensue. Emphysema of the lungs may be complicated with chronic bronchitis, winter cough, asthma, and affections of the heart.

If the chest is examined there is found increase of resonance throughout, but most marked at the summits of the lungs and on their anterior borders (*vide* Plate, p. 29). There is also heard a short faint sound when the breath is drawn in, and a prolonged sound when it is expelled.

*Treatment.*—When the lung cells have broken into each other the condition is incurable. But much may be done to alleviate by careful diet as mentioned under Asthma (p. 63), especially avoiding articles which cause flatulence; by pure air; by residence in a climate neither too hot nor too cold (the Riviera for instance); by avoiding violent exercise; by warm clothing, especially for the feet; and by tonics, the best of which are iron and quinine (Recipe 70). If asthmatic attacks occur, they should be treated as mentioned at p. 61.

**MEASLES.**—A contagious eruptive fever which usually attacks early in life, and seldom occurs more than once to the same person. The period between exposure to infection and the commencement of the symptoms is from eight to fourteen days. The malady commences with chilliness, feverishness, and cold in the head. The eyes are red, sore, watery, and the throat may feel sore. The glands under the jaw may be enlarged; there are sneezing, running from the nose, cough, and probably pains in the limbs. The tongue is white, with red edges. At the end of the third day or beginning of the fourth day of the above symptoms, the rash appears first on the forehead, face, and neck, then on the trunk, and lastly on the arms and legs. The rash at first appears as small round, red, velvet-like spots, somewhat resembling flea-bites, but not feeling raised above the surface of the skin. These extend and merge into each other, assuming semicircular or crescentic outlines of a crimson or dark brick-red colour, and slightly raised above the surface of the skin. If pressure is made with the finger the eruption disappears, returning when pressure is removed. The fever and cough continue, but the latter becomes loose. Three or four days after its appearance the eruption begins to fade, first on the face, then on the limbs. In about two days it disappears, with scurfiness of the skin. Often there is intolerable itching, especially when the eruption is at its height and when it begins to decline. The fever does not diminish temporarily on the appearance of the rash, as is the case in small-pox, but continues until the fading of the rash commences, when it gradually subsides. If the temperature rises above 103° the case must be regarded as a severe one, when there is usually a peculiar characteristic odour. Great debility, the tongue becoming dry and brown, and the eruption purple, is indicative of danger.

In some severe cases of measles there is not only cough but also bronchitis, or even inflammation of the lungs, when symptoms present as described under such heads (pp. 102, 328). Sometimes towards the termination of the attack, *ophthalmia* (*vide* p. 227) may occur. In other cases the cough continues, and often there is delicacy of the chest, from which the patient is long in recovering.

The principal distinctions between the earlier stages of measles and of small-pox, scarlet fever, or roseola are as follows:—Measles is known by the catarrhal affection, or appearance of a cold, with which it is ushered in, and by the crescentic peculiarity of form and crimson colour of the rash, which first appears as red spots, not raised above the surface of the skin. In small-pox there are no catarrhal symptoms, and there are generally vomiting and pain across the loins before the rash comes out, which shows as raised red spots. Scarlet fever begins with a sore throat, and the vivid scarlet rash appears early. In roseola there is no prior cold, or watering of the eyes, and the rash appears suddenly, in patches of various sizes and shapes. For further distinctions *vide Scarlet Fever*, p. 377; *Small-pox*, p. 404; *Roseola*, p. 387; *German Measles*, p. 334.

*Treatment.*—The patient should be kept indoors—if a bad case, in bed—as this is the best method by which a more equable temperature may be maintained, draughts avoided, and tendency to bronchial or lung affection lessened. It is generally advisable to give a hot bath at the onset of the disease, then dry the surface of the body and put the child to bed directly. If the necessary precautions are used no chill need be feared, and the hot bath will probably tend to bring out the rash. While great care is taken that the patient should not be exposed to draught and chill, the room should be airy and well ventilated. The room should also be darkened, as the eyes are sensitive. Dryness or tingling of the skin may be relieved by bathing with tepid water, taking care that only one portion of the body is exposed at one time. Rubbing the hands and feet with salad oil will relieve the sensations of heat and tightness produced by the rash. At first no solid food will be cared for, but the patient is always thirsty, and may drink milk-and-water, toast-water, chicken broth, and lemonade or tamarind whey (*vide Addendum*). If the bowels are confined, castor-oil or senna, but after they have been thoroughly opened purgatives should be avoided, as the bowels are liable to become irritable. Citrate of magnesia (*vide* p. 15) may be given to diminish feverishness; if there is cough, Recipe 57. The inhalation of the steam from a mixture of 1 part of vinegar and 3 of water is also useful. If the breathing becomes hurried, a mustard poultice or the mustard leaf, or for young children a linseed-meal poultice, should be applied to the chest. As a general rule stimulants are not desirable, but in cases where there is much exhaustion a little port wine may be allowed. If cough continues after the rash is gone, it should be treated by giving Recipe 57. If the eruption suddenly disappears, and there is great depression and distress, a warm bath will generally revive the eruption and afford relief.

Measles is very contagious, and during the illness all offensive *excreta* or dirty linen should be immediately removed and disinfected. All the rules given regarding disinfecting (*vide Appendix*, No. 121) should be carried out. Measles is most contagious when the rash is out, but it may also be contracted by another child during the catarrhal stage before the rash appears; and it is not safe for other children to mix with affected patients until three weeks after the rash has disappeared, and then only if all clothing has been disinfected and washed. Isolation of a patient is the only way to prevent the disease spreading.

**MEASLES, GERMAN** or **RÖTHELN.**—Difference of opinion exists as to whether this is a mild form of measles or a distinct disease. It commences in the manner mentioned under measles, but the symptoms are less severe. The rash terminates sooner than that of measles, the itching is less, and scurfiness of the skin is almost limited to the face and chest. Fever and cough are present as in measles, but to a lesser degree. From the above it will be seen that German measles is a much less severe disease than ordinary measles. The *treatment* given for measles is equally applicable to German measles, so that practically it does not signify if the one is mistaken for the other.

**MOLES** and **MOTHER'S MARKS** are discolorations found in some part of the skin at birth. The *skin is not raised* or rough, but more or less discoloured, and often called 'port-wine mark.' Such marks are of no consequence, although if on the face disfiguring. Unfortunately they are irremediable. The term 'mother's mark' is often erroneously applied to a NÆVUS, which is a collection of small blood-vessels *raised above the surface of the skin.* This may be of various sizes, from that of a pin's head to the circumference of a crown piece, or larger. When the child cries the colour of these patches becomes deeper. Although not painful, they may grow to a large size, and be the source of periodical bleeding. Generally a surgical operation is required.

**MOON**, Diseases supposed to be caused by the.—The deleterious influence of the moon has been credited from the earliest times, for we have a passage in one of the Psalms, 'The sun shall not smite thee by day, *nor the moon by night.*' That the rays of the moon are injurious has received support from the fact of meat becoming tainted sooner on a moonlight night. This does not occur if the meat is well protected. When meat becomes tainted during a moonlight night it is from the operations of insects, which the moonlight lures from the retreats they pass the dark nights in.

The maladies most credited to the influence of the moon are as below:

*Swollen face, toothache, deafness, earache,* and *rheumatism.* But these are the natural results of exposure to damp from dew, or to cold winds, which must be the consequence of lying without any protection from the rays of the moon; for the absence of protection from the latter must also entail want of shield from the former. Moreover, similar results occur from exposure on dark nights, not only to human beings, but also to animals, when they are said to have a 'stroke of the land wind.'

*Moon paralysis* is a misnomer. After persons have slept in the open, either in the moonlight or otherwise, it has often occurred that they have found themselves unable to move the eyelids, or an arm, or a leg properly. But the loss of power thus occurring is not true paralysis. It is rheumatism, and it will be found the person is able to move the part affected, but refrains from doing so in consequence of the attendant pain. It is not consequent on the moon's rays, but arises from chill or cold. The malady should be treated as rheumatism, with hot baths, liniments, and colchicum (Recipe 52).

*Paralysis of the bladder*, or inability to make water, may result from night chill, and has been erroneously attributed to the moon. This is more likely to occur in men suffering from stricture or irritable bladder, especially if they have been drinking. A hot bath will probably afford relief; if not, the catheter is required, and the case must be treated as *retention of urine* (*vide* p. 421).

*Dropsical effusions* sometimes result from exposure to damp, chill, and cold land winds (*vide* p. 187), and are not attributable to the moon-rays.

*Mental Excitement* or *Insanity*.—Lunatics are more excitable and noisy in the brilliant moonlight of the tropics than at other periods. Not only does the light interfere with sleep, but a tropical moonlight night is more noisy than a dark night. Animals, birds, and insects are more restless and noisy. As mental excitement is thus caused to the confirmed lunatic, so those predisposed to insanity are kept awake and excited.

*Moon-blindness* arises from the rays of the moon. The *retina* or expansion of the nerve of the eye becomes paralysed from lengthened exposure to a brilliant moonlight, even although the eyes are covered by the lids; just as sometimes occurs to men working in front of a blazing furnace, or to arctic voyagers from the glare of snow. Sometimes there is total blindness both by day and night, or loss of vision may be only partial. The treatment is blisters behind the ears, purgative medicines, and confinement in a darkened room.

*Paroxysmal Fevers*.—It is a very general impression that these diseases are more prevalent and more likely to recur at the lunar changes. Statistics do not confirm such impressions. Nevertheless, persons subject to fever will often assert their malady returns at the new and full moons; or, if the fever does not recur, they feel uncomfortable, and suffer from various anomalous and ill-defined sensations, evidencing some deviation from health. That the moon *per se* exerts such influence may be questioned; but at the lunar phases there are atmospheric changes which may affect the sensitive constitutions of those disposed to disease. Thus the barometer suffers a depression of about the tenth of an inch at the new and full moon; while there may be other more subtle influences at work, with which we are unacquainted. In the description of intermittent fever it has been noted what apparently slight causes (errors of diet, cold, mental emotions, &c.) will induce a return of fever in those who have suffered from the complaint, and the atmospheric changes consequent on the lunar phases seem to be sufficiently powerful to induce a similar result. However this may be, the practical application of the present knowledge of the matter results in the desirability of those subject to fever taking precautionary measures, such as a dose of quinine, and avoidance of exposure, just previous to the changes of the moon.

**MORTIFICATION, or GANGRENE.**—This signifies the death of any part of the body. There are three varieties, *dry*, *moist*, and *senile*. *Dry gangrene* is marked by the part affected assuming a pale white appearance, here and there mottled brown. The part is cold, and there is loss of motion and sensation. Soon the skin is converted into a black mass.

*Moist gangrene* is characterised by swelling at first red, then becoming purple or black, on which blisters form. The part is cold, with much pain. *Senile gangrene* is often preceded by very cold feet, and commences as a blackish spot at the inner side of the great toe, or on the smaller toes, surrounded by an inflamed circle which extends up the limb. Mortification of various parts may occur from old age; from debility, poverty, starvation, excessive cold, disease of the arteries of the part; or from injury to the nerves or arteries. When any part mortifies it emits an offensive odour. Surgical advice is required. If this cannot be obtained, chloral should be given to relieve pain, and poultices made of powdered charcoal will be the best applications.

**MUMPS.**—An infectious disorder, consisting of inflammation of a gland called the 'parotid gland,' situated behind the jaw below the ear. It generally occurs in children, but sometimes in adults, and seldom attacks the same person twice. It commences with slight fever. After a few hours, or perhaps in a day or two, a swelling, often of almost stony hardness, is noticed before and under the ear, extending along the neck towards the chin. This lump is exceedingly painful, and continues swollen for four or five days, while the skin is often red. It then gradually disappears, leaving no trace. The swelling of mumps seldom gathers. It may affect one or both sides of the face. It is contagious, and sometimes runs through a whole family or school. In severe cases swallowing is difficult from the pressure of the swelling on the throat, and but little food can be taken. Occasionally during the course of the disease, but generally at its subsidence, a similar swelling may affect the breasts or the testicles.

*Treatment.*—If mumps is severe, causing difficulty of swallowing or of breathing, leeches to the part may be required; but usually hot fomentations will be sufficient. Flannel wrung out of hot poppy-head decoction (*vide Appendix*, No. 81) is the best application. During the intervals of fomentation the parts should be wrapped in flannel. The patient should be debarred for a few days from meat; and aperient medicines, as senna or castor-oil, should be given. Citrate of magnesia, in doses according to age, should be used as a cooling mixture, and rest and quiet should be enjoined. If the inflammation migrates to the breast or to the testicle, the treatment proper for inflammation of those parts should be employed (*vide* pp. 94, 438).

**NAILS, DISEASES OF THE.**—Sores near the toe-nails are often very troublesome, especially when accompanied by what is popularly termed 'ragnail,' or 'the growth of the nail into the flesh.' It does not, however, arise from any alteration in the nail, but from the soft parts being pushed up against the edge of the nail by tight or ill-fitting boots. If this continues, an ulcer is formed at the root of the nail.

*Treatment.*—The objects are to remove the irritation caused by the nail. In many cases, after soaking and softening the nail in hot water, it may be filed or scraped so thin, and so much of the corner may be cut away, that the soft parts are no longer irritated. Or, by filing the nail thin in the middle, the offending edge may be caused to rise into its situation. To aid this, the soft parts should also be carefully pressed away from the sharp edge of the nail, by introducing beneath the overhanging skin a small piece of lint, and pressing it well down towards the bottom of the sore. Persons disposed to this affection should wear their shoes loose, square at the tips, and keep their nails scraped rather thin, so that they may be more flexible. A V-shaped piece cut out from the middle of the nail, the apex going down as far as possible without pain, is a means of prevention.

[If the nail is very tough and thick, the lint mentioned above should be first soaked in a mixture of two drachms of *solution of potash* in one ounce of water. This will soften both the nail and the skin, which may be afterwards easily scraped, or even wiped away. If the means as above do not suffice, and the edge of the nail still presses into the parts, the corner must be cut away with a sharp pair of scissors, which is a very painful operation, and should be performed by a surgeon.]

An ulceration, technically termed '*Onychia*,' sometimes forms about the finger-nails of unhealthy children. It commences as a deep red swelling, in which matter forms, succeeded by an ulcerated condition. Poulticing and letting the matter out by means of a lancet are the remedies. Laxatives and tonics will also be required.

The nails are affected in certain diseases, viz., gout, psoriasis, ringworm, scrofula, and syphilis, as mentioned under such headings. Telegraph operators are liable to breakage and dropping off of the nail, caused by continual tapping on the telegraph key, for which rest is the cure.

**NERVOUSNESS.**—There is an irritable state of the nervous system, most common in women, but occurring in men.

There are two systems of nerves. One called *cerebro-spinal*, passing from the nervous centres, viz. the brain and spinal cord, to all parts of the body. These nerves consist of two sets of fibres, one of which (sensory) convey impressions to the brain and spinal cord, the other set (motor) conveying mandates to the muscles. The other nervous system, called the *sympathetic* or unconscious system, consists of a number of ganglia or centres (being enlargements in the course of the nerves) placed at intervals throughout the body, and being connected with each other and with the other system of nerves by numerous filaments. Nerve force and the nervous system resemble electrical force and the telegraphic system. Electrical force originates in the battery, and nerve force in some nerve centre. Electricity must pass from the battery through the wire to the instrument before the click of the sounder is heard, and nerve force must pass from a nerve centre through the nerves to a muscle before that muscle can move, and it must pass from a nerve centre to the cells, of which internal organs are composed, before such organs can perform their functions.

The causes which may interfere with the vital process carried on by the nerves, and with the complicated mechanism of the nervous system, are multitudinous. The nervous system of some people is, probably from heredity, more prone to disturbance than that of others. In addition to heredity or constitutional tendency, the causes of nervous affections may be classed under two heads: (1) *mental* impressions, such as anxiety, excessive study, shocks of all kinds, &c.; (2) *defective nutrition* from any cause, but chiefly from dyspepsia, or worms. The nerves, like all parts of the body, require suitable nourishment. When food is not properly digested, the nerves, like other parts of the body, suffer in consequence. Thus a vicious circle is established. The indigestion affects the nerves, and the disordered nerves affect the indigestion.

Nervousness is characterised by numerous symptoms, such as causeless irritability, flushing from slight emotion, tremblings, sudden attacks of faintness or palpitation, frequent desire to make water, a variable and excitable temper, fits of low spirits, a tendency to weeping. When aggravated it constitutes *hypochondriasis* (*vide* p. 304) in men, and *hysteria* (*vide* p. 305) in women. It requires attention to the general health, and tonics.

**NEURALGIA.**—The term is applied to nervous pain which may occur in any part of the body. The principal local neuralgia are *brow-ague* or *brow-ache, hepatalgia pleurodynia, sciatica, tic-douloureux, toothache,* which are elsewhere described (*vide Index*). For neuralgia make a small muslin bag and fill it with salt, heat it hot, and place it against the aching spot; it will retain the heat for a long time, and will greatly relieve.

Many neuralgic affections are benefited by the injection of different agents beneath the skin. Hypodermic tabloids containing a certain amount of the agent required are prepared by Messrs. Burroughs & Wellcome. A person subject to neuralgia may, with the sanction of a medical man, learn to use the hypodermic syringe. A fold of the skin should be lifted, and the syringe needle should be introduced with a slight rotatory motion parallel with the surface. This is better than putting the skin on the stretch and then thrusting the needle through at right angles.

**OXALURIA** is the name given to a condition of urine when octohedral or 'dumb-bell' shaped crystals of oxalate of lime are passed in the urine. It is often associated with hypochondriasis, nervousness, insomnia, and atonic dyspepsia. Persons so affected are usually 'below par.' But others passing such crystals are apparently in good health, or sleepiness by day may be the only complaint. Exercise, good food, freedom from brain-work, and tonics (Recipe 75, or if in a malarious district, 76) are the requirements.

**PAIN.**—Pain is a symptom of disease (*vide* p. 37). There are two distinctive pains: *inflammatory* and *irritative*. Inflammatory pain is *increased* by pressure; irritative or spasmodic pain is *relieved* by pressure. Thus the pain of inflammation of the bowels is distinguished from that of colic, gravel, or gall-stones, being *increased* by pressure; while the pain of the latter maladies is *relieved* by pressure. Pain of the chest may arise from cold, consumption, inflammation, rheumatism, indigestion. Pain in the joints suggests rheumatism, gout, scrofulous or other inflammation, or hysteria. Pain in the stomach or bowels indicates wind, acidity, dyspepsia, colic; or, if long-continued and increased by pressure, inflammation. Pain in the back and limbs ushers in fevers and small-pox. Pains all over the body mark simple cold, influenza, or dengue fever. Pain in the face or other parts of the body, when periodic and without fever, is generally neuralgic. Whenever pain is dangerous there is generally fever.

**PARALYSIS**, or **PALSY**, signifies loss of power of motion of a limb or of one-half of the body. Sometimes sensation, or the power of feeling, is also lost, but this more rarely. The following are the principal varieties:—

1. *Paralysis from Disease or Injury of the Brain.*—Paralysis of one kind or other very often follows an attack of apoplexy, and sometimes occurs from disease of the brain, without any prior apoplectic fit (*vide* p. 53).

2. *Paralysis from Injury of the Spine.*—(*Vide* p. 557).

3. *Paralysis from Disease of the Spine.*—This form of paralysis, called *progressive locomotor ataxy, creeping paralysis*, or *tabes dorsalis*, depends on disease of the spinal cord. The symptoms are gradual, commencing with feelings of

fatigue in the loins and legs, tingling in the feet, and sometimes coldness of the bowels. Then pains occur in the thighs and legs of a boring paroxysmal character, sometimes described as like electric shocks, and often at first supposed to be rheumatic. There is frequently a history of preceding venereal affection. As the disease advances the muscles of the limbs waste, which has led to the affection being also termed *progressive muscular atrophy*. In some cases there is disordered vision, inability to retain urine at night, perhaps discharges from the privates, and a feeling of constriction about the waist. As the pains increase the patient finds he is losing control over his legs; that he staggers, particularly when commencing to walk; and that he cannot walk firmly without support. He lifts his feet unnecessarily high, throws them forwards and outwards, and brings the heels down with a stamp. He walks best when looking at his feet, and if he shuts his eyes or walks in the dark he probably falls. Sensation also becomes impaired, and the patient feels as if he were standing on wool or sand. At length walking is impossible, and the hands may be affected. Chronic inflammation of the bladder (p. 71) may result, but death usually occurs from chest affection. The duration of the disease may be some years. Treatment consists in nutritious diet and tonic medicines.

Paralysis of any of the above kinds is rarely cured, the most that can be done being attention to the general health and *massage* of the limbs, (*vide Appendix*, No. 116).

4. *Paralysis, Alcoholic.*—Paralysis from immoderate use of spirituous liquors chiefly affects females. The onset is gradual, with pain, followed by numbness in the feet and legs, weakness of the knees, loss of power, and uncertain gait. As the disease advances the legs waste, and the person becomes bedridden. The arms are rarely affected. The malady is generally ascribed to an accident

or chill, the habit of drinking being concealed. The brain and spinal cord are not implicated, the malady being in the local nerves. The treatment is strict abstinence from fermented drinks, good diet, massage, galvanism, tonics, and carriage exercise.

Alcoholic paralysis is often permanently benefited by Faradism or Voltaism. As a medicine, pills containing one-fiftieth of a grain of phosphorus, one-fourth of a grain of extract of nux vomica, and one grain of precipitated carbonate of iron. Dose—one, thrice daily.

5. *Paralysis, Lead.*—Painters and others who work with lead are subject to paralysis of the wrists, and the hand *drops.* A blue line on the edge of the gums close to the teeth generally accompanies wrist-paralysis from lead. This appearance and paralysis (also lead colic, *vide* p. 134) has resulted from lead in the colouring of room-paper. The treatment is removal from the cause and Recipe 49, with aperients if there is constipation. Afterwards Recipes 21 (*vide* p. 134, small type).

6. *Paralysis, Facial,* or paralysis of some of the muscles of the face, may be part of a general paralysis (*vide* p. 342), or it may arise from cold, unconnected with serious internal disorder. A person, after exposure to a draught, may not be able to move one side of the face, which appears blank and expressionless, and saliva may trickle from the mouth. It is often supposed the patient has had a 'stroke,' or that he has been affected by the moon (*vide* p. 335); but this is not the case. It is a species of rheumatism, and will gradually disappear under the influence of fomentation with hot poppy-head water (*vide Appendix,* No. 81) and Recipe 30.

7. *Paralysis, Infantile.*—Paralysis sometimes occurs to infants when teething, especially if being brought up by hand, or if suffering from improper feeding, or from debility, or from worms. It is usually met with when the double teeth are coming through. After some days of

feverishness, which, however, may not be noticed, the child goes to bed apparently as well as usual, but after probably a restless night the mother is alarmed to find one arm, or perhaps one arm and both legs, helpless. Generally the affection lasts only a few days or weeks, passing away as the child's feeding and nutrition improve.

Or the paralysis may happen as a *result of fevers*, or after *diphtheria*, only becoming evident when the child begins to walk. *Diphtheritic paralysis* generally commences in the muscles of the throat with some difficulty of swallowing, and children after diphtheria should be closely watched for such signs. These forms of paralysis are longer in getting well. The patient should be constantly in the fresh air, the limbs should be frequently shampooed, and iodide of iron (Recipe 74) should be used in doses according to the age of the child (*vide* p. 6).

8. *Paralysis, Hysterical,* has been referred to under *Hysteria* (*vide* p. 305). It generally affects a joint, as the knee or the legs, and may be accompanied by tenderness about the middle of the spine or between the shoulders. It is known from real paralysis by presenting in hysterical patients, generally young girls; and if tenderness of the back exists, by the skin being more sensitive and the tenderness more marked (*vide Hysteria*, p. 305) than is found in real disease of the spine. Although not much benefited by medicines, it generally gets well under the influence of hygienic measures.

**PALSY, SCRIVENER'S**, or **WRITER'S CRAMP**, and **TELEGRAPHIST'S CRAMP**, is a local spasm, or, in bad cases, a local palsy. In the spasmodic variety attempts to write call forth uncontrollable movements of the fingers or wrist, so that the pen starts up and down, and a mere scrawl results. In other instances the pen cannot be held, and the wrist is almost powerless. There is a tired feeling in the latter part, and particularly in the ball of the thumb and in the little finger. Occasionally the arm is painful to the elbow. The causes are too much writing, aided often by an irritable constitution. The only means of relief is perfect rest from the accustomed work, frequent shampooing in all directions, and strengthening the system by tonics, fresh air, and exercise. As prevention is better than cure, the first warnings of this malady, viz. a tired feeling in the thumb or little finger after writing, should be accepted as a hint that the parts are being used too much.

*Among telegraph clerks* the same kind of cramp occurs. *Pianists*, *bricklayers*, and *nailmakers* suffer from a very similar affection, caused by continual strain on the wrists, involved by their employments. The remarks under 'Writer's Cramp' regarding prevention and cure are applicable.

**PARAPHYMOSIS.**—A condition of the private parts often occurring in male children. It consists in the foreskin being drawn back from the end of the penis, where it remains and cannot be returned. The result is swelling and redness of the parts, attended with considerable pain and sometimes by difficulty in making water, or even complete inability to do so. The parts should be returned to their natural positions as soon as possible. They should be first bathed with ice-cold water. Then the 'glans,' or head of the penis, should be compressed with the fingers and thumb, so as to squeeze the blood out of it; at the same time it should be pressed backwards while the foreskin is drawn forwards. If this does not succeed after several trials, a slight cut will probably be necessary, for which the child should be taken to a surgeon.

**PHYMOSIS** signifies the opposite condition to the above, and consists in an unnaturally long foreskin, with a small opening, so that it cannot be drawn back to expose the head of the penis. This condition is often congenital;

but it may result from sores or ulcers. It causes much local irritation from retention of secretions between the head of the penis and the foreskin. It causes difficulty of micturition, the urine distending the foreskin like a bladder. From the straining efforts required in passing water, rupture or protrusion of the bowels may be produced. It may be the cause of nervous affections, as epilepsy and chorea. A surgeon should be consulted as soon as possible as to the propriety of operations; circumcision being required in bad congenital cases. When it occurs in connection with sores and ulcers, rest, fomentations, and Recipe 2.

**PILES** or **HÆMORRHOIDS.**—To understand piles it must be recollected that the blood is carried by the arteries *from* the heart to all parts of the body, and it returns by the veins *from* all parts to the heart (*vide* p. 500). The rectum or lower gut is a *terminal* point surrounded by a large amount of loose tissue in which a number of arteries and veins meet. It is also a *dependent* part, from which the blood must rise against the force of gravity. Hence it is a locality in which blood is liable to stagnate, especially if any obstruction occurs above, as so frequently offered by liver affection.

Piles may be either *external* or *internal*; or partly internal and partly external. *External piles* consist *at first* of an enlarged vein, which appears at the very verge of the orifice in the shape of a dark-coloured tender swelling, usually about the size of a hazel-nut. In a little time the watery part of the swelling is absorbed and the swelling disappears, leaving some thickening where the skin joins the gut. External piles are very tender and painful, causing much heat and pain about the fundament, especially when calls to stool occur; but they seldom bleed.

*Internal piles* are composed of an enlarged vein pushing the membrane of the gut before it, and to such an extent that they often assume a pear shape. Internal piles are very insidious in their growth, and sometimes it is bleeding which first attracts notice. A small and unsuspected internal pile may cause anomalous symptoms, such as mentioned under nervousness (*vide* p. 340), the cause of which is not recognised until blood is noticed in the stools. When piles increase in size they cause weight and burning in the gut, straining at stool, frequent desire to make water, sometimes inability to make water, pain in the loins and down the thighs, and whites (*vide* p. 462) in females. Internal piles may also ulcerate, giving rise to dysenteric symptoms (*vide* p. 194). Or they may protrude externally, when, if not returned, they may be constricted by the muscle round the orifice of the gut, when they first swell and afterwards mortify. Internal piles frequently bleed more or less, sometimes profusely. Bleeding from piles takes place as a rule *after* the action of the bowels, and the blood covers the motions; more rarely it precedes the stool; in exceptionally severe cases it occurs independently of the action of the bowels, on the person suddenly standing up, or without assignable cause. If the loss of blood is not excessive, it appears at first to have a salutary effect on stout and robust persons, not, as popularly supposed, by the discharge with the blood of some deleterious matters from the system, but by relieving other organs, especially the liver, of fulness and congestion. In time, however, the loss of blood being repeated, perhaps even daily, the debilitating effect far counterbalances any healthy tendency, rendering the person weak and anæmic, exciting many of the symptoms detailed under nervousness (p. 340) and anæmia (p. 46), and also rendering the person more liable to various diseases, especially ague and scurvy. On the other hand, the *sudden* cessation of bleeding from piles has been followed by apoplexy (*vide* p. 53) and liver congestion (*vide* p. 318).

Both external and internal piles may appear at the

same time. At first they present during a short period, and then, becoming smaller, cease to give trouble probably for months. At length, if not properly treated, they become permanent, and if not always bleeding or inflamed, they are the source of continual discomfort. Both varieties are also liable to become inflamed and ulcerated. When piles become inflamed, there is much heat, pain and swelling, which last result may be seen in the case of external piles. There will also be an aggravation of all the symptoms previously enumerated.

The *causes* of piles are numerous. Constipation and the consequent straining at stool, sedentary pursuits, and too long sitting on soft seats have a tendency to excite them. Too much horse exercise or camel-riding, riding in a jolting vehicle, the immoderate use of strong purgatives, especially aloes, are all exciting causes. Warm, moist, and miasmatous climates, by inducing relaxation generally, and of the veins in particular, are also causes. Congestion of the liver is a fertile source of piles, also the frequent occurrence of bowel complaints. The connection between piles and chronic dysentery is noticed at p. 194. Piles are often associated with, or cause, *fissure* or *ulcer of the anus* (*vide* p. 272). Less frequently they are accompanied by *polypus* (*vide* p. 355).

*Treatment.*—The treatment of piles must be divided into that proper during the painful or inflammatory stage and that necessary when the parts are quiescent. When *external* piles are inflamed, fomentations or poultices should be applied, and the bowels should be maintained open by castor-oil or by sulphate of soda (Recipe 2), which produces watery stools. The patient should be kept at rest in bed, and, if feverish, citrate of magnesia (p. 15) should be administered. After the sore or inflammatory condition has passed away the parts should be bathed frequently with cold water or cold alum water, while tolerably active exercise must be taken, and the bowels prevented becoming costive by laxative medicines, or perhaps by brown bread. The utmost cleanliness is necessary, as dirt may cause the piles to ulcerate, from the irritation it excites.

In the treatment of inflamed *internal* piles, or those not protruding outside the verge, the bowels should be at once thoroughly moved by castor-oil, after which, as poultices or fomentations cannot be applied to the part, injections of warm water may be used. The patient should be kept quiet in bed, and, if feverish, should take citrate of magnesia draughts (*vide* p. 15). When piles are inflamed, whether internal or external, the diet should consist chiefly of broth, toast, eggs, or milk, and no stimulants should be allowed.

When internal piles protrude after stool, they should be sponged with cold water or with alum water (Recipe 100) before being returned. When they do not return, the person should lie down for a time, when perhaps the protruded substance will be drawn back by the action of the bowels. If not, they must be returned by gentle pressure, otherwise they may become constricted and inflamed by the pressure of the verge of the anus. Persons subject to internal piles should acquire the habit of visiting the closet at night instead of the morning, that the piles, if protruding, may be returned when the recumbent posture is about to be assumed, rather than previous to the active business of the day. *Excessive bleeding* may be stopped by injections of cold or iced alum water (Recipe 100).

A host of medicines have been lauded as beneficial in piles; but the cure of piles consists more in hygienic measures, and in attention to diet, than in medicines. The patient should restrict himself to a carefully regulated and temperate diet, with plenty of vegetable food and little meat, abstaining from highly seasoned dishes, pastry, and spirits. He should also take care that his bowels are kept open, for which Recipe 2 may be used. After each motion the parts should be well bathed with cold water. Regular exercise is desirable. Change of climate to Europe will often relieve piles when other means fail. But frequently a surgical operation is required.

[Of local applications for *external* piles, the best is probably compound gall ointment (Recipe 25). Or a preparation from the American witch hazel, known as 'hazeline,' may be used, being a more cleanly application than ointment. The piles should be bathed with hazeline three or four times a day, and a piece of linen or absorbent cotton dipped in it should be kept applied during the intervals. The best applications for *internal* piles, when not inflamed, is injection of Recipe 100, cold, night and morning; or an ounce of hazeline with a similar quantity of water. When there is tendency to inactive or congested liver, Friedrichshall or Hunyadi Janos mineral waters.]

Plague, or Pestis.—As the disease prevails periodically on the shores of the Euphrates, and as communication with India is frequent and rapid, it is fortunate that plague has not yet been added to the list of ever-present Indian diseases; which, however, might occur at any time. In fact, an epidemic, which, if not true plague, was certainly very similar to plague, has several times prevailed in various parts of Western India. The first symptoms are lassitude, shivering, vomiting, often of black material, and a heavy, stupid expression of countenance, with redness of the eyes. Then there is high fever, and darting pains in the groins or armpits, where large boils quickly form. There is also often an eruption of mulberry-coloured spots or watery blisters on the body. Profuse perspirations are regarded as favourable; diarrhœa, bleeding from the nose or bowels, and delirium are unfavourable signs. The duration of bad cases is only two or three days, but less severe cases may be protracted two or three weeks. The disease may develop in a few hours after exposure to contagion. It may be communicated through the medium of the atmosphere, or by clothes or other articles which have been in contact with the sick. The conditions under which plague arises are a warm, moist, semi-tropical atmosphere; a low-lying alluvial soil, near the banks of rivers; crowded or badly ventilated dwellings; putrescent emanations from decaying animal or vegetable matters; insufficient or unwholesome food. When thus originating it may spread among other populations less influenced by the conditions named. The *treatment* consists in affording a pure atmosphere, in giving light but nourishing food, with stimulants, and in treating the boils as indicated under that heading.

**PLEURISY.**—Pleurisy is inflammation of the membrane covering the *outside* of the lungs and the *inside* of the chest, and separating one from the other. At the commencement of acute pleurisy there is generally shivering followed by fever, and by sense of weight, or 'stitches' in the chest. This in a few hours becomes acute *stabbing* pain, and is most felt in the side about the level of the nipple, shooting to the front of the chest, to the collar-bone, or to the armpit. There is short dry cough, the breathing is short and 'catching,' being frequently attended by an *expiratory* groan, and the pain is increased by coughing, by taking a long breath, or by lying on the affected side. The pulse is frequent and hard, feeling under the finger like a tense vibrating string. The tongue is furred white, the urine scanty and high-coloured, and the skin hot, rising in temperature to 100° or 102°.

Pleurisy may be caused by cold or by injuries, and often arises during the progress of fevers. If not checked, the result is the effusion of a watery fluid in the membrane placed between the lungs and the inside of the chest, forming dropsy of the chest. In favourable cases the acute pain and fever subside about the fourth or fifth day; but if there be any fluid effused, the cough and difficulty of breathing may persist indefinitely.

Pleurisy may be distinguished from *inflammation of the substance of the lungs* by, *first*, the character of the pain, which is *stabbing* or *lancinating* in pleurisy, but dull and aching in inflammation; *secondly*, by the cough, which is hard, dry, and short in pleurisy, and unattended with expectoration. In inflammation of the lungs the cough is more prolonged, and the expectoration is frothy and 'rusty,' or brown-coloured from admixture with blood. Mild cases of pleurisy may also be mistaken for the neuralgic pain in the side known as *pleurodynia* (*vide* p. 355), and *vice versâ*. *Pleurodynia* is distinguished by its generally affecting the left side of females, and by there being no attendant fever.

*Treatment.*—The patient should be kept in bed, warm and free from draughts. He should move and talk as little as possible, as motion accelerates the breathing and increases the pain. The diet should consist of eggs, beef-tea, broth, jelly, and fish. As a rule leeches are desirable and they may be applied over the painful part, one for each year of the patient's age, up to thirty in number. If they cannot be obtained, hot bruised poppy-head poultices should be applied over the painful part. As medicine, 3 or 4 grains of Dover's powder every four hours. Restlessness at night may be relieved by chloral. During convalescence care against cold and chill is urgently necessary, and if there is any remaining cough, Recipe 57.

[In young robust persons, if there is much feverishness, tartar emetic mixture (Recipe 59). When pain is relieved or ceases, this medicine must be discontinued. If the mixture produces sickness, the quantity given as a dose should be lessened. If the pain is *very severe*, and the patient a strong robust person, bleeding from the arm may be required, after which the pain is much relieved, and a long breath may be taken with more ease. But bleeding cannot be attempted except under medical advice. The pain may also be combated by the injection of morphia, a procedure requiring the supervision of a medical man.]

Pleurisy, Chronic.—Chronic pleurisy is generally a consequence of the acute form, but occasionally it commences as a sub-acute disease. In either case feverishness at night, a permanently quickened pulse, emaciation, difficulty of breathing increased on exertion, and inability to lie on the healthy side are the principal symptoms. These symptoms may be more or less severe according as the pleurisy is of greater or smaller extent. Such a condition is apt to alternate with symptoms of the more acute form, such as more severe pain, and fever of a *hectic* nature (*vide* p. 269). Chronic pleurisy may exist for months or years, the person so affected sometimes feeling little of the ailment, at others suffering from repeated sub-acute attacks. But in such patients the breathing is generally difficult, particularly on exertion, and there is tendency to night fever and night sweats. The *treatment* consists in supporting the patient's strength and in promoting the absorption of any effused fluid. The *first* indication should be fulfilled by liberal diet and by tonics, as Recipe 66; the second by the frequent application of some counter-irritant, which, in the absence of the remedy mentioned in the small type below, may be mustard poultices to the painful part. The chief means by which increase of the disease may be guarded against is care to avoid cold, for any slight cold is very liable to attack the chest as the weakest part, and to result in an accession of the more acute form of the malady. Intermittent fever or ague must also be guarded against by the use of quinine, for when fever occurs it is very liable to induce an increase of the pleuritic affection.

[The best local application is iodine paint, which should be applied to the side by means of a feather or brush every day, or less frequently after the first two or three days, so as to maintain an irritation of, but not to blister the skin (*vide Appendix*, No. 111). Iodide of potassium (Recipe 21) should also be administered internally. These measures, particularly the iodine paint, should be had recourse to immediately on every fresh attack.]

The ultimate results of either acute or chronic pleurisy may be accumulation of *water* in the cavity of the *pleura*, or membrane between the lungs and walls of the chest, which condition is called *Hydrothorax*, or accumulation of pus in the same position, called *Empyema*. These conditions may be suspected when, after pleurisy, night fever and pain remain, when the person grows emaciated, and when one side of the chest appears more prominent than the other. Such conditions require careful treatment by an experienced surgeon, and are often fatal.

**PLEURODYNIA** means nervous pain generally occurring in the left side, and especially to debilitated females suffering from chlorosis (*vide* p. 50), or flatulent dyspepsia (p. 204), amenorrhœa (p. 468), whites (p. 462), neuralgia (p. 341), or nervousness (p. 340). For distinction from pleurisy *vide* p. 352. Pain in either side may also be due to rheumatism of the muscles, when the pain is more diffused and movement is painful. A severe pain on either side may also be the precursor of shingles (*vide* p. 396). In either case a mustard leaf or poultice is a good local application. But medicines should be given with the view of remedying the condition with which the pain appears to be associated.

**POLYPUS.**—A polypus is a pear-shaped tumour, growing from a pedicle or stem. The most usual positions are the ear, the nose, the lower gut, the female privates, and less frequently the throat. Polypi may be soft, gelatinous, and light in colour, or comparatively hard, fleshy, and red. *Polypus of the ear* is noticed at p. 215. *Polypus of the nose* causes a feeling of stuffing in one or both nostrils, sneezing, and discharge, and snoring during sleep when the mouth is kept wide open. Taste and smell are impaired, and the speech becomes thick and nasal, all the symptoms being aggravated by damp weather. When one nostril only is affected, on stopping it by pressure with the finger, the person breathes well through the other. As the polypus grows it may present as a more or less reddened tumour at the entrance of the nostril; or it may hang through the posterior nostrils into the throat, causing constant hawking and spitting. Sometimes the patient feels the tumour flapping to and fro with the breathing, or it may be heard moving. It may cause bleeding from the nose (*vide* p. 510). *Polypus of the rectum*, or lower gut, causes the sensation of the presence of a foreign body in the part, or a feeling of weight and irritation which may be mistaken for piles. There is also frequently acute pain on going to stool very similar to that caused by *fissure* (*vide* p. 272). As the polypus grows it may present at the orifice, and, sometimes partially passing during stool, gets nipped, giving rise to much suffering. Polypus of the rectum is sometimes associated with piles, but the latter are much more common, and bleed much more than a polypus. When polypus of this part occurs, as it sometimes does, to children, it is generally of the red variety, and, presenting at the orifice like a red strawberry, may be mistaken for *protrusion of the bowel* (*vide* p. 84). But polypus is not common, and usually bleeds in children, while protrusion of the bowel is common, and does not usually bleed. *Polypus of the female private parts* gives rise to feelings of local weight and irritation, and the sensation of a foreign body. But polypus is comparatively rare, and such symptoms are mostly due to *displacements of the womb*, for which malady polypus may be mistaken (*vide* p. 478). As it grows it may present at the orifice, and may still be mistaken for a womb affection, so that persistent symptoms of the kind demand professional advice. The only cure for any kind of polypus is remova. by surgical operation.

**PREGNANCY, DISEASES OF.**—The most usual complaints during this period are as below.

1. INDIGESTION DURING PREGNANCY is generally marked by constipation, by heartburn, and by flatulence. The urine is also altered, often forming a filmy deposit on the surface when allowed to stand. The countenance occasionally becomes sallow, and there are sometimes eruptions on the face. The treatment consists in maintaining the bowels moderately loose by castor-oil, by senna, or by Recipes 1 and 2; in the use of remedies mentioned under *Flatulence* (*vide* p. 273), and in attention to diet, which should be nourishing but easily digestible.

2. Fainting Feelings and Palpitation are more common about the period of quickening, or between the end of the twelfth and the sixteenth week of pregnancy. Fainting feelings, or palpitations, often accompany the first movements of the child, and will be the more persistent and severe if indigestion prevails, or if the person exposes herself to the ordinary causes of fainting, as hot rooms, fatigue, or excitement. Often the least thing affects the patient, and there is frequently a dread felt of something unpleasant happening. A stimulant, as sal volatile or wine, and the recumbent posture are the immediate treatment required. All tight articles of dress should be discarded. But unless care is taken to avoid excitement this nervous condition is liable to result in abortion, or premature labour.

3. Alterations in Disposition and Temper show in various ways. The pleasant-tempered woman may become irritable, and *vice versâ*. There is often capricious appetite and 'longing' for improper or unobtainable articles of diet. Longings, if practicable, may be generally complied with.

4. Morning Sickness.—This generally sets in about the sixth week, ceasing after the third month. But it may commence earlier, and it may continue to the termination of the pregnancy. Most women suffer more or less from nausea and vomiting, especially in the morning, but with some women it continues more or less during the entire day, and may be extraordinarily violent. A minor degree of nausea during child-bearing is popularly supposed to be a good sign, and if only present to a slight degree in the morning, treatment is not required. In other cases great attention must be paid to diet, one article after another being abstained from, in order to discover any offending material. For it sometimes happens that substances taken by women with perfect im-

punity at other times cannot be eaten during pregnancy. Rich, indigestible food, as pastry, made dishes, and salt meat, should be avoided. The bowels must be kept open by castor-oil. Quinine with an aperient if the bowels are confined, as Recipe 66, with the addition of six drachms of sulphate of soda, may be tried. A little tea and toast should be taken in the morning, before the erect posture is assumed. If *acidity* of the stomach is present, the medicines mentioned under such head should be employed. Some women find it a good plan to drink a glass of warm water, and so encourage the sickness for a few minutes, which then passes off, leaving them free for the day. *When vomiting or nausea is very distressing, continuing all day*, nourishment in the shape of good soup and brandy should be administered at intervals of half an hour, but not more than two or three spoonfuls at once. Champagne and soda-water sometimes afford relief. Sal volatile in a little water may be tried. Ipecacuanha wine given in one-drop doses, in a teaspoonful of water, every hour, has sometimes a very good effect. Sucking ice is also often useful, and a mustard poultice to the pit of the stomach should not be neglected. The wet compress may also be tried. This is made by placing several folds of wet linen over the stomach, covering with oiled silk, and then applying a bandage from eight to ten inches wide. This should be drawn moderately tight, and worn for two or three hours every morning. When vomiting is very uncontrollable, an injection of forty grains of chloral in six ounces of lukewarm water may be given.

[Other remedies are effervescing draughts of citrate of magnesia (*vide* p. 15) with two or three drops of chloroform; magnesia in peppermint water, as Recipe 61; also Recipes 6, 16, 22, 36, and 37, any of which sometimes suit one person but not another, nor even the same person at different times. The inhalation of the steam from hot water in which a little laudanum has been mixed in the proportion of 1 ounce of the latter to 2 quarts of the former may be advisable.]

5. Toothache or Salivation.—The pain is sometimes confined to a decayed tooth; occasionally it attacks a sound one. The first, if far gone, may be extracted, although this is not always advisable, as the shock has been in nervous women followed by miscarriage; but a sound tooth should never be taken out. Local applications may be used, as mentioned under *Toothache*, p. 448. But more benefit will be derived from attention to the general health as regards the state of the bowels, of the digestion, and of manner of life in matters of regimen and early hours. Washing the mouth with a tea-spoonful of salt in a tumbler of water is beneficial.

*Salivation*, or the profuse secretion of saliva, is less common than toothache, but sometimes occurs either in connection with the latter ailment or alone. Astringent gargles may be used (Recipe 100), or a piece of alum may be sucked occasionally. Attention must be paid to the general health, and constipation must be avoided.

6. Swelling of the Legs.—Occurs during the latter months of pregnancy. This condition, and *varicose* or enlarged veins, with which it is often associated, are due to the pressure exercised by the distended womb on the blood-vessels passing from the body to the lower extremities. When the legs are swelled, they 'pit,' or show an indentation when pressed with the fingers. The swelling is much less in the mornings, sometimes totally disappearing after lying down, but soon returning on the erect posture being reassumed. No kind of medicine is of avail; as, until the pressure is removed by the birth of the child, the results must continue. But the condition may be lessened by frequently lying down, by keeping the legs up on a stool when sitting, and by applying bandages, or wearing an elastic stocking.

*Note.*—If swelling of the face or of other parts of the body takes place, especially if there is *albumen* in the urine (*vide* p. 101), medical advice should be obtained, as it may be the commencement of some serious disease. In the absence of medical assistance the person should be treated as for dropsy from exposure (*vide* p. 187).

7. Cramps of the Legs.—(*Vide* p. 409.)

8. Varicose Veins.—(*Vide* p. 456.)

9. Irritation of the Breasts.—About two months after conception there is an uneasy sensation of fulness, with throbbing and tingling pain, or perhaps pain *below* the breast on the left side. The breasts increase in size, feel knotted, and there is a dark circle round the nipple. There is sometimes a milky or watery secretion from the nipple. These symptoms may cause annoyance, but they may be relieved by keeping the bowels open and by bathing the breasts with warm water.

During the latter month of pregnancy, and especially before the first confinement, the nipples should be bathed twice daily, with equal parts of brandy and water, or with alum water, or with infusion of green tea, and they should be pulled out and elongated with the fingers. Any flannel covering worn over the nipples should be dispensed with. It is also a good plan to expose the nipples to the air for two or three hours daily, which has a similar effect. These measures prevent 'cracking' during suckling, and render the nipple harder and longer, and therefore more easily accessible to the child's mouth. The pain *below* the breast, mentioned above, often depends on constipation, and may be relieved by aperients. When the breasts are tender, heavy, and enlarged, much benefit is experienced by supporting them by a pad of wadding attached to the stays, or by a handkerchief passing under the breast and tied over the opposite shoulder.

10. Piles.—Piles are very common during pregnancy; they are caused by the pressure of the distended womb, and medicines do not much benefit. After confinement

they generally disappear. Avoiding standing about, and lying down frequently, washing the parts with cold water and applying gall ointment (Recipe 95), or hazeline, is the proper treatment (*vide* p. 349).

11. Irritation of the Bladder and Private Parts. Depend on the pressure exerted by the distended womb. *Irritation of the bladder* manifests itself by 'scalding,' by frequent desire to make water, or by inability to retain the water, which frequently passes even against the will of the patient. Some relief may be obtained by drinking freely of barley-water, linseed tea, or lime-water and milk, by relieving constipated bowels, by aperients, and by maintaining the recumbent posture for several hours during the day, lying on either side instead of the back. But often nothing will relieve this condition, until the womb rises sufficiently high, so that the pressure from its bulk on the bladder is removed.

Occasionally not only irritation of the bladder, but even *retention of urine*, or *inability to make water*, is caused by women in the early months of pregnancy neglecting to pass water until the bladder becomes much distended, so that its muscle loses the power of contracting to expel the contents. Females travelling by rail, or in other positions where they are unable to obey the calls of nature, are exposed to this accident. When retention of urine occurs, the person should as soon as possible take a warm bath. If this does not produce the desired effect, she should go to bed, take 10 grains of Dover's powder, and be covered with blankets to produce perspiration, and so relieve the bladder until urine passes naturally, or a doctor can give relief by passing a catheter. Drinking meanwhile should be abstained from, and no medicines, as spirits of nitre or gin, calculated to increase the secretion of urine should be taken, for by such means the distension of the bladder would be increased, while its power of expulsion would be decreased. The bladder, when paralysed in this way, does not recover its tone immediately, and therefore may require to be again relieved by the warm bath or the instrument. When cases of this kind are neglected, and the bladder is distended to its greatest limit, the water may begin to flow off by drops *without the will or even knowledge of the patient.* Nurses are often deceived by this appearance, and fancy that the water having commenced to come will soon flow naturally. But the reverse is the fact, and when this occurs the case demands constant medical aid.

For *irritation of the private parts, vide* p. 365.

12. JAUNDICE.—Usually occurs about the fifth month, and probably passes away before the end of pregnancy, as the pressure causing it is removed by the alteration in the position of the womb. An occasional dose of castor-oil is desirable.

13. MISCARRIAGE.—Miscarriage occurs some time before the sixth month of pregnancy. If the child is born after that time it is called *premature delivery.* The most usual period of miscarriage is about the third month, and it is more likely to happen about the time corresponding with what would have been the natural monthly period had not pregnancy occurred. When it has once occurred it is very likely to happen again. The causes are various, often depending on debility, and often brought on by imprudence in horse exercise, dancing, or from excitement, from passion or fright. It also frequently results from blows, falls, or concussions, such as missing a step coming downstairs, bumps in a carriage, jolting in a palankeen, &c. In other instances it is due to local weakness or disease of the womb. Attacks of dysentery often lead to miscarriage. There is in some women an inherent weakness of constitution, which prevents pregnancy passing on to the full time. Attacks of

malarious fever add to this weakness, rendering miscarriage in such persons an ordinary sequence of conception.

*Symptoms.*—When threatened with a miscarriage the patient experiences a sense of uneasiness, languor, and weariness, with aching pain in the back, loins, and hips, and a slightly bloody discharge. After these symptoms have lasted a variable time, there are pains very like those of labour, often vomiting, and sometimes profuse bleeding, the blood passed being of a vivid red colour. This may continue for several days, the pain and bleeding recurring at intervals; or the miscarriage may commence suddenly, and the whole be over in a few hours. The *ovum* or *fœtus* is expelled in the shape of a reddish-white ball, the size of a pigeon's egg at three months, and larger in proportion afterwards. After the *ovum* or *fœtus* has passed away the pain and bleeding cease. The danger and after-injury are in proportion to the amount of pain and of attending bleeding.

*Treatment.*—If the bleeding is slight and the pain trifling, the abortion may sometimes be prevented by *perfect* quiet and rest on a hard bed in a cool room, aided by a dose of 30 drops of chlorodyne in 1 ounce of water, followed by alum mixture (Recipe 42). But if increased pain and bleeding occur, the miscarriage will certainly take place, when the danger to be guarded against is profuse loss of blood. The alum mixture should be continued, the patient should not be allowed to move from the bed, and cloths saturated with cold water should be applied to the external outlet. As before mentioned, the bleeding ceases directly the abortion passes, but it is sometimes necessary to remove the mass with the fingers. The after-treatment requires as much care as after confinement. The patient should rest in bed seven or eight days and then return gradually to her employments, while the diet should be simple, and the bowels be maintained moderately open. Getting about too soon after a miscarriage is not unfrequently the origin of some malady of the womb, from which the woman may long suffer.

[A better medicine than the alum mixture mentioned above is Recipe 43, which, if possible, should be procured and used.]

**PRIVATE PARTS, FEMALE, DISCHARGE OF THE.**—This may arise from *gonorrhœa* (*vide* p. 281) or from *whites* (*vide* p. 462). Discharge may also occur in children, as a result of the irritation caused by *worms*, especially by *thread-worms* (*vide* p. 487), or from *constipation* (*vide* p. 138); particularly when little balls of hard fæcal matter are allowed to collect in the lower gut. Discharges occurring to female children may arouse suspicion of unfair usage; but they are commonly due to the causes indicated. The treatment consists in finding out and in removing such causes; in cleanliness; and, as the malady mostly occurs to weakly children, in giving good nourishing diet, and, after removal of the causes, tonic medicine (Recipe 66).

**PRIVATE PARTS, MALE, DISCHARGE FROM THE.**—Generally occurs from *gonorrhœa* or *gleet* (*vide* p. 281). But a glairy, clear, ropy discharge may present when there has been neither gonorrhœa nor gleet, when it will probably be due to irritation of the parts, consequent on *Piles* (*vide* p. 347), or on *Worms* (*vide* p. 487), or on *Varicocele* (*vide* p. 454), or on *Constipation* (*vide* p. 137).

Another malady of the kind is known technically as *spermatorrhœa*, and consists of nocturnal discharges of a milky appearance. Occasional discharges of this description are of no consequence. In severe cases similar discharges may occur during the day. Often this depends on certain bad habits, and the result will cease when such practices are discontinued. Such discharges are often associated with dyspeptic symptoms, and the patient is frequently out of health, his system below par, and influenced by some disappointment or mental anxiety. The recurrence of the symptoms tends to exaggerate the depressed condition, the mind of the patient dwells needlessly upon it, and he erroneously supposes the malady to be of great importance. This, however, is not the fact. If there are piles, or varicocele, or constipation, these maladies must be treated, and not the effect they cause. If there are dyspeptic symptoms, treatment must be directed towards them (*vide* p. 197). If the spirits are depressed, change of employment, or relief from mental occupation, and change of locality are indicated. In the meantime the bowels should be kept open, and the closet should be visited in the evening, so that the lower bowel may be emptied before the person retires to rest. Late suppers should be avoided, and no spirits should be taken. The patient should sleep on a hard bed, and be lightly covered, and he should not lie on his back. To prevent this, some solid substance fastened with a handkerchief on the back, a little below the loins, is a good contrivance. As medicine, if there are no prominent dyspeptic symptoms requiring treatment, and if the bowels are sufficiently open, quinine and iron (Recipe 70), with double doses of bromide of potassium (Recipe 19) at night.

The following pill is very beneficial. Phosphorus *one-fiftieth* of a grain, extract of nux vomica one-fourth of a grain, precipitated carbonate of iron 1 grain. Dose—one, thrice daily.

**PRIVATE PARTS, IRRITATION AND ITCHING OF THE.** —Irritation of the private parts often takes the shape of intense itching or smarting, which prevents sleep, and so destroys the health. It may depend on thread-worms (*vide* p. 486), or lice (p. 613), or irritable bladder (p. 73), or whites (p. 462), or eczema (p. 396), or gout (p. 282), or diabetes (p. 164); or it may be sympathetic with cancer of the womb (p. 111), and it often occurs during pregnancy (p. 362). The itching may or may not be associated with an eruption of minute watery vesicles. The treatment must depend on the cause. As a local application for intense itching, bathing with cold or iced water is the best remedy. If the itching is accompanied by the eruption of vesicles mentioned above, alum water should be used. Sometimes much relief may be obtained by bathing with cold poppy-water (*vide Appendix*, No. 81).

A good lotion is made as follows: borax, a tea-spoonful; hot water, a pint; peppermint oil, 5 drops; to be used frequently with a sponge. Shake well before using.

**PRIVATE PARTS, FEMALE, OCCLUSION OF THE.**—This consists in the apparent formation of a skin at the orifice, uniting the two sides, which seem thus grown together. It depends on the collection of the natural discharge near the orifice, and although of some strength and thickness, it is not a new growth. The urine of children thus affected often squirts in a backward or forward direction, which may first attract attention. It chiefly occurs to children who are not kept properly clean. The remedy consists in breaking the obstruction down with a probe or a quill, in applying a little salad oil to the parts, and in perfect cleanliness.

**PROSTATE GLAND, ENLARGEMENT OF THE.**—The prostate gland surrounds the *urethra*, or urinary passage at the neck of the bladder, and is liable to several diseases. The most important disease of the gland is *slow enlargement.* This is most common after middle age, and is characterised by frequent calls to make water, especially during the night, increasing slowness and difficulty in making water, and straining. But straining does not much increase the flow of urine, which falls directly forward and is not ejected in a stream. There is a sense of weight in the fork so that the patient often imagines he has piles. The enlarged gland mechanically prevents the bladder being perfectly emptied, and the urine remaining decomposes and becomes ammoniacal, setting up chronic inflammation of the bladder (*vide* p. 71). Then the urine is loaded with sticky, tenacious mucus, or purulent matter, which adheres to the bottom of the utensil, and is frequently tinged with blood. There may also be fits of complete retention of urine (*vide* p. 420). Bleeding, sometimes copious and sudden, may also occur. The early symptoms of enlargement of the prostate are sometimes very like those arising from other causes, as *stone in the bladder* (p. 73) and *stricture* (p .419), so that physical examination is usually necessary to decide the point.

*Treatment.*—This disease is seldom cured, although much may be done to retard its progress. The patient must avoid irregular diet, fatigue, and exposure to cold. The bowels should be kept open, so that there may be no straining at stool. Enemas of warm water will prove beneficial for the relief of occasional fits of spasmodic pain.

The urine should be frequently tested with litmus paper (*vide* p. 288). If the urine is acid, Recipes 35 and 37 may be tried in succession. If the urine is ropy and thick as well as acid, Recipes 27, 28. If the urine is neutral, known by no change in the colour of the paper, Recipe 31. If it is alkaline, and especially if also thick and ropy, Recipes 33, 34; the former being advisable if the liver is not acting. The passage of a peculiarly shaped catheter may be also necessary, so that the malady is one requiring the daily attention of a surgeon.

**RHEUMATISM, ACUTE.**—Acute rheumatism, often termed *rheumatic fever*, is more common in young than in old persons; it commences usually after exposure to damp cold, with fever, a full quick pulse, hot skin, coated tongue, and scanty urine which deposits a dusky reddish sediment. The pain generally comes on in one of the larger joints, which is highly inflamed, red, and swollen, so that it cannot be moved, and the slightest touch is shrunk from.

The inflammation may attack several or all the joints, but more commonly two or three are affected one day, and then others are suddenly attacked, the first joint implicated growing, almost as suddenly, comparatively well. There are also frequent sour perspirations, which do not afford relief. These perspirations are often accompanied by an eruption of small vesicles known as *sudamina* (*vide* p. 399), which is caused by the heat and moisture, and is of no consequence. The duration of the disease may be a fortnight to three weeks, when complete recovery may occur, or stiffness and pain in the joints may remain. If the temperature of the body rises to 105° Fahr. it is an alarming symptom indicating *heart affection*, as described below.

A frequent accompaniment of acute rheumatism is *affection of the heart*, the disease extending inwards and attacking that organ. Sometimes the symptoms are very faintly pronounced, but there will be more or less sharp cutting pain in the left side, increased by taking a long breath, a feeling of distress or tightness of the chest, short hacking cough, and more or less difficulty of breathing. There may also be occasional palpitations and irregularity of the heart's action, manifested by the pulse being irregular, feeling *small* under the finger, and affording a peculiar jar or thrill to the touch. During an attack of rheumatic fever such symptoms should be daily watched for, as they denote a serious aggravation of the illness, from *inflammation of the membranes* covering or lining the heart. Of the latter membrane are formed the delicate valves guarding the portals of the four chambers of the heart. When these valves become inflated there is tendency to deposit of material from the blood upon them, or they may be contracted, or their action otherwise interfered with. Then there is an impediment to the easy passage of the blood, which even years afterwards may evidence itself by alteration in the sounds of the heart, and by the result—*dropsy*—from which death sooner or later occurs. Acute rheumatism, from its tendency to affect the heart, must always be regarded as serious.

*Treatment.*—In ordinary cases clothe the patient in flannel, keep him at rest during the whole period of the disease, and apply a hot alkaline lotion to the affected joints. The lotion should be composed of half a pound of common carbonate of soda dissolved in one quart of hot water, or, if obtainable, of poppy-head water (*Appendix*, No. 81), with which cloths should be well saturated, wrapped round the parts, and the whole covered with oiled silk, or other waterproof material. If the pain from movement is not too great, a hot bath at 98° Fahr. should be given daily, a couple of pounds of common carbonate of soda having been previously dissolved in the water. If the bowels are not moved naturally, they should be acted upon occasionally by Recipes 1 and 2, and citrate of magnesia draughts (*vide* p. 15) should be taken three times daily. Dover's powder in 10- or 15-grain doses may also be given at night when sleeplessness from pain is complained of. When the symptoms indicate extension to the heart, mustard leaves or poultices should be applied over the seat of pain, the patient should be forbidden to talk much, the Dover's powder should be continued at night, and Recipe 50 should be given very frequently, or every three hours. Low diet, no meat, and abstinence from stimulating liquors are necessary.

[If procurable, give the following: salicylate of soda, 3 drachms; distilled water, 12 ounces. Dose—two table-spoonfuls every three hours. Or if the case is very severe, with much pain and swelling of the joints, salicylic acid and morphia, Recipe 29. Either of these medicines often does much good; but if so the relief is experienced within two days, in which case it should be given less frequently. But salicylate of soda, or salicylic acid, in exceptional cases, or given in larger doses, may produce nausea, noises in the ears, deafness, delirium, or albumen in the urine (*vide* p. 101). When using these medicines the urine should be examined twice daily, and if any albumen presents, or if symptoms as above occur, the medicine should be stopped. If no relief is obtained the colchicum and alkaline mixture (Recipe 52) should be used. If the heart becomes affected a blister should be applied if obtainable, instead of mustard.]

**RHEUMATISM, CHRONIC.**—Is most frequent in elderly persons, especially in those classes exposed to vicissitudes of weather, and who are ill-fed. Chronic rheumatism may attack the joints, when it is termed *Rheumatoid Arthritis*. Or it may attack the muscles, when it is termed *Muscular Rheumatism*. There is pain in the larger joints, accompanied sometimes with swelling, but the smaller joints, as the knuckles of the fingers, do not always escape. It is to this form of the malady that the term *Rheumatic Gout* is often applied. In old cases of joint affection, cracking or grating sounds may be heard when the limbs are moved. With chronic rheumatism there is generally neither fever nor perspiration. Sometimes the pain is relieved by warmth, in other cases warmth increases it. The first thing to attend to is the removal of the causes by which the malady is kept up. Rooms with damp floors and walls, insufficient clothing, especially want of flannel, and absence of nourishing diet, are among the most prominent. As medical treatment, warm clothing, generous living, Dover's powder occasionally at night, and rubbing the parts with grass oil may be recommended.

Lumbago (*vide* p. 324) is a form of muscular rheumatism; *Sciatica* (*vide* p. 378) is frequently combined with muscular rheumatism. *Stiff Neck*, which is also muscular rheumatism, may often be much relieved by spreading a layer of cotton-wool over the part, and then ironing it with a hot flat iron.

[As internal remedies, Recipes 30 and 52 may be procured and tried in succession. As external application, Recipe 80.]

**RICKETS.**—This disease is an imperfect development of the bones, which, being deficient in earthy salts, become soft and yielding. It is a disease of early infancy, and sometimes exists at birth, although often not recognised till the child begins to walk. Rickets is most likely to occur from six months old till all the teeth (which are always backward) have appeared, but it may present up to seven years old. It usually occurs to scrofulous or to delicate children, particularly if they have suffered much from bad nutrition consequent on repeated or long-continued *disorder of the stomach* (*vide* p. 417); or if they have been fed too exclusively on farinaceous foods (*vide* Chapter V., *On the Feeding of Children*; or *Index*). Unhygienic conditions, as damp residences, want of ventilation, and unsuitable clothing, add much to the liability to the disease. The first symptoms are common to several diseases of children, viz. fretfulness, irritability, capricious appetite, disordered bowels, with lead-coloured stools, thick urine, and emaciation. Probably the first thing which attracts the attention of the mother or nurse, beyond the fact that the child is peevish, and that its food does not appear to do it good, will be sweating of the head at night. There is also slight fever, followed by swelling of the bowels, which often feel knotted; the condition, in fact, described as *atrophy* (*vide* p. 66) being established. Then there is profuse perspiration at night of the whole body, with a tendency to kick the clothing off. The joints, especially the knees, ankles, and wrists, now grow tender, and become swollen, thickened, and knotted in appearance; or as if surrounded by a ring of bone. To this the term 'double-jointed' has been applied. The legs may bend outwards or inwards, with the results, perhaps, of permanent 'bow leg' or 'knock-knee.' The child cannot stand, is unable to turn itself in bed, and dreads to be touched. There may also be a thinning of the bones of the head, especially at the back; and the *fontanelles*, or spaces between the bones at the top, do not close, giving the head a large appearance. Sometimes the head is incessantly rolled from side to side, often making a bald place on the back of the head. Sometimes the spine or bones of the chest become affected, and there may be permanent deformity of the spine, or the condition known as 'chicken breast.' Before this occurs, if the fingers are passed carefully down the front of the chest, two rows of little bony knobs may be felt. A child with rickets always looks prematurely old and careworn, and there is an unnatural brilliancy of the eyes. The disease may last months, and may terminate from exhaustion, from diarrhœa, or from some affection of the chest supervening, or less frequently from convulsions. The first signs of recovery are the child being able to move better, decrease of emaciation, and natural stools.

*Treatment.*—Recipe 66 may be used. Also lime-water (Recipe 25) and milk in equal parts. Animal broths should also be given freely, but vegetable food more sparingly. A little port wine may be usually taken with advantage. Plenty of fresh air, ventilation of sleeping-rooms, freedom from damp, and warm clothing are imperative. Sea- or salt-water baths, or, if movement is painful, salt-water sponging, are beneficial. The child should sleep on a good even mattress, and should sit up as little as possible. He should also be kept from walking till the bones are able to bear the weight. If the spine is affected he should lie mostly on the back.

Cod-liver oil, and citrate of iron and quinine (Recipe 70) are required, or iodide of iron (Recipe 74) if the bowels are enlarged.

**SALIVATION.**—This term signifies an increased and unnatural flow of saliva. The salivation occurring to pregnant women is referred to at p. 359. But salivation may occur from inflammation of the gums and mouth, as the result of cold, of debility, of indigestion, of teething, and of taking mercury and some other substances. In such cases there are swelling of the cheeks, tongue, and gums, enlargement of the glands under the jaw, stiffness of the latter, shooting pains in the face, fœtor of the breath, and a profuse discharge of saliva. *When salivation has been caused by mercury*, the fœtor is more marked and peculiar, and there is a more or less distinct red line on the gums near the teeth. As the swelling becomes greater the tongue and cheeks are indented by the teeth, and ulcers form. The usual duration of mercurial salivation is from ten days to a fortnight; in some cases the inflammation may be more prolonged, and the resulting ulcers slower in healing. The treatment should consist in the use of astringent gargles, of which alum is one of the best (Recipe 100), or port wine and water in equal parts may be used, sometimes one, sometimes the other appearing to suit best. The patient's strength must be supported by fluid but nourishing and easily digestible diet. Afterwards, or *when salivation has occurred from debility from the first*, tonics, as quinine and iron (Recipe 73), will be advisable, while remaining ulcers should be daily touched with a concentrated solution of alum (3 drachms of powdered alum in 1 ounce of water), or with vinegar applied by means of a feather or camel-hair brush.

[Recipes 102 and 103 should be procured and used if the alum gargle is not satisfactory.]

**SCARLET FEVER or SCARLATINA.**—The latter word signifies the same as scarlet fever. It is not a diminutive, and is not properly employed to denote milder cases. Scarlet fever is not so common in India as in England, but becoming more so, consequent on successive importations from Europe. Scarlet fever is a contagious eruptive fever, generally occurring early in life. It seldom happens twice to the same person. The *cause* of scarlet fever is the conveyance in some way or another of the germs of the disease from the sick to the healthy. The active poison is believed to be an organism or *microbe* which has been found in the blood of the patient, in the scurf or peels of skin cast off, and in the breath. It has also been found that cows affected with small vesicles on a red and swollen teat, and with shedding of the hair in patches, develop a similar microbe, which, impregnating the milk, is believed to give rise to scarlet fever in those drinking it. The disease has also been supposed to be conveyed through the medium of books from circulating libraries, and it may be carried in any article of clothing. The germs may also adhere to the walls and furniture of rooms, giving rise to the malady in fresh occupants after a lengthened period, even of months. In the earlier stages especially the exhalations from the mouth and throat may convey the disease, if such exhalations are incautiously inhaled by a healthy individual; but in the latter stages the scurf or flakes of skin cast off are more likely to convey the malady if inhaled or swallowed by another person. The time at which the disease ordinarily appears after exposure to infection is from seven to ten days, although there are many instances when it showed itself much quicker, within twenty-four hours, and when it developed later, up to fourteen days. The time at which a patient ceases to be capable of conveying infection is not less than ten weeks after the appearance of sore-throat and rash. Complete freedom from scurf and scales is not, as often assumed, sufficient evidence of a patient being free from infectious material. After five weeks the danger is very much lessened; but complete safety cannot be assumed in less than ten weeks.

*Symptoms.*—The symptoms of an ordinary case of scarlet fever are as follows. For twenty-four hours there are chills or shivering, followed by fever, sore-throat, nausea, pains about the limbs and body, and often vomiting and diarrhœa, the urine being scanty and high-coloured. Sore-throat is the main characteristic of scarlet fever, as cough is of measles. The throat is vivid red, the redness being equally diffused over the tonsils and back of the throat, which distinguishes it from ordinary inflammation of the tonsils (*vide* p. 444), which usually affects one side. In young children convulsions, or premonitory symptoms of convulsions (p. 144), occasionally occur. The rise of temperature is very marked, often, as tested by the clinical thermometer (p. 34), rising to 105° on the first day, while the pulse may be 120 or much quicker in children (*vide* p. 31). On the second day the rash appears, spreading from the face and neck, over the breast, trunk, and limbs. But the rash is not (as in small-pox) attended with any diminution of the fever. First there are a multitude of minute red points. Then these run together, or others appear, until the whole surface of the skin is uniformly scarlet, without (as in measles) patches of intervening healthy-looking skin. The skin now begins to itch intolerably. The whites of the eyes may also become scarlet. The tongue presents characteristic red spots with white fur between, looking as if powdered with cayenne pepper. If not previous to, then accompanying the eruption, one or more glands in the neck may enlarge, causing increased difficulty of swallowing. The tonsils are now often coated with specks of white mucous deposit, which is different from the harder yellowish patches of exudation in diphtheria (*vide* p. 177). The rash generally lasts till the fifth or sixth day, when it begins to decline, disappearing on the eighth or ninth day with much scurfiness of the skin, which sometimes comes off the hands and feet in large flakes or scales. Occasionally this scaling commences earlier, or it may be delayed, and not be entirely completed for some weeks. When the attack is severe there is always much fever and often delirium at night, and in children there may be convulsions. The duration of an ordinary case is fourteen or fifteen days.

*There is great variability in the symptoms of scarlet fever.* During epidemics, cases occur, in which sore-throat is the *only* recognisable symptom, but the malady is nevertheless scarlet fever, and infectious. On the other hand, it is liable to assume aggravated forms. The tonsils or the glands of the neck, or both, may 'gather.' The throat affection may extend to the ears, causing violent pain, or inflammation in those organs. In another variety the face is dusky, the rash livid in colour, discharges occur from the female privates, and the fever is typhoid in character. The danger is then extreme, and the patient requires stimulants most urgently. In a third form of the disease the fever and sore-throat may appear without any rash. This variety is often fatal, and may be mistaken for diphtheria. The urine may become dusky and contain albumen (*vide* p. 101), symptoms which should be watched for, as they may be indicative (especially in children) of supervening convulsions, of head affection, of nephritis (*vide* p. 314), or of other future kidney malady.

*Sequelæ.*—After almost any variety of scarlet fever, the person often shows much debility for some time, and is liable to different kinds of dropsy. The whole body may become swollen (*Anasarca, vide* p. 187), the urine scanty and smoke-coloured, and the kidneys affected as in Bright's disease (*vide* p. 100); or there may be swelling of the abdomen only (*Ascites, vide* p. 188), or enlargement of one or more of the joints. Discharges from the nostrils, or from the ears, ophthalmic affections, permanently enlarged tonsils, and troublesome diarrhœa, are also frequent sequelæ.

Scarlet fever may be mistaken for measles. The prominent symptoms of each are therefore contrasted.

| Measles | Scarlet Fever |
| --- | --- |
| Cold in the head. | None. |
| Hoarse cough. | None. |
| Eruption crimson-coloured. | Vividly scarlet. |
| Eruption raised in crescent-shaped patches. | Not raised, not crescent-shaped. |
| Affection of the chest or bronchitis accompanying. | Affections of the throat accompanying. |
| It is very common in India. | Seldom occurs in India. |

Scarlet fever may be further distinguished from the eruption of measles, or from erythema, or erysipelas, by the production of a white line on the skin by scraping it with a pencil or the back of the finger-nail. This white line lasts a minute or so and then disappears—a condition not produced in the other forms of skin affection mentioned.

*Treatment.*—The diagnosis of scarlet fever from measles is important, as in the latter disease the patient should be at first kept warm, in order to guard against affections of the chest. In scarlet fever the patient should be at first kept moderately cool until after the eruption shows, when more clothing should be allowed. The patient should be placed in a well-ventilated room, and isolated to prevent the spread of the disease to others. During the preliminary fever, cooling draughts, as citrate of magnesia (*vide* p. 15), should be given, and the bowels should be opened by castor-oil or senna for a child, and by sulphate of soda (Recipe 2) for an adult. When the eruption has fairly come out the use of violet powder, or sponging gently with tepid water, is often both grateful and beneficial, or, if possible, a warm bath should be given every night. The diet should consist of good broths and gruels, and when convalescence is established a more generous diet, with iron and quinine, should be allowed. When the throat is much inflamed or ulcerated, a poultice of linseed meal, or hot moist flannels, or sponges, may be applied externally, and a solution of alum of the strength of five drachms to the ounce of water should be brushed over the tonsils, or three or four grains of finely powdered alum may be blown into the throat from several quills joined together or from a long glass tube. The throat should also be well steamed internally several times daily, by permitting the steam of hot water to pass into the mouth. Sucking ice generally relieves the thirst, and sometimes the throat also. The ventilation of the sick-chamber, the prompt removal of *excreta*, the support of the patient with nourishing diet, especially in those cases where the throat is very inflamed, or when little or no eruption appears, and the avoidance of all causes of nervous or mental excitement, especially when there is albumen in the urine, are the principal measures of cure.

*Scarlet fever is very infectious.* The patient, therefore, should be isolated from the first. The sick-room should be cleared of all needless furniture or drapery, and all the rules given regarding 'disinfection' should be strictly carried out. (*Vide Appendix*, Nos. 121 to 130.)

If after scarlet fever any portion of the skin peels off in flakes, anointing with sweet oil or glycerine will relieve the soreness. Dropsical swellings, or other after-effects of scarlet fever, must be treated as mentioned under the heads of the different ailments.

If obtainable, disinfect the throat twice daily by painting it inside with boracic acid—2 drachms dissolved in 1 ounce of glycerine. Also, after the sponging or warm bath, when the eruption begins to subside, apply the following ointment to the whole body: carbolic acid 30 grains, thymol 10 grains, vaseline 1 drachm, simple ointment 1 ounce.

**SCIATICA.**—Sciatica is a painful affection of the large nerve passing down the back of the thigh. There is acute agonising pain extending from the buttock to the ham. It is known from rheumatism by the pain, being limited to the course of the sciatic nerve, and by being little if at all aggravated by motion, although increased by pressure. But sometimes the muscles near the nerve are also affected with rheumatism, when the distinction is not so clear, as the pain is felt in the whole of the back part of the limb instead of in a line nearly in the centre. It may originate from cold, or from sitting on a wet seat; or in more rare cases it is a consequence of constipation, being then produced by the direct pressure of fæcal matter in the bowels on the sciatic nerve, before it passes by the nates. The *treatment* consists in rest, wearing warm flannel drawers, hot fomentations, the use of the hot flat iron as recommended for stiff neck (*vide* p. 370), or mustard poultices or small blisters over the more painful parts. Purgatives, as Recipes 1 and 2, in full doses, should also be given. In cases connected with rheumatism the treatment appropriate to chronic rheumatism should be employed.

[Galvanism may also be tried; and the subcutaneous injection of morphia is often most beneficial.]

**SCROFULA.**—This is a depraved condition most frequently hereditary, and is indicated by two different but common types, both of which are very liable to tubercular affections (*vide* p. 88). The *dark* type is characterised by coarse black hair, a thick upper lip, wide nostrils, frequently ill-shaped features or hands, clubbed nails marked with lines, and ill-proportioned body and limbs. The scrofulous child thus indicated may be weak in intellect, and is particularly liable to *enlargement of the glands* of the neck, often ending in abscess; to *enlarged tonsils*; to *discharges about the ear*; to *ophthalmia* and *ulcers of the cornea*; to certain skin diseases, especially *eczema*; to *atrophy*; to *disease of the joints*; and less frequently to *rickets*. If the child grows up it is pale, ill-nourished, and still prone to eruptions, to swelling of the glands in the neck, to unhealthy ulcers, and to affections of the joints. The second or *light* type of scrofula often exhibits what many call beauty. There are a thin skin, clear complexion, rosy cheeks and lips, blue bright eyes, large pupils, long eyelashes, silken hair, oval face, delicately chiselled features, small bones, and the veins are distinctly visible through the skin. The intellect is often powerful, and sometimes precociously developed. Children thus characterised are more liable to *bronchitis*, to *atrophy*, to *water on the brain*, and, as they grow up, to *consumption*, than to the maladies mentioned above as most frequently associated with the *dark* type. Scrofula is in many instances dependent on some hereditary constitutional taint, but it may be excited by poor living and damp lodging, by unventilated apartments, combined it may be, with drunkenness and venereal taints. Matches between near relations are also supposed to engender scrofulous children. Good air, good food, cod-liver oil, and exercise may eradicate the taint.

**SCURVY** is popularly supposed to be a scab or scurf on the skin, which is erroneous, as it consists of an alteration in the blood and tissues of the whole body. Scurvy may be either *declared* or *latent*. *Latent* or *hidden* scurvy is much more prevalent in India than is supposed, arising from a difficulty experienced in many positions into which residents are thrown, of obtaining a sufficient amount of fresh vegetable diet possessing anti-scorbutic properties, and which no indigenous vegetable does possess in any useful degree. There is another cause why, among Europeans, the scorbutic taint frequently exists, either hidden or declared. Even those with a table well supplied with fresh vegetables often insensibly acquire a habit of eating less vegetable material as part of their daily food than they would do in

Europe. This partly arises from loss of appetite during the hot weather, and partly from soups and curries being mainly composed of animal constituents, resulting in a diminution of vegetable matter in food which is consumed. Another cause predisposing to scurvy in India is the darkened dwellings in which so many persons exist during half the year. The hot wind, and with that the light, are shut out by many Europeans, while most natives live in a hut, or even the better classes in a house, probably with only small external openings. As plants when deprived of light become white, so human beings become pale, weak, spiritless, unhealthy, and anæmic.

LATENT SCURVY.—1. A minor degree of the degeneration constituting scurvy may exist for an indefinite period without any appreciable symptoms. 2. It may cause what at first appears to be simple anæmia. 3. It may manifest its presence by delaying convalescence from other diseases, by causing a slight bruise to become an ulcer, or by retarding the healing of sores, such sores often not presenting the usual spongy appearance and propensity to bleed of the confirmed scorbutic ulcer. 4. Maladies, as the Delhi and other boils and sores (*vide* p. 77), may be frequently traced to those conditions under which scurvy arises. 5. Scurvy sometimes develops itself by such premonitory symptoms as *malaise*, wandering rheumatic pains, a little puffiness under the eyes, ulcers of the mouth and soreness of the tongue, the gums being unaffected and no other symptoms of scurvy being present. In children the latent scorbutic condition is favourable to the development of aphthæ (*vide* p. 446). 6. Natives suffer considerably from chronic inflammation of the roots of the teeth, which is mostly scorbutic. 7. Debility and palpitations of the heart with dropsical swellings, especially of the abdomen, may exist in badly fed people, apparently partly as the result of starvation and partly as the result of scurvy. 8. A diarrhœa with chocolate-coloured stools may be the only manifestation of the scorbutic condition. 9. A chronic ophthalmia may be the result. 10. It may cause the development of gout. 11. It may appear as beri-beri (*vide* p. 384). 12. It may cause *purpura*; a condition in which the skin, especially of the legs, becomes studded with dark-coloured spots of various sizes, originating from the rupture of little blood-vessels in the skin.

Declared Scurvy.—The symptoms of scurvy *when the disease has passed the latent condition* are—soreness of the gums, weariness, dejection of spirits, dull pains in the limbs, palpitation, and shortness of breath. The tongue becomes pale and flabby, the complexion muddy, the lips bluish or livid, the eyes surrounded by a dark circle. The gums grow more affected, swollen, spongy, and bleeding on the slightest touch. The teeth are often loose, the breath foul, and as the disease advances blue spots, like bruises, appear on different parts of the body. Slight pressure or injury now produces a bruise, scratches become ulcers, and old wounds or scars open afresh. The joints become swollen and stiff, great emaciation takes place, 'puffy' dropsical swellings appear, diarrhœa or dysentery sets in, bleeding may occur from the gums, nose, or bowels, and the patient dies exhausted.

*Treatment.*—In all cases of scurvy, whether simply manifested by obscure premonitory symptoms, or when evident and confirmed, the use of fresh vegetables and of fresh meat is the great remedy. But the meat should be quite freshly killed, as certain chemical changes occur after a few hours, rendering it less anti-scorbutic. Plenty of salt should be eaten with the food. Milk should also be taken *ad libitum*, and if fresh milk cannot be obtained, preserved or condensed milk may be used. The *fresh* milk of the cocoa-nut is esteemed anti-scorbutic, and if available several pints may be drunk daily. Lemon-juice should also be taken to the extent of two or three ounces daily, or, if this is unobtainable, nitrate of potash (*vide* p. 26), in 10-grain doses, may be given twice a day. As adjuncts, fruits (especially oranges, lemons, limes, apples, grapes, and pummaloes), sugar and molasses, cocoa, pickles, vinegar, onions, all the *cruciferous* vegetables (as broccoli, kale, cabbage, turnips, mustard, cress, watercress, radishes, spoonwort or scurvy-grass), and potatoes will be the most beneficial. Wine (as sauterne, grave, claret), ale and beer, and a fresh infusion of malt, should also be given. If aperients are required, fresh infusion of tamarinds or sulphate of soda may be used. Ulceration of the gums requires astringent gargles of alum, or of port wine and water, or of decoction of pomegranate (*vide* p. 25). If diarrhœa persists, a milk diet is advisable, and syrup of bael (*vide* p. 22) should, if procurable, be taken as a medicine. When debility is very marked the recumbent posture should be maintained, or faintings, which have proved fatal, may occur.

If fresh meat cannot be procured, 'Liebig's extract of meat' is recommended, as it contains in a condensed form those substances (salts of potassa) which are required. If the aperients mentioned are not satisfactory in action, cream of tartar may be used in 1- to 3-drachm doses.

The *cure* of scurvy is more difficult than its *prevention*, and the latter should be constantly held in mind by those placed in such positions as to be exposed to scorbutic influences. The diet should contain a proportion of anti-scorbutic material, and if fresh meat and vegetables cannot be obtained in sufficient quantities, vegetables which may be kept—as potatoes, onions, or preserved vegetables, or bottled lime-juice, or vinegar and milk—should be used daily. *Amchur* or *kuttai* (dried unripe mangoes) may be powdered and mixed with soup or vegetables, the dose being an ounce daily. Other preventive measures, whether on board ship or on land, consist in great attention to cleanliness, in ventilation, in a suitable degree of warmth, and especially in freedom from damp.

THE FORM OF SCURVY KNOWN AS BERI-BERI.—*Beri* is the Cinghalese for weakness, and the repetition of the word implies great weakness. The symptoms of beri-beri are great debility, stiffness of the legs and thighs, succeeded by numbness and swelling of those parts, with great difficulty in using the limbs. In the course of a few days, or even hours, the body becomes swollen, the breathing quick, and the pulse feeble, while the urine is very scanty, and the thirst great. Diarrhœa and insensibility terminate the illness. The causes are exposure to cold, damp, and night land winds, particularly when the person is debilitated by declared or latent scurvy. Beri-beri frequently occurs to natives living on the damp sea-coasts of Western India, or in persons long confined on board ship, or in others who, proceeding into the semi-desert districts of the west, cannot procure the more liberal diet and fresh vegetable material to which they have been accustomed. Europeans seldom suffer from the malady. Medicines to promote the flow of urine and to increase the action of the skin should be used. Half a drachm of sweet spirits of nitre may be given in a little water three times a day, and 8 or 10 grains of Dover's powder at night. A mustard poultice should be applied daily over the loins. Lime-juice and fresh vegetables should form a main feature of the diet. Wine and brandy will probably be required from the first, and should be freely given, to the extent of 6 or 8 ounces of wine, and half that quantity of brandy, daily.

[Other medicines which may be procured are—Recipe 11 if the bowels are confined, and the person has not been previously in a weak state of health; Recipe 15 to relieve constipation in a weakly person. Then Recipe 53 may be substituted, as preferable to the spirits of nitric ether alone.]

**SCORBUTIC ULCER.**—Trivial injuries in those affected with scurvy frequently cause ulcers, of foul, spongy, ill-conditioned appearance, and inclined to bleed. Eating into the flesh, they may produce great injury and disfigurement. They have often prevailed epidemically among troops and sailors who had become more or less scorbutic. These ulcers may attack any part of the body, and are attended with impaired appetite, foul tongue, spongy gums, and debility. Treatment consists in anti-scorbutic remedies internally, and the external application of various lotions or ointments, as Recipes 86 or 97.

[But a better application for a scorbutic ulcer is Recipe 96, or, if the sore is painful, Recipe 93, which should be procured for use.]

**SEA-SICKNESS.**—There are many remedies of doubtful efficacy; none decidedly curative. Cold brandy and water benefits some persons. Champagne suits others. Making a continuous expiratory effect as in whistling, when sinking sensations are felt, is sometimes beneficial. So is a tight belt or bandage round the body with a pad, so as to produce pressure on the stomach.

[Two drops of creosote on a lump of sugar will sometimes check the sickness. Five drops of chloroform on a lump of sugar, or in a glass of sherry, with half a tumbler of cold water, is often successful. Or chloroform globules, each containing about 5 minims of chloroform, may be procured from the chemist. Cocaine tablets containing one-twentieth of a grain of cocaine hydrochlorate are portable and efficacious, and may be tried. Applying ice-bags to the spine will check vomiting for a short voyage, as across the English Channel. A belt, which may be inflated so as to excite pressure over the stomach, has been invented.]

But the best means are, on commencing a sea voyage, to empty the stomach, and to remove acidity by an emetic, composed of a teaspoonful of soda and a table-spoonful of mustard, in a large tumblerful of warm water; or several good purgative doses should be taken. This will render the person much less liable to sea-sickness.

**SHIVERING, or RIGORS.**—Shivering, or cold feelings, not amounting to actual shivering, are very important symptoms of many diseases. Nearly all acute diseases, and especially fevers and inflammations, commence with chilliness or actual shivering. Shivering occurring *during the progress* of a malady is generally significant of the formation of matter in some part.

**SKIN DISEASES.**—Practically, diseases of the skin may be divided into the five following forms :—

1. RASHES; or alterations of the colour of the surface of the skin, generally of a reddish hue, and which do not proceed to the formation of watery matter.

2. VESICLES; which, commencing as little pimples, eventually contain a globule of watery fluid in the summit.

3. PUSTULES; which also, commencing as little pimples, eventually discharge matter.

4. SCALES, or SCALY ERUPTIONS; so called in consequence of flakes of diseased upper skin being cast off.

5. TUBERCLES; commencing as round bodies under the skin, which may eventually ulcerate.

1. RASHES.—The principal rashes are as follows :—

FRECKLES, or EPHELIS, are little coloured patches, caused chiefly in fair people by exposure to the sun. They are not painful, nor injurious. They may be got rid of by avoiding exposure to the sun, wind, and dust.

*Applications for Freckles.*—A wash made by beating twenty sweet almonds into a paste in a mortar, adding a pint of warm water, and then straining the emulsion ; or a wash composed of equal parts of lime water and milk may be employed. The face should be sponged with the wash, which should be allowed to dry on the skin. The latter should be cleansed with glycerine soap and water in half an hour, and prepared white fuller's-earth (called *cimolite*) may be applied. A mixture which has some repute for dispersing freckles is—2 ounces of lemon-juice, half a drachm of borax, and a drachm of white sugar, applied occasionally.

ERYTHEMA, OR THE BLUSH.—This consists of light red patches of various size and form, appearing in different parts of the body, and generally passing away in three days or a week. There is considerable itching or tingling. It frequently occurs previous to the monthly flow, on the legs of girls. It may follow drinking cold water when the body is heated. It may accompany teething, and in infants generally attacks the thighs and genitals. It is not dangerous, and is rarely attended with fever. The bowels should be acted upon by a gentle purgative, the patient should be careful in diet, and *white* fuller's-earth or violet powder may be applied.

Roseola, Rose Rash, Tooth Rash, or Red Gum.—It is distinguished from measles by its occurring suddenly, without any prior cold, sneezing, or watering at the eyes, and by the eruption being in irregular patches of various sizes and forms, and not crescentic or half-moon shaped, as the eruption of measles presents. It is distinguished from scarlet fever by the absence of sore-throat. It is known from erythema by its more rosy tint. There are several kinds of roseola, only one of which need be particularly mentioned, viz. *roseola annulata*, which appears in rosy rings, inclosing a portion of healthy skin. Sometimes the eruption of roseola precedes the eruption of small-pox, and when this latter disease is in the neighbourhood, and rose rash occurs to a child, it must be regarded as a suspicious circumstance, as the possible forerunner of small-pox. If it presents in children, the gums, if swollen and painful, should be lanced; if the bowels are costive, they should be opened with a little castor oil or senna; and if there are symptoms of acidity of the stomach a few grains of citrate of magnesia may be given. When the malady occurs to adults there is generally one or other form of dyspepsia, for which appropriate treatment will be needed.

Uticaria, or Nettle Rash.—An eruption resembling in appearance, and in the accompanying stinging pain, the condition of the skin produced by nettles. But sometimes the rash commences as long white wheals, surrounded by a red band or margin, as if the part had been struck by a cane. The rash frequently appears suddenly; may last only a few minutes, or for a day or two, and may disappear as suddenly; or it may vanish in the daytime, returning at night. There is severe itching or tingling, which may be alleviated by applying sal volatile 1 part, water 2 parts. From the sudden manner in which it occurs, sometimes attended with vomiting and feverishness, it often excites alarm; but it is not dangerous, and often depends on improper diet. In some persons it follows eating shell-fish, strawberries, cucumbers, or mushrooms. A very similar rash has also followed taking copaiba, or quinine (*vide* pp. 18, 281). It often succeeds drinking cold water when the body is heated. If there is reason to suppose the stomach contains indigestible matter, as will probably be the case if the rash comes on after a full meal, particularly after a hearty supper or a late dinner, and especially if there is nausea and vomiting, an emetic should be given (Recipe 54). In other instances aperients, as Recipes 1 and 2.

LEUCODERMA, or WHITE SKIN.—This consists of white patches on any part of the body, giving when numerous a piebald appearance to the skin of the native. It depends on deficiency of colouring matter. When general it constitutes the condition known as *albinism*, the eyes being discoloured, and the body becoming a tawny red. There is no known cure. It is mentioned here because it is often mistaken for leprosy, to which it has no relation. It is not contagious, and a good servant need not be discharged because he develops white skin patches.

Leucoderma is not scientifically a rash, but it has as good a claim to be described under rashes as freckles, which dermatologists always place under rashes; freckles being an excess of pigment or colouring matter, leucoderma a deficiency.

2. Vesicles.—The principal vesicular affections are as follows:—

Tinea Tonsurans, or Ringworm.—A *contagious* skin disease, commonly attacking the heads of children, but frequently appearing on the face, body, or limbs, or in the roots of the nails, or in the beard. It is caused by the growth of a fungus (*Trycophyton tonsurans*) which belongs to the lowest species of vegetable organism.

*Ringworm of the Head.*—The earliest symptoms are a little redness or scurfiness on some part of the scalp, but these early symptoms most usually escape notice. Then in two or three days there are circles of minute pimples, which also may not be recognised until they, in the course of a few hours, turn into minute vesicles. These break and discharge their contents, producing a thin scab, which may be mistaken for scurf. Fresh circles of pimples and vesicles quickly form on the *outside* of the first crop, the disease spreading in more or less circular-shaped patches. As the malady goes on, from the discharge consequent on the eruption, and induced by scratching, larger and thicker scabs form. Neglected ringworm may thus involve nearly the whole of the scalp, these latter stages being very similar to *Scald Head*, p. 399. There is, however, a peculiar condition of the hairs in the part affected, which distinguishes ringworm from any other head affection. With a good magnifying glass the hairs over the affected spot appear as if rubbed off close to the scalp; the short portions remaining looking dry, lustreless, bent or twisted, split, and running in a line different from that of the healthy hairs, affording a fancied resemblance to a stubble-field. The hairs thus affected are dead; and when attempts are made to extract them they often break. When the root comes away, and is placed under the microscope, the distinctive fungus may be recognised in the shape of bright, round, cellular bodies, about $\frac{1}{7000}$ to $\frac{1}{5000}$ of an inch in diameter, collected in chains or groups. The most minute redness or scurfiness on the head of a child should always be regarded with suspicion, as the possible commencement of ringworm. When there is a scurfy spot although the place is *not* red; or when there is a red spot although the place is *not* scurfy, examination with a strong glass will often show either minute vesicles, or if at a later stage lighter-looking portions of hair-shafts, which have escaped observation by the naked eye. If redness or scurfiness present on the heads of children who have been exposed to infection, the safest plan is to conclude ringworm may be present, and to use appropriate remedies.

*Treatment.*—In a case of ringworm the child should wear a skull-cap, and the head should be washed twice daily with carbolic acid solution (Recipe 118), or with carbolic acid soap. If this does not remove the suspicious appearance in two or three days, the head for one inch round should be thoroughly shaved, not shaving the part affected. After which the great object is the removal of diseased hairs, which should be carefully extracted, one by one, with a pair of broad-nibbed forceps. Unless this is done very gently, but at the same time firmly, the hairs will break, and the roots remain. The hairs removed should be burnt. Then every particle of scaliness should be washed away with soap and water. Then strong vinegar, or strong alum water (alum 4 drachms, water 1 ounce), or ink may be applied to the part. Ink is a popular and useful remedy, the good effects resulting from the iron and tannin it contains. Whatever remedy is used should be rubbed on the scalp with the finger, so as to insinuate it into the holes from which the roots of the hairs have been plucked, and in which the fungus vegetates. The application may be repeated for five or six days, once daily; a search for and extraction of broken hairs, not previously observed, being first instituted. This may cut the malady short; if not, the remedies mentioned in the small type should be procured. As the fungus grows most luxuriantly on weakly children the diet should be liberal, constipated bowels should be relieved, and tonics (Recipe 67) will be required. The cure of ringworm is accomplished when the bad hairs have vanished, and when new, silky, downy hairs begin to spring up, and *not before*.

Ringworm is highly infectious, spreading both by direct contact and through the air. Other children must be kept as much as possible away from the patient, and separate combs, brushes, towels, soap, and washing utensils must be provided. Clothing and bedding used by the patient should be disinfected (*vide Appendix*, No. 122), and the soiled things should be washed separately. If ringworm occurs in a school, or large family, the first thing is to institute a regular and periodical search on all heads, and the next thing is to *isolate* those affected. If this is impossible the healthy should have their heads washed daily with carbolic acid solution (Recipe 119), and the hair should afterwards be anointed with some kind of greasy pomade. Plenty of brushing is also a precautionary measure of value; and extraordinary attention should be given to ventilation of both living and sleeping rooms.

If practicable 'Goa powder' should be obtained, which is the powdered pith of a tree (*araroba*) growing in the Brazils. A few grains of the powder should be mixed with vinegar or lime-juice to form a paste of the consistency of cream, which should be rubbed on with the fingers night and morning for eight or ten days. Under the action of the Goa powder the part affected becomes whitish, while the surrounding skin is stained brown. A preparation of Goa powder known as *chrysarobin* is made, a solution of which may be applied with a brush. Goa powder is often adulterated. It is a fine yellowish powder without smell or taste, and it is well to see the powder, and not trust to a prepared solution. Care should be taken that neither the powder nor the solution touch the eyes, as it may cause much irritation. Goa powder is reputed an infallible remedy for Indian parasitic ringworm, but it sometimes fails. Other remedies for ringworm which may be tried in obstinate cases are—*iodine paint* applied with a feather once daily, until the skin is blistered or very tender. A solution of carbolic acid (10 grains to the ounce of water), applied with a brush, often cures the disease. This application may be repeated once or twice according to the effect it produces, desisting as soon as the skin is tender or blistered. If these measures are not successful, an ointment composed of equal parts of simple and mercurial ointment should be well rubbed into the part for half an hour twice daily. Recipe 70 is a better tonic than Recipe 67 mentioned in the large type. But if the child is thin, feeble, and badly nourished, it should have cod-liver oil twice daily, in which 5 or 6 grains of carbonate of iron may be mixed, instead of Recipe 70.

Ringworm of the Body is known in the vernaculars as *dad, dadru, majees dad, denaii*, and among Europeans as 'dhobee's itch,' 'washerman's itch,' 'Malabar itch,' 'Burmese ringworm,' &c. It commences as a small itching scurfy spot, and, enlarging at the circumference, shows a line of minute vesicles. As this advances in semicircular patches, the skin over which the disease has passed gets well. It frequently develops round the fork and waist, being determined to the latter part in natives, by the irritation of the clothing worn round the body. But it may appear on the face, or in the roots of the nails, or in the beard. Ringworm of the body causes much itching, especially at night, which keeps the person awake and tends to destroy the general health, while the scratching induced causes a scaly or cracked condition of the skin, when it has been mistaken for *eczema*. *Treatment* depends considerably on the extent of the disease. When, at first, the parts affected are small, the remedies mentioned for ringworm of the head may be used. But if early treatment has been neglected, and the disease is extensive, or the skin inflamed, the part should be sponged four or five times daily with a mixture of half an ounce of sal volatile in 6 ounces of water, until the remedies mentioned below can be procured.

Wash twice daily with carbolic acid soap. Then sponge with a solution of 2 drachms of bicarbonate of soda in 8 ounces of water. Afterwards rub the following ointment well in: sulphate of zinc 60 grains, lanolin 1 ounce. If this is not successful after six or eight days, use iodide of lead 1 drachm, lanolin 1 ounce. In proportion as the general health is improved, the more readily is the parasite destroyed by local measures.

Scabies, or Itch.—Itch commences as small vesicles less than the size of a pin's head, generally between the fingers, afterwards spreading to other parts. It is caused by an animalcule, which burrows under the skin. This insect is called *Acarus scabiei*, and is round in shape, varying from one-seventh to one-quarter of a line in length and breadth. The female, being larger than the male, is sometimes visible to the naked eye as a greyish-white moving atom. Under the microscope it presents a tortoise-like shape, and is found to be studded with hairs and bristles, the head terminating with two pairs of mandibles. With these it burrows through the thinnest part of the upper layer of the skin, selecting such spots as the space between the fingers, or the inside of the wrist, where the structure is thinnest and softest. Once buried it does not come out again, but burrows within the skin, where other insects are produced, which in their turn burrow and reproduce their kind. These burrows may usually be seen in the shape of dotted or zigzag marks on the skin, looking like faint needle-scratches. The itching produced is intolerable, especially at night. After itch has continued some time, and been neglected, it discharges matter and may become open sores. A person with itch should be isolated. The parts affected should be first *well* washed with ordinary soap and water, which opens the burrows, and then *well* rubbed twice daily with compound sulphur ointment (Recipe 92). After three days the patient should take a hot bath and be well washed with carbolic soap. Then the sulphur ointment should be again employed. When the hands are affected, they should be well washed and rubbed with the ointment, and then inclosed in a bag of oiled silk all night, and the rubbing repeated in the morning, after a good washing with soap and water. Beyond opening the bowels if confined, no internal treatment is necessary. The clothing of persons with itch should be disinfected by baking in an oven at a temperature of 140° Fahr., or by the fumes from burning sulphur (*vide Appendix*, No. 129); or if this cannot be done the clothes should be boiled.

Lichen Tropicus, or Prickly Heat.—This is probably the first complaint a new-comer to India suffers from, and, although unattended with danger, it is very annoying. The symptoms are itching, tingling, pricking, and sweating, while the skin is covered with a bright red eruption, eventually presenting little watery heads or vesicles, some of which afterwards contain a little white matter. The eruption is deepened in colour by exercise, or by hot drinks. The eruption should not be suddenly checked. As an external application, equal parts of sal volatile and water will be found to allay itching. Rubbing the skin with a rough towel tends to stop the itching, the heads of the little vesicles being broken, after which they do not itch. Light clothing, temperate diet, and an occasional aperient are necessary. Children suffering from prickly heat should be fed on bread, rice, sago, arrowroot, milk, and only a little meat broth. If thirsty and feverish, citrate of magnesia may be used as a drink (*vide* p. 15).

Twenty grains of sulphate of copper dissolved in an ounce of water, the solution to be sopped lightly on the parts, is much recommended. Or 2 drachms of bicarbonate of potash in half a pint of water.

Prurigo, or Itching.—Intense itching, always worse at night, is the prominent symptom. It generally attacks the posterior parts or privates, but sometimes occurs in the flexures of the limbs, or on the shoulders and back.

At first the parts implicated are covered with pimples or vesicles, raised above the surface of, and redder than, the skin. But afterwards there is no evident deviation from the natural state, except redness or scabs produced by scratching. It is common among old people, it occurs in diabetes, and in other feeble conditions. It is also a frequent complaint of pregnant women.

A variety of the malady is *Prurigo formicans*, when there is not only an intolerable itching at one or more parts, but the patient also complains of a feeling like the creeping of ants or the stinging of insects (hence the specific name) over the whole body. These latter sensations are more generally complained of by natives than by Europeans, and are sometimes so distressing as to prevent sleep. The principal causes of this affection are debility, want of cleanliness, and friction or irritation of the skin.

Another variety is *Prurigo hyemalis*, or 'frost itch,' which may be general or local. It occurs to some people whenever the air is clear, dry, and frosty, and although more frequent in temperate climates, it may present, in those predisposed, during the cold season of Northern India.

*Treatment.*—When *local* itching occurs, stimulating drinks should be forbidden, and only easily digested food allowed. Internal remedies are seldom of much use, excepting chloral, which may be required to procure rest. Local applications recommended are numerous, but probably cold lotions (Recipe 97) or ice-cold water are the best. When troublesome local itching occurs, the absence of lice should be ascertained, for it sometimes arises from their presence, and can then only be cured by destroying the insects (*vide Lice*, p. 613). For *general* itching tonics, cleanliness, and unirritating clothing.

HERPES, or TETTER.—There are varieties of this eruption. It often occurs on the lips, accompanying a common cold, in the shape of five or six little vesicles on an inflamed base, which burst and form a scab. The foreskin is another part not uncommonly attacked. The number of vesicles, sometimes ten or a dozen, and the attendant itching, which is often very troublesome, serve to distinguish *herpes* of this part from more important affections (*vide* p. 457). Less frequently, *herpes* occurs on the forehead, when there is much stinging pain and numerous rings of vesicles, which when healing may leave a mark for life. The most serious variety is that called *Herpes Zoster*, or 'Shingles.' In this form of herpes a line of vesicles rises, reaching from the spine round the lower part of the chest to the breast-bone, usually on one side. There is a popular but erroneous idea that if it occurs on both sides it terminates fatally. The eruption is often preceded, and always accompanied, by severe shooting pain and feverishness. The vesicles burst about the fourth day, when scabbing takes place, the whole process lasting about one fortnight. Indigestion is the most usual cause of all varieties of herpes. The *first two forms* rarely require medical treatment. For the *two latter* the bowels should be kept open, the diet regulated, and an alum lotion (Recipe 97) applied. If the pain is great, a strip of lint, wet with poppy water (*vide Appendix*, No. 81), may be placed over the part. In all cases scratching should be refrained from.

ECZEMA, or RUNNING SCALL.—There are various degrees of eczema. It occurs as an eruption of small raised vesicles crowded together on broad irregular patches of bright-red skin, accompanied by much itching, tingling, and smarting, and usually presenting in the flexures of the limbs, as the groins or armpits. The fluid in the vesicles soon becomes milky and turbid, and in four or five days the vesicles burst, when the fluid is discharged and dries into thin yellowish-green scabs. Fresh vesicles form on the surrounding skin, while the parts already affected remain sore. The duration of this malady may be from a week to months, or more, and in prolonged cases the scabs become detached, leaving a sore raw surface, or they crack, exuding a clear watery fluid, which has led to the term 'salt rheum.' When the discharge resembles matter it isoften called *impetigo,* or *pustular eczema,* also 'crusted tetter, and 'cowrass.' In children it may be connected with teething, and may appear behind the ears; in females it may be connected with irregular and painful monthly courses; and it sometimes appears near the nipples of suckling women. In many cases it appears to be caused by indigestion; it also may arise from heat, on a fair and tender skin, when it is called *eczema solare,* or 'heat spot.' When there is a predisposition to the malady, its appearance seems to be determined to different spots from the heat or irritation of clothing. It also arises from the handling of dry powders, or certain metals. From its affecting the hands of grocers, who handle sugar, it has been called 'Grocer's Itch.' It is sometimes induced on the hands of bakers by flour; and on the hands of bricklayers by lime: hence it has been called 'Baker's' and 'Bricklayer's Itch.' Eczema often recurs in different parts of the body at certain seasons, as the spring and fall. In such cases the cause is obscure; but it is often found there is some latent scrofulous taint in those affected. *Treatment* consists in the removal of indigestion, and in measures adopted against any irregularity in the monthly courses of the female. As a local application, olive or salad oil should be smeared on the parts, and if there are scabs or crusts a hot linseed-meal poultice should be applied at night. The scabs will come off with the poultice in the morning, and oil may be again applied. The parts may be occasionally sponged with hot water and glycerine soap, but only when cleanliness requires it. All irritating applications should be avoided, and if any application increases the itching and tingling, it does not agree. As scratching irritates the parts, it should be refrained from.

[If the above-mentioned applications are not satisfactory, glycerine should be procured and used instead of the oil. If the malady still persists, lead ointment (Recipe 96) may be applied. If there is very much itching and smarting the following ointment: iodide of lead 12 grains, chloroform 40 drops, glycerine 1 drachm, lanolin 1 ounce. In some cases an ointment composed of 30 grains of sulphate of zinc, mixed in half an ounce of lanolin, is more beneficial: an ointment composed of white precipitate 1 drachm, lanolin 1 ounce, is successful in many instances; in others greasy applications do not suit, and the lotion (Recipe 97) may then be used. When eczema attacks children behind the ears an alkaline wash (Recipe 99) is often very useful, but in such cases attention to teething, if in progress, will be also necessary. When in adults the eczema persists after the acute stage has passed away, the malady becoming what is called 'chronic eczema,' the *liquor arsenitis potassæ* (Recipe 75) should be given three times a day, *after* meals, until the characteristic effects of arsenic are produced (*vide* note to Recipe 75), when the medicine should be stopped. Sulphur baths are also advisable, as those of Harrogate or Aix-les-Bains.]

PEMPHIGUS, or POMPHOLIX, or BLEBS.—These names have been given to a peculiar blister or *bleb*, which forms on different parts of the body, especially of children. The first change consists in the appearance on the back, belly, or limbs, of red circular spots, which itch and burn. In a few hours, at the middle of the spots, small transparent vesicles arise, which enlarge, and soon cover the whole of the red patch, excepting a narrow margin. The blebs are round or oval in shape, and may attain the size of a pea, or even of a hen's egg. The contents, at first transparent, gradually become turbid, and in two or three days the blebs burst; the place then becoming covered with a scab, under which the skin heals. Before the first blebs heal, new ones form, and the disease may continue in this manner for days or weeks. In infants, *pemphigus* usually appears to depend on *disordered stomach*. In adults it may be preceded by dyspepsia or debility from various causes; but sometimes the patient looks and feels well throughout the attack, until exhausted by the loss of sleep caused by the itching. The *treatment* consists in attention to the general health, and in the remedy of any digestive disorders. The diet should be liberal. Local treatment consists in puncturing the blebs with a fine needle, and in protecting the parts from injury from the clothing sticking to them, by simple dressing (Recipe 86). For some time afterwards a stain remains on the skin, but there is no permanent scar.

SUDAMINA, or MILIARIA.—An eruption of numerous minute watery vesicles, seldom attaining the size of a pin's head. *Miliaria* is the term generally given to this affection when the skin appears also reddened. It occurs during most diseases which are accompanied by much perspiration, as fevers, acute rheumatism, and inflammation of the lungs. From the eruption so frequently accompanying 'milk fever,' that malady is sometimes termed 'Miliary Fever' (*vide* p. 629). It is caused by the little ducts from which the perspiration oozes becoming clogged by the secretions of the skin, and it is usually seen on the bodies of patients who have been kept too warm, or whose skins have not been sufficiently cleansed. The eruption presents principally about the neck, chest, and armpits. It is of little consequence, but indicates that the patient requires a cooler regimen, and greater cleanliness of the skin. It is important that it should not be mistaken for the specific eruptions of certain fevers (*vide* pp. 242, 247).

3. PUSTULES.—The principal pustular affections are as follows:—

FAVUS, or SCALD-HEAD.—Scald-head is a contagious disease, caused by a parasite (the *Achorion Schönleinii*) which usually grows near the roots of the hair. Under the microscope the parasite differs considerably in appearance from the fungus of ringworm, being more jointed and smaller. The first symptoms are scarcely distinguishable from those of ringworm. It first causes slight itching and a red-coloured eruption, palpable also to the touch. As the eruption spreads it is not circular in shape like ringworm, but of irregular and undecided form. In about twelve hours each little red point of which the eruption is composed contains a small globule of yellowish watery fluid. This and the subsequent thicker secretion drying on the surface of the skin assume a honeycombed appearance, some part of the scab being depressed or 'cup-shaped,' and some elevated, or presenting the appearance of a series of concentric rings. The crust emits a mouse-like odour, and is often perforated by hairs, which do not break off so readily as in ringworm, and are consequently more easily extracted by the roots. As the disease advances the secretion becomes more thick and copious, until there may be a layer of yellowish-looking scab or crust over the whole head. When the malady has been neglected, sores and ulcers form on the scalp, underneath its scabby covering. The disease is sometimes called 'crusted ringworm,' or *porrigo favosa*. If the malady is recognised early, the *treatment* for 'ringworm' (*vide* p. 390) should be employed. If nothing has been done until scabs have formed, the head should be poulticed and bathed with hot water, until the whole of the scabby matter is removed, and the surface is quite clean. Then olive oil or glycerine should be applied, and the scalp should be covered with a close-fitting skull-cap. The remarks under ringworm, as regards diet, medicine, and preventive measures, are applicable. The parasite of scald-head may be conveyed by cats from one child to another, involving an obvious precaution.

[For scald-head it will be desirable to use carbolic acid ointment (Recipe 93). On this not being successful, an ointment composed of one drachm of tar and one ounce of simple cerate may be employed.]

ACNE, OR COPPER NOSE.—This consists of isolated pustules, forming on a hard red base in the small glands of the skin, sometimes very long in coming to a head, and most frequently seen on the nose, but sometimes on the cheeks, forehead, or chest. Acne pustules are sometimes called 'blackheads,' and the contents are erroneously supposed to be 'grubs'; being in reality compressed matter, the end of which has become blackened by exposure to the air. It is due to a stoppage in the glands of the skin by such matter accumulating there. It is generally connected with dyspepsia, with excess of eating or drinking, especially over-indulgence in alcoholic liquors, and in women with uterine disorders, or with the 'change of life.' The *treatment* consists in proper regulation of the diet and the mode of life generally, particularly as regards exercise, and in the relief of dyspeptic symptoms, or of symptoms referable to the womb.

SYCOSIS, or CHIN WHELK, commences with redness or smarting of the skin of the lips or chin, on which pimples appear, which slowly come to a head and discharge matter. Fresh crops occur for many weeks, until, in bad cases, the beard falls off in patches. Sycosis has been confounded with ringworm of the beard (*vide* p. 389), and has been erroneously attributed to a parasite. The causes are the same as those of *acne*. The hair should be cut close, poultices applied till the surface is clean, and afterwards olive oil. Aperient and alterative medicines, as Recipes 1, 2, 35, should also be given.

Steam the chin every night by holding it over hot water. Then rub for three minutes with terebene soap and flannel. Afterwards apply a lotion composed of precipitated sulphur half an ounce, glycerine 2 drachms, spirits of wine 1 ounce, rose water and lime water each 3 ounces. Allow this to dry on and remain all night. In the morning clean with terebene soap. If not successful after a few days, use carbolic acid ointment (Recipe 93) instead of the lotion.

4. SCALES, or SCALY ERUPTIONS.—The principal scaly eruption is *Psoriasis*, or *Dry Tetter*, of which there are three varieties, all non-contagious. The *first* form begins as small round shining, itching spots, soon becoming covered with thin white scales, which, falling off, leave the skin beneath slightly tender and reddened. The spots

increase in size, but retaining the circular shape until they attain several inches in circumference, when they become broken and assume the form of irregular scaly patches. This circular form is sometimes called *lepra*, and may be mistaken for ringworm; but lepra is scaly, while ringworm is not; it always appears on the body, while ringworm usually affects the head; and there are generally several or many patches of lepra, while ringworm is usually single. In the *second* form the disease commences as *irregular* scaly patches without the prior ring-like appearance. Both these varieties frequently attack the flexures of the limbs, and the inner surface of the thigh and armpits, the palms of the hands, and the nails, which become white speckled, irregular, and brittle. When the palms are affected by the non-circular form, it is often confounded with eczema of such parts, and has also been called 'Grocer's Itch' (*vide* p. 397). The *third* form is known as *pityriasis* (vernacular *senwha* or *chulee*). It differs from psoriasis in consisting of much smaller scales, which are sometimes almost microscopical in minuteness; and in being more diffused, occasionally even universal over the whole body. Boatmen who expose their naked backs to the sun are especially liable to pityriasis. As it does not cause much inconvenience, and as the scales glisten in the sun, giving rise to an appearance like tortoiseshell, pityriasis is often considered as a mark of beauty. The causes are not well understood. At some times it seems to depend on exposure or on digestive disorders, appearing and reappearing with such conditions. The *treatment* requires attention to the general health, as the avoidance of any article of diet known to induce dyspepsia, and the relief of constipation if present by laxative medicines, as Recipes 1 and 2.

[It will be desirable to take Recipe 35, and, after the acute stage has passed away, arsenical solution (Recipe 75). Itching may be relieved by a lotion, containing half an ounce of spirits of wine, half an ounce of tincture of opium, with 12 ounces of water. Equal parts of tar, spirits of wine, and soft soap, is a favourite formula. The patent 'Pearl Ointment' may be rubbed in with advantage. Sometimes mercurial ointment diluted with a similar quantity of simple ointment is beneficial. At other times sulphur ointment (Recipe 92). In chronic psoriasis, sulphur baths.]

5. TUBERCLES.—The principal tubercular forms of skin disease are tubercular *leprosy* (*vide* p. 317), *fibroma*, and *lupus*.

FIBROMA consists of the growth of numerous pendulous tumours in the skin. They are not painful, do not gather, remain during life, and are incurable.

LUPUS often commences with distinct tubercular elevations on the cheek by the side of the nose. Sometimes these are preceded by a red patch. In most cases pustules form which are succeeded by an ulcer. To this condition the term *Noli me tangere* has been applied. The ulcer is liable to spread. Lupus is most common in young scrofulous individuals. Surgeons destroy the ulcer with caustics, but until this can be done soothing applications are best.

**SLEEPLESSNESS** is technically known as *Insomnia*. There may be no desire to sleep, or a dread of going to sleep, or the slumber may be restless or disturbed, or a person may be sleepy during the daytime but unable to sleep at night. In the absence of any special disease, such as anæmia (*vide* p. 46) from any cause, or latent gout, sleeplessness may arise from dyspepsia, mental anxiety or excitement, late meals, taking tobacco or strong tea or coffee at night, want of exercise, close unventilated rooms, too soft or too hard beds, from cold feet, and in India from heat and mosquitoes. Every case must therefore be treated on its own merits. The dyspeptic should not go to bed with an undigested meal on the stomach, and should avoid tobacco, tea, and coffee at night. Regular hours of retiring should be adopted, so that the force of habit may be enlisted. Exercise is necessary, and should be taken to the verge of fatigue. The work of the day should be dismissed from the mind, and any excitement, such as reading works of fiction at night, should be avoided. Intervals of relaxation must be insisted upon, and in bad cases entire mental rest. When the tone of the system is lowered, a moderate supper of plainly cooked and nutritious food frequently predisposes to sleep. In other cases a glass of water taken before retiring often does good, but a 'night-cap' in the form of stimulants, is only of temporary benefit. In all instances the bedroom should be well ventilated, the bed should be in the middle of the room, and curtains should not be used. A hot bottle to cold feet is desirable. Bromide of potassium (Recipe 19) may be taken in double or even treble doses at bedtime—a medicine especially useful in cases of sleepiness by day and wakefulness at night. When the digestive organs are in good order and the bowels freely open, an occasional dose of chloral may be used; but the habit of taking chloral must not be indulged in (*vide* p. 11).

*Bromidia* (*vide* p. 62, small type) may be tried.

**SMALL-POX.**—A contagious eruptive fever, generally occurring but once in life. From the period of the formation of matter, until the skin has become quite free from scales, is the time during which the disease is most contagious, although a person may convey the affection up to ten weeks after the appearance of the first symptoms. Infection may also be conveyed by various articles, especially by clothing and bedding. The period from exposure to infection to the appearance of the disease is ordinarily twelve days. The early symptoms are shivering, alternating with burning heat, drowsiness, nausea, often vomiting, headache, pain in the back and loins, and occasionally sore throat. Then fever sets in, the pulse becoming quick, and the skin hot, the temperature (*vide* p. 33) perhaps rising to 104° or 105°. If now the finger is pressed on the forehead, a shotty feeling may be noticed before the eruption is visible. After two, or perhaps three days, an eruption of raised red spots appears on the face and forehead, and this is usually attended with some diminution of the fever, the temperature falling to 101° or 102°. The longer the eruption is in appearing, the less serious does the disease prove. On the third and fourth days the eruption spreads over the body; on the fifth day each pimple becomes a vesicle with watery head, round base, *central depression,* and inflamed margin. This *central depression* is characteristic, and distinguishes the malady from *modified* small-pox or chicken-pox. During the next three days matter forms in the vesicles, and they are more prominent. When matter has formed, the peculiar and unmistakable *smell* of small-pox is present. If the case is severe the face is much swollen, and the eyes are closed by the swelling. About the tenth day the pustules, first on the face, later on the hands and feet, begin to dry up, and about the fourteenth day they form scabs; these fall off from the twentieth to the twenty-third day, leaving the skin of a reddish-brown colour. Frequently scars or 'pits' are left by the healing of the pustules. As the eruption attains its height the fever generally for two or three days very much increases, the temperature again rising to 104° or 105°; this is called the *secondary fever* of small-pox, and usually occurs on or about the eleventh day, which is the period in bad cases of *the greatest danger from exhaustion.* The tongue is furred white throughout, and sometimes swollen. In adults the bowels are most frequently constipated during the whole time; in children there is frequently diarrhœa at the commencement. As mentioned at p. 387, the eruption called *roseola* sometimes precedes small-pox. For distinction from measles *vide* p. 332.

In very bad cases the pustules are so thick that they almost or quite join; the disease is then said to be *confluent*. In such instances the fever is much more severe, there is delirium, and the patient may die insensible. In severe cases the eruption appears in the nostrils, in the eyes, on the tongue, and in the mouth and throat, and there is profuse flow of saliva and great swelling of the hands and feet. Children, especially if teething, may be *attacked by convulsions, generally at the commencement of the eruption.*

Small-pox frequently leaves after-effects, such as a succession of boils, disease of the eyes, affections of the ears, formation of matter about the joints, or a weakened condition from which the patient is long in rallying.

*Treatment.*—The sick person should be as much as possible isolated, if practicable in a separate building. The room should be well ventilated, but not kept too cold, and *all* the rules given regarding 'Disinfection' (*vide Appendix*, Nos. 121 to 130) should be strictly carried out, both *during the disease and afterwards*; for small-pox germs retain vitality for a very long period, not only in clothing and bedding, but even in the paper and crevices of walls. Attendants should avoid inhaling the breath of patients. The bowels should be kept moderately open by aperient medicines, and cooling citrate of magnesia draughts (*vide* p. 15) should be given. The legs and arms may be sponged daily with warm water. The eyes should be carefully washed and bathed several times daily with warm milk and water, or, if affected, with warm alum lotion (Recipe 97), and after each bathing salad oil should be applied to the edges of the lids. The diet should consist of milk, tea, gruel, beef tea, or chicken broth. When the pulse is weak and the strength fails, symptoms most likely to present with the secondary fever about the eleventh day, stimulants, as wine and ammonia, may be required.

During the drying up period frequent changes of clothing, and if the patient is not very weak, a daily bath. During convalescence quinine is useful.

There have been many experiments tried with the view of preventing *pitting* or scars. The surface must be maintained as cleanly as possible, by *gently* sponging away the discharge. Then flour or starch may be abundantly dusted over the face and body, which will relieve itching. Olive oil and cold cream are also good applications. A better is carbolic acid 1 part, salad oil 10 parts, to be well mixed and applied over *one-half* the body daily. The carbolic acid tends to destroy the unpleasant fœtor, and also moderates the violence of the suppurative process. When the pustules have burst, the consequent itching and irritation may be relieved by sprinkling the parts with violet powder, or oxide of zinc, or a mixture of both. But in bad cases of small-pox, notwithstanding any application, there will always be some marking left. The patient should be prevented from scratching, and if a child, the hands should be muffled, as the irritation from scratching increases the after-marks.

Vaccination.—Although the cure of small-pox is not practicable, its prevention is sufficiently easy by vaccination. Vaccine matter is small-pox matter deprived of its virulence by passing through the system of the cow. It produces no ill effect, and yet the person who has been vaccinated is as much protected against small-pox as if he had had that disease. If the latter affection is taken after cow-pox, which sometimes happens, it is always mild, scarcely ever leaving any injurious results on the constitution. Experience and statistics show that vaccination protects the individual, and greatly diminishes the amount of small-pox in the community. The vast majority of ailments which have been ignorantly attributed to vaccination have no possible connection with it. The most likely ailment to occur after vaccination is erysipelas, if in the neighbourhood. But erysipelas may occur after any trivial injury, and is entirely unconnected with the use of cow-pox matter.

Vaccination should be performed in infancy, and about the age of seventeen. Healthy children should be vaccinated within three months after birth, or prior to the commencement of teething; and when small-pox prevails, at a much earlier period. If, however, a child suffers from disordered bowels, or from eruptions of the skin, or is weakly, and there is no small-pox about, it may be desirable to postpone the operation till after most of the teeth have appeared. In India the cold season is the best time for vaccinating.

On the second day after vaccination a small red spot may be observed at each scratch of the lancet. On the fifth day there are circular pearly vesicles containing a limpid fluid. On the eighth day these are fully developed, the centre of each being *depressed*, with an inflamed red ring around, of the breadth of from one to three inches. There is probably slight fever, often some swelling of the arm, and sometimes enlargement of the glands in the armpits. On the eleventh day the pustules burst, leaving a scab. About the twentieth day the scab falls off, leaving permanent scars or 'pits.' If these symptoms (excepting the enlargement of the glands in the armpit) do not present, particularly if the red ring or *areola* is not well developed, the operation is not successful, and confers no protection.

During the progress of the vaccine pustule great care should be taken lest the child rubs or scratches the part. If this occurs there may be a troublesome sore, and much redness about the armpit. Under such circumstances it may be necessary to apply a bread poultice until the sore is clean and healthy, after which simple ointment (Recipe 86) is the best application. Shields have been devised for the protection of the part, but they are not recommended, as they may not be kept clean, and if lent may convey erysipelas.

Vaccination is usually performed on the arm, but there is no reason why the arm should be preferred, excepting that it is perhaps a more convenient place than any other part of the body; and the same side should be chosen as that on which the mother generally nurses, as there will afterwards be less liability to friction.

Modified Small-pox.—This is the term applied to small-pox occurring after vaccination or after small-pox. There is generally for three days more or less feverishness and headache. Then the eruption shows itself, and the protective value of previous vaccination, or of previous small-pox, becomes evident. In a case of unprotected small-pox, the progress of the eruption is attended by aggravation of the feverish symptoms; but in modified small-pox, when the eruption shows itself, the patient feels better. The eruption of modified small-pox consists of a few pimples, or a few vesicles (containing water only), or a few pustules. Often the vesicles dry up about the fifth or sixth day without becoming pustular, a condition which has given rise to the popular terms 'Horn-pock' and 'Wart-pock.' The small-pox pustules, on the contrary, pass through a definite course, and, instead of subsiding as pimples or vesicles, always suppurate. Lastly, modified small-pox does not emit that peculiar nauseous odour of small-pox, and there is no *secondary fever*, or increase of fever on the subsidence of the eruption. Chicken-pox (*vide* p. 117) is by many considered to be modified small-pox. Modified small-pox is contagious. The *treatment* of modified small-pox consists in free ventilation round the sick person, who should be isolated as much as possible. Aperient medicines, as Recipes 1, 2, and cooling medicines, as citrate of magnesia (*vide* p. 15), may be given.

**SOMNAMBULISM.**—A clear explanation of sleep-walking has not yet been given, but the condition is the power of movement remaining with apparent mental rest. Avoiding heavy meals at night, or mental excitement before going to bed, or thinking of the day's occupations, are the principal means of prevention. Freedom from worms should be assured.

**SPASM**, or **CRAMP.**—Spasm is the sudden, involuntary contraction of a muscle; which contraction may be *continuous*, or more or less *relaxing*, or altogether *ceasing*, during intervals. Spasm may be *general*—that is, numerous muscles may be affected—as occurs in *convulsions*; in *epilepsy*; in *tetanus*; in *hydrophobia*. Or spasms may be *local*—that is, confined to one muscle or set of muscles—of which spasmodic *asthma*, spasmodic *colic* (often called spasms or cramps of the stomach), spasmodic *stricture*, *hiccough*, *squinting*, *club-foot*, and *cramps in the legs* during cholera are examples. The treatment of spasms will therefore be found under the headings of the different maladies of which they form a part.

*Spasm or cramp in the legs* requires special mention. The attack is sudden, and most frequent in the night. The muscles of the calf are drawn into knots which may be felt; there is intense pain; and the parts frequently feel sore afterwards. Sometimes the thighs are attacked.

The malady is most prevalent in elderly people, but it also occurs to pregnant females. It is often caused by constipation, when a collection of fæcal matter in the lower gut presses on the nerve (*sciatic*) which afterwards divides into various smaller nerves to supply the legs.

When it occurs to pregnant females it is usually caused by the pressure of the enlarged womb on the nerve. For such cramps constipation must be avoided by the appropriate remedies (*vide* p. 135), and any dyspeptic symptom present should also be treated (*vide* p. 197). Locally the best plan is *brisk* rubbing with salad oil and brandy in equal parts, or, if available, with soap and opium liniment. But in cases where the cramps depend on pregnancy the rubbing should be *gentle*, as the enlarged veins generally also present during pregnancy might be ruptured by hard rubbing (*vide* p. 457). A bandage or garter tied tightly round the leg above the seat of pain will often relieve cramp, but the bandage should not be permitted to remain on for longer than four or five minutes, and should not be used if there are enlarged veins. The garter should be disused, and the stockings may be suspended by a tape buttoning to the corset.

**SPINE, CURVATURE OF THE.**—There are three principal varieties of spine-curvature, viz. to either side, forwards, and backwards, but the lateral curvature is most common. It occurs chiefly to young females, and the first sign is probably one shoulder being observed higher than the other. Preventive measures are—care against constrained positions, as during writing, for instance, so frequently fallen into by children. Also against the practice of raising children by placing the hands under their armpits, and letting the whole weight of the child's body drag on the shoulders. Children should be ordinarily raised by placing one arm under the buttocks; and they should never be hauled about by one arm. In all instances of threatening spine-curvature, exercise short of fatigue, avoidance of strained positions, much rest in the recumbent posture, attention to the general health, with liberal diet and tonic medicines, are the requirements.

**SPITTING OF BLOOD.**—Blood proceeding from the mouth may come from different sources. *It may be from the throat or tonsils*, in which case the quantity brought up is small, and the bleeding part, probably an ulcer of the tonsils, may be easily seen. This bleeding is of little consequence, and requires no particular treatment. *Or blood may come from the gums*, as during scurvy, when it should be treated by the remedies proper in that disease. *Or blood may proceed from the socket of a tooth* which has been extracted (*vide* p. 512), or it may come *from the back part of the nose* (*vide Bleeding from the Nose*, p. 510).

SPITTING OF BLOOD FROM THE LUNGS, or HÆMOPTYSIS, is a more serious form, and is often a symptom of consumption. Frothy bright-coloured blood is coughed up, and there may be pain and a sensation of 'bubbling' in the chest. *Perfect* quiet is necessary, and half a tea-spoonful of salt in a little water may be given every five minutes till nausea is induced. Or, if at hand, five grains of ipecacuhana in an ounce of water till the patient feels sick. Afterwards cold or iced acid drinks, of which the best is fresh lime or lemon water.

Recipes 43 and 44 should be procured if possible.

HÆMATEMESIS, *or vomiting of dark-coloured blood from the stomach*, must be distinguished from *hæmoptysis* or coughing up *bright frothy* blood from the lungs. *Hæmatemesis* is in some cases dependent on disease of the liver or spleen, and it occasionally occurs when the menstrual flow is scanty or suppressed. But in the great majority of instances it occurs in consequence of an ulcer of the stomach eating into a blood-vessel. In all such cases the blood is *vomited, not coughed up*, and its colour is almost *black*, like coffee-grounds—*not red*; and blood is often passed by stool. It is generally preceded or accompanied by burning boring pain in the stomach, and if the ulcer is large the loss of blood is sufficient to cause alarming faintness, which may be felt before any blood is vomited, and for which stimulants must *not* be given. The great point is to keep the stomach at rest, so as to allow the ulcer to heal, or, at least, the ruptured vessel to become plugged up. This will not take place if the stomach is excited to action by food, or if the circulation is excited by stimulants. Ice should be swallowed in little lumps, *cold* fluid food, as broth or milk, should be given in spoonfuls at intervals of a few minutes, alum mixture (Recipe 42) should be administered, and perfect quiet should be insisted upon. In very severe cases *all food* should be given as cold nutrient injections, thus affording the stomach perfect rest (*vide Appendix, Digested Enemas*). In cases of either *hæmoptysis* or *hæmatemesis* medical aid should be sought.

For vomiting of blood (*hæmatemesis*) obtain Recipe 46 if possible.

The distinctions between bleeding from the lungs and bleeding from the stomach are placed in comparison below:—

| *Hæmoptysis, or bleeding from the lungs* | *Hæmatemesis, or bleeding from the stomach* |
|---|---|
| Usually difficulty of breathing, pain in chest. | Nausea, pain, and tenderness at the pit of the stomach. |
| Blood coughed up in mouthfuls. | Blood vomited profusely. |
| Blood frothy. | Blood not frothy. |
| Blood of a florid red colour. | Blood dark-coloured. |
| Blood mixed with saliva. | Blood mixed with food. |
| No blood passed by stool. | Blood often passed by stool. |
| Cough and bronchial symptoms. | None. |

**SPLEEN DISEASE.**—The spleen is covered by the stomach in front and by the ribs behind (*vide* p. 29), and in health is not easily felt. Most diseases of the spleen are regarded as due to malaria, and are often the sequelæ of attacks of ague. The principal kinds of spleen disease are *acute* and *chronic congestion.*

*Acute congestion of the spleen* most frequently arises suddenly during ague. In the cold stage of ague the blood is driven from the surface, the spleen becomes extraordinarily full of blood, and its tissue is stretched and strained. There is pain and tenderness on pressure under the ribs on the *left* side, the pain sometimes extending to the *left* loin or to the *left* shoulder, and the person cannot lie comfortably on the *left* side. There may also be nausea and vomiting. There may be blood in the vomit, but more usually blood appears in the stools. Bleeding from the nose may occur. When the congestion is less there are feelings of fulness and distension in the side, without actual pain, which are also aggravated by pressure. In persons subject to attacks of ague, congestion of the spleen, sometimes occurs *instead* of the ague fit, but in such cases there will usually be some heat of skin and quickened pulse. More rarely acute congestion presents in persons who have not suffered from ague. Acute congestion generally terminates in a few days with perspirations, diarrhœa, and thick sediment in the urine. At first the congestion of the organ subsides, leaving no trace; but after repeated attacks the strained tissue does not resume its natural dimensions, as deposits from the blood take place in it. Then *permanent* enlargement results, when the spleen may be easily felt under the ribs, by placing the thumb in front towards the stomach, and the fingers behind towards the back, on the left side of the body.

*Chronic congestion,* or enlargement of the spleen, may be the result of attacks of acute congestion. But often chronic enlargement of the spleen comes on so gradually, and painlessly, that it is long unattended to, until at length the enlarged organ excites fulness, weight, and dull pain in the left side. When the organ is much affected the enlargement, popularly known as 'ague cake,' is sometimes so great that the spleen may be both seen and felt, filling up and rendering protuberant half the cavity of the bowels, thus forming the condition so often seen in native children, and known as 'pot-bellied.' With enlarged spleen it will usually be fouud, especially in children, that the temperature as tested by the clinical thermometer (*vide* p. 33) rises in the evening to above 100°. If this rise is persistent, there is evidence that the disease is gaining ground. Whether in children or adults, when the spleen is enlarged, it becomes tender and brittle, and is easily ruptured (*vide* p. 595).

The spleen is concerned in the elaboration of the blood, and when there is chronic disease of the organ it is always associated with a deficiency of red globules in the blood, and hence the person becomes pallid and sallow, there is a peculiar pale tremulous tongue, the whites of the eyes become pearly or lemon-coloured, there are frequent attacks of diarrhœa, and, in short, the condition known as *anœmia* becomes established (*vide* p. 46). Up to a certain point this state may terminate in recovery, but a stage of splenic blood-deterioration is at length reached, when medicines are useless. The spleen-enlargement increases, the person becomes more debilitated, dropsical swellings of the belly and legs occur, and diarrhœa or dysentery becoming permanent, the person sinks.

*Treatment.*—In cases when the spleen has become *suddenly* painful, hot fomentations are required. In all cases if there is no diarrhœa, the bowels should be acted upon by the sulphate of soda, quinine and iron (Recipe 3). If there is diarrhœa, the same recipe should be taken without the sulphate of soda. When intermittent fever or ague is present, treatment mentioned under that head must be adopted. When enlargement of the spleen occurs *gradually* without fever, or without pain and tenderness, tonics are required, and in the absence of other medicines Recipe 3 may be taken, with or without the soda salts, as the bowels may require. It should, however, be recollected that in all varieties of spleen disease a free action on the bowels is generally desirable. Children should be encouraged to take plenty of milk, with which a little lime water (Recipe 25) may be mixed; they should be clothed warmly, the bowels should be kept open if necessary by citrate of magnesia (*vide* p. 15), and small doses of sulphate of iron may be given (*vide* p. 24). Moderate pressure by a wide flannel bandage round the body is advisable.

[When obtainable, instead of the medicines mentioned above, *for acute cases*, 2 scruples of compound jalap powder with 5 grains of snlphate of iron every morning, and iron and quinine (Recipe 70) three times a day. In more chronic cases Friedrichshall or Hunyadi Janos water, and pills containing arseniate of iron one quarter of a grain, strychnine one-fortieth of a grain, quinine one grain, thrice daily. The part may be painted externally with iodine paint (*vide Appendix*, No. 111). Afterwards ointment of iodide of mercury (Recipe 94) may be rubbed in daily. For children Recipe 16, if the bowels are confined, and Recipe 70 in proportionate doses. The skin over the enlarged spleen may be gently rubbed with soap liniment.]

Spleen enlargement in Europeans eventually requires change to Europe. Removal to a cold climate will in most instances, if not too long deferred, result in recovery. When European children suffer from enlarged spleens their removal from India is imperatively demanded. If this is impossible, removal from the locality to the sea, if practicable; if not, to the hills.

**STOMACH, DISORDERS OF THE.**—The stomach may be disordered by a multitude of causes, the principal of which are improper food, alcoholic liquors, fevers, and (especially in children) other exhausting diseases. When disorder of the stomach arises from improper food or drink, there may be *headache* (*vide* p. 291); or there may be a *bilious colic attack* (*vide* p. 131). But the disorder may not terminate in such ailments. There may be increasing pain and tenderness at the pit of the stomach, with constant hiccough, nausea, and vomiting, even water being rejected. The vomit consists of fluid, often tinged with bile; the breath is sour, the tongue furred in the centre, with great thirst and much feverishness, and the mouth may be sore. It is to this condition that the term *gastric fever* has been applied. But a disordered stomach will recover itself in the course of two or three days. If the symptoms continue longer, there is reason to fear either *typhoid* or *remittent fever*, or, in children, *hydrocephalus*. All these diseases may commence with disordered stomach; and in some cases it is not, at first, possible to say whether such symptoms are referable to disordered stomach, or are the results of a commencing fever. If the stomach symptoms come on after indulgence or improper food, and if there is no *typhoid* fever in the neighbourhood, it may be safely concluded that the ailment is not *typhoid*. But it may be *remittent fever*, and this the more likely if there has been no prior cause for disordered stomach, or if the person has been exposed to the sun, or sleeping in damp malarious localities. If the attack is *remittent fever* the stomach symptoms will continue longer than two or three days, while fever will prevail as under 'Remittent' (*vide* p. 258).

*Treatment.*—If the disorder of the stomach assumes the form of headache, or of a bilious attack, the treatment mentioned at pp. 292, 131, should be pursued. If the disorder has arisen without evident cause, and the bowels are constipated, a laxative, as Recipe 2, should be given. Then *the main point is to allow the stomach perfect rest*; and only milk and lime water (Recipe 25), or, if preferred, milk and soda water, should be given in table-spoonfuls every half-hour. Sometimes weak beef-tea, or arrowroot, suits the irritable stomach best. If the stomach rejects a table-spoonful of fluid, the quantity should be reduced to a tea-spoonful. The patient should not drink quantities of water, which he will crave for, but suck pieces of ice. Chloral (Recipe 64) may be given at night. Fomentations should be applied over the pit of the stomach.

STOMACH DISORDER IN INFANTS AND CHILDREN.—Is much most common in infants being brought up by hand. It may be caused by uncleanliness of the feeding bottle, especially about the cork; by overfeeding, or by improper food. Very sour breath, vomiting after food, flinching when slight pressure is made on the pit of the stomach, flatulence, sometimes aphthous mouth and fever (*vide* p. 446), are characteristic. Children thus affected also usually suffer from diarrhœa, and the stools may be light of colour, and containing lumps of undigested milk. Disorder of the stomach most usually in children subsides in a few days; or it may terminate in *infantile diarrhœa*, or in *dysentery*, or in *remittent fever*, or in *thrush*, or in *convulsions*, or in *rickets*, or in *water on the brain*, or in *atrophy*, or, if the child has been exposed to the specific contagion, in *typhoid fever*.

*Treatment* is more dietetic than medicinal. The condition is often induced, and frequently kept up, purely by improper feeding. Giving milk or other food whenever the child cries is a fertile cause. Although much may be rejected by vomiting, enough remains to decompose in the stomach. The best treatment is abstinence, so that the stomach may have time to recover itself. Children with disordered stomach will not suffer from hunger, even if given water only, for a day or two. The milk should be given sparingly, and lime-water (Recipe 25) should be given several times daily; or, if the infant is being fed, lime-water should be mixed with the milk in one-third proportion. In severe cases it often happens that milk is injurious, because it so quickly decomposes in the sour stomach of the child. It is therefore often advisable to stop milk, or farinaceous foods if being used, and to give instead, at hourly intervals, tea-spoonfuls of raw meat soup, or of beef-extract; sometimes one, sometimes the other being best retained (*vide Addendum*).

[If obtainable, peptonise the milk with Fairchild's peptonising powders, when it may perhaps be retained. In severe cases, when there is no natural colour in the stools, it is advisable to give some medicine to act on the liver, when podophyllin and rectified spirit mixture, as recommended at p. 142 for some forms of constipation, may be tried. If the desired effect is not produced, for a child one year old, 1 grain of calomel, with one-sixth of a grain of ipecacuanha every three hours for six doses. When nothing can be retained on the stomach, and the child appears sinking from want of food, the limbs should be rubbed with cod-liver oil; small pieces of sponge, soaked in cod-liver oil, should be placed in the armpits, and injections of beef-tea may also be used.]

The diseases for which gastric disorder in children are most likely to be confounded are *hydrocephalus*, or *water on the brain*, and *enteric fever*. The chief characteristics are therefore placed in comparison:—

| *Gastric Disorder* | *Hydrocephalus* | *Enteric Fever* |
|---|---|---|
| Common in young children. | Common in young children. | Not common in young children. |
| Vomiting continual and severe. | Vomiting continual and severe. | Vomiting occasionally present, but not severe and continued. |
| Disgust for food after vomiting. | Asks for food after vomiting. | Disgust for food. |
| Vomiting ceases after the stomach is empty. | Continues after the stomach is empty. | Continues. |
| Pain and tenderness at the pit of the stomach. | Pain in the head. | Pain and tenderness over the bowels at the sides. |
| Bowels loose; stools light, with undigested food. | Bowels usually constipated. | Diarrhœa, with yellow-coloured stools. |

| Gastric Disorder | Hydrocephalus | Enteric Fever |
|---|---|---|
| Bowels variable, often distended by flatus. | Bowels shrunken and contracted. | Bowels drum-like. |
| No delirium. | Delirium. | Delirium. |
| No eruption. | No eruption. | Eruption of mulberry-coloured spots about the twelfth day. |
| No rolling of the head. | Rolling of the head. | Not. |
| Origin from improper feeding. | Origin often constitutional. | Origin from a specific poison. |

**STRICTURE.**—Stricture, or contraction of any of the natural passages of the body, may occur as the effects of disease or of injury.

Stricture of the Gullet.—This prevents the passage of food into the stomach, and is characterised principally by gradually increasing difficulty of swallowing, noticed probably during years, and occasionally aggravated by fits of spasm. There is also pain in the chest and between the shoulders, and if an instrument is passed into the gullet it meets with an obstruction. Hysterical females may also suffer from symptoms of stricture of the gullet, but in such cases the difficulty of swallowing often appears suddenly and vanishes as quickly. Hysterical females should be treated for hysteria. When symptoms as above occur to others, general and surgical treatment under professional superintendence is required.

Stricture of the Rectum.—The symptoms are pain, straining, and difficulty in passing the fæces, which are voided in small narrow flattened pieces. There are also cramps and pains in the thighs, frequent desire to make water, and dyspeptic symptoms. A medical man should be consulted as soon as possible.

Stricture of the Urethra.—The urethra, or channel by which the urine passes, is subject to both *permanent* and *spasmodic* stricture.

*Permanent Stricture* signifies a contraction of the canal

of the urethra in one or more places owing *generally* to attacks of gonorrhœa, but caused *sometimes* by injury. The symptoms of stricture of the urethra are frequent desire to pass water, especially at night, a little urine dribbling out after micturition and wetting the clothes, increasing difficulty in making water, a small, forked or twisted stream of water, and that stream diminished in bulk. There is often itching at the end of the penis, and a gleety discharge. As symptoms much resembling those of stricture occur from stone in the bladder (*vide* p. 73), or enlarged prostate gland (*vide* p. 366), examination by passing an instrument (*vide* p. 493) is the only certain test.

*Treatment.*—Any stomach disorders, or acidity of the urine, must be removed by aperients and antacids, and temperance, rest, and early hours must be adopted. But mechanical treatment is of most importance, and consists in the periodical passing of an instrument, only to be performed by a surgeon. When the stricture has been dilated, the passage may be kept open by the patient, if instructed how to use a bougie of the proper kind.

*Spasmodic Stricture* usually occurs to persons who have some slight permanent stricture. The exciting causes of spasm of the part are indulgence in drink, especially of an acid nature, retaining the urine too long, exposure to wet, horse or bicycle exercise, irritation from piles, or some unnatural condition of urine. The symptoms are now those of *Retention of Urine.* The patient has a great desire to pass water, and on straining finds himself unable to do so; the bladder becomes distended, and appears as a globular tumour in the lower part of the belly. The suffering is great and the person grows feverish, and, if not relieved, the continued efforts at evacuation may terminate in rupture of the bladder or urethra, and in *extravasation*, or escape of the urine into the surrounding tissues. When this serious complication results, the patient during a violent effort of straining feels something give way; his painful sense of distension becomes immediately less, and he thinks himself getting well. He probably now makes a little water, as the stricture relaxes when the pressure behind is removed, and this further adds to his satisfaction. But in a very short time smarting pain occurs about the anus, in the fork, and in the privates; for the irritating urine has penetrated into all these parts, which rapidly become red, much swollen, and inflamed. Blackish spots and blisters, significant of *mortification*, soon appear, the tongue becomes black, the pulse feeble, and muttering delirium and hiccough precede a fatal termination.

When the escape of urine is not great, as occurs if the patient is relieved at the critical period, an abscess forms in the fork behind the scrotum. Or sometimes an abscess forms without any escape of urine, simply as the result of irritation. This, called *perinæal abscess*, is known by throbbing pain, tenderness, hardness, and a globular swelling, with hot skin and feverishness. Frequently a *perinæal* abscess results in *fistula* (*vide* p. 44), through which often urine finds its way from the bladder.

*Treatment.*—When stricture causes *retention of urine*, the first thing is to relieve the patient. If the symptoms are not very severe, and if the stoppage of water has succeeded a debauch or exposure to cold, a hot bath followed by fomentations to the fork and lower part of the bowels, and a full dose, as 12 or 15 grains, of Dover's powder, will generally afford relief. If the bowels have not been recently opened, an ounce of castor oil should be taken one hour after the Dover's powder. If these measures do not succeed in the course of three hours, a full dose, as 30 grains, of chloral may be given, and leeches to the number of thirty should be applied *behind* the scrotum. If urine does not pass, the catheter should be introduced (*vide* p. 493), which may be very difficult, and will require the aid of a surgeon. *The treatment of extravasation of urine*, and of abscess from this cause, urgently require skilled aid, in the absence of which it will be best to apply poultices made of finely powdered charcoal, and poppy water (Recipe 81).

[In addition to the remedies mentioned above for the relief of *retention of urine*, tincture of iron mixture (Recipe 71) should be procured, 1 ounce of which should be given every quarter-hour. It will also be advisable to give a morphia draught (Recipe 65).]

When *extravasation* of urine occurs, a free incision, three inches long and one deep, should be made in the middle line of the swollen scrotum, and any other parts of the scrotum or perinæum which are swollen and prominent should also be pricked. Then a poultice should be applied, and a catheter should be introduced into the bladder and retained there, to allow of the escape of urine. When abscess forms in the perinæum or fork, it should be opened without delay. The diet should consist of nourishing broths and soups, and, if *extravasation* occurs, wine or brandy should be freely administered.

**ST. VITUS'S DANCE.**—This disease, technically termed *chorea*, generally affects children, especially female children, and is most common from eight to fourteen years of age. Children badly fed, or living under bad hygienic conditions, are especially liable. Antecedent illness, as scarlet fever, measles, whooping-cough, or rheumatism, predisposes. Other causes are intestinal irritation from constipation, or from worms; it has been known to arise from the irritation caused by a decayed tooth or from teething; it is sometimes a consequence of debility or *anæmia*; it is frequently associated in young girls with irregularities of the menstrual flow. It has followed frights occurring to weakly children. Mental over-work is a predisposing cause. Immoral practices may induce it. It occasionally seems to be hereditary without special cause.

Chorea generally comes on very insidiously, and is

often preceded by night terrors (*vide* p. 145), or by vague pains of a rheumatic nature, which may be regarded as 'growing pains.' Other premonitory symptoms are moping and melancholy combined with fidgetiness and restlessness, bad temper, and inability to sleep. Then there are slight contortions of the face, or slight convulsive movements of the legs. When fully formed there may be convulsive movements of all the limbs. In walking the leg is suddenly thrust to one side, or pulled backwards; or in conveying the hand to the mouth it is snatched towards the forehead or shoulder, or above the head. Occasionally there may be difficulty of speech, or paralysis of one limb, or fainting fits, or palpitation of the heart. The valves of the heart are also liable to become affected, especially in those who have previously had rheumatism. In exceptionally severe cases the convulsive movements are so violent and continued that the patient may die from exhaustion. The ordinary duration of chorea is two months, but it may last six.

*Treatment.*—The probable cause of the malady must be studied. If from worms, they should be expelled (*vide Worms*, p. 482). If from constipation, this condition must be relieved. If from decayed teeth, they must be removed. If from teething, the swollen gums must be lanced (*vide* p. 434). If from anæmia, that condition must be treated (*vide* p. 46). If from menstrual irregularity, this must be treated (*vide* pp. 468, 470). If from simple debility, tonics are necessary, of which the most successful is arsenic (Recipe 75) in doses according to age (*vide* p. 6). If from immoral practices, such habits must be abandoned. In very severe cases perfect rest and quiet should be ensured, the patient should be placed in bed in a darkened room, all causes of excitement should be avoided, the limbs should be shampooed several times daily, and for adults bromide of potassium (Recipe 19) should be given thrice daily, and chloral (Recipe 64) at night to procure sleep. For children, the same medicines, in the doses mentioned at pp. 9 and 11. As soon as possible in severe cases, and immediately in mild cases, change of air and surroundings is most desirable. The heart-affection sometimes accompanying chorea usually remains for some time afterwards, but gradually gets quite well.

**SUNSTROKE**, or **INSOLATIA**.—There are several forms, presenting considerable variety of symptoms, as below:—

1. *Heat Fainting*, or *Syncope*. 2. *Heat Apoplexy*, or *Coup de Soleil*. 3. *Sun Fever*.

Sunstroke of all kinds is due to nervous disturbance from prolonged high temperature,[1] either with or without direct exposure to the sun's rays. The liability to sunstroke is increased by fatigue, mental excitement, depression of spirits, living and especially sleeping in crowded apartments; by want of ventilation, by want of water, by constipation of the bowels, and by the abuse of alcoholic drinks.

*Premonitory Symptoms of Sunstroke.*—Frequently previous to an attack of sunstroke, the person affected becomes irritable, restless, and complains of headache. He feels dull and listless, and is unable to make much exertion without a great effort. The appetite fails, and a feeling of nausea, and constipation of the bowels are often present. An absence of perspiration may also be noticed, the skin may be unusually hot and dry, there may be slight sensations of giddiness, and there may be more frequent desire than usual to make water, although little fluid is passed. Confusion of ideas, confusion of vision, loquacity, fits of laughing and crying may occur. Such premonitory symptoms may prevail for hours or for days previous to the fully developed attack, or they may not occur; or, occurring,

[1] For the manner in which elevated temperature acts, *vide* Chapter VI., 'Heat.'

may pass away. When anything of the kind is noticed in persons exposed to a high temperature, every means possible should be used to secure ventilation and movement of air, shade and coolness should be sought, cold water should be plentifully drunk, and the body should be well sponged with water, or a bath should be taken. A purgative (Recipes 1 and 2) will generally be desirable, and citrate of magnesia draughts (*vide* p. 15) should be given every two hours.

1. Heat Fainting, or Syncope.—Either after the foregoing premonitory symptoms, or without such symptoms, *heat fainting*, or *syncope*, commences with feelings of faintness, sickness, giddiness, shivering, cold extremities, frequent desire to make water, and sometimes drowsiness. The face is pale, the surface of the body is cold, and often bathed in perspiration. The breathing is of a sighing or gasping character, the action of the heart and pulse are weak, sometimes intermittent, the pupils of the eyes are contracted, and there may be more or less insensibility.

2. Heat Apoplexy, or Coup de Soleil.—Heat apoplexy may be preceded for a variable time by the *premonitory symptoms* as above detailed. Or, *secondly*, it may commence as *heat fainting*, or *syncope*, which condition, after a few minutes, or perhaps a few hours, passes into another state, characterised by *flushing of the face, heat of body and head, bloodshot eyes, strong quick pulse, stertorous snoring, or puffing breathing (marking the brain most affected), or noisy, irregular, and incomplete breathing (marking the lungs most affected). In a very short period insensibility ensues, and sometimes convulsions. Or, *thirdly*, *coup de soleil* may occur suddenly, without either premonitory symptoms or the fainty feelings of heat syncope. In such cases the person falls down as suddenly as if struck with apoplexy, and the symptoms are as above (*commencing at *flushing of the face*). Sometimes

there may be convulsions, but in the majority of these cases the patient does not move again. According as the malady appears to expend itself on the head or chest, the terms *Heat Apoplexy* and *Heat Asphyxia*, or *Heat Suffocation*, have been applied.

*Treatment.*—The form in which the disease attacks should be recognised. When the patient is faint, sick, giddy, shivering, and cold, lay him on his back in the shade, rub the limbs, loosen the clothing, and give wine or brandy and water. But the case must be treated with caution, on account of the tendency of the malady to run on to that condition marked by flushed face, heat of skin, bloodshot eyes, and quick, strong pulse. When such symptoms are observed stimulants should be withheld, cold water should be poured on the head, punkahs should be used to cool the surrounding atmosphere, and, if the patient can swallow, a quick purgative, as 1 ounce of sulphate of soda in three ounces of water, should be given. If available, 8 or 10 grains of quinine should be added to this draught; or it may be given afterwards. Recipe 105 should also be used cold as an injection; or, if not at hand, an injection of cold water. The extremities should be rubbed, mustard poultices or turpentine stupe should be applied to the nape of the neck, and, if insensibility and puffing breathing ensue, the injection should be repeated, and twenty leeches may be applied at the roots of the hair above the temples. The patient may also be wrapped in a wet sheet.

When the symptoms point to lung affection (known by the irregular, noisy, laboured, and incomplete breathing, but neither sighing nor stertorous or puffing), in addition to cold affusion, quick purging, and friction to the extremities, a large mustard poultice should be applied to the chest. If doubt is felt as to which is most affected (the head or the chest), or if, as often occurs, both are affected, mustard poultices or turpentine should be placed both on the back of the neck and on the chest (*vide Appendix*, Nos. 108, 109).

In all varieties of sunstroke the patient should be encouraged to drink plentifully of cold water, to supply the place of the evaporation of fluid constantly taking place from the skin.

If the patient has previously suffered from venereal, iodide of potassium (Recipe 21) should be given as soon as possible. Venereal sometimes produces a condition of the blood-vessels of the brain which may predispose to sunstroke and to its after-effects, and which condition the iodide tends to correct.

Although recovery is often rapid and complete, more commonly fever and oppressed breathing prevail more or less for some days. All forms of sunstroke are frequently followed by periodical headaches, by fever, by neuralgic affections, by dysentery, and sometimes by paralysis. They occasionally leave permanent injury of the brain, which may terminate in softening of that organ, or in insanity. Often, when recovery seems complete, the person is afterwards unable to bear any exposure to the sun, and is unfitted for active life in the tropics.

[As noted above, in the great majority of cases of sunstroke, quick purging is most desirable. Therefore, if obtainable, two drops of croton oil mixed in a little sugar should be given instead of the sulphate of soda. If the patient cannot swallow the croton oil and sugar, it should be placed, by means of a feather, on the back of the tongue. Subcutaneous injection of quinine is also advisable.]

3. Sun Fever.—May be very trivial or very severe. Probably most people who are exposed to the sun during the day experience some feverishness afterwards, and often take no notice of it. It may disappear in a few hours, or it may cause a restless night, and perhaps diarrhœa. Or it may continue with languor, weakness,

loss of appetite, &c., presenting precisely the same symptoms as described under *continued* or *ephemeral* fever at p. 239. It seldom lasts more than twenty-four hours, and then declines, or develops into a condition known as ARDENT SUN FEVER. This severe form of sun fever chiefly prevails in the months of April and May, and in seasons when the temperature is unusually elevated. The attack, or development from a minor degree, is generally sudden, commencing with premonitory chills. There is pungent heat of skin and great thirst, the tongue is parched, red, and dry, the pulse quick and strong. There is much headache, flushed face, throbbing of the temples, restlessness, nausea, and bilious vomiting. The duration of the disease is about sixty hours, after which, if amendment does not take place, insensibility precedes death.

*Treatment.*—For a minor degree of sun fever, or for irritability after exposure, a cold or tepid bath according to habit, rest and quiet under a punkah, and, if the bowels are confined, an aperient dose are desirable. For *ardent sun fever*, leeches to the head (one for each year of the patient's age up to thirty), shaving the head, and the application of cold to the head, a darkened room, rest, quiet, and repeated purgatives (Recipes 1, 2). In the latter stages, if great exhaustion occurs, ammonia, wine, brandy and water, and nourishing broths.

[Whenever the temperature rises suddenly to 103° or 104° Fahr. (*vide* p. 34) *cold* baths are very serviceable, but in the absence of a medical man are not advised.]

*The means of prevention* of sunstroke and sun fever are considered in Chapter VI., under 'Heat.'

**SWELLING OF THE LEGS.**—Occurs from causes specified under dropsy (p. 186); and under diseases of pregnancy (p. 359); or at the change of life (p. 481); or in connection with amenorrhœa (*vide* p. 468); or from scurvy (p. 380); or from enlargement of the spleen (p. 414); or as a consequence of debility, or of heat. Swelling of the feet is common in India, especially towards night; but, unless connected with obvious derangement of the health, does not need medical treatment.

**TEETHING, or DENTITION.**—The intimate connections which exist between the nerves supplying the stomach (*pneumogastric*), the nerves supplying the teeth-pulp (*the fifth pair*, or *trifacial*), and the nerves supplying the general system (*the sympathetic*), are so extensive and numerous that functional interference with any part of one set is liable to act upon the others. Hence the frequent association of stomach or bowel complaints, of fever, of skin diseases, and of other derangements, with teething, especially when children are improperly fed.

When the teeth appear naturally, and the child is in good health, they do so in the order shown by the following plates. The two lower central incisors, or front

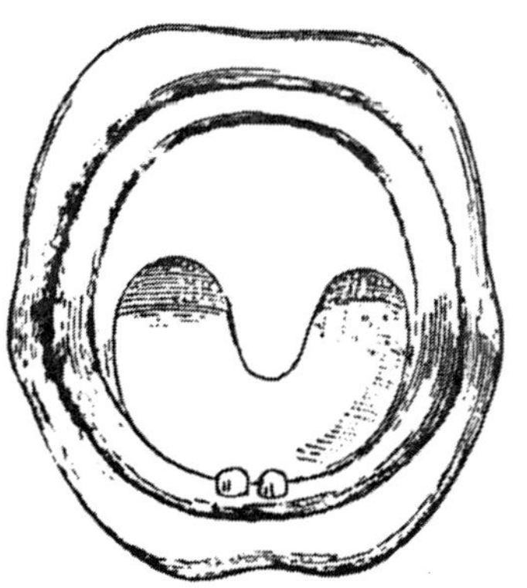

teeth, penetrate the gums between the sixth and seventh months (plate 1); the corresponding upper central incisors

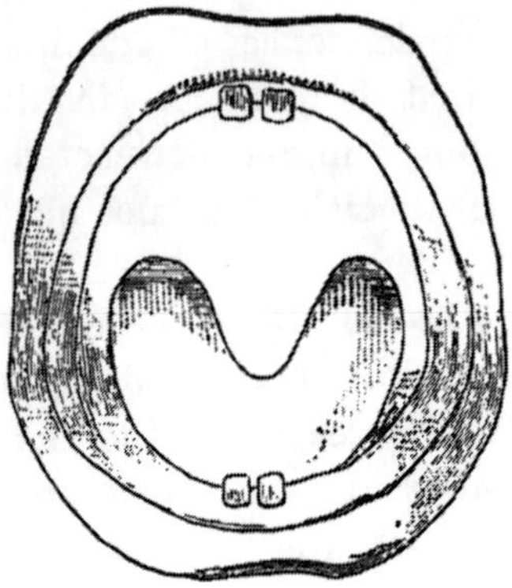

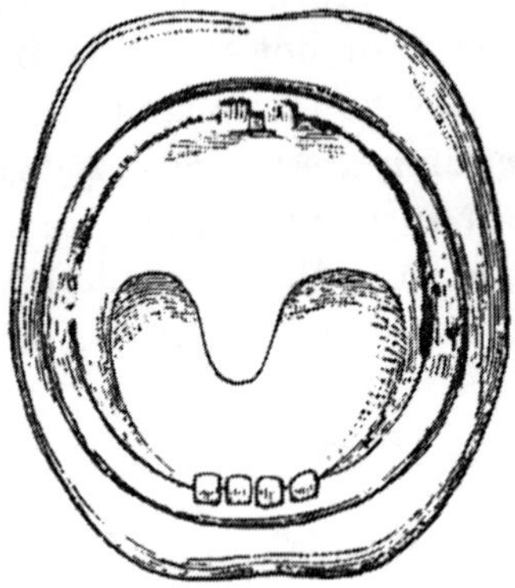

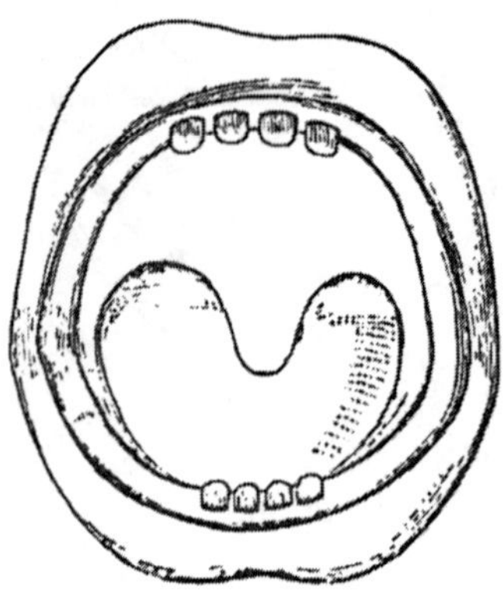

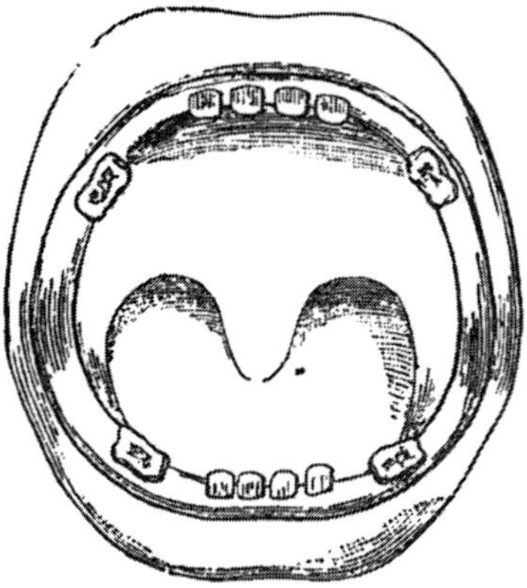

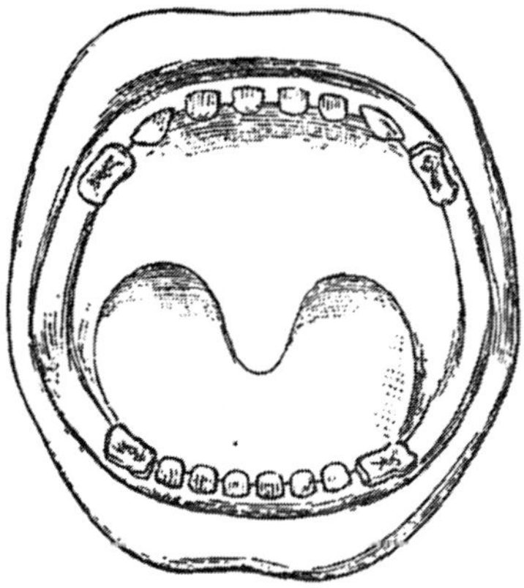

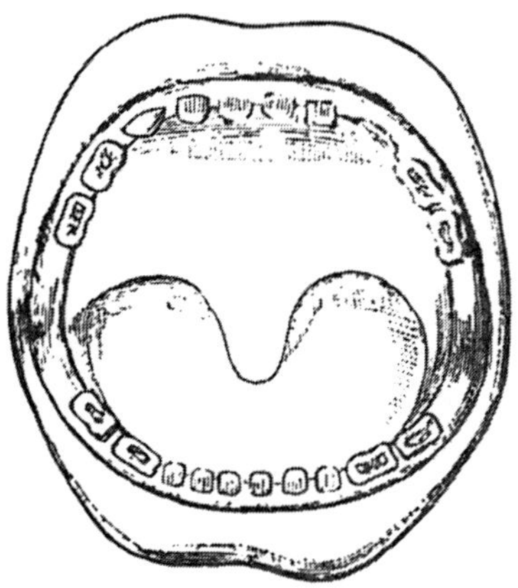

in from three weeks to a month afterwards (plate 2); the two lower lateral incisors about the eighth or ninth month (plate 3); the two upper[1] lateral incisors generally soon or a month afterwards (plate 4). The anterior molars or grinders of the under jaw make their appearance between the twelfth and fourteenth months, those of the upper jaw following shortly afterwards (plate 5). The canine or eye teeth are cut between the sixteenth and twentieth months (plate 6). Last of all, the second molars are cut between the twentieth and thirtieth or thirty-sixth months (plate 7).

Thus, the cutting of the twenty temporary or 'milk teeth,' as they are called, is completed, as a general rule, at the age of two and a half to three years.

Formation of the Teeth.—At birth the teeth consist of pulpy substance buried in the gums, and it is not till the *third or fourth month* that they assume shape and hardness. Infants at this period may suffer from symptoms of teething. The mouth may be hot; there may be restlessness, flushings of the face, heat of hands and surface generally, with loss of appetite, and perhaps vomiting and diarrhœa. But the gums do not show *localised* irritation, and the condition is often attributed to some other cause. The same occurs during the intervals between the appearance of the teeth, and is vulgarly called 'the breeding of the teeth' in the gums. It arises from the pressure made below the surface of the gums by the growing teeth, which have not yet risen sufficiently to render the skin of the gums tense and prominent. A little of a preparation of sixty grains of bicarbonate of soda, well mixed with one ounce of honey, should be rubbed on the gums two or three times daily, and cooling medicine, as citrate of magnesia (*vide* p. 15), should be given. Remedies for diarrhœa, or for constipation, or for flatulence (*vide*

[1] The upper lateral incisors often precede the lower ones.

pp. 172, 138, 273), as such conditions may prevail, should also be prescribed.

Cutting of the Teeth.—Most people will, doubtless, remember feeling pain when the wisdom teeth appeared, and infants, probably, often experience the same annoyance. This, however, is not always the case, for sometimes it is discovered that an infant has cut a tooth who had not yet shown any indication, excepting an increased flow of saliva, that dentition had commenced. But more frequently the mouth becomes hot, and the gums look tense, tumid, and shining, while the position of each tooth is marked some time before its appearance by an increased prominence of the gum. If teething is going on naturally, and there are no symptoms beyond a little feverishness, dribbling from the mouth, or occasional diarrhœa, interference is not necessary. Preventing the dribbling from the child's mouth saturating the clothing and producing cold is all that is required. The most common complaints during teething are restlessness, and feverishness at night. The child's temper is cross, the flesh becomes soft, and there is loss of colour, all improving on the day the tooth comes through. But the liability of infants to illness at such period should be borne in mind; and care should be taken not to make any alteration in the infant's food while it is actually cutting the teeth; but rather, if change of diet be necessary, to take the opportunity afforded by one of those pauses of dentition to which reference has been made. Should the child grow suddenly hot and feverish, or wake screaming at night, cooling medicine, as citrate of magnesia (*vide* p. 15), may be given every two hours, while the bowels, if confined, should be moved by castor oil. An india-rubber *ring*—the best shape, as it cannot be thrust into the eye—may always be given to the child to suck. The pressure against the gums of the elastic india-rubber substance is agreeable to the child, and, moreover, tends to increase the rapidity with which the gum above the rising tooth is absorbed. Giving sweet things to children to suck during teething must be condemned, as the 'barley sugar,' or other material sometimes used for this purpose, being swallowed, turns acid in the child's stomach and disorders the bowels. When a tooth is near the surface, there is a prominent, shining, and sometimes white appearance of the gum, and the child who before was pleased to have the gums rubbed, does not willingly permit them to be touched. If the child is feverish or otherwise suffering, the gum may be lanced. But the gum-lancet should seldom be used unless there is evident irritation or prominence of a gum, or when it appears the gum will certainly burst in a day or two. Under such circumstances lancing the gum will spare the infant much suffering. In a smaller number of cases it may be necessary to lance a red and swollen gum when the tooth is not so near—as when a child has convulsions, or is attacked with other serious ailment. But this is done to scarify and relieve the turgid gums, *not* to divide them down to the tooth.

LANCING THE GUMS OF CHILDREN.—This is very easily managed, and any intelligent person seeing it done once or twice may do it effectually. The operation may be performed with a gum-lancet (*vide* p. 491), the edge of which must be placed vertically on the top of the inflamed gum, and moved along, pressing firmly at the same time, till the edge of the instrument grates on the tooth. Care must be taken that the instrument does not slip.

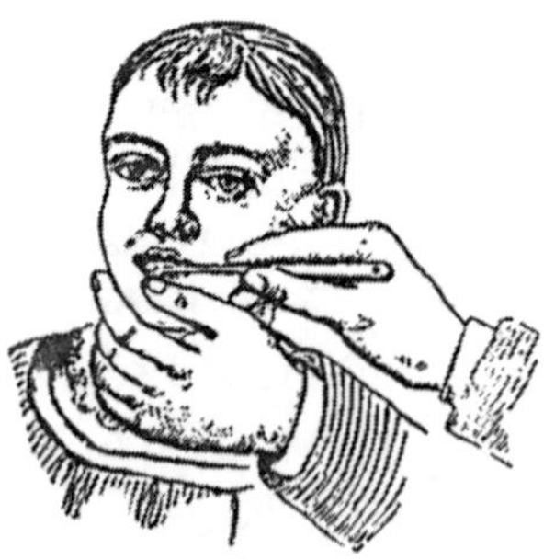

The best way to lance the gums of infants is to place two chairs near a window, so that the light falls on the operator. The child's nurse, sitting on one chair, should allow the head of the child to fall gently backwards on the operator's knees. Then the lancet may be easily used as mentioned above. If the child is restless, a shawl may be wrapped round its body to prevent the hands being raised to the mouth.

During teething there is a demand in the system for certain mineral matters, of which the principal is lime, which plays a considerable part in the construction of the teeth. Therefore, when teething is difficult, or when the maladies mentioned below supervene, a little lime-water may be given (*vide* Recipe 25). A few spoonfuls may be mixed daily with the food of the child if being fed by hand. Or if 'phosphate of lime' is procurable, a couple of grains should be given in a little water with each meal, instead of lime-water.

The principal maladies occurring during, or excited by teething, are as follows:—

1. VARIOUS FORMS OF SKIN DISEASES.—Almost any variety of skin disease may occur during dentition. Most frequently skin affections at such times take the form of 'breaking out,' or *eczema*, near the ears; or of 'rose rash,' or *erythema* (*vide* pp. 386, 396); or of *pompholix* (*vide* p. 398); or the glands underneath the chin may swell. It frequently happens that, in spite of any treatment, these skin affections persist during the whole period of teething, then getting well. They are seldom dangerous, and rarely need much medical treatment. They frequently serve as a relief to the system, and if they are suddenly checked, disease of some internal organ may manifest itself. It is generally better to abstain altogether from external medicinal applications. The parts affected should be kept perfectly clean by washing frequently with glycerine soap, after which a little cold cream or simple ointment may be applied. Maintaining the bowels freely open by castor oil or by citrate of magnesia, together with the careful regulation of the food, are the best means of curing these

eruptions. They are often increased by acidity of the stomach, and are then much benefited by 2 or 3 grains of bicarbonate of soda, or magnesia, given daily. If there is debility or feverishness, a grain of quinine may be added.

*Rose rash, roseola,* or *red gum,* and *erythema,* all skin affections occurring during teething, are described under *Skin Diseases*, pp. 386, 387.

2. Thrush, or Aphthæ (*vide* p. 446).

3. Flatulence (*vide* p. 273).

4. Vomiting.—Vomiting during teething is common, and may be connected with skin maladies, or with diarrhœa, or be a symptom of disordered stomach (*vide* p. 415), or may occur unassociated with other ailments. It may depend on indigestible food, or on too frequent feeding; or it may arise from that intimate communication between the different nerves supplying the teeth and stomach, as before noticed (p. 429), and by which the irritation arising in one part is conveyed to, and reacts on, another part of the body. Vomiting, therefore, is to be relieved by attention to the food, giving particular care to the cleanliness of the utensils used, if the child is taking other sustenance than human milk; by relieving constipation or diarrhœa by appropriate remedies; and by lancing the gums if they present the appearances described as indicating the use of the instrument (*vide* p. 434).

5. Diarrhœa (*vide* Infantile Diarrhœa, p. 172).

6. Cough.—Cough of a short, dry, hacking character, often commencing soon after the child is put to bed, is caused by sympathetic irritation of the upper part of the air-passages, is of a nervous nature, and will be best relieved by bromide of potassium (Recipe 20). But cough of a different character, accompanied by wheezing of the breathing, and feverishness occurring during teething, must be looked upon with suspicion as the possible com-

mencement of *bronchitis* or *inflammation of the lungs*, and Recipe 57 should be given immediately.

7. BRONCHITIS AND PNEUMONIA (*vide* pp. 105, 328).
8. CONVULSIONS (*vide* p. 145).
9. PARALYSIS OF INFANTS (*vide* p. 344).
10. DISORDERS OF THE STOMACH (*vide* p. 417).

TEETH, SECOND OR PERMANENT SET.—The advance of the second set of teeth causes the absorption of the roots of the temporary or milk teeth, and thus facilitates their shedding, the crowns falling off and leaving room for the permanent teeth to come forward and supply their places, in which process the following order is usually observed. First, between five and six years of age, the *first permanent molars* or grinders (four in number) appear, *immediately behind* the milk molars, and for a short time the child has four permanent and twenty temporary teeth. The front teeth, *middle incisors* (four in number), are next shed and renewed, usually when the child is between seven and eight. Then a year or so later the side or *lateral incisors* (four in number) are replaced by others. The anterior double teeth *molars* (in number four) are replaced about the ninth year by the *bicuspids*, or small or false permanent molars, and about the tenth year the posterior double teeth *molars* (four in number) are replaced by similar teeth. About the eleventh year the *canine* teeth (four in number) are replaced, these being the last of the milk teeth to be exchanged. Near the twelfth year four more true or large *molars* arise, and the appearance of these teeth is regarded as a sign that the child is twelve years old. The third double teeth (molars), or wisdom teeth (*dentes sapientiæ*), four in number, seldom appear until three or four years subsequently, and often later. The number of the second set of teeth when complete is thirty-two.

As a rule, no trouble attends the appearance of any of the permanent teeth, excepting the wisdom teeth. But sometimes the front teeth are too crowded, and the side teeth may grow so out of line as to irritate the mouth and require extraction. In many cases the individual may, by constantly pushing with the tongue, do much towards maintaining the teeth in an even row.

The cutting of the wisdom teeth is often attended with pain. The difficulty arises from the teeth appearing so close to the curvature or angle of the lower jaw that the mucous membrane of the mouth, where passing from the cheek to the jaw, is caught by the rising wisdom tooth, and nipped every time the mouth is closed. Ulceration is produced, and a troublesome sore may result. Sometimes there is stiffness, or even closure of the jaw in consequence. The best *treatment* is to nip away, with a sharp pair of scissors, any overhanging fold of membrane, so that the teeth may not press upon any part of the texture of the mouth when the jaws are closed. The ulcer will then heal, particularly if touched occasionally with a camel-hair pencil charged with strong alum water, or with vinegar.

**TESTICLE, INFLAMMATION OF THE.**—May arise from various causes, as injury, mumps, and gonorrhœa. The whole organ may be affected, or the posterior part may be chiefly implicated. The symptoms are heat, swelling, redness, great tenderness, pain between the legs, aching and dragging sensation in the loins, feverishness, nausea, and sometimes vomiting. If discharge has been coming from the penis, it ceases when the testicle inflames. Both testicles may be affected, but usually the right is attacked.

*Treatment.*—If an injection is being used it should be stopped. Perfect rest in bed is desirable, and the inflamed part should be raised on a small pillow. It should be assiduously fomented with hot poppy-water (*vide Appendix*, No. 81), and if the inflammation is violent, and the pain and tenderness unbearable, leeches should be applied (one for each year of the person's age up to thirty), not on the testicle itself, but along the course of the cord in the flexure of the groin. Magnesia draughts (*vide* p. 15) should be given to relieve feverishness. If necessary, the bowels should be well opened by successive doses of Recipe 2, and chloral (Recipe 64) should be given at night to relieve pain and afford sleep. The attack runs its course in about ten days, after which the testicle will require to be supported until all remaining hardness and swelling subsides, which may not be for some weeks. If a person with swelled testicle is unable to keep at rest, as advised above, the great thing is to support the parts well by a suspensory bandage, or with the handkerchief as described below. In severe cases the person is totally unable to move about, however much he may wish to do so, and in all cases the less he does so the more quickly will a cure be brought about.

*When swelled testicle occurs to boys with mumps,* the pain and swelling are usually moderate, and beyond raising the organ and fomentations, no treatment will be required. This form of swelled testicle subsides rapidly, without leaving any permanent swelling.

[If a suspensory bandage is not obtainable, a substitute may be formed by a broad bandage and a handkerchief. The bandage should be passed round the waist like a belt, and fastened. Then the handkerchief should be folded into a triangular form. The centre of the base of the triangle is to be passed under and behind the purse, as far as possible. Then the two lateral ends of the handkerchief are to be drawn up, and passed (on each side) first in front, and then over and behind the waist-belt, each end being then brought in front of that part of the handkerchief passing over the bandage. The two ends are then tied together. The front end of the handkerchief is then brought up, passed under the bandage, carried over it, and attached to the knot formed by the other two ends. In this manner a bag may be formed.]

**TETANUS.**—The disease usually commences with stiffness of the neck and about the jaws, which are opened and closed with difficulty. The person frequently regards this as due to cold, and thinks it rheumatism. There is often difficulty of swallowing, leading to violent ejection of fluids from the mouth or through the nose. In some instances the malady does not proceed further, and the patient may recover. But in other cases, in the course of a few hours or days the jaws become firmly closed, constituting 'lockjaw.' *Spasms* of the limbs and body also supervene, by which the patient may be bent like a bow, resting on his heels and the back of the head; or the body may be bent to either side. Sometimes the hands and forearms to the elbows escape these spasms. The face is contorted into a frightful grin, known as the *risus sardonicus.* There is agonising pain in the limbs during the spasms, and also at the pit of the stomach, shooting through to the back. The spasms recur at periods varying from a few minutes to hours; but during the intervals between the spasms the muscles remain hard, and do not thoroughly relax unless the patient sleeps. During the spasms the breathing is laborious, the skin is hot, and drenched with perspiration. The patient may die from suffocation, in consequence of spasm of the top of the windpipe (*glottis*), or from spasms fixing the muscles of the chest and preventing breathing, or he may die from exhaustion. The *causes* of tetanus are not well understood. It sometimes follows exposure to cold; in females, cold bathing during the monthly period has excited it; and it often follows wounds or injuries; but it would seem some peculiar irritable condition of the constitution must be present when tetanus occurs from such causes. It has been noticed at p. 438 that stiffness of the jaws may be caused by cutting a wisdom tooth, so that when symptoms of the kind present in young people, it will be well to ascertain if this is the case.

Tetanus may be mistaken for *hydrophobia* (*vide* p. 300), and *vice versá.* But in hydrophobia there is generally *fear of water*, in tetanus there is no such fear. In hydrophobia there is no lockjaw, in tetanus lockjaw. In hydrophobia there is constant 'hawking' and spitting, in tetanus none. In hydrophobia there is complete relaxation of the muscles after any convulsive seizure, in tetanus the limbs remain more or less hard between the struggles. There is generally the history or mark of a dog-bite in the one case, and not in the other; but probably the mark of some other injury.

Tetanus may also be mistaken for poisoning by *strychnine* (*vide* p. 586). In tetanus some exciting cause, as a wound, is often present. In tetanus the muscles of the jaws are first affected, which is rarely the case in poisoning by strychnine. In poisoning the spasms chiefly affect the extremities, and in tetanus the hands and forearms often escape. In poisoning, although the jaws may be firmly closed, the mouth can be opened during the intervals between the spasms, and there is no real 'lockjaw' as in tetanus. Tetanus comes on more gradually than the effects of strychnine, which presents in a few minutes after a poisonous quantity has been taken. In tetanus the spasms do not thoroughly relax even between the paroxysms; in poisoning the periodical relaxation is complete.

*Hysterical convulsions* have been sometimes mistaken for tetanus; but a reference to the description of hysteria (*vide* p. 305) will at once show the difference.

*Treatment.*—Chlorodyne, or chloral, to relieve pain and spasm, supporting the strength with good soups and stimulants (to give which a tooth must often be removed), are the requirements. Ice, if procurable, may be pounded, put in a bag or cloth, and applied over the spine.

[If the above remedies do not relieve the spasm, 5 drops of chloroform with 20 minims of tincture of opium in an ounce of water; this not seeming efficacious, morphia (Recipe 65), that medicine being repeated every four hours, which appears most soothing.]|

INFANTILE TETANUS, or *tetanus neonatorum.*—Lockjaw, or even complete tetanus, sometimes occurs to infants, generally between the third and tenth day after birth, and when slight is spoken of by nurses as 'nine-day fits' (*vide* p. 145). It is usually preceded by premonitory symptoms, such as restlessness, whimpering, broken sleep, yawning, and hasty snatches at the mother's breasts, which are soon relinquished; but often such symptoms are not noticed, or referred to some other cause. Probably the first thing which attracts attention is inability of the infant to take the breast properly, which may be attributed to some fault of the mother's nipple, or to tongue-tie of the infant, until at length the infant's jaws are noticed to be stiff. When an infant has taken the breast properly and then does not do so, suspicion of lockjaw should arise, and the jaws should be examined for stiffness. *Roseola* or 'red gum' (p. 387) is sometimes associated. If the disease goes on, the symptoms as detailed at p. 440 present. The causes of the tetanus of infants are exposure to impure air, or chill, or mismanagement and irritation of the navel-string. The treatment consists in giving nourishment, the best being the mother's milk. The jaws must be gently separated by the end of a spoon protected by a little linen rolled round it; and then milk, diluted with one-third the quantity of lime-water (Recipe 25), should be given cautiously. If there is difficulty in swallowing, not more than half a teaspoonful, or even less, should be given at one time, but the attempt should be hourly repeated. An enema half milk, half lime-water (*vide* Recipe 25) should also be given thrice daily, and a warm bath (*vide Appendix*) twice daily. As medicine half a grain of chloral, and 1 grain of bromide of potassium dissolved in half a teaspoonful of water, every five or six hours.

**THIRST.**—Thirst is a symptom of disease (*vide* p. 37), and is always an accompaniment of fevers. Thirst also attends certain forms of dyspepsia, and is a prominent symptom of diabetes. Pure water may always be used to allay thirst. Citrate of magnesia is often beneficial (*vide* p. 15).

**THROAT, DISEASES OF THE.**—Sore-throat occurs as a symptom of various maladies, viz., diphtheria, scarlet fever, mumps, consumption, syphilis, inflammation of the windpipe, croup, thrush, small-pox. The principal affections of the throat itself are—1, *hoarseness*; 2, *elongated uvula*; 3, *inflammation and its results*; 4, *enlarged tonsils*.

1. HOARSENESS.—Hoarseness arising from cold depends on irritation about the top of the windpipe and back part of the throat. It is usually more pronounced in the morning, passing off as the day advances. For simple hoarseness unconnected with serious symptoms, flannel round the throat, a mustard poultice, the feet in mustard and water at night, and an expectorant (Recipe 57) are sufficient.

*Hoarseness*, caused by over-exertion of the organ by singers or public speakers, or by clergymen, is so common in the latter class as to be named 'clergyman's sore-throat.' It most frequently arises from straining of the voice by too long or too frequent speaking. The stiff band-like collar many clergymen wear presses on the throat when the head is bent, and produces constriction of the parts. The forward and downward inclination of the head when preaching, necessitated by the position of clergymen, is another cause, for barristers, who from their position when speaking look upwards, rarely suffer. Cold and damp churches, or passing from hot churches into the cold air, also tend to congest the throat. But in many instances of clergyman's sore-throat there is evidence from their anæmic appearance of constitutional debility. Clergyman's sore-throat is rarely connected with any inflammatory action. But the throat may be red and congested and feel sore. The only effectual remedy is *rest*, and then gradually bringing the voice into play, while avoiding the band-like stock and also looking down as much as possible. But a few days' rest is insufficient, some cases requiring weeks or months. When 'clergyman's throat' is feared, it is well for the throat to be 'hardened' from the first. While the beard is allowed to grow, as a protection against sudden chills, the throat should be rather exposed to the air than wrapped up in woollen 'comforters.' An alum gargle (Recipe 100) may always be used with advantage.

A piece of *borax of soda*, about the size of a pea, allowed to melt in the mouth, before speaking, often affords temporary relief. *Chlorate of potash* tabloids may be used for hoarseness, and have the advantage over gargles that they are gradually dissolved in the saliva, and are thus constantly brought into contact with the affected parts. Children take the tablets readily, as they have no unpleasant taste; while the convenience of carrying them in the pocket commends them to travellers. Burroughs and Wellcome's 'voice tabloids' of cocaine with potash and borax are recommended. When, in addition to huskiness or hoarseness, the tonsils are red and swollen, a solution of nitrate of silver (strength 8 grains to 1 ounce of water) may be applied to the tonsils, with a camel's-hair brush, twice daily. Quinine and iron (Recipe 70) may generally be taken with advantage.

2. Throat, Elongation of the Uvula of the.—The *uvula* is the appendage to the soft palate, which may be seen hanging in the centre of the back of the throat. Its office is to prevent fluids regurgitating by the nostrils during swallowing. When the uvula is affected by cold, or from public speaking, or sometimes participating in a deranged state of the stomach, it becomes relaxed and *elongated*, so as to extend down to the back of the tongue. This produces irritation, with huskiness of voice, and a peculiar hacking cough, especially when air is inhaled through the mouth in reading or speaking, and often also nausea or even vomiting. Alum powder, or nitre, may be applied night and morning with a brush, and attention should be paid to the state of the bowels.

[If this does not succeed, 10 grains of nitrate of silver dissolved in an ounce of water should be applied with a camel's-hair brush or feather twice daily. These means failing, one-third of the length of the uvula should be cut off by the surgeon.]

3. Throat, Inflammation of the.—Dangerous forms of inflammation of the throat are mentioned as occurring in *Scarlet Fever* and *Diphtheria*. Sore-throat is also a symptom of venereal disease. But when the throat is affected by such causes, other symptoms will be present, as detailed under the headings mentioned. Here is considered that inflammation of the throat which arises from cold, and to which fatigue, anxiety, and depression, and the foul air of sewers and drains predispose. Sore-throat from cold may be mild or severe. When moderate it constitutes a common sore-throat; and may or may not

be attended with some degree of hoarseness of the voice, which shows that the parts behind the throat are more or less implicated. When sore-throat is severe it constitutes *quinsy.* In this case generally one, but sometimes both, tonsils are affected. The part attacked becomes much inflamed and swollen, and often either *ulcerates* or '*gathers.*' When ulceration takes place, there is increasing soreness, swallowing is painful, and the ulcers may be seen as raw deep sores on the tonsils. When 'gathering' or suppuration occurs, there is increasing swelling, much *throbbing* pain in the throat, pain in the ears, headache, great difficulty of breathing and of swallowing, constant desire to swallow, while fluids put into the mouth may run through the nose. The process of 'gathering' occupies three or four days, when the abscess breaks, discharging thick fetid matter, which affords immediate relief.

*Treatment.—Mild cases of sore-throat* are sufficiently met by a mustard poultice applied externally, an occasional aperient (Recipes 1 and 2), and an alum gargle (Recipe 100). *Ulcerated sore-throat* requires touching with concentrated alum solutions (powdered alum 3 drachms, water 1 ounce). *When the tonsils gather,* fomentation should be used outside; the throat should be frequently steamed; ice may be given to suck; *calmative* doses of chloral (*vide* p. 10) may be used to allay pain and procure rest; and, if possible, the abscess should be lanced by a surgeon.

[Nitrate of silver solution (strength 10 grains to an ounce of distilled or boiled water) may be used in preference to alum solution.]

4. Throat, Enlargement of the Tonsils of the.—Enlargement of the tonsils is frequently the result of repeated attacks of inflammation. But enlargement of the tonsils often occurs gradually to children and young persons, and more commonly if there is any constitutional scrofulous taint. Residence in marshy damp localities

favours this affection. The tonsils become enlarged and hardened; there is some difficulty in swallowing, heavy breathing, and often more or less indistinctness of speech, with a peculiar nasal twang. Some degree of deafness may be present, and the person sleeps with the mouth open, snoring loudly. The patient is liable to acute attacks of sore-throat, from slight exposure to cold. This enlargement of the tonsils is more common in cold than in tropical climates; but it often presents in children during the cold season of the northerly provinces of India where the nights are characterised by a low temperature. It also occurs in the colder climates of the hill stations. The *treatment* consists in avoiding cold and chill, and in improving the general health by tonics, of which probably citrate of iron and quinine (Recipe 70) will be the most beneficial. The diet also should be nutritious. Alum gargle (Recipe 100) may be used; but local applications do little good. As a rule, enlargement of the tonsils will decrease as the patient grows older and stronger.

Painting with solution of nitrate of silver, or of iodine, as frequently recommended, has in some instances appeared to irritate, and thus favour the growth of the tonsils. Excision, or cutting off the tonsil, is sometimes advocated. This operation is, however, seldom really necessary, and never so unless the parts become white, hard, and so enlarged as to interfere distressingly with swallowing or speech.

Great caution ought to be exercised in taking a child from India to Europe with enlarged tonsils. Unless other ailments forbid, enlargement of the tonsils would afford a good argument for keeping the child in India for 'another year.' In any case, care and warm clothing on passing out of the tropics are essentially necessary; for an increase or recurrence of the malady is very likely to take place as the colder climate is entered, or even after some length of residence therein.

**THRUSH, or APHTHÆ.**—This is a disease sometimes called 'white mouth,' and generally affecting children, especially those brought up by hand, and particularly if there is a scurvy taint (*vide* p. 381). It commences with peevishness, feverishness, and often disordered bowels. It consists of an eruption on the tongue, lips, cheek, and gums, of small *white* vesicles, which discharge a whitish mucus like morsels of curd, for which they are often mistaken, and which consist of microscopical vegetable *parasitic* growths (named *Oïdium albicans*). This mucus adheres for some days, and, then falling off, discloses small ulcers. As a rule, thrush is not dangerous; but it sometimes spreads into the throat, inducing difficulty of breathing and of swallowing; and occasionally, in very weakly children, spreading ulceration, *gangrene*, or mortification of some part of the mouth, may result. The *parasite* noted above is probably generated in a dirty, sour condition of the feeding-bottles. Then such causes as debility, improper food, sour milk, impure air, irritation from teething, produce a disordered state of system, from which originates an unhealthy condition of the mouth suitable for the lodgment and grôwth of the parasite. *Treatment* should be directed towards the recognition and removal of the causes. If the bowels are costive, citrate of magnesia should be given (*vide* p. 15); but if, as more usually happens, there is diarrhœa, Recipe 18. If there is great debility, Recipe 66, and as soon as procurable Recipe 70 instead. The source and preparation of the food must be specially investigated (*vide Feeding of Children, Chap. V., or Index*), and a little lime-water (Recipe 25) should be given with the food. The child should be removed from any source of impure air, and if it is teething and the gums are swollen, they should be lanced (*vide* p. 434). The child should be fed frequently, as sucking is painful, and the pain causes the child to refuse the breast. Cleanliness is most essential, and after every meal the mouth should be washed out with warm water. The secretion in the mouth should be removed by frequently, but gently, washing the mouth with a piece of lint, firmly fixed on a stick of whalebone, and moistened with hot water. No force should be used to detach the flakes, only those loose being taken away. Afterwards alum, 1 drachm mixed with honey 4 drachms, should be applied, which will tend to destroy the parasite.

Sometimes an appearance resembling thrush is found at the outlet of the bowels, when the thrush is popularly said to have 'passed through.' The parts should be washed with alum solution (Recipe 97).

[If this does not succeed, the eruption should be brushed, twice daily, with a solution of *hyposulphite* of soda 1 drachm, water 1 ounce, which is reputed to destroy parasites.]

**TOOTHACHE.**—Toothache is generally caused by irritation or inflammation of the nerve of the tooth. Decay of the tooth until the nerve is exposed is the most frequent cause. The decay commences on the outside of the tooth and saps inwards. Frequently a slight chip or injury of the enamel initiates the decay. But the decay of food undergoing decomposition between the teeth, or in the natural depressions of the teeth, chemically affects and destroys the enamel, acting much in the same manner as acids. A fungoid growth (*Leptothrix buccalis*) found in the mouth attacks carious teeth, and helps the decaying process. Decay is often very insidious, and the fact of it being present is frequently only known by the occurrence of pain. It would be well if the teeth were systematically examined several times a year. A warning of pain, however slight, should never be neglected, and should lead to investigation and to such measures—stopping or otherwise—as may be required. The teeth of women during the period of pregnancy (*vide* p. 359) are apt to decay rapidly, and are peculiarly sensitive—a good reason for having them put in order previous to that event. In young people decay runs a more rapid course in consequence of the structure being softer, the shell thinner, and the pulp larger than in the teeth of older persons—an additional reason why the teeth of young people should be especially attended to. The great preventive of decay is keeping the surfaces of the teeth clean of the food, tartar, and mucus that lodge between and about them, and the use of the tooth-brush should be taught as soon as there are teeth. As a rule, and especially when there is a thick, sticky saliva, a saponaceous tooth powder, or soap, should be used. Many tooth powders are not only useless but actually injurious.

A *tooth powder* should be alkaline; finely pulverised, that it may not mechanically abrade the teeth; antiseptic, to destroy microbes; should contain nothing irritating to the gums; and should be pleasant to the taste. Pumice powder is too gritty; camphorated chalk makes the gums spongy. The following is a good recipe:—Precipitated chalk 1 ounce, powdered Castile soap 1 drachm, oil of eucalyptus 1 drachm, and, if no objection to the taste, carbolic acid half a drachm.

Although decay of a tooth is the most common cause of toothache, it may present without any deterioration of the kind. Toothache is sometimes *neuralgic*, coming on at regular intervals, and then sound teeth are attacked. This will require purgative medicine, followed by quinine. In some cases the crown or body of the tooth is unaffected, but the fangs or roots are diseased, causing the tooth to feel big and tender. This is usually associated with a succession of gum-boils (*vide* p. 290), and extraction of the tooth is generally necessary.

A large number of nostrums are sold as cures for toothache. But there is no specific cure. A hollow tooth may often be kept easy by filling it with beeswax. When there is a large hollow, and pain is severe, a good application is a mixture of camphor and opium, of each one grain, made into a paste, with which the hollow tooth should be filled, the cavity having been previously dried by means of lint or cotton-wool. Or a few drops of spirits of camphor (*vide* p. 24) may be applied on a small roll of lint. Strong snuff, or a small quantity of black pepper, snuffed up the nostrils, often affords temporary relief.

In addition, the following may be procured. For application to the inside of the tooth on lint, a drop or two of creosote, chloroform, laudanum, oil of peppermint, oil of cajeput, or oil of cloves. Cotton-wool wet with chloroform, placed in the ear, often gives relief. A mixture of 10 grains of alum dissolved in half a drachm of chloroform may be applied to the tooth by means of lint or cotton-wool. Equal parts of chloral and camphor form a syrupy liquid, which may be used both to put in the tooth and to rub the face with. Collodion is also a good application. The cavity in the tooth is first to be carefully dried by means of a little lint, or the collodion will not adhere. One or two drops are then introduced, which, while liquid, exactly fill the cavity. As the ether contained in the collodion evaporates, the pain is assuaged, and a protective layer of collodion is formed in the hollow. A mixture of creosote three parts and collodion two parts forms a kind of jelly. Placed in the tooth it dries and forms a hard mass, which protects the decaying parts from the air, and thus relieves the pain. Nitrate of silver scraped to a point and applied to the interior of the tooth will, if well managed, be sure to afford relief. Burroughs & Wellcome's 'Cocaine Tabloid,' containing one-sixth of a grain, placed in the cavity of the tooth and covered with cotton-wool, is much recommended. Liniments, as Recipes 89, 90, applied externally, are also often useful. But if a tooth is too far gone to be stopped, and is the site of periodical pain, the only certain relief is extraction.

**TOOTH-DRAWING.**—To be able to draw a tooth moderately well would often prove a useful knowledge. A few plain directions may enable the amateur to relieve a class of sufferers often glad to incur some risk rather than endure the continuance of the pain.

The front and eye teeth may be best pulled out with straight forceps. The gum should be first separated from the neck of the tooth, by passing a gum-lancet to the extent of less than a quarter of an inch between the gum and the tooth. Then the blades of the forceps are to be placed, one before and one behind the tooth, and the ends made to clip just where the tooth dips into the gum. The right hand then grasps the handles of the forceps, while

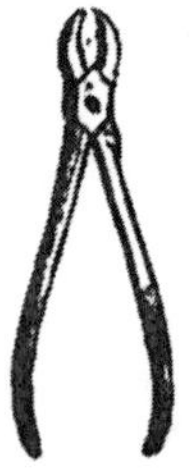

the forefinger is at the same time thrust in between the

handles, thus preventing too great pressure being made, by which the tooth might be snapped off. If it be an upper tooth, the operator may steady the patient's head by getting it beneath his left arm, and then pulling down, giving the tooth a lateral twist at the same time, by which it is soon drawn if the pull be steadily made. If it be a lower tooth, the operator steadies the head in the same way, but with the thumb of his left hand on the sound teeth, presses the jaw down, whilst his right hand pulls up, twisting as he pulls the tooth. The mode of extracting from the upper jaw is here shown.

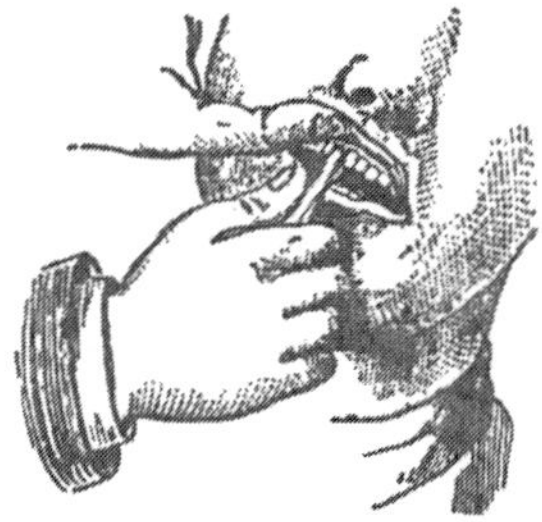

Drawing a back tooth is a more difficult matter, and is effected with forceps of different shapes, the claws being turned downwards instead of being straight, as shown in the following diagram of the forceps clasping an extracted molar or back tooth. The forceps must be applied round

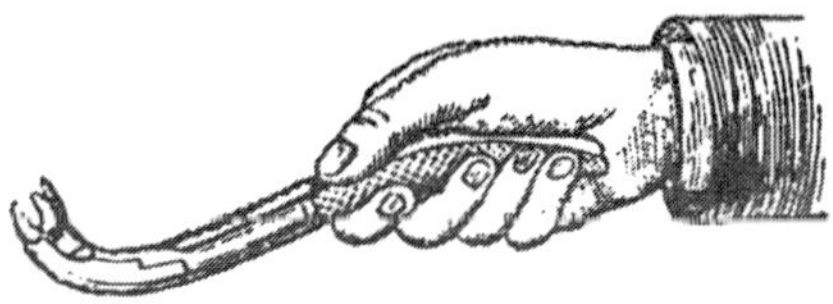

the neck of the tooth, as described for the front teeth. The forceps should be grasped firmly, the tooth moved from side to side with a twisting motion, and then pulled straight out. In extracting teeth with the forceps, three things should be kept in view: *first*, to prevent the forceps pressing too heavily round the neck of the tooth, by which it is liable to be broken; *secondly*, to loosen the tooth by a twisting or lateral motion; *thirdly*, to pull it straight out. But the pull should not be made with too great violence or suddenness, otherwise, the tooth escaping from the socket suddenly, the forceps may hit against and perhaps break other teeth.

It may be desirable to draw back teeth with the 'key' when they are much decayed and cannot bear the pressure of the forceps, or when, the crown being lost, there is little hold for the claws of the forceps. But the key is an instrument with which more harm may be done than with the forceps, and therefore its use is not described.

**TONGUE AND MOUTH, ULCERS OF THE.**—May arise from *salivation*, *aphthæ*, *scurvy*, *venereal disease*, *cancer*, *debility*, or from *dyspepsia*. When ulcers arise without any evident cause they are usually dyspeptic, and the best application readily obtainable is a concentrated solution of alum (powdered alum 3 drachms, water 1 ounce), applied several times daily with a feather or brush; or, this not succeeding, strong vinegar may be used in a similar manner. Accompanying dyspepsia or other ailments should receive appropriate treatment.

[*Dilute* sulphuric acid, applied with a feather to the ulcer, will be found a better remedy than alum. It causes acute pain for a few moments, but the ulcers are much less sore afterwards, and heal more quickly.]

**TUMOURS.**—The term is applied to almost any swelling, and does not, as popularly supposed, signify any particular disease. There are therefore many kinds of tumours, some of which are mentioned under the maladies of which they form parts. A common form is the *fatty tumour*, which may occur in any part, and frequently developes in the scalp. *Rhinophyma*, or 'hammer nose,' is the term applied to a swelling which sometimes forms on the nose, usually in the shape of a front and two lateral lobes. The term *aneurism* is applied to a pulsating tumour resulting from the rupture of an artery. Aneurism most frequently occurs in the artery of the thigh (*vide* p. 502). When firm pressure is made in the course of the artery *above* such a tumour the pulsation stops, which is a distinctive sign. The only cure of most tumours is by surgical procedure.

**ULCERS.**—Ulcers are raw open sores, generally hollowed out lower than the surrounding skin, which may result from any inflammation of the surface of the body, as, for instance, from boils, or from injuries. Ulcers of a peculiar kind are caused by scrofula, venereal disease, scurvy, cancer and gout. Chronic ulcers of the legs are common in elderly people, and are frequently caused in the first instance by varicose veins (*vide* p. 456). Ulcers require different treatment according to their cause or condition. The most universally suitable application is water dressing (Recipe 85), or, if procurable, carbolic acid lotion (Recipe 119). When an ulcer will not heal readily, unless it be the chronic ulcer of the leg of old people, some constitutional taint may be suspected.

**URINE, DISEASED CONDITIONS OF.**—The *quantity* of urine passed by a healthy adult in twenty-four hours is from thirty to forty ounces. But it varies with the amount and influence of fluids, and of some solids consumed. Also with the weather, being more copious in cold weather, when there is less sensible and insensible perspiration from the skin. The *quantity of urine is increased* in diabetes, also often in hysteria. It is *scanty* in inflammation of the kidneys, in albuminuria, and in most fevers. It is *retained* in stricture, sometimes in hysteria, and sometimes by infants. It is *suppressed* (i.e. there is none secreted) in collapse, and in cholera. It is *passed more frequently* when there is enlarged prostate, gravel, stone, irritable bladder, or inflammation of the bladder or kidneys. It is *passed painfully* in most maladies connected with the urinary organs, excepting diabetes and Bright's disease.

The *colour* of healthy urine is a pale straw or amber, and it should show but a very slight quantity of mucus, which appears as a filmy cloud. A heavy whitish deposit, clinging to the utensil when turned, indicates much mucus, which forms in chronic affections of the bladder. A yellowish-brown colour is characteristic of bile and jaundice. A smoky hue denotes the presence of a small quantity of blood; a dark brown colour more blood; and a distinct red colour much blood. Blood in the urine (or *hæmaturia*) may occur from a great number of causes. Such causes may be either local affections of the urinary organs themselves, as stone or tumour in the kidneys or bladder; or such causes may be general, as scurvy, the presence of a parasite in the blood, fevers, &c. In the fevers of Africa blood in the urine occurs so frequently that it has been specially designated *hæmaturic fever*. Blood in the urine has been noticed as occurring in Indian fever (*vide* p. 260), but it is not ordinarily present. High-coloured urine attends most fevers, which may be difficult to distinguish from blood without the aid of a microscope. A *milky appearance* indicates the condition known as *chyluria*. Matter, or *pus*, renders urine turbid, and it does not clear on boiling. The *smell* of urine is faint and peculiar. In diabetes there is a sweetish whey-like odour. In various chronic maladies of the urinary organs there is an ammoniacal smell. Blood or bloody discharge causes a smell like that of faintly tainted meat.

The principal salts seen as deposits in the urine are given under *gravel*, p. 285, and *oxaluria*, p. 341. The methods of detecting invisible unnatural conditions, chiefly albumen and sugar, are given at pp. 101, 164.

*Caution.*—On standing healthy urine undergoes change. After a variable time, according to the temperature, it becomes cloudy, and emits a characteristic odour. This is not indicative of disease.

**VARICOCELE.**—An enlarged condition of the veins within the *scrotum* or purse, which feel soft like a bag of worms. The swelling is irregularly pyramidal, the base resting on the testicle, and the apex pointing upwards.

It is most common on the left side, and it is accompanied by a dull aching pain, by a sensation of weight, by a dragging pain in the back and loins, and sometimes by glairy discharge from the privates. If the person lies down the swelling *gradually* subsides, with relief of the painful feelings. It is worse if the bowels are constipated, and is in some cases caused by constipation. Often no particular cause is evident, but bicycle-riding tends to induce it in those constitutionally predisposed. After it has existed some time, it is apt to cause neuralgia of and wasting of the testicle. Varicocele may be mistaken for *rupture* or for *hydrocele*, and the distinguishing features are given at p. 593. The disease may be palliated by wearing a suspensory bandage (*vide* p. 439), by bathing the scrotum daily with cold water, and by regulating the bowels to avoid constipation. Such measures are generally sufficient, although sometimes a surgical operation is necessitated.

**VEINS, INFLAMMATION OF THE.**—This, technically termed *phlebitis*, may occur in any part of the body, but the limbs are most frequently affected. It may originate from injury, from exposure to wet and cold, or from *thrombi* or clots of blood forming in a vein. The veins of the part affected are hard, swollen, knobbed, painful and tender. There is stiffness and difficulty of moving the part, and often swelling of the whole limb. There is also fever, and the temperature may be 100° or upwards. If the superficial veins are affected, they may be seen of a red or purple colour. In severe cases abscesses may form in the course of the veins, or absorption of putrid matter may take place producing blood-poisoning (*vide* p. 587). Perfect rest should be enforced. Hot poppy-head fomentations (Recipe 81) should be used assiduously, and Dover's powder and quinine (Recipe 17) should be given twice daily. If necessary chloral at night to relieve pain. The bowels should be kept open by Recipe 2. If abscess forms it should be treated as given at p. 41. The diet should be strengthening from the first.

**VEINS, VARICOSE.**—This term is applied to an enlarged, dilated, and tortuous condition of the veins. Varicose veins of the leg are noticed at p. 360, as a result of pregnancy. *Varicocele* (*vide* p. 454) is also a form of varicose veins. *Piles* (*vide* p. 347) is a similar condition of the vessels of the part. The cause of varicose veins is some sluggishness of the, or impediment to the circulation of, the blood through the veins, which (*vide* p. 500) *return* the blood from the extremities of the body *to* the heart. Hence the veins of the legs, which have the largest columns of blood to support, are most likely to become varicose. Sluggishness or feebleness of the circulation may depend on debility from many causes. Impediments to the circulation, particularly of the legs, are various; such as pregnancy, or constipation. Occasionally varicose veins are found in other parts of the body. The part affected is attacked by dull aching pain, and the varicose veins may be seen—looking dark-coloured—and may be felt—like soft, prominent cords—ramifying under the skin in different directions, or clustered in raised knots. The leg swells, particularly in the evening or after exertion. Often the veins appear at the point of bursting, and, if the disease is neglected, the skin may give way, and a copious bleeding may take place, which continues until it is stopped by pressure, or until the person faints, after which an *ulcer* may form on the leg.

*Treatment.*—The part affected should be frequently sponged with cold water; if the leg, *it should be kept raised*, and friction with soap liniment should be used for ten minutes three times daily, the leg being rubbed *gently upwards*, from the ankle towards the knee, so as to assist the venous circulation. Moderate walking exercise may be taken, but only after the precaution of a well-applied bandage (*vide* p. 495), which should be put on when the limb is elevated and not swollen, over a thin angola or silk stocking. If there is debility, generous diet and tonics, of which iron is the best, should be given (*vide* p. 24). If the varicose veins appear connected with constipation, Recipe 2; or if with inactive liver, Recipe 1 is required. In such cases mineral waters (Friedrichshall or Hunyadi Janos) are often of great value. If the varicose veins are connected with *pregnancy*, while the precautions as above are taken, it will not be desirable to give any medicines except castor oil for the relief of constipation. Varicose veins from pregnancy usually disappear after the birth of the child, but varicose veins from other causes, if neglected, may increase to such an extent as to require surgical treatment. If a vein should burst, *vide* p. 512.

If procurable, Recipe 71; and Recipe 12 instead of Recipe 1 if the liver is inactive. For sponging instead of cold water, tincture of hamamalis one ounce, in one pint of water. An elastic stocking should be procured. The measurements required are. 1. Round the thickest part of the instep. 2. Round ankle bone. 3. Round small of leg. 4. Round thickest part of calf. 5. Round leg just below knee. 6. Length of leg from heel to just below knee. The measurements should be taken when the veins or leg are least swollen.

**VENEREAL DISEASE**, or **SYPHILIS**.—This disease is the consequence of contagion, and there are two kinds of sores. One usually presents in about ten days, but may appear at any time up to a month after exposure. It first shows, on some part of the genitals, in the shape of a small red pimple, which about the fourth day becomes a watery vesicle with an inflamed base. Then a little matter forms, and, discharging, leaves a *painless* sore or ulcer, with a hard margin, elevated edges, and depressed centre. The other kind of sore usually appears within four or five days after exposure, commencing as a pustule, or containing matter from the first. It is not hard, but more painful than the first description of sore.

Next, about fifteen to thirty days after the commencement of the sore, or after the sore has healed, there may be swelling and tenderness of the glands in the groin, eventually forming a *bubo* (*vide* p. 109). If this occurs, it may either subside or form matter, which then points like an ordinary abscess. The bubo is most likely to form into an abscess if it occurs after the softer description of sore. The *secondary symptoms*, referred to below, are most likely to present after a hard sore. The sore on the privates, and the swelling in the groins, complete the symptoms of *primary syphilis*.

But the person affected is not free from disease. Weeks, months, or years afterwards, *secondary symptoms* may occur. On an average, the period of their appearance is in about six weeks, and in the majority of cases the sequence is much as follows. The person grows dispirited, is probably troubled with rheumatic pains, particularly in the shin-bones, and complains of loss of appetite and want of sleep. Then either skin diseases, or sore-throat, or ulcers of the tongue or mouth, or all these affections, appear. The mildest variety of sore-throat is simple redness, or soreness; but very often there are ulcerations. The patient has a hoarse, guttural way of speaking, and may complain of pain in the ears. Next, or at the same time as the sore-throat, appear eruptions of the skin, of various descriptions. Perhaps the most common venereal skin affection is a scaly eruption very much as psoriasis is described (*vide* p. 401), and which often attacks the palms of the hands. The nails may also be affected, loosening for some distance from their extremities, and becoming rigid transversely, or marked with faint oval spots longitudinally. But these are not the only results of secondary syphilis. It not unfrequently attacks the internal nostrils, producing a foul discharge, and it may ultimately destroy the bones of the nose. Or it may attack the shin-bones, the surfaces of which swell, become very painful, and form what is termed *nodes*. These *nodes* sometimes gather, burst, and leave deep foul ulcers, at the bottom of which is *carious* or diseased bone. The windpipe may also be implicated, producing huskiness or loss of voice, which may become permanent. Internal organs, as the brain, spine, or liver, may also become diseased, giving rise to various anomalous symptoms, only to be recognised by the experienced practitioner.

But even this is not the end of venereal. Women frequently miscarry as a result of syphilitic poison in the system. Children of diseased parents are often born diseased. When a child is born syphilitic, it is weakly and shrivelled, with hoarse cry, snuffling respiration, discharge from the nostrils, and copper-coloured blotches on the skin, especially about the privates. It has a prematurely aged look, and often suffers from *pemphigus* (*vide* p. 398.) In other cases such symptoms appear a month or so after birth. If the child of syphilitic parents escapes such maladies in infancy, it is more liable than other children to suffer from *atrophy* (*vide* p. 66), and when growing up the individual is much more likely to become consumptive or scrofulous.

*Treatment.*—If the means mentioned in the small type are not at hand, the parts should be kept perfectly clean, an alum lotion (Recipe 97), or if available carbolic acid lotion (Recipe 119), should be applied, and the patient should be kept as quiet as possible, taking aperient medicine, as Recipes 1 and 2. Then if the sore is not a syphilitic chancre it will get well; and if it is, the best method, in the absence of medical aid, will have been pursued. For the treatment of bubo, *vide* p. 109.

[If the pimple is observed *before* it becomes a sore, or *chancre*, it will be advisable to destroy it by the careful but thorough application of nitrate of silver. Then the part should be treated with water dressing (Recipe 85). If, however, the ulcer or *chancre* has formed without this being done, black-wash (Recipe 88) should be applied with lint, and, provided the patient is not broken down in health by previous disease, blue pill should be given, in 3-grain doses, three times a day, until there is a metallic taste in the mouth, or the gums become slightly sore. If the blue pill acts on the bowels, one quarter of a grain of extract of opium should be combined with each dose. Meanwhile the patient should live regularly, but not too low; the clothing should be warm, and but little exercise should be taken.

For *secondary* symptoms, the best remedy is iodide of potassium in five or eight-grain doses. But the Protean varieties of secondary syphilis demand the advice of a surgeon.

A syphilitic infant should be brought up by hand, so that it may not imbibe further poison from its mother, nor infect a nurse. Half a drachm of mercurial ointment may be spread on a piece of flannel, to be tied round the child's waist every morning till the symptoms disappear.]

**VOMITING.**—Vomiting is a symptom of disease rather than a disease itself (*vide* p. 37), and consists of an inverted action of the stomach, accompanied by faintness. It may be caused by unwholesome food, or by intemperance. It is an ordinary symptom of disorders of the stomach and bowels, but it is also often indicative, especially in children, of some head affection. It often occurs at the onset of fevers, and especially at the commencement of small-pox. It is a symptom of rupture, of dyspepsia, of colic, of gravel, and of cholera. It also occurs from the violence of whooping-cough; it may be produced by poisonous agents, as arsenic; it occurs in sea-sickness, and is often very troublesome to pregnant women. The colour, smell, and taste of vomited material are instructive and characteristic. Thus, in *cholera* the fluid vomited is whitish. In *hæmatemesis*, or bleeding from the stomach, it is black. In certain diseases implicating the *urinary* organs the odour is ammoniacal. When there is *stoppage of the bowels*, fæcal matter is often vomited. When *bile* is vomited, the taste is acid and bitter, and the colour yellowish. In some forms of *dyspepsia*, fluid looking and tasting like sour water is brought up.

**WARTS.**—Warts are growths from the skin, often occurring without assignable cause, particularly on the hands of the young. Frequently if left alone they gradually disappear. When warts grow with a thin neck a piece of strong waxed thread may be tied tightly round the narrow part. After a day or two the wart will fall off, and the part should be afterwards daily touched with alum.

[Pure acetic or nitric acid carefully applied every day to a wart will destroy it. The acid may be applied with a stick of cedar wood, and care must be taken that it does not touch the healthy skin, or it will act as a caustic and destroy that also. The use of the acid may be continued daily, so long as no pain follows the application.]

**WETTING THE BED BY CHILDREN.**—Sometimes it depends on thread-worms; less frequently on the presence of a stone in the bladder; sometimes from a long foreskin, under which dirt and discharge accumulate. It often depends on irritability of the bladder, perhaps caused by a too acid condition of the urine; it is sometimes connected with irritable condition of the nervous system, causing the child to wake frightened and screaming, as described under *Convulsions* (*vide* p. 146). It sometimes occurs from idleness and indisposition to get out of bed. The *treatment* consists in attacking the cause. If there is no evidence of other maladies, but there is night screaming, bromide of potassium (Recipe 20) may be given with advantage. The urine should be examined with litmus paper. Healthy urine is slightly acid, and should turn blue litmus paper slightly red; but if the paper becomes instantly of a bright red colour the urine is too acid, and it will be advisable to give citrate of magnesia (*vide* p. 15), which should be continued until the urine only colours litmus paper slightly. When there is no assignable cause, the child should be made to empty the bladder immediately before going to bed, and he should be provided with a little vessel which may be taken into the bed. If the practice be persisted in, either idly or unconsciously, the child should be roused in the middle of the night for the purpose of emptying the bladder. He should also be induced to hold the water as long as possible in the daytime, so that the bladder may become accustomed to being full, and no fluid should be allowed for two or three hours before bedtime. The child should also be induced to lie on the sides and not on the back, in which latter position any urine in the bladder presses on the most sensitive part of that organ, and induces desire to make water. This may be accomplished by fixing a cotton reel behind by a string passed through the hole in the reel and round the waist, the pressure from which will cause the child to turn on his side.

[Instead of citrate of magnesia obtain Recipe 35. Benzoic acid may be obtained and tried in one-grain doses up to two years old, and in two-grain doses above that age, thrice daily. Electricity to the spine is sometimes useful.]

**WHITES.**—This signifies an increased secretion from the female private parts. The discharge is of a white or faintly yellow colour, and may amount to several ounces daily. Sometimes it assumes a glairy appearance, more like white of egg. The appetite is impaired, the bowels generally constipated; there are often palpitations, giddiness, fainting, or neuralgic pains, with flatulence, pain in the back or in the left side, pallor, and hysterical symptoms. The causes are difficult menstruation, chronic inflammation of or displacement of the womb, frequent childbearing, want of exercise, luxurious living, and other causes of general debility. The *treatment* consists in attention to any menstrual disorder, or womb affection, which may be present. But if such causes are not evident, and the discharge appears to result from debility, treatment must consist in attention to the general health, to diet, and to the state of the bowels, in regular hours, proper exercise, and change of air. Cold bathing, or at least pouring cold water down the spine, is also advisable, except when the woman is pregnant. To arrest the discharge, alum lotion (Recipe 97) may be used as an injection. Infusion of green tea is a good injection, and may be made by pouring a pint of boiling water on half an ounce of green tea, macerating, straining, and using the injection cold. For the method of giving a female injection, *vide Appendix*, 'Injections.'

[Recipe 107 may be used if the alum lotion or tea infusion is not beneficial.]

**WHITLOW.**—There are several kinds of whitlow. The slightest form occurs on one side of the root of the nail, beginning with a little inflammation and throbbing. By degrees a whitish semi-transparent bladder is formed extending more or less round the nail. If not opened the fluid separates the scarf-skin from the true skin underneath, through which it bursts, discharging watery matter, when the finger may get well. But if the matter has been pent up for some days it frequently ulcerates the true skin, and a little red body sprouts up through the opening in the scarf-skin, which is excessively tender, and is vulgarly called 'proud flesh.' If this increases the nail may be destroyed. The blister should be snipped with scissors, and a bread poultice applied, followed in a day or two by simple dressing or oiled rag. If red proud flesh forms, the dead scarf-skin should be removed, and alum should be lightly applied to the part.

*The Second Form of Whitlow* occurs in the bulbous ends of the fingers. This is much more severe, and the matter is deeper seated beneath the true skin. No blister forms, but the finger swells and is red, afterwards becoming white as the matter approaches the surface. The pain extends into the hand and arm, and the nail is usually destroyed. The finger should be deeply lanced on the inside, in the direction of its length, and a poultice applied. When matter ceases to flow, the part should be plastered.

*The Third Form of Whitlow*, called *thecal abscess*, is the most severe. The sheath containing the tendons of the finger inflames, becoming hot, red, and terribly painful; the finger swells, and unless quickly attended to, the inflammation spreads into the hand and arm, and the tendons, or one or more bones of the finger are injured, and may slough out. Leeches, bathing the part in hot water, and hot linseed-meal poulticing should be used. The inflamed part should be lanced *to the bone early*, within twenty or thirty hours from the beginning of the attack. To secure perfect rest the finger should be placed on a splint, which may be cut out of any soft piece of wood, or made from a piece of perforated zinc. The splint should extend from the end of the finger to the wrist, and under the finger should be the breadth of the finger, but it will be more comfortable if made wider under the palm. It should be wrapped in cotton cloth, to be changed daily, when the splint should also be well washed. After the lancing, poultices should be applied till the matter ceases to flow, and afterwards plasters. However skilfully treated, either from a piece of bone being lost, or from contraction of the tendons, some deformity often results. In *all* cases of whitlow the hand should be kept in a sling, with the fingers pointing to the opposite shoulder.

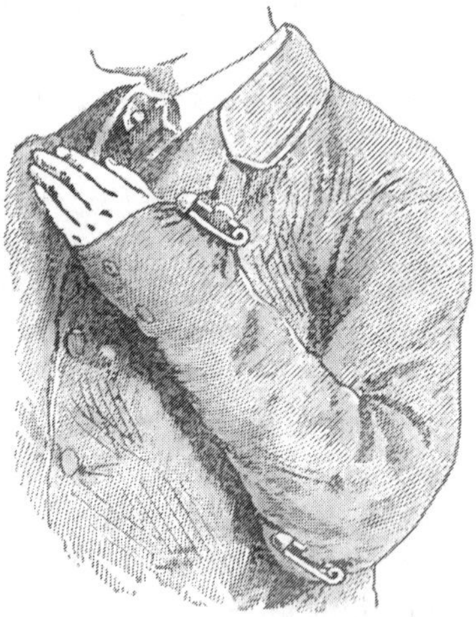

An excellent plan to secure the advantages of position and immobility in such cases is to bend the elbow at an acute angle, and raise the hand towards the opposite shoulder. Then, pinching up the top of the coat-sleeve at the wrist, fix it to the coat with a strong safety pin. The sleeve then acts as a sling. If greater immobility is required attach a fold of the sleeve to the coat, just under the elbow, with another safety pin, and attach the inside of the arm sleeve to the body of the coat with a third safety pin (*vide* plate).

**WHOOPING-COUGH.**—Whooping-cough is called also *Kink-cough* and *chin-cough*. It is a contagious cough, happening generally to young children, but sometimes to adults, and usually only once in life. It has been thought to depend on a microbe, which breeds on the membrane of the throat and nose. It commences as a common cough, but after some days the cough comes on in fits, after which the breath is drawn in with a long effort, and accompanied by a peculiar 'whoop.' In bad cases there may be twenty paroxysms in a day, and several fits of coughing without the whoop being heard. A child with whooping-cough soon learns when the paroxysm is commencing, and is frightened. He rushes to the mother or nurse; or, if of a more advanced age, stamps his feet in a state of agitation, and clutches some article of furniture by which to steady himself. Vomiting frequently attends the fits of coughing, and the suffocation of the child may appear threatened, when suddenly the characteristic whoop is heard, which terminates the paroxysm, and the child returns to its play. From the vomiting, children with bad whooping-cough frequently cannot retain sufficient food in their stomach to supply the wants of the system, and may suffer from starvation. Simple whooping-cough is never fatal; but unfortunately whooping-cough may excite other maladies. The force of the cough may cause blood-shot eyes, bleeding from the nose or from the ears, and sometimes *rupture of the drum* of the ear (*vide* p. 214). Occasionally also *rupture* (*vide* p. 589) is caused by the force of the cough. In most cases there is some degree of *bronchitis* attending the complaint, shown by hurried breathing, feverishness, and by wheezing heard in the chest (*vide* p. 105). In some cases *inflammation of the lungs* is induced (*vide* p. 328). In other instances, from injury to the lungs from the force of the cough, the foundation of *asthma* or emphysema is laid (*vide* pp. 60, 330). Or there may be, especially in weakly children, tendency to *hydrocephalus*, marked by sudden startings from sleep and rolling of the head (*vide* p. 88). *Convulsions* may also be excited, the approach of which is indicated by contractions of the fingers or toes, or by turning in of the thumb to the palm of the hand (*vide* p. 145). Lastly, *diarrhœa* may supervene (*vide* p. 172). The ordinary time after exposure to infection that the disease presents is fourteen days. The average duration of whooping-cough is about six weeks, but it may get well in a few days or weeks, or continue for months. The danger of infection lasts six weeks after recovery.

*Treatment.*—During the paroxysms of cough the child's back should be supported with one hand, and the forehead should be supported with the other. Mucus coughed up, or anything vomited, should be wiped away from the mouth, and the back should be gently rubbed. In the intervals between the cough the chest and back should be daily rubbed with equal parts of brandy and salad oil. The bowels should be regulated by castor-oil or senna; and ipecacuanha wine in small doses according to the age of the child (*vide* p. 15) should be given. If the child is old enough to understand, half a drachm of salt dissolved in an ounce of water snuffed up the nostrils may be beneficial. If the spasms of cough are severe, and there is no chest complication, a bath at 98° Fahr. for ten minutes every night will be salutary. This will strengthen the child, by increasing the action of the skin and enabling it to do its part towards throwing off the disease, while it allays irritability and causes better nights. In those cases where the cough appears principally of a dry spasmodic character, bromide of potassium (Recipe 20) will be advisable, and this may be given with the ipecacuanha wine or at different times. To lessen the depression caused by the fits of coughing, 4 drops of sal volatile should be given to an infant one year old, and 8 drops to a child three years old, after each fit of coughing, in a little milk-and-water. The diet should also be well attended to, and no indigestible food allowed. In cases where vomiting is a prominent symptom, strong broth or soup should be given immediately after the paroxysm of coughing, so that there may be time for some digestion of food to take place before the next attack. In the latter stage of obstinate whooping-cough nothing is so serviceable as change of air. But in the earlier periods there is often feverishness and tendency to bronchitis. When such conditions prevail the patient should be kept warm, and the exposure which change of air necessitates should not be thought of. Complications, as bronchitis, convulsions, affections of the head and bowels, must be treated as mentioned under such headings.

[Instead of brandy and oil, procure soap and opium liniment to rub the back with; and remember it is *not for internal use.* Instead of ipecacuanha wine procure Recipe 57. Numberless remedies have been tried to cure whooping-cough, but none will always succeed. In very bad cases 20 drops of chloroform may be placed on a handkerchief, which is to be held *half a foot* from the child's face *during the fit.* Recipe 60, 61, 62, 63 may be procured and tried in succession. Inhaling the spray from an atomiser of a solution of 1 drachm of carbolic acid in 14 ounces of water may also be tried. A solution of Condy's fluid, 1 drachm to a pint of water, may be snuffed up the nostrils from the palm of the hand. Whooping-cough frequently causes great debility, and tonics, as quinine and iron (Recipe 70), should then be given, in doses corresponding to the age of the child (*vide* p. 6).]

**WOMB, DISEASES OF THE.**—Many causes combine in inducing a great tendency to womb disease in the European female in India—some preventable, others less so, inasmuch as the latter consist of climatic influences. One of the first effects of hot tropical climates on the system of the European is a greater tendency to affections of the abdominal organs, in which condition the womb partakes. Hence the necessity of increased care, especially as regards exposure to cold, or injudicious exertion, during the monthly period. *The most common maladies* which arise from these various influences affecting the womb are as follows.

AMENORRHŒA, *Scanty* or *Suspended Flow*, or *Failure of the Monthly Courses.*—The monthly affection of women commences about the age of fifteen, and ceases about forty-five. In the natives of India it generally commences and ceases a couple of years earlier. It may be suspended or fail under the following circumstances:—1st, *it is not present as a general rule during pregnancy or suckling;* 2ndly, *instead of appearing at the usual age, it may be retained or delayed;* 3rdly, *the menses may be secreted for a time, and their recurrence prevented;* 4thly, *the non-appearance of the discharge may depend on some mechanical obstruction, or on disease of the womb;* 5thly, *it may be concomitant with 'change of life.'*

1st, *when the cause of the failure of the monthly course is pregnancy*, there will be other symptoms of such condition, and nothing is required to be done. When the flow is not present during *suckling* it is in accordance with nature, and nothing is required to be done. If the flow appears during suckling it is a sign that suckling should be discontinued, as the system cannot bear two drains (*vide Over-nursing*, p. 655).

2ndly, *when, instead of appearing at the usual age, the discharge is delayed*, the girl will probably be pale, weakly, and debilitated, the bosoms will be little developed, and there may also be dropsical swellings of the legs, arms, or face. Periodical pains in the back and loins, irregular recurring headaches, white discharges, palpitations of the heart after slight exertion or on any agitation of mind, capricious appetite leading the patient to eat such articles as chalk or cinders, and irritability of temper are also usually noted. The face may appear 'grubby' from pustules of *acne* (*vide* p. 400); or there may be small elevations or pimples which do not contain matter, and *eczema* or *erythema* (*vide* pp. 386, 396) may appear on the legs. In bad cases the complexion becomes sallow, dark, or greenish, the condition of the patient soon becoming that described as 'green-sickness' (*vide* p. 50). Under such circumstances tonics are of the greatest service, especially those preparations which contain iron; and in the absence of other medicines, 3 or 4 grains of sulphate of iron (*vide* p. 24) may be given in an ounce of water three times a day during the intervals, but not for three days before or after the expected period. Moderate exercise in the open air, especially on horseback, but without tiring the patient; a generous but wholesome diet, with a little wine; cheerful society without excitement or late hours; the avoidance of close rooms, and cold bathing during the intervals between the monthly periods will do much good. Change of scene by unfatiguing travel, and salt-water bathing, are also often beneficial. The bowels should be regulated by aperients, especially Recipes 1 and 3. Such medicines, together with hot foot or hip baths, to which a little mustard may be added with advantage, should always be taken a day or two before the expected period, at which time cold baths should not be used, and all kinds of excitement should be carefully avoided. If baths cannot be conveniently procured the patient should sit over hot water. When pain of back or loins indicates that nature is making an effort, and the hot baths are not successful, a mustard poultice may be applied over the lower part of the bowels for two or three nights in succession.

[Recipe 15 should be procured for use previous to the expected period, instead of Recipe 1; and Recipe 71 for use during the interval. If this does not succeed, permanganate of potash 2 grains, extract of gentian 2 grains, made into a pill, to be taken three times daily, commencing a week before the expected period.]

*The above indicates the treatment when amenorrhœa occurs*

*in pale weakly girls*, but sometimes the menses are tardy in appearing, the patient being rosy and robust, and the bosoms and form well developed. In such cases there will probably be roughness or sometimes scaliness of the face, and often at each period pain of the back and loins, flushing of the face, giddiness, and headache. Before this comes on the patient should take Recipes 1 and 2 for two or three nights and mornings in succession, and a mustard poultice should be applied to the lower part of the bowels. If these measures do not succeed, three or four leeches should be applied to each groin, the bleeding from which should be encouraged by fomenting. These means should be repeated every four weeks until the menses do appear; and after this occurs, a warm bath should be taken at night at the approach of each period, for some time afterwards. The food should be principally farinaceous; and ale, porter, and wine should be avoided. Exercise both on foot and horseback may be freely taken.

3rdly, *the menses may have been secreted for a time and their recurrence prevented.* The discharge at an early period often does not occur regularly at the end of every four weeks. The constitution seems to require the influence of habit, and for some time slight causes will induce suppression. Damp feet, sitting on damp ground, cold bathing, standing in a draught, fatigue, passion, excitement of any kind, fright, or severe mental work, will often suddenly check the discharge if present, or prevent its reappearance. When the discharge is suddenly checked or prevented, there is usually headache, lassitude, and probably pains in the lower part of the bowels; and it has been noted at p. 440 that the sudden check of the discharge by cold bathing has been known to cause tetanus. If there is repeated failure of the monthly flow, the constitutional condition becomes the same as, or even worse than, the state occasioned by the non-appearance of the flow at the usual time of life (*vide* p. 468).

The *interruption* of the menses may be caused by the debilitating effects of other diseases, such as consumption, Bright's disease, and some forms of hæmorrhage. But such stoppages are less abrupt, and are not followed by the peculiar symptoms above detailed; while there are the symptoms of the other disease which may be present, which will serve to point out the cause of the prevention.

*Treatment.*—When the stoppage of the monthly flow occurs as a consequence of other debilitating diseases, no special treatment directed to excite the flow will be desirable. But when the stoppage occurs to otherwise healthy women, the following measures may be adopted. Females of full habit require means that deplete or lower the circulation; and, on the contrary, delicate patients must be invigorated by means which inprove the state of the blood and give tone to the system. If sudden suppression or stoppage of the menses occur after they have been established, a hot bath at 106° Fahr. is suitable for every constitution, and, if taken immediately after exposure to cold or other cause of obstruction, would often prove successful. In other respects the treatment detailed for delicate or plethoric persons under the second heading may be adopted (*vide* pp. 468, 470).

4thly, *the non-appearance of the discharge may depend on some mechanical obstruction*, or on disease of the womb. Obstruction chiefly occurs in young girls; disease to older women. The means directed in the foregoing remarks having failed, after a fair trial, to produce the desired effect, no delicacy of feeling should prevent application to a medical man in order that it may be ascertained if any anatomical obstruction is in the way, or if any disease exists. If such is the case, medicine may increase the evil, and delay will increase the difficulties.

5thly, *stoppage of the monthly courses from 'change of life'* is considered under that heading (p. 481).

CAUTION.—In any kind of delayed or suppressed discharge, medicines which excite the flow of the menses are best dispensed with excepting under medical advice. Some may prove dangerous, and, when administered by quacks or well-meaning but ignorant friends, have often done much injury. Suspended flow may usually be overcome without the use of such medicines, and, if the individual is otherwise in good health, need not be the subject of much anxiety, and should not be rashly interfered with. The fear of 'decline' or other malady, as the *consequence* of delayed menstruation, is not well founded. The delay is more frequently the *result* than the *cause* of such maladies being in the constitution.

DYSMENORRHŒA, or *Painful Menstruation.*—This is even more common in India than the former condition, and is generally symptomatic of congestion about the womb or ovaries. In *exceptional* cases it results from the womb being flexed, or otherwise out of place, or from narrowness of the mouth; and in some few instances it appears to be connected with a gouty condition. The symptoms are—tenderness and pain in the lower part of the bowels, especially a little above the groin, and often most felt on the left side. Frequently the pain is of a very acute, darting character, shooting down the thighs, coming on in severe paroxysms, sometimes so violent as to cause the person to roll about as if suffering from colic. There may also be nausea, vomiting, diarrhœa, sudden desire to void, and pain when passing, water. When the pain and tenderness in the groins are prominent, it indicates that the *ovaries* are principally implicated, and the malady is known as *ovarian dysmenorrhœa.* The patient is also frequently hysterical. Such symptoms may precede the monthly period by a few hours, or sometimes days; often twenty-four hours previously is the most painful time. The symptoms may disappear on the first flow of the discharge, or they may continue with the passage of clots of blood or membranous shreds until the discharge ceases. As a rule there is most pain when there is least discharge. Females who suffer thus at the monthly periods are frequently dyspeptic during the intervals; or they may suffer from cough, palpitation, face neuralgia, fixed pain in the head, or from pain in the left side, or under the lower part of the left blade bone, or in the very lowest part of the spine. They may have attacks of menorrhagia (*vide* p. 474), and *whites* (*vide* p. 462) are frequently present.

The *treatment* consists in maintaining the bowels moderately open (Recipes 1 and 2), in avoiding all exposure to damp and chill, or excitement of any kind, for three or four days previous to the expected period; while at the same time guarding against idleness and want of occupation, which, especially in young women, tend to induce a mental and nervous condition favourable to the malady. When pain occurs, a warm bath at the commencement of the attack seldom fails to give relief. After leaving the bath the patient, being well dried, should go to bed, and keep up the soothing effects of the bath by the application of flannels wrung out of hot water over the lower part of the bowels and privates. Or, if the bath is not available fomentations should be applied to the lower part of the bowels, and chlorodyne in 30-minim doses may be given. If nervous or hysterical symptoms are present, sal volatile may be used, or, if not obtainable, wine or brandy-and-water will prove temporarily beneficial. But it is not desirable to give either wine or brandy if it can be avoided, and the dose should not be repeated, but bromide of potassium (Recipe 19) should be given every second or third hour. If the pain assumes a neuralgic periodical character, returning daily, or twice daily, quinine (Recipe 66). During the intervals exercise short of fatigue should be taken, and the patient may walk or drive out in a carriage, but horse exercise is improper. Late hours should be avoided, and a generous but wholesome diet should be adopted, with great attention to the ventilation of the sleeping apartment.

[Instead of Recipe 1, obtain Recipe 15 as an aperient pill. Instead of sal volatile or wine, Recipe 39. If not successful, *four* drops of tincture of Indian hemp may be taken in a little water every two hours for seven or eight times for the relief of pain. Recipe 73 should be obtained for use during the intervals, with or without the sulphate of soda, according as the bowels require aperient medicines or not. But if the iron in Recipe 73, as is sometimes the case (*vide* p. 25), appears to induce nervous irritability, or other unpleasant symptoms, Recipes 74 and 75 may be taken *together* instead. If there is any suspicion of gout, Recipe 52.]

When *dysmenorrhœa* is persistent and not relieved by medicines and regimen as above, it should be ascertained if any displacement or obstruction exists.

MENORRHAGIA, or *Excessive Menstruation.*—This is when the flow returns with unusual frequency, or continues longer than ordinary, or is more abundant than natural at the proper period. The flow should naturally occur once in every twenty-eight days; the average time of its continuance is three days, and the amount of fluid lost is about four ounces. There are exceptions to these general rules, but usually when such conditions are interfered with something wrong will have occurred. *Excessive, too frequent, or too long-continued menstruation* may be the result of two quite opposite states of the system, viz. *plethora* in some instances, and *debility* in others. *An immoderate flow arising from plethora* is usually preceded by shivering, pains in the head and loins, flushed countenance, and febrile symptoms. *An immoderate flow from debility*, which is most usually met with in India, is attended by paleness, languor, feeble pulse, fainty feelings, neuralgic pains, depression of spirits, flatulence, and disordered bowels, with dull aching pain in the back, loins, and thighs. Excessive menstruation is very likely to occur to women who have suffered much from over-nursing, or from frequent pregnancy, and sometimes when a doubt of pregnancy exists, it may be difficult to distinguish this affection from miscarriage (*vide* p. 362). Soft, luxurious beds, heavy skirts hanging from the waist, much standing about, and moist warm rooms predispose to menorrhagia.

*Treatment.*—In all cases of profuse menstruation, *rest in the horizontal posture is indispensable,* with perfect quietness; and in severe cases cold wet cloths laid over the lower part of the bowels and between the thighs. If the patient is of plethoric habit, indicated by a florid countenance and considerable muscular development, the diet should be low, consisting chiefly of milk and light puddings, the drink being a little weak claret-and-water, or lime-juice-and-water flavoured with sugar. If the patient be of a delicate constitution, indicated by pallid countenance and deficiency of muscular development, a more liberal diet, with a little claret or port wine, may be allowed. *But excepting in rarely severe cases, when there is very profuse bleeding,* stimulants should not be given with the view of combating faintness, as their action, by exciting the circulation, would tend to increase the discharge, and fainty feelings will pass away if the person keeps lying down. Everything should be given cold or very cool, taking hot drinks when the discharge is on being calculated to increase it. Quinine (Recipe 67) should be always used, as quinine has an action on the womb (*vide* p. 17), and would tend to correct any injurious malarious influence so often present. The liver is generally inactive, and the bowels are often costive. Constipation, if prevailing previously to the attack, should be removed by sulphate of soda (*vide* p. 20) for plethoric persons, and castor-oil for more weakly persons. Provided that movement does not cause renewed bleeding, the patient should as soon as possible get into the open air, taking at first only carriage exercise and not walking at all. During the intervals the greatest attention should be paid to ventilation of the sleeping apartment; the bed should be hard and the clothing light; the bowels should be kept moderately open (Recipes 1, 2), and usually sulphate of iron (*vide* p. 24) will be advisable.

[If the immoderate discharge arises from a plethoric state, in addition to low diet and purgatives recommended above, Recipe 4 should be procured and taken, *with the quinine*. In severe cases astringent medicines combined with sedatives (Recipe 45 or 47) should be used, the latter being the more powerful. In still more violent cases it may be necessary to use injections of ice-cold water to stay the bleeding; or if this does not suffice, astringent injections, as Recipe 98.

If during the interval hysterical and nervous symptoms are present, bromide of potassium (Recipe 19) may be used. If the loss of blood occurs only at the monthly period, the medicine should be commenced the week before, and when the discharge ceases it should be discontinued. If the loss of blood occurs at irregular periods, the medicine should be given continually until the loss is controlled, and after the first five days the dose should be doubled. If symptoms such as pallor, debility, and palpitations seem to require iron, *ferrum tartaratum* may be procured and taken in 6-grain doses *with* the bromide of potassium.]

**WOMB, INFLAMMATION OF THE.**—Inflammation of the womb may be either *acute* or *chronic*. It may occur in connection with disorders of menstruation, or without such prior ailments. When acute, the malady commences with cold or shivering, followed by quick pulse and fever. There is pain, increased by pressure, over the lower part of the bowels, which sometimes spreads over the whole of the bowels, the patient lying in bed with her knees drawn up as described under *Inflammation of the Bowels* (*vide* p. 79). There is pain about the loins and thighs, difficulty and frequency in making water, which is hot and scalds and becomes turbid as it grows cool, a sense of weight or 'bearing down,' swelling of the abdomen, more or less fever, and often nausea and vomiting. After the first two or three days there is a light-coloured discharge, which gradually becomes darker, imparting a yellowish-red stain to the linen. There is also often diarrhœa, and if the person is subject to piles they may inflame and add to the distress. The *causes* of inflammation of the womb are cold, particularly cold taken after confinement or during the monthly period, blows or falls, menstrual irregularities, the use of too strong injections, or the use of unsuitable pessaries, too frequent sexual intercourse, injuries during childbirth, too much exercise on horseback, or too long standing, walking, or dancing.

The *treatment* consists of leeches (one for each year of the patient's age) over the tender part of the belly, followed by fomentations; or in less severe cases counter-irritation by mustard poultices. Saline medicines, as citrate of magnesia (p. 15), should also be used, and the bowels should be opened by castor-oil. Unless there is diarrhœa, which sometimes accompanies, castor-oil should always be given, as hardened fæces in the lower bowel may press against the womb and mechanically irritate that organ. The diet should be chiefly fluid, and the drink toast-water, or rice-water. Rest in bed is indispensable, as walking, standing, or even sitting in the erect position is injurious, and has often caused a relapse. If neglected, inflammation of the womb may terminate in the formation of matter somewhere in the neighbourhood of the organ, which will be very injurious to the constitution. This may be suspected if a recurrence of shivering takes place during the existence of pain and tenderness as above described. In such a case it will be well for the patient to take a warm bath at 100° Fahr., this temperature being kept up for half an hour or longer, until faintness supervenes, as the best means of checking the inflammation. After the bath, the patient, being well dried, should be covered by blankets, take 10 grains of Dover's powder, and two hours afterwards drink freely of toastwater to promote perspiration. The bowels should also be again opened by another dose of oil. Perfect rest, attention to diet, and maintaining the bowels freely moved are the main points to be afterwards attended to; but the opinion of a surgeon should be sought.

**WOMB, CHRONIC INFLAMMATION OR CONGESTION OF THE.**—This is a minor degree of the acute form described above. It may come on gradually, or it may remain after the acute form has subsided. There is more or less pain and tenderness about the lower part of the bowels, with 'whites,' a sense of 'bearing-down' pain in the loins, and painful monthly periods; the condition being often more or less associated with *ovarian dysmenorrhœa* (*vide* p. 472). More or less dyspepsia is always present. If long continuing, it may lead to structural alterations about the womb, such as enlargement, displacement, suppuration in the neighbourhood, or ulceration of the mouth. The person should apply mustard leaves or poultices to the lower part of the bowels daily, or as often as can be borne. The recumbent posture should be maintained for several hours daily; tendency to constipation should be watched for and relieved; piles, if present, should be treated; cold hip-baths should be taken, or cold water should be poured down the spine daily. Tonics, as iron and quinine, and generous diet will generally be required. In this, as in all affections of the womb, horse exercise should be forbidden. When symptoms as above are persistent, it should be ascertained if there is falling, or displacement, which requires treatment by a surgeon.

[It will be desirable to procure iodide of potassium mixture (Recipe 21). Instead of mustard poultices, iodine paint should be applied as often as can be borne (*vide Appendix*, No. 111).]

**WOMB, DISPLACEMENT OR FALLING OF THE.**—This consists most usually of a falling of the womb below its natural position. But the womb (which is pear-shaped) may be bent either *forwards*, or *backwards*, or to *either side*.

In such cases the thin neck bends, and the heavier body inclines in one or other of the directions mentioned. Displacement of the womb is most frequent in women who have borne large families, or who have got up too soon after confinements. Tight-lacing, which produces forcible downward pressure on the womb, is a fertile cause. It may occur in the first instance suddenly after exertion, as lifting heavy weights, or from retention of urine (*vide* p. 361), or it may come on gradually from local weakness of the ligaments of the womb, or from weakness of the general system. It happens in *every degree*, from very slight falling to the protrusion of the womb externally; or from a slight inclination from the proper position to injurious pressure against the adjoining bladder, rectum, nerves and blood-vessels. The symptoms are feelings of weight and bearing-down pains, with a sensation of fulness of the belly, tenderness or aching about the groins and thighs, and 'whites,' the painful sensations being much relieved by lying down. There is often frequent desire to make water, or in some cases inability to do so, caused by pressure on the bladder, when the womb is displaced in the direction of that organ. Constipation may occur from a similar cause, when the womb presses on the rectum. All these symptoms are more or less severe as the organ is more or less displaced. The digestive organs are influenced injuriously by falling of the womb, so that the ailment is frequently associated with liver and stomach derangements, and this, reacting on the nervous system, produces a depressed and impaired state of general health. Displacement is often associated with *dysmenorrhœa* (*vide* p. 472). It may also be complicated by *ulceration*. Displacement, especially when combined with these two latter ailments, is a frequent cause of sterility.

*Treatment.*—This varies with the degree of displacement. In the less severe cases medicines should be administered with the view of strengthening the system (Recipes 66, 67). Prolonged rest in the horizontal posture should be enforced, and about a pint of cold water should be injected night and morning, the patient being in the recumbent position at the time. If this treatment is insufficient, injections of other kinds, as mentioned under the head *Whites*, should be tried. If *dysmenorrhœa* is present, it should be treated (*vide* p. 473). If the displacement of the womb is considerable it may require replacement by the hand. When displacement of the womb has occurred it is liable to return, and instruments may be necessary to retain the part in position. But pessaries are used too often, and their continued use often gives rise to a nervous irritable condition of system which is erroneously supposed to be due to the malady. Pessaries may also become the cause of ulceration.

[When chronic affections of the womb are attended with various dyspeptic symptoms, acid (Recipe 34) taken before meals, pepsine with the meals, and soda-mint tablets after the meals, will prove serviceable. If the flavour of soda-mint tablets is objectionable, 5 or 6 grains of bicarbonate of soda may be substituted.]

**WOMB, ULCERATION OF THE.**—Signifies a sore at the mouth of the womb, which may be a mere abrasion or a deep ulceration. It arises from numerous causes, the most common being chronic inflammation or displacement. The symptoms of a mere abrasion are unrecognisable, and when there is deeper ulceration the symptoms are not well defined, ranging from nervous irritability to those detailed as characterising chronic inflammation or displacement, with which it is usually associated. It cannot be positively stated that ulceration exists without examination, and a great deal too much has been made of ulceration as a separate ailment. It very rarely exists as a separate ailment, and if it does it will get well without treatment. If it exists in connection with other ailments, they should be treated, and not the ulceration they cause.

CHANGE OF LIFE.—The monthly discharge of females commences about the fifteenth year, terminating about the forty-fifth. It is to the period of cessation that the term *change of life* has been applied. This period is popularly supposed to be fraught with danger to the female, and there is doubtless often considerable suffering at such times, and in some women a more than ordinary liability to various ailments. Other women pass through this period of their life without any sensible derangement of health; the monthly flow gradually becoming more scanty until it ceases altogether. Other females may, when about forty-two or forty-three years of age, begin to suffer from periodical fainting fits, from palpitations of the heart, from despondency, from swelled legs, from swelling of the bowels, from nervous headaches, from flushings, or from night perspirations, from pain in the breasts or in the left side, from eruptions, especially *eczema*, from numbness of the extremities, from bleeding at the nose, or from bleeding piles. Drowsiness by day and sleeplessness at night are common complaints. There may also be hysterical symptoms, or hysterical fits. Some suffer from frequent desire to pass water, and from inability to hold it, a little escaping on any exertion, or even on sneezing or coughing. The temper, formerly the reverse, may become irritable, and the disposition may appear temporarily changed. Then the monthly flow may either be scanty or it may not appear for several months, and then it may return in considerable quantity. The course to adopt is first to ascertain if there is any special disease, such as chronic inflammation, displacement, or falling, which may give rise to the symptoms. If the patient has not begun to suffer until the period of change of life, the idea of such causes existing may generally be dismissed. Then the symptoms should be treated as they arise, and as detailed under the headings named. Care should be taken to keep the bowels regular, more especially when women of plethoric habit are the patients, in order to guard against any tendency to 'fits' or other maladies sometimes supervening. For such purpose, for plethoric women Recipes 1 and 2 may be recommended. For more feeble patients citrate of magnesia and tincture of ginger (*vide* p. 15).

[When there is no special disease to account for the symptoms, they may be treated as follows. For headache and drowsiness, eau de Cologne saturated with camphor may be rubbed on the forehead and temples; or the head may be sponged with the following Recipe:—solution of ammonia 2 ounces; salt 2 ounces; spirits of wine, 3 drachms; water 32 ounces. Sleeplessness and despondency indicate the use of bromide of potassium (Recipe 19). Palpitations and flushings require tonics (Recipe 70); hysterical symptoms, valerianate of zinc, in 2-grain doses.]

**WORMS.**—There are three common varieties of worms infesting the human intestines.

*Tape-worms* are most common in adults, *round-worms* in children: *thread-* or *maw-worms* may occur in either children or adults. The variety of worms present can only be *positively* ascertained by actual observation, the symptoms arising from either class being very similar. The stools should be carefully washed and examined daily, when either joints of the tape-worm, or a round-worm, or maw-worms, will eventually be discovered if the unhealthy state arises from such parasites. It should be a rule not to give any medicines for worms until their presence has been actually ascertained.

TAPE-WORM, of which there are several varieties, lives in either the large or small intestines, sometimes stretching throughout their whole extent. Its length is therefore sometimes very great, varying from six to twenty feet or more. It is a flat, ribbon-like worm, of a white colour, from one-third to one-half of an inch broad at the widest part, and composed of segments or pieces about an inch long, each segment fitting into the preceding one, and a fully developed worm numbers 1,100 of these joints.

Each joint possesses a male and female organ, and each worm is therefore a chain of individuals. Towards the head the worm tapers very much, and the segments are shorter. The head is triangular in shape, about the size of a pin's head, and is further known by four black spots which are the suckers by which the worm clings to the bowels. The worm increases in length by fresh segments, developed at the neck, while the fully formed segments at the tail drop off, and pass away with the stools. The pieces thus expelled contain myriads of ova in which are embryos provided with a boring apparatus. On the extrusion of the joints putrefaction sets in, liberating the ova, which are carried by wind, water, or other agencies, wherever accident may determine. These ova may be taken into the stomachs of animals (such as rabbits, pigs, or oxen) with their food. When thus swallowed by an animal the egg breaks, and the embryo, by boring, lodges itself in the flesh, there developing into a bladder-like substance or 'cyst,' and causing the affection known as 'measles.' The measle when eaten with meat attaches itself to the human intestine, and there grows into a tape-worm. Several animals—as, for instance, the dog—are subject to tape-worm, and help to propagate the disease in the manner described. The tape-worm embryo may also be eaten with vegetables on which it has been accidentally deposited.

The principal *cause* of tape-worm is eating very underdone meat, which from unclean feeding may contain numerous germs. It is also believed to be conveyed into the human system by using some kinds of fish, especially pike, and in India the 'singharee,' as food. It has been ascertained that fair cooking destroys the vitality of any ovum, although it may escape destruction when meat is only half-cooked.

The *symptoms* of any kind of worms vary greatly, some persons being unaware of the presence of worms until attention may be directed to the passage of pieces by the stool. The indications commonly present are uneasiness in the bowels, sometimes amounting to pain of a gnawing character. There is frequently irregularity of the bowels, straining at stool, fœtid breath, furred tongue, nausea, variable appetite, irritable bladder, and itching at the nose and fundament. The patient grinds his teeth when asleep, and children often awake frightened and screaming. There is frequently headache and giddiness, dry cough, palpitation, fainty feelings, a depressed or hypochondriacal condition, and, in women, hysterical symptoms. Pieces of the worm are occasionally passed with the stools, and are the most certain, and only conclusive, proof of the existence of the parasite; but caution is necessary that pieces of white *mucus* sometimes passed should not be mistaken for worms.

*Treatment.*—Tape-worm is best treated by some specific remedy as mentioned below. The reason of success or failure of worm medicines depends much on the manner of taking them: if they reach the worm they kill, or at least expel it; if not, they fail. In the case of tape-worm it is particularly necessary that they should reach the head of the worm, for, although many yards of tape-worm may be voided, if the head remains it will grow again, and the old symptoms will return. But the head is exceedingly tenacious of its hold, and is protected by the thick mucus which the irritation of its presence causes the intestines to secrete. It is therefore necessary that preliminary steps should be taken before giving worm medicines. Three days previously the patient should be put on a light diet of meat, eggs, milk, toasted bread, and green vegetables; avoiding such articles as potatoes, pastry, puddings and farinaceous food generally. The third day only beef-tea or thin soup should be allowed. Then on the third night an aperient should be taken, which may be castor oil for children, and Recipes 1 and 2 for adults. Next morning, or after these medicines have operated, the specific remedy is to be taken on an empty stomach. In the absence of the medicines mentioned in the small type, this may be decoction of pomegranate-root bark, prepared as detailed at p. 26. Two fluid ounces should be taken fasting, and a similar dose should be repeated every half-hour, until six draughts have been taken. For children, doses according to the table of proportions at p. 6. If it excites nausea or vomiting, a mustard poultice or leaf may be applied to the pit of the stomach, and this should not prevent repetition. Then, if the bowels are not freely acted upon after four hours, a dose of castor oil should be used. The worm will probably pass away with the motions thus produced. But the head of the worm should be sought for, and if it cannot be found the treatment should be repeated, after intervals of three days, until the head is found, or until all symptoms disappear.

[Better remedies are oil of male fern (also called liquid extract), spirits of turpentine, and Kossou. The dose of oil of male fern for an *adult* is one drachm, one-third part to be given at intervals of half an hour in some thick gruel, congee water, or mucilage. Of spirits of turpentine half an ounce, of which half should be given first, and the remainder thirty minutes afterwards in some thick fluid. Of powdered Kossou half an ounce after steeping for five minutes in a tumbler of hot water, the whole of which should be taken when lukewarm, first well stirring, that the powder also may be drunk. These remedies should be taken on an empty stomach after preliminary treatment as detailed above, and only liquid food should be allowed for twelve hours, but a dose of castor oil should be taken three or four hours afterwards. Kossou is not recommended for *children*; the best medicine for a child of four or five years old being from twenty to twenty-five minims of oil of male fern divided into three doses, and taken at intervals of half an hour, as recommended for adults. Or sixty minims of spirits of turpentine may be taken in three divided doses. Or santonin may be used as directed for round-worms: the precautions regarding liquid diet and a following dose of castor oil (as for adults) being taken. It is advised that if one remedy fails the others should be employed, in the order named both for adults and children.]

ROUND-WORMS.—May exist in any part of the intestines, and even in the stomach, from which they may be vomited or passed by the mouth. They are most common in children from three to ten years of age, who may be infested with one or many. In shape they resemble the common earth-worm, and are of a pale pink or white colour, and semi-transparent. There is a circular depression behind the head, and the latter presents three small elevations, between which lies the mouth. The symptoms they produce are very similar to those of tape-worm. The certain proof of the existence of round-worms is the sight of one passed with the stools.

Round-worms do not require, like tape-worms, to complete their life cycle by passing through the body of an intermediary animal. The ova of the worm, being discharged, is conveyed again into the system chiefly through the medium of insufficiently washed vegetables.

*Treatment.*—In the absence of the remedies mentioned below, the treatment by decoction of pomegranate-root bark, as detailed for tape-worm, may be pursued.

[If obtainable (after preliminary treatment as for tape-worm, *vide* p. 484) give for an *adult* 6 grains of santonin powder at bedtime, the same quantity early next morning, and a table-spoonful of castor oil one hour afterwards. This failing, turpentine may be used, as for tape-worm. For *children*, the best plan is to give a dose of castor oil the first thing in the morning, and to allow nothing but liquid food during the day. In the evening another dose of oil should be administered, and then santonin, for a child of two years old, in two-grain doses, three times during the next day; increasing the quantity by a quarter of a grain for each year of age. The santonin may be mixed, and taken as a powder, with white sugar. While taking the santonin still only liquid food should be allowed. Lozenges containing various quantities of santonin can be procured from the chemists.

Santonin should be kept in a bottle protected from the light by being pasted over with brown paper, as exposure to light deteriorates the medicine. Peculiar effects have followed taking santonin. The urine may acquire a reddish tinge, giving rise to suspicion of blood in that fluid. Or vision may become affected, every object appearing yellow or green. These effects pass off without leaving permanent ill-result. Should santonin fail, oil of male fern and turpentine may be used as for tape-worm.]

THREAD-WORMS.—Thread-worms, also called *maw-worms*, are about one-third of an inch long, slightly bent, white and semi-transparent. They almost invariably infest the lower part of the bowels near the fundament, where they create much itching and irritation; but their headquarters, where they principally breed, is much higher, in or about the cæcum (*vide* pp. 29, 81). They are not only passed with the fæces, but crawl out during the night on the clothes, in large numbers; they also excite mucous or bloody stools. In females they may crawl into the private parts, creating irritation and discharge (*vide* p. 364). They may also crawl under the foreskin of males, with a similar result (*vide* p. 364). Their presence is sometimes attended in children with a milky appearance of the urine. They may also originate protrusion of the bowel (*vide* p. 84). They are most common in weakly, dirty children who may pass hundreds, or even thousands, of worms.

*Treatment.*—Thread-worms are best expelled from adults by giving some saline aperient with iron, as Recipe 3, and by injecting the lower gut daily with 20 grains of quinine dissolved in 8 ounces of lukewarm water, or with a table-spoonful of common salt in 8 ounces of water. Children should be given a dose of castor oil in the evening, and an enema containing 6 or 8 grains of quinine, or a tea-spoonful of salt, the next day after the action of the oil has ceased. (For the method of administering enemas to children, and the quantity to be injected, *vide Appendix, Injections.*) It is not advisable to give specific remedies, as santonin or turpentine, for thread-worms, which inhabit the lower part of the intestines, and which, therefore, are not so much exposed to the action of remedies given by the mouth as other kinds of worms having their habitation in the upper portion of the bowels. Personal cleanliness is essential, especially avoiding putting the hands to the mouth after application to the anus, which the itching induces, as the ova may be thus directly re-transferred to the system.

[It is also desirable to apply round the anus, salad oil and carbolic acid, in the proportion of a drachm of the latter to 2 ounces of the former, which will tend to destroy any ova deposited outside. If the injections mentioned above are not quite successful, an enema of infusion of quassia may be used. This not destroying the worms, an enema composed of two drachms of tincture of the sesquichloride of iron in 6 ounces of water may be employed. If these measures fail, turpentine given by the mouth should be tried.]

*Other effects of Worms.*—In addition to the distressing symptoms previously enumerated which they usually excite, tape-worm especially may be the concealed cause of anæmia (*vide* p. 46), of hypochondriasis (p. 304), and of nervousness (p. 340). In children round-worms especially may cause a progressive emaciation (the food, although taken in fair quantity, not doing any good), with swelling and hardness of the bowels, a condition which may be mistaken for atrophy (*vide* p. 66). Convulsions (p. 145), paralysis (p. 344),St. Vitus's dance (p. 422), and infantile remittent fever (p. 263) may all be excited in children by worms, generally round-worms. Round-worms have also crawled into the air-passages and caused suffocation, and into the gall-bladder and caused liver disease.

*Prevention.*—The means of prevention of all kinds of worms is avoiding underdone animal food, especially beef and pork, from which tape-worms originate ; and avoiding eating imperfectly washed vegetables, from which other varieties may be introduced. A liberal allowance of salt with the meals is desirable. The stools of those suffering from worms should be disinfected (*vide Appendix*, No. 126) and buried, to prevent the ova being taken into the bodies of animals used as food. Persons with worms should occupy separate beds, or the malady may be immediately communicated.

**WORMS IN THE NOSE.**—The affection generally described as worms in the nose, or *Peenash*, is in reality maggots in the nose. It is a malady almost entirely confined to the lower class of dirty natives. A fly enters the nostrils and deposits larvæ or eggs within, which eventually become maggots. If any disease causing discharge from the nostrils exists, the flies are attracted, and are most likely to effect entrance. Anyone may daily notice flies clustering about the eyes and nostrils of dirty natives, particularly children, the latter taking little trouble to rid themselves of the nuisance. At such times, or during sleep or weakness from disease, the flies enter the passage and maggots in the nose is the result. Sometimes one or two maggots are passed daily, at others several dozens may be passed or extracted. They sometimes consume not only the interior of the nostrils, but even eat their way through the skin of the nose and into the mouth. A good application is lime-water (Recipe 25), injected by means of a syringe. When visible, the maggots should be extracted with forceps. Maggots may also present *in the ears*, the symptoms and treatment being the same.

[But better injections are 'black wash' (Recipe 88) and carbolic acid lotion (*vide Appendix*, No. 119), which may be obtained and used alternately several times daily.]

## CHAPTER III

### *ACCIDENTS AND INJURIES*

**INSTRUMENTS REQUIRED.**—The instruments and appliances required in ordinary surgical practice are—

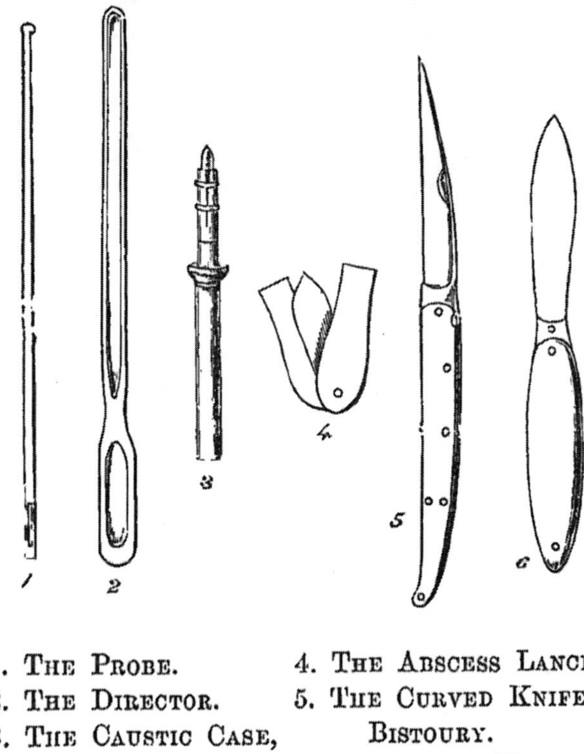

1. The Probe.
2. The Director.
3. The Caustic Case, or Holder.
4. The Abscess Lancet.
5. The Curved Knife, or Bistoury.
6. The Blunt Knife.

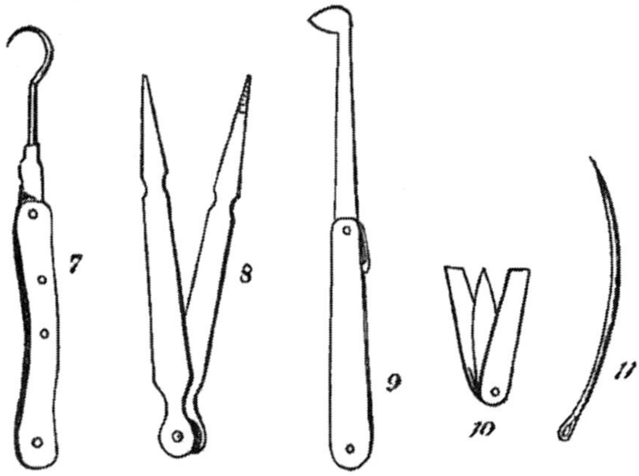


7. The Tenaculum.
8. The Forceps.
9. The Gum Lancet.
10. The Vaccinating or Bleeding Lancet.
11. The Curved Needle.
12. Scissors.

These instruments may be contained in a small leathern case, in which also a little lint, ligature silk, and plaster should be carried.

1. The Probe is a piece of silver wire, sufficiently flexible to bend without breaking, and used to ascertain the depth of wounds, or if foreign bodies are present or not.

2. The Director is a thicker piece of silver wire, deeply grooved on one side, and used to guide the surgeon's knife when opening sinuses or *fistulæ*. The director is first passed where it is wished to cut, and the knife is then thrust in the groove of the director.

3. The Caustic Case, or Holder, is a silver tube for holding caustic.

4. The Abscess Lancet is a large lancet, with broad-shouldered blade, used for opening abscesses.

5. The Curved Knife, or Bistoury, is a thin knife, approaching the semicircular shape, used with the director for opening deep sinuses or *fistulæ*.

6. THE BLUNT KNIFE, or SPATULA, is chiefly used for spreading ointments or plasters.

7. THE TENACULUM is a curved piece of steel wire, set in a handle, and used for seizing bleeding vessels.

8. THE FORCEPS are pincers, with or without a spring, used for taking off dressings, seizing foreign bodies, &c.

9. THE GUM LANCET has a small cutting surface projecting from the end, used for lancing the gums.

10. THE BLEEDING or VACCINATING LANCET is used as its name implies; also for opening small abscesses. But the instrument employed either for bleeding or vaccinating should not be applied to any other purpose.

11. THE CURVED NEEDLE is a bent, flat-shaped needle, used for applying stitches to wounds.

12. THE SCISSORS should be sharp and pointed.

In addition to the ordinary instruments described above as contained in the pocket-case, the following articles will be required in the medicine-chest for use in surgical cases:—

1. CATHETERS, FLEXIBLE.
2. BANDAGES.
3. PLASTERS.
4. LINT.
5. SPONGE.
6. TOURNIQUET.
7. LIGATURE SILK.

1. CATHETERS, FLEXIBLE.—Catheters are instruments for drawing off the urine, and three of different sizes of the flexible—not metallic—kind should be carried in the medicine-chest. The use of silver or metallic catheters, or of flexible catheters *with the wire inserted*, requires special surgical skill, and should not be attempted. The sizes of the catheters recommended for the travelling-chest are those known as Nos. 2, 4, and 8. But as flexible catheters are liable to get stiff and break from age and heat, their condition should always be carefully examined before being used. It sometimes happens after accidents, as, for instance, fractured thigh, or from spasmodic

stricture (*vide* p. 420), that the person cannot make water and may require the catheter passed. And although this is an operation demanding surgical skill, it will be better for it to be attempted without special skill than for the patient to be left without endeavours towards relief, and exposed to the risk of the urinary passages bursting, with often fatal consequences.

By attention to the following directions, and with a flexible catheter, injury can scarcely be inflicted. The wire should be taken out of the tube of the catheter, and the latter should be warmed in *tepid* water, then dried and oiled. If the water is too hot the instrument will become too soft to pass without the wire. The patient should lie on his back with the head and shoulders raised, and the knees elevated and separated. The operator should stand on the left side of the patient. Next, let the head of the penis be grasped with the fingers and thumb of the left hand, and the organ extended upwards and forwards. Next, hold the catheter in the right hand, and insert the point into the orifice of the urinary passage; then press steadily on, and the instrument, in the absence of permanent stricture, will pass into the bladder, and urine will probably flow. The passage is between eight and nine inches long, and if, when the instrument has been passed so far, urine should not flow, the catheter should be withdrawn for about an inch. If urine is still absent, the probability is that the eye of the instrument is stopped up and requires cleansing. After use the instrument should be carefully washed with hot water and carbolic solution (*vide Appendix*, No. 119).

A condition known as *catheter shock* or *collapse* (*vide* p. 520) sometimes follows the passing of an instrument. The person may be merely faint, or there may be more decided symptoms of collapse. The treatment should be as for collapse (*vide* p. 521). Sometimes a shivering fit occurs after the passage of an instrument, followed by fever, pain in the back, loins, and limbs, and perspiration. To this condition the term *catheter fever* has been applied. Treatment as for ague (*vide* p. 255).

2. Bandages, or Rollers, are made of strips of linen, calico, or flannel, or of porous or solid rubber. A bandage for the arm should be about two inches wide by eight yards long; a leg bandage two and a half inches wide by ten yards long; and a bandage for the body five inches wide by twelve yards long. A bandage ought to be made

of one continuous piece without any joinings, and the selvedges should always be torn off. The surfaces and

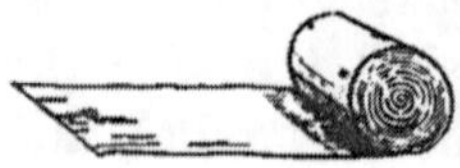

edges should be smooth and even, and there should be nothing which can press unequally on the skin. Bandages should be kept ready tightly and longitudinally rolled up; hence their name 'rollers.' This may be done perfectly well by hand, another person

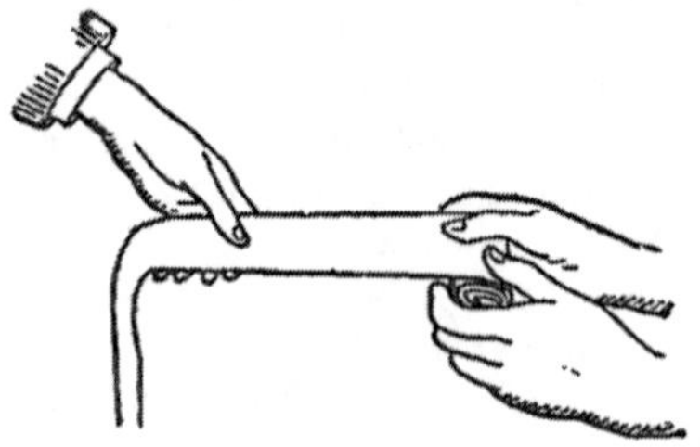

holding the end of the strip of cloth; or it may be fastened to the leg of a table, or at any fixed point. Unless this is done, there is a difficulty in rolling the cloth smoothly. Besides the roller there are compound bandages, as the T-shaped bandage, described under *Protrusion of the Bowel* (*vide* p. 85), the figure of ∞ shaped bandage, described under *Fractured Collar-bone* (p. 560), and in another form under *Bubo* (p. 109); the four-tailed bandage, described under *Fracture of the Jaw* (p. 559), and various other forms. The principal uses of bandages are

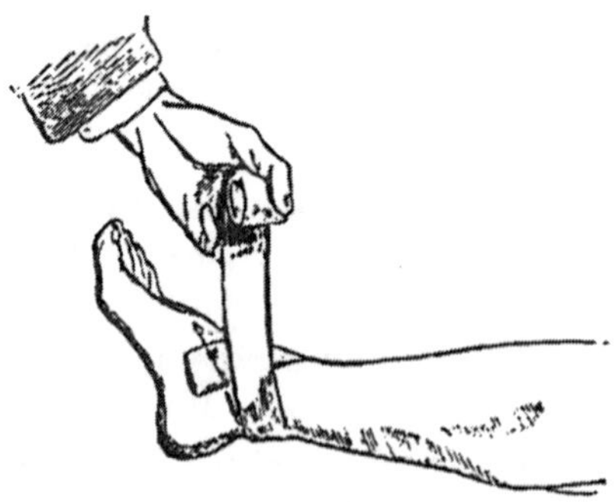

to keep on dressings, to protect diseased or wounded parts from injury, to place restraint on motion of injured parts, and to afford support to muscles and vessels. In applying a bandage the first thing necessary is to obtain a point on which the required traction may be made. Therefore a turn round the *arm* or *ankle* should be taken before the bandage is applied symmetrically to the *hand* or *foot*.

Then the roll should be held in the manner represented below, and it should be passed from one hand to the

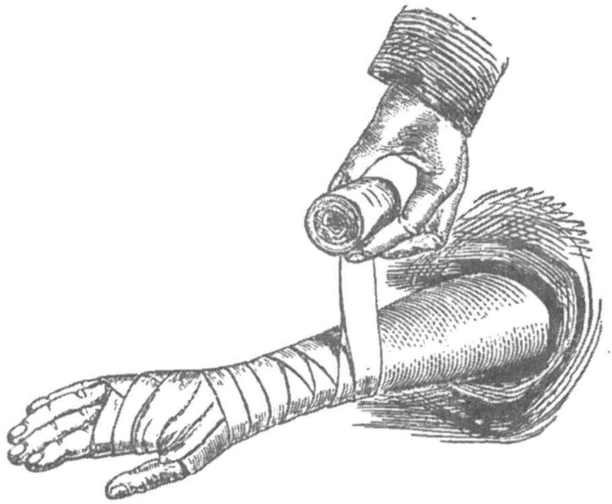

other as it encircles the limb. A bandage should always be first applied to the extremity of the limb, where it should be tightest, gradually becoming more slack as it ascends, and each fold should overlap about one-third of the previous one. No part must be 'skipped' or left uncovered by the bandage, or swelling of such part will very probably occur, and the roller will become loosened and easily detached (*vide* figures above and the one opposite).

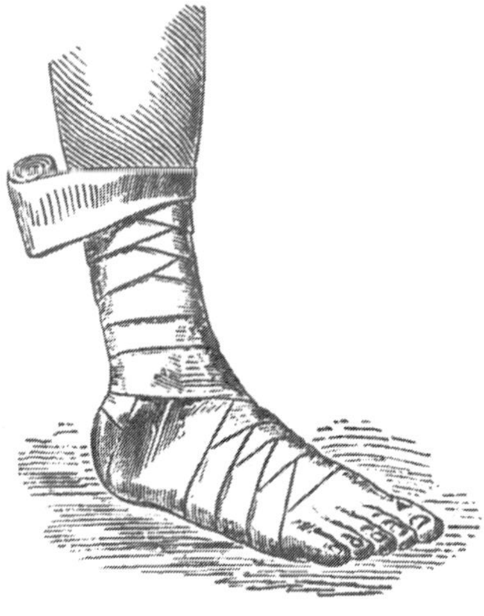

Where the limb increases in size the bandage must be turned on itself, as represented in the sketches. When a bandage is changed, the part over which it has been applied should be sponged with soap and water and then dried, both for cleanliness and also to prevent irritation from the bandage. When a bandage has to be applied to the head, the hair ought to be combed, so that it may lie flat, and not make unequal pressure on the scalp. When a bandage is used to give support, or to make pressure, great care should be taken that it is not too tight in any part of its course, as mortification of the limb has been caused by too tight a bandage. It is particularly necessary to bear this in mind when applying a bandage to a limb that has been recently fractured. In such cases the parts are liable to swell, and a bandage which at the time of its application was sufficiently easy may soon become so tight as to cause a dangerous constriction, and this is especially liable to happen if the limb is allowed to hang down. In cases of bad fracture, or any severe injury, the bandage should be applied loosely in the first instance, particularly in the neighbourhood of the injury, and as the swelling decreases the bandage may be tightened. As the nails are always left uncovered in the application of bandages, it is a good test of the state of the circulation to make pressure upon them. If the circulation is free, the white mark which is made by pressing upon the nail ought to disappear at once when the pressure is removed. But if it lingers and fades away slowly, the injured limb is too tightly bound, and bandages and splints should be loosened.

3. PLASTERS are made by spreading the material on calico or on leather. Plasters are spread on leather when it is required to afford more support to the part affected than would be given by calico—as, for instance, to fractured limbs after the splints are dispensed with. Adhesive plaster is the variety generally used for wounds. Plaster may be carried ready spread, but should be rolled up with oiled paper to prevent sticking.

4. Lint is required for cleansing wounds, for making small pads, and for spreading ointment on when a thicker substance than linen is desirable as a covering for wounds.

5. Sponge is useful for the purpose of conveying a stream of water to a wounded or diseased part. But sponge should *not* be used for cleansing wounds, as it is liable to become contaminated by the discharge. Lint, tow, or linen rag, which should be afterwards destroyed, may be used for cleaning away discharges. The artificial antiseptic sponge prepared by Messrs. Burroughs & Wellcome is recommended for all long cases.

6. Tourniquet.—This is a strip of strong cloth about an inch and a half wide, furnished with a buckle and pad,

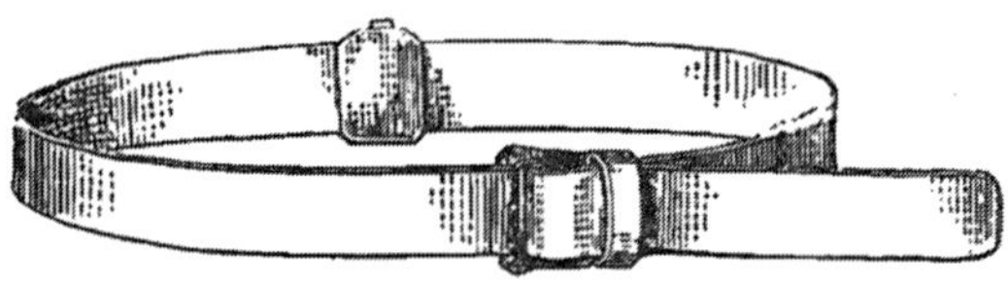

as here shown. It is used to stop bleeding or *hæmorrhage* by being buckled round the limb *above* the bleeding part, the pad being placed *over* the main artery. Or a tourniquet may be extemporised as figured at p. 509.

7. Ligature Silk.—This is used for sewing up wounds and tying bleeding blood-vessels. Prepared catgut is the best, but both hemp ligature and silver wire are used. In the absence of prepared catgut, strong well-waxed thread or silk may be substituted.

**THE IMMEDIATE AND GENERAL TREATMENT OF ACCIDENTS AND INJURIES.**—1. The history of the accident should be ascertained by a few clear questions, addressed to the patient if he is sensible and able to speak, or otherwise to the bystanders.

2. If the patient is insensible, place him on the ground or floor, lying rather on the right side, and with the head raised to the level of the body by a pillow, folded coat, or

other soft substance. This will render the breathing more easy than it would be if the patient lay on the back. Then split open or unbutton any clothing pressing upon the neck, chest, or bowels.

3. The face and chest should be sprinkled with cold water and then wiped dry, and some cold water may be drunk if the power of swallowing remains. Wine or brandy should not be hastily given, without evidence of their being needed, even if there is bleeding.

4. Examine the head and limbs one by one. If there is bleeding, note where it comes from, and follow the directions given under *Bleeding* (*vide* p. 504). The prominent parts of the limbs may be examined with very little movement of the body, and any change of form will probably be recognised by the eye, after the clothing has been taken off, which should be accomplished by cutting open, not pulling off. If necessary to remove clothing, do so first from the uninjured side.

5. If there be local injury, it should be treated, if possible, at once, as described under the different headings.

6. Allow no useless talking to, or in the hearing of, the patient, and send away all except those necessary for his attendance. See that he has plenty of fresh air.

7. In all cases of serious injury aid should be procured immediately. When sending for a surgeon the message should be as clear as possible, and if practicable a written one.

8. If it is necessary to move a person after injury, especially of the head, the patient should be carried while lying down. He should not be allowed to mount a horse, to sit upright in a vehicle, or to walk. *An exception to this rule is injury to the arm or forearm* (*vide* p. 499). A hurdle, or shutter, or door, or *charpai* covered with straw, coats, or blankets, may be converted into a litter. If poles are procurable they may be fixed beneath each end

of the litter, which will thus be carried long distances more easily. If neither hurdle, door, *charpai*, nor shutter can be obtained, a good substitute may be made by fastening four stout poles together, and tying a blanket securely to them, as shown below.

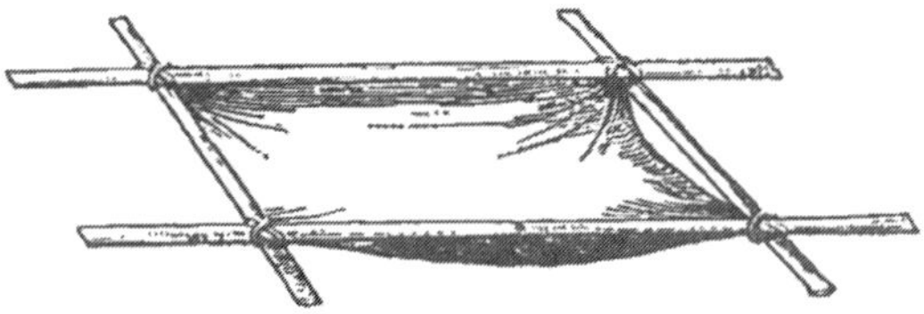

The foot of the litter should be placed at the patient's head in a line with his body. Two people should then place themselves one on either side of the patient, and join hands underneath the body and hips. Another person should take charge of the injured part. The patient should be then lifted, carried backwards over the litter, and then lowered on to it. The litter should be carried by the hand, and not on the shoulders, as the patient would be out of sight. The front and rear bearers should start with opposite feet, which prevents lateral motion. In ascending a hill the patient's head should be in front, in descending behind, except in the case of a broken leg, or thigh, when such a course would throw the weight of the body on the injured part. Much harm is often done by moving a person, without taking any means to protect an injured limb, and especially so in fracture of the lower extremities. If the leg or thigh is broken, the person should be placed on the other side, the broken limb should be placed exactly on the sound one with straw or something soft between, and the two limbs should be tied together with handkerchiefs. The sound limb then acts in some degree as a splint for the broken one and prevents motion.

*When the arm or forearm is broken*, the least painful

and injurious position is resting the forearm in a broad handkerchief slung from the neck with the elbow bent, and with a small pillow or pad between the arm and the side. A person so injured will be able to walk with less pain than he would suffer from movement in a carriage.

**COURSE OF THE BLOOD-VESSELS.**—The circulation of the blood throughout the body is carried on by the heart, as the central receiving and propelling organ, and by blood-vessels connected with it. These blood-vessels consist of two distinct divisions, named ARTERIES and VEINS: the *former* carrying *bright red* arterial blood *to* the different parts of the body *from* the heart, and having a *distinct pulse* at each beat of the heart; the *latter* carrying *dull red or dark blood from* the various parts of the frame *back* to the heart, and *not possessing any distinct pulsation.* The main *arteries* pursue a tolerably direct course to the various limbs, and are placed, as a rule, not very near to the surface of the body; the position they occupy is the sheltered one on the *inside* of each limb. The *veins* run in two sets: *superficial,* which are abundant in number, communicate freely with each other, and run a tortuous course; *deep,* which for the most part are situated side by side with the large arteries, and are more direct in their course. The veins and the arteries are connected in the skin and in the other textures of the body, by a system of very minute vessels termed *capillaries.* A knowledge of the course of the principal blood-vessels may be obtained by seeking out their course on the living subject by the pulsation they afford; and an outline of the course of the main vessels will not be difficult to remember, and will be a necessary guide to the ready arrest of bleeding.

In the following drawings (Figs. 1, 2, 3, 4, and 5) the *dark* vessels represent veins, and the *light* vessels arteries. The letter *a* in the drawing signifies artery, the *v* signifies veins.

There is on each side of the neck a large artery (*carotid*, Fig. 1) which carries blood *from* the chest *to* the neck and head. It runs in a line from the inner end of the collar-bone to the angle of the lower jaw, and the pulsation is throughout fairly evident to the finger. The *deep jugular vein* lies very nearly parallel to the artery; the *superficial jugular vein* is near the surface, and can be seen under the skin.

The large artery (*subclavian*, Fig. 2) which supplies the arm and hand with blood *passes out of the chest directly over*

Fig. 1

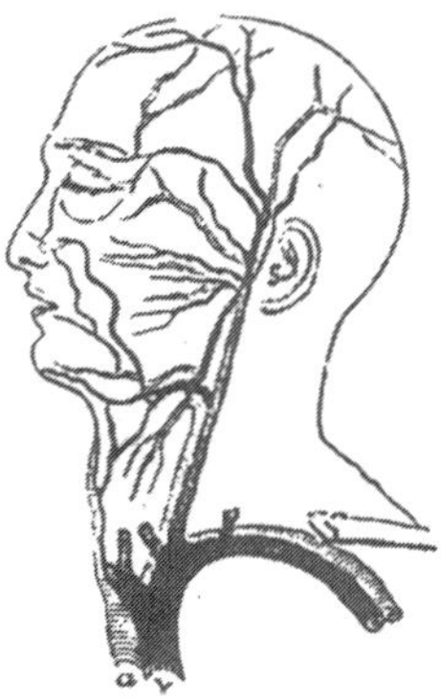

Fig. 2

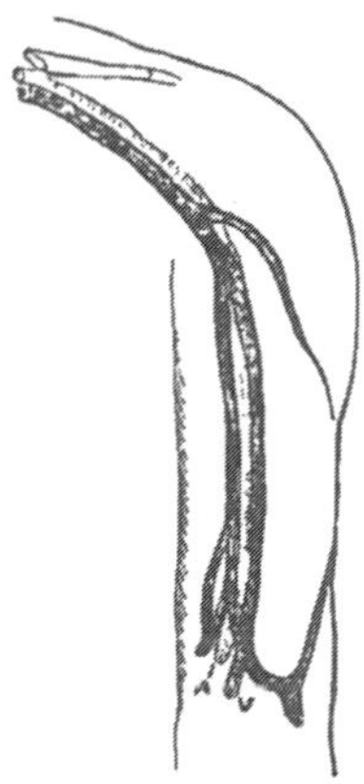

Fig. 3

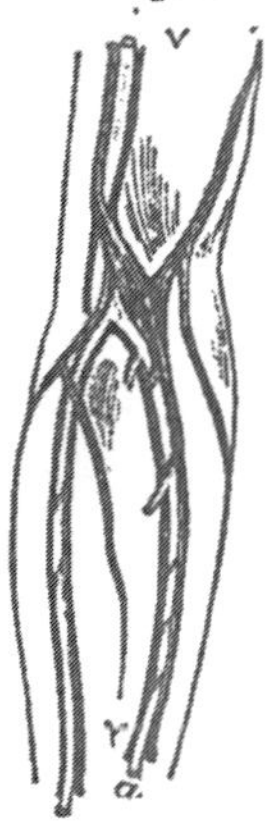

*the uppermost or first rib*, and then curves downwards. In the armpit the artery (here termed *axillary*) may be felt beating by pressing against the arm-bone near the top of the hollow of the armpit. From this point it runs onwards to the elbows, *keeping on the inside of the arm*, and to the inner side of the prominent muscle (*biceps*) of the arm (where it is termed *brachial*). It is accompanied by parallel veins.

*Just below the bend of the arm* the artery (Fig. 3) divides into two; one (now called *radial*) taking the line of the *outer bone of the forearm*, the other (*ulnar*) *lying almost parallel with the inner bone.* In the upper part of their course pulsation is not well felt, as they are covered with muscles. At the wrist joint both vessels may be felt beating.

Fig 4

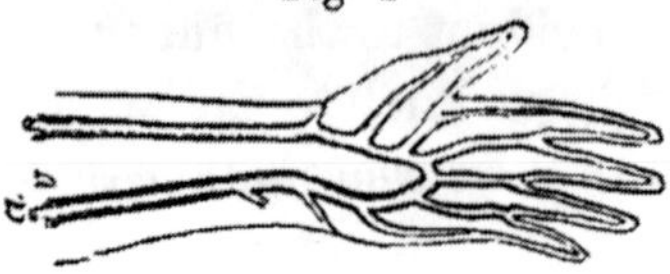

Other branches pass onwards (Fig. 4), forming arches in the palm of the hand and in the ends of the fingers.

Fig. 5

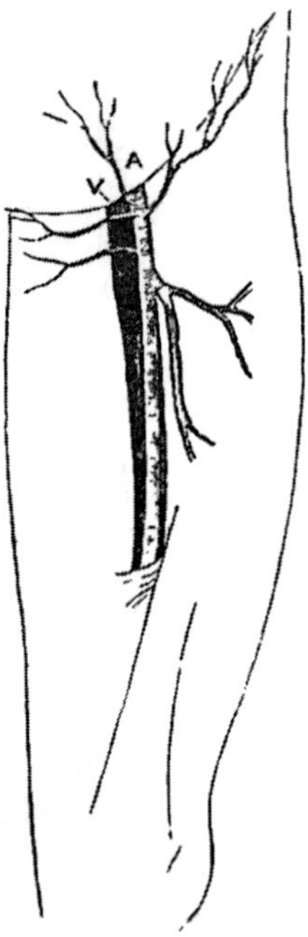


The large artery for the thigh, leg, and foot (*femoral*, Fig. 5) passes *out from the groin, lying about the middle of the crease of the groin,* and almost at rightangles to it. From this point it runs onwards, *inclining to the inside,* and turning round a *little below the middle of the thigh-bone* into the ham. A line drawn from the centre of the fold of the groin to the inner side of the knee marks its course. In the upper three inches of its course the artery lies very superficial, and may be felt pulsating. It then becomes deeper-seated, but may still be compressed against the thigh-bone. The artery is accompanied by a large vein which lies at first to the inner side, but afterwards behind. Several smaller and one large branch are given off as the artery passes through the thigh (*vide* Fig. 5).

The main artery at the knee divides into two (called the *anterior* and *posterior tibial*); one passing down the inner front of the leg, the other through the calf. Both are deeply seated and covered with muscles, and their pulsation, except near the ankle joint, is not easily detected.

The foot, like the hand, is supplied with small branches from the two arteries.

**BLEEDING or HÆMORRHAGE, VARIETIES OF.**—*Bleeding from arteries* is ordinarily recognised by *vividly scarlet blood rushing out in jets, or jerks. Bleeding from veins is known by the black appearance* of the blood, and by its *flowing in a continuous stream,* and not in jets. When, however, an artery is wounded deep in the substance of a limb, the jet, or jerk, may be absent, and from retention in the deep wound the blood, although arterial, may become darker than it would otherwise be. At p. 500 it is stated that arteries carry blood *from* the heart to all parts of the body, while veins take the blood *back* to the heart. The practical application of this knowledge is, that bleeding from arteries is further distinguished by the facts that *pressure on the side of the wound nearest the heart stops the flow of blood from arteries; while pressure on the side of the wound furthest from the heart stops bleeding from veins.* In other words, bleeding from arteries *in the limbs* is to be stopped by pressure above the wound, and bleeding from veins by pressure below the wound. But for bleeding in the head or neck the reverse obtains. Bleeding from a large artery is dangerous, and will not stop without surgical treatment; but bleeding, except from a wounded artery of considerable size, is seldom dangerous to life. It generally stops on the application of pressure to the part (as afterwards described), or when the person becomes faint. Bleeding from veins is not often dangerous, and will generally stop without surgical treatment. The reasons why arteries continue bleeding and veins do not are found in the difference of structure, and in the manner of circulation of the blood.

As the matter is important, the distinctions between bleeding from arteries and from veins are placed in contrast.

| *Bleeding from Arteries* | *Bleeding from Veins* |
|---|---|
| Blood scarlet. | Blood dark. |
| Rushes out in jerks. | Flows in a continuous stream. |
| Pressure on the side of the wound nearest the heart stops the flow. | Pressure on the side of the wound furthest from the heart stops the flow. |
| Dangerous from a large artery, and will not stop. | Not often dangerous, and generally stops. |

**BLEEDING, MEANS OF STOPPING. WHEN NOT VIOLENT.**—*Bleeding from a wound when not violent* may generally be stopped by sponging the part with *cold* water; or, if more copious, by *pressure* with the finger, or with a bit of cork or a hard linen pad; especially if the wounded part is over a bone, where pressure can be made against the bone. At the same time the bleeding part should be raised as high as possible above the level of the heart. But if this does not succeed, each edge of the wound must be lifted up, carefully examined, and the mouth of any bleeding *artery* should be seized obliquely with the forceps, or with a pair of pincers out of a pocket knife, so that the whole is in the grasp of the instrument, and then *twisted* round, but not so completely as to cause the end of the artery to be broken off. If the bleeding is not thus stopped, the artery will require *tying* as described and sketched below. When the artery can be seen by turning up the flaps of the wound, the point of a tenaculum (A) should then be applied as nearly as possible to it, and the spouting mouth (B) drawn up sufficiently to pass a strong catgut ligature, silk, or thread round it below the tenaculum.

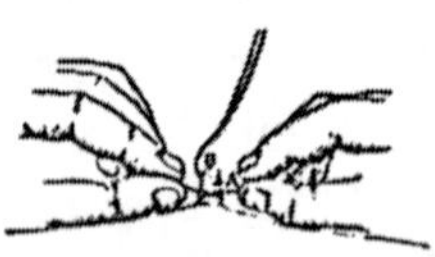

One end of the ligature should then be passed through the other, and both ends drawn steadily till the blood ceases to flow from the vessel, the mouth of which is then seen gaping, open, and white. The knot should then be completed. After which, if the bleeding cease, the wound may be brought together by plaster, the ends of the ligature remaining *outside* at the most dependent point of the wound. The ligature will come away with the discharge in five or six days' time, or at an earlier period if on a small vessel. Instead of the tenaculum, forceps may be used to take up the mouth of the artery, or even a strong piece of wire sharpened at the end.

If a small bleeding vessel cannot be stopped by cold, pressure, twisting, or tying, a *graduated pad* should be placed over the wounded part. This is made by rolling a small piece of lint or cotton cloth into a pad to fit into the wound, then placing four or five increasingly larger pads over one another. The whole should be secured by a bandage, which will probably stop the bleeding, at least till surgical aid arrives. The whole should remain for twenty-four hours, when the dressing may be cautiously soaked with lukewarm water and removed, after which plaster may be applied; or, if there is no plaster, a soft rag wet with cold water.

**BLEEDING, MEANS OF STOPPING WHEN VIOLENT.**—*When blood is flowing fast*, or when if *not* violent it cannot be stopped by cold, pressure, twisting, or tying, the first thing to do is to compress the artery supplying the part with blood as shown in the following sketches. The procedure after the flow of blood has been commanded by pressure of an artery, is given at p. 510.

**BLEEDING FROM A WOUND IN THE HEAD OR NECK.** Moderate bleeding from any part of the *head or face* may be stopped by placing a *graduated pad* (*vide* p. 505) over the wound and bandaging firmly. If very copious or from the neck it will be from some branch of the carotid artery. Firm pressure should be made in the neck over the course of this artery (*vide* p. 501), in a direction rather inwards and backwards, so as to press the vessel against

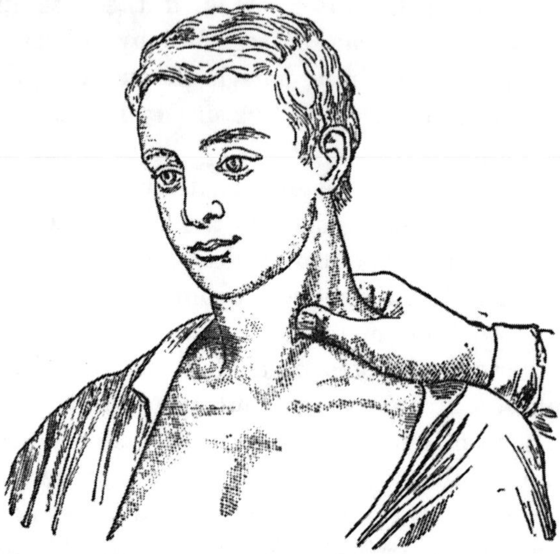

the side projections of the bones of the neck. The pressure is best accomplished with the fingers or thumb.

**BLEEDING FROM THE ARM, NEAR THE ARMPIT.**— A bystander should press his thumb firmly into the neck

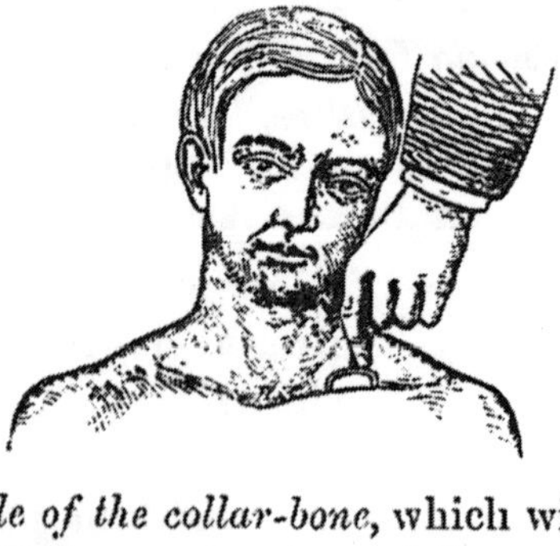

*behind the middle of the collar-bone*, which will stop the flow of blood through the great artery of the arm as it is first coming out of the chest. As, however, the pressure thus made soon tires the thumb, the handle of a large key, or other object of similar shape, *wrapped in three or four folds of linen*, may be pressed behind the middle of the collar-bone, and held without fatigue for an indefinite time till surgical assistance can be obtained; or, if the bleeding comes from a small artery, until the blood ceases to flow, which may be ascertained by slightly and gradually diminishing the pressure.

**BLEEDING FROM THE LOWER PART OF THE ARM, OR FROM THE FOREARM BELOW THE ELBOW.**—The brachial artery may be controlled by compression with the fingers on the inner side of the arm in the position of the

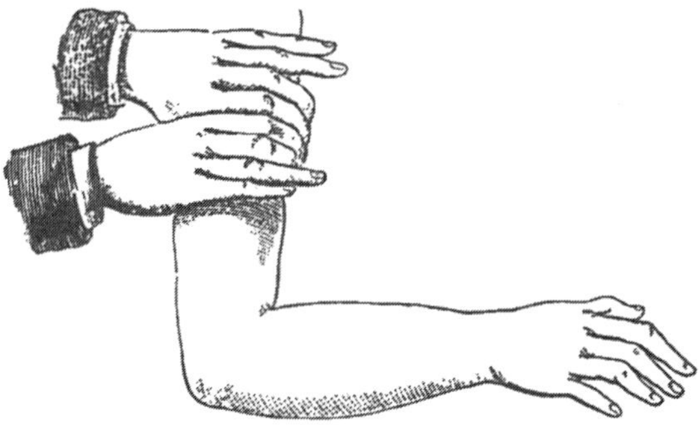

artery as shown above. More permanent compression may be made by the tourniquet if at hand (*vide* p. 497); or by the handkerchief and stick, as figured at p. 509, round the thigh; or by placing a thick ruler or stick *in the armpit* and then binding the arm tightly to the chest.

**BLEEDING FROM THE PALM OF THE HAND.**—A pad should be placed over the radial artery at the wrist (where the pulse is felt), and another pad over the ulnar artery on the other side of the front of the wrist (*vide* fig. 4, p. 502) and bandaged tightly. If this does not stop the bleeding, a *graduated pad* (*vide* p. 505) should be placed over the wounded part. Another thick piece of lint or cloth should be placed on the back of the hand. Then two pieces of wood, or two paper-knives, should be laid transversely, one across the front and one across the back of the hand, and their ends should be tied firmly together. The forearm should then be bandaged, the elbow bent, and the hand bound to the opposite shoulder. Or the pin sling may be used (*vide* p. 464). The whole should be allowed to remain for twenty-four hours, after which the part should be dressed as an ordinary wound. If pieces of wood, such as paper-knives, are not at hand, the bleeding may be stopped by binding the fingers over a ball of wood, or tightly rolled cloth, placed in the palm, then bending the elbow, and binding the hand to the opposite shoulder.

**BLEEDING FROM THE UPPER PART OF THE THIGH.** The great artery which supplies the limb should be pressed

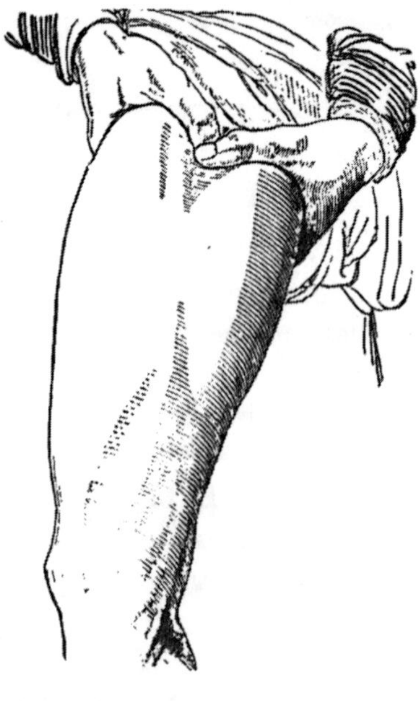

so as to prevent the flow, by applying the thumbs with some force immediately below the middle of the crease of the groin. This pressure is made with less difficulty than when necessary behind the collar-bone, but the door-key or other convenient instrument may be used (*vide* p. 506).

**BLEEDING FROM BELOW THE MIDDLE OF THE THIGH, or FROM THE LEG.**—When bleeding is below the middle of the thigh, and a tourniquet (as figured at p. 497) is not at hand, a good substitute may be used, composed of a stout pocket-handkerchief and a piece of tough stick, which is to be applied as follows :—Pass the handkerchief once or twice round the limb, some distance,

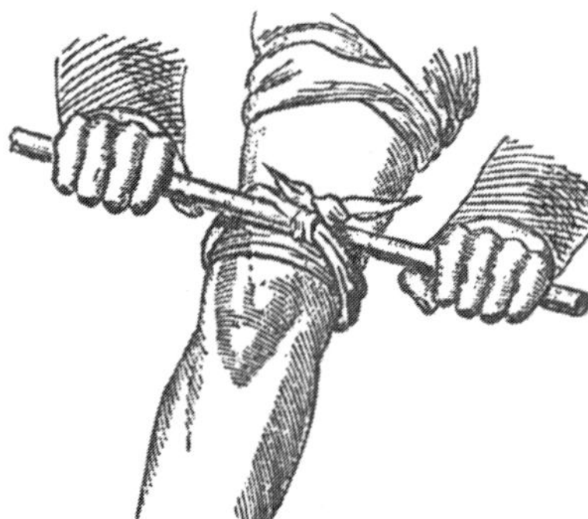

if possible, above the wound. Then push the stick between the handkerchief and the skin, and twist the stick so that it screws the handkerchief until the blood ceases to flow. The twisting should only be continued till the bleeding stops, as the application of more pressure than is necessary to effect this may bruise the limb. A pad, or wine cork, placed underneath the handkerchief, over the course of the vessel, will lead to more direct and therefore more efficient pressure, without so much tightening of the bandage.

**BLEEDING FROM THE SOLE, OR FRONT OF THE FOOT.**—When there is bleeding from *the sole* a pad should be placed in the hollow behind and below the inner and outer ankles, and bandage tightly. If this does not stop the bleeding, a *graduated pad* should be applied to the wound as for bleeding from the palm of the hand (*vide* p. 507). When the bleeding is from the *front of the foot*, a pad and bandage should be tightly applied. In all cases of bleeding from the foot, it should be raised on a pillow above the level of the body.

**BLEEDING, HOW TO PROCEED AFTER COMPRESSING THE ARTERY.**—If the flow of blood has been commanded by compression of a distant artery, all clothing, bandages, or dressings should be removed from the wound, and all clots of blood should be washed away, with *cold* water, so that it may be seen exactly where the bleeding comes from. When the wound is quite exposed, the tourniquet or other means used for applying pressure *should be slightly relaxed.* The sides of the wound should be turned up, and any bleeding vessel seen should be sponged with *cold* water, *pressed*, *twisted*, or *tied*, and the wound should be dressed as described at p. 504.

**BLEEDING FROM THE NOSE.**—This may result from injury; or it may occur from a plethoric or too full condition of system; or, on the other hand, from a thin, poor state of the blood, as happens in scurvy, or as the result of venereal, fevers, malarious poisoning, and kidney or liver disease. It may also occur as a consequence of polypus (*vide* p. 355). If the bleeding arises from a blow, it will probably stop after a few minutes, and the application of cold water to the face and back. If it continue from any cause, a pinch of powdered alum dissolved in a couple of table-spoonfuls of cold water may be thrown up the nostrils with a syringe; or powdered alum may be snuffed up if a syringe is not at hand. In all cases of obstinate bleeding from the nose, the body should be kept in the upright posture, and the hands should be raised and held by other persons above the head. A bladder of ice or a cold wet cloth may be applied to the forehead and back of the neck; a piece of cold metal, as a door-key, to the back; and pressure should be made over the facial artery, by placing the finger in the angle formed by the side of the nose and cheek. The nostrils should also be pressed together with the thumb and fingers for half an hour. The feet and legs may be placed in hot mustard-and-water. If these measures do not succeed, plugging the nostrils will be required. The anterior part of the nose is easily plugged by inserting a roll of lint into each nostril, but the posterior nostrils can only be plugged by a surgeon acquainted with the anatomy of the parts, who would probably use an inflatible elastic tube. In some cases the blood may not pass from the nostrils, but, proceeding from the back of the nose, may trickle into the throat and be swallowed or spit out. In such instances plugging the posterior nostrils is still more necessary, as serious injury to the constitution, or even death, has occurred from prolonged bleeding from the nose.

If bleeding from the nose depends on too full a condition of system, recurring perhaps periodically, low diet, purgatives (Recipes 1 and 2), especially if costiveness is present, and astringent medicines (Recipe 42) are the proper remedies. Moderate bleeding from the nose may be regarded as salutary, when the person is red-faced, plethoric, and subject to headache or giddiness. It is then an effort of nature to relieve herself, and, unless violent, should not be suddenly restrained. If the bleeding appears to depend on too low a condition of the system, tonics are necessary, and the diet must be liberal; while any scorbutic, malarious, or venereal condition should be treated (*vide* pp. 380, 266, 458). Bleeding from the nose frequently occurs to children, and in the majority of cases a thin, depraved condition of blood is the cause, and the complaint must be treated accordingly. If bleeding depends on a polypus the growth should be removed (*vide* p. 355).

[Hazeline may be used with a syringe. A cotton-wool plug saturated with a strong solution of antipyrin (antipyrin thirty grains, water a teaspoonful) may be inserted into the nostril. When the bleeding is connected with a plethoric condition of system, sulphuric acid (Recipe 43) is a better remedy than the alum mixture (Recipe 42) mentioned above. When the bleeding depends on simply a feeble state, without special taints as referred to above, iron mixture (Recipe 71).]

**BLEEDING FROM THE SOCKET OF A TOOTH.**—This is sometimes very troublesome or profuse after the extraction or accidental loss of a tooth. It may be stopped by applying a plug of lint to the part, shutting the teeth close, and running a bandage round the chin and head to prevent the mouth being opened for several hours, during which time the pressure thus exerted stops the bleeding. Or the extracted tooth may be returned to its socket to act as a plug, the chin being bandaged as above.

**BLEEDING FROM VARICOSE VEINS OF THE LEG.**—Profuse bleeding may occur from the bursting of enlarged or varicose veins in the legs, especially of pregnant women. The person should lie with the leg higher than the body, and pressure should be made on the bleeding part with a pad of lint or cotton cloth soaked in cold water, till the bleeding stops. Afterwards a pad, and bandage from the foot upwards, should be applied (*vide* p. 495).

**BLEEDING FROM LEECH-BITES.**–Leech-bites, whether made for curative purposes or by leeches attaching themselves to travellers or sportsmen, sometimes give much trouble from bleeding. If the person is moderately strong, and the loss of blood is only from one or two wounds, it may be allowed to go on, and it will stop in a few hours. But if in delicate people or children, the loss of blood must be stopped at once; more especially if the patient is to be left during the night. This is usually effected by the application of cold water, or by pressure with the finger, through which bleeding cannot take place, continued, if necessary, for an hour. If this does not succeed, a pinch of powdered alum should be pressed into the bites.

[Other means, are pledgets of lint dipped iu spirits of wine, which may be pressed into the bite; or the latter may be touched with a finely pointed stick of caustic. Occasionally, it has been found necessary to pass a needle through the skin under the bite, and to tie a ligature below the needle in the form of a figure of ∞ knot.]

**BLEEDING, INTERNAL.**—This occurs from injury or disease of internal blood-vessels. The bleeding may take place into the lungs, when the blood is *coughed up*; into the stomach, when the blood is *vomited up*; into the bowels, when it is *passed by stool*; into the bladder, when it *escapes with the urine*; or into other cavities of the body, from which there is no outlet, as, for instance, within the skull. Internal bleeding, excepting when into the cavity of the skull, is accompanied by great depression and faintness, by cold perspirations, by feeble intermittent pulse; the condition described as *collapse* (*vide* p. 520) being present. When bleeding takes place within the head, laboured breathing and insensibility, as described under *Apoplexy*, are the chief results. Perfect rest, acid drinks, as lemon juice and water, keeping the body cool and the feet warm, are the principal requirements.

**BLEEDING, CONSTITUTIONAL,** or **HÆMOPHILIA.**—This is a disease, often hereditary, to which males are most liable. It is characterised by immoderate bleeding after very slight injuries; and it sometimes occurs without any injury, especially from the gums or nose. The joints often swell when bleeding takes place. It may commence in childhood, and several of a family may be subject to it. A rag spread with powdered alum should be pressed on the bleeding part, and Recipe 67, or, if obtainable, 71, should be given internally.

**BLEEDING, GENERAL TREATMENT OF, AND WHEN TO GIVE STIMULANTS.**—Stimulants, as wine and brandy, should not be hastily given even if there is faintness. Faintness is nature's method of staying bleeding, and stimulants, by exciting the circulation, tend to increase bleeding. On the other hand, if faintness passes beyond a certain limit, it may be fatal. When faintness occurs in a case where there *has not been much bleeding*, and when *no large wound exists*, if there is no internal bleeding the faintness will probably be more from fright than loss of blood. The person should *keep the recumbent posture*, and he should be placed between blankets, bottles of hot water, or hot bricks, wrapped in flannel, being placed near the feet and in the armpits, taking care that the heat is not sufficient to burn the patient. Warm brandy and water should be given frequently in small quantities, the brandy being diluted with an equal quantity of water. *But if there is profuse bleeding, brandy must not be administered so freely*, and it should be given cold. With respect to the actual amount of brandy to be given, no positive rule can be laid down. A table-spoonful every half-hour, if there is no bleeding, and a tea-spoonful if there is, may be accepted as some guide. If brandy is not at hand some other spirit, as whisky or rum, should be used. Until the bleeding has been stopped, warmth should only be applied to the feet; and while faint, *the person must not be raised to an upright position*. Under all circumstances milk or broth may be given, but while there is any fear of bleeding everything must be given cold.

**BLISTERS.**—This term signifies the formation of watery fluid between the upper and middle layers of the skin. They generally result from friction, as of an ill-fitting boot, on the toes or heel. Or they may be produced by irritating substances applied to the skin, or arise from burns or scalds. The proper method of treating a blister, however produced, is, if very small, to smear it with a mixture of spirits of wine and tallow or mutton fat, and then to let it alone, when the contained fluid may be absorbed, and the upper layer of the skin will eventually peel off, leaving a healed surface below. If the blister is large, it should be pricked at the most dependent position, and the water should be allowed to drain out, and a piece of worsted may be passed through the blister and tied in a loop, which will prevent the aperture closing up before the water has drained away. The loose skin above should be preserved as long as possible, as it forms the best covering for the tender surface below. It should be protected by simple ointment (Recipe 86), or olive oil spread on lint, and the part should be carefully guarded from any injury.

To prevent blisters on pedestrian excursions, thin woollen hose and a well-made boot with broad sole, so cut that the upper leather does not unduly compress the foot, are desirable, and the socks should be well soaped previous to long walks. After some hours on the road, changing or turning the socks is desirable. If walking must be performed while blisters are present, take all pressure away from the part by cutting a hole in the leather of the shoe over the blister.

Ulcers of the Toes and Heels may result from neglected blisters, or from a bad state of health. These are troublesome to heal, requiring perfect rest of the part, great cleanliness, dressing with simple ointment (Recipe 86), and attention to the general health.

[Often such ulcers require a stimulating dressing, and when simple dressing does not suit, procure the ointment (Recipe 93).]

**BRUISES.**—Bruises are injuries in which the skin is not broken. They may be slight or severe. In the first variety the surface of the skin only is injured, but the little blood-vessels therein contained being ruptured, blood becomes effused in the skin, and discoloration occurs. This is at first bluish-black, then it passes through shades of violet, green, and yellow, until, by the end of ten days or a fortnight, it disappears. The familiar instance of a 'black-eye' will illustrate this description of bruise. If the injury is more violent, a similar rupture of blood-vessels, and escape of blood, takes place in structures beneath the skin. Or, as sometimes happens, the skin may escape injury, and the deeper parts alone suffer. In this case discoloration does not become apparent until twenty-four hours, or longer, after the injury. For slight bruises, such as occur to children falling down, the old-fashioned remedy of brown-paper steeped in brandy is not a bad application, or spirits of camphor, or tincture of arnica may be painted over the injured surface. For more severe bruises, keep the bruised part well raised, if practicable, lying on a pillow, and fomented continually with hot water and flannels. If the bruise is of a serious nature, blisters will now probably form on the surface of the skin. These must be snipped with sharp scissors at the most dependent part, and the contained water allowed to drain out. But the raised skin or cuticle should *not* be taken away. After the first two days hot fomentations may be *gradually* discontinued, and a cold lotion, composed of 1 ounce of vinegar in 4 ounces of water, may be employed. At a still later period, rubbing the part with brandy and salad oil in equal parts, or, if obtainable, with soap liniment, may be adopted.

Sometimes bruised parts are so injured as to inflame, or a large blood-vessel may be ruptured, and much blood escapes into the tissues. Abscess may form, the skin may burst, and mortification may occur. Poultices of bread and charcoal (*vide Appendix*) should be applied, until the mortifying parts separate, and the wound becomes clean. Surgical interference, in the form of incisions to promote exit of matter, is not unfrequently necessary.

*Bruises or contusions of the head* are frequently followed

by effusion of blood beneath the skin, which is called a *blood-tumour*. This is frequently seen on the heads of newly-born children (*vide* p. 638), caused by the pressure during a prolonged or difficult labour. A blood-tumour, occurring to an adult after an injury, may give rise to a suspicion of a fracture with depression of the bone, as the blood-tumour has generally a hardened base, with a softness or depression towards the centre. There will, however, be an absence of the symptoms of fracture (*vide* p. 556), and firm pressure with the finger on the hardened part will discover the uninterrupted surface of the harder bone beneath. In ordinary cases of bruised scalp, followed by blood-tumour, time and the application of a cold lotion (Recipe 83) will effect a cure.

**BURNS AND SCALDS.**—The effect of burns and scalds on the skin is, in the first instance, the same.

Three different degrees of burning or scalding include all varieties. *1st.* When the contact with fire or water has been slight and the injury is that of redness, or inflammation of the skin. *2nd.* Where blisters have formed from a greater amount of heat. *3rd.* When there is destruction of the skin or underlying structures, or where they are changed into a black or yellow mass, and all vitality destroyed.

*A slight burn or scald* may be treated by the application of lint, or cloth, or plantain leaf soaked in salad oil; or ice pounded or scraped, made as dry as possible, mixed with lard or butter or oil, spread on cotton cloth, and kept on until it melts; or if not available, the part may be covered with a layer of cotton-wool secured by a bandage. Severe burns most frequently happen from the clothing catching fire. The sufferer should not run about, as every draught of air will fan the flame. He should lie down on the floor, and roll, or be rolled in a rug, table cover, carpet, or any convenient article sufficiently voluminous and thick to stifle the flames. Or, such not being available, the person should roll on the floor, until the flames are mechanically put out. If water is at hand, it should be dashed on the person. Then the patient should be laid on a bed, and if there is much shock (*vide* p. 520), which always follows severe burns, and is indicated by cold, shivering, pallor, and faintness, some hot coffee, or wine and water, or brandy and water, whichever may be first available, should be given at once, and bottles of hot water should be applied to the feet. After the first shock has passed away, chloral may be given to relieve pain, in doses according to age (*vide* p. 10). The clothing should be removed by cutting it away from the injured parts. If the skin adheres to the dress, the piece of the latter should be left, rather than the skin be torn in taking it away. The stockings must be removed with great care, lest the upper layer of the skin separate with them, which would increase the sufferings of the patient. It will facilitate the removal of the stockings if they are first soaked with salad oil. In the case of burns or scalds of the hands or feet, it is a good plan to immerse them, with the gloves or stockings on, in cold water. After a few minutes they should be removed, and partially dried with a towel. A mixture of equal parts of tepid milk and water should then be frequently dropped on the glove or stocking. After five or six hours the coverings may be cut carefully away, and the blisters may be snipped. Then, in the absence of the *carron oil* mentioned below, the parts may be covered with lint wet (preferentially) with salad oil, or with milk. But severe burns should, as soon as possible, be dressed with carron oil (Recipe 87), which should be warmed, and then spread thickly on lint or linen rag. Cold applications to extensive burns or scalds should be avoided as most injurious. The first dressings should not be removed for two days, after which the part should be dressed daily, and 5 grains of crystallised carbolic acid should, if obtainable, be added to and well mixed with every 4 ounces of the carron oil. At each removal of the applications the parts must be well cleansed by permitting a stream of warm water to flow over them from a sponge, but the injured parts should not be wiped with the sponge. All blisters should be snipped, but no wrinkled skin or raised cuticle should be removed. In dressing extensive burns, care should be taken to avoid exposing more than a small part at one time, or the cold will be injurious. The cotton-wool dressing, or the plan of dusting burns with fine flour, frequently employed in Europe, is not recommended for severe burns or scalds in India. As such applications are used on the principle of excluding air, they must be suffered to remain *in situ* several days, becoming hard, dry, irritating, and liable to harbour maggots. When the surface becomes red, healthy, and clean-looking, nothing will be more beneficial than simple water dressing, *id est*, lint soaked in tepid water, laid on the part, and the whole covered with oil-skin. If granulations become exuberant, growing above the surrounding skin, and forming what is popularly called 'proud flesh,' they must be lightly touched with alum.

*Superficial burns and scalds, although only producing redness of the surface, are, if extensive, and particularly if occurring to children, very dangerous*; stupor and insensibility are especially liable to occur to children after extensive burns; burns of the body are more dangerous than those of the limbs; shivering is a bad symptom; insensibility to pain, stupor, and twitchings of the limbs, are the usual precursors of death. Persons with bad burns are peculiarly liable to attacks of bronchitis, or inflammation of the lungs; to diarrhœa, accompanied by ulceration of the intestines; also to *pyæmia* (*vide* p. 587).

Burns or Scalds of the Fingers and Toes must be treated with great care, that the different parts may be kept separate, so as to prevent the raw surfaces of the fingers or toes touching each other. This may be readily effected by different dressings.

INTERNAL SCALDS OF THE THROAT, affecting the upper part of the windpipe or *glottis*, are very dangerous, from the swelling they occasion inside the throat. Such injuries most frequently occur to children, the symptoms being suffocative cough and difficulty of breathing. Ice to the throat, ice to suck, water and milk to moisten the mouth and throat, and a tea-spoonful of salad oil every three hours are the best remedies. But such cases frequently require the windpipe opened by a surgical operation.

BURNS FROM CORROSIVE LIQUIDS, as oil of vitriol and mineral acids, should be treated in the first instance by copious washing with water, or if available with soda and water; and afterwards as ordinary burns.

BURNS AND SCALDS, SEQUEL OF.—As burns heal, there is always tendency to contraction of the parts, especially if the injury is about the neck or joints. During healing every endeavour should be made, by bandaging, pads, and splints, to keep the parts in their natural position, and thus oppose the tendency to deformity. Cicatrices, disfiguring scars, contracted joints, and deep ulcers, sometimes the results of burns and scalds, require treatment by a surgeon.

**COLLAPSE, SHOCK,** or **PROSTRATION.**—This is an accompaniment of severe injuries, as gunshot wounds, laceration of joints, blows on the stomach or privates, bad burns or scalds, and great losses of blood. Collapse may also be produced by fear, by cold, and from large doses of certain poisons. The condition is very similar in appearance to fainting (*vide* p. 234). In some cases there are nausea, hiccough, and vomiting from the first. Occasionally the person is bewildered and incoherent, as if intoxicated. Vomiting is often a prelude to recovery, the first sign of which is called the *reaction.* Favourable signs are, returning warmth of the surface of the body, and slight restlessness on the part of the patient, with inclination to lie on the side. After a few hours there may be fever indicated by a hot skin, a flushed face, and rapid pulse. These symptoms in favourable cases soon pass off. In unfavourable cases the febrile symptoms increase, and after a few hours signs of nervous excitement and of *exhaustion* appear. There is trembling of the tendons of the wrist, restlessness, and generally delirium. The pulse becomes feeble, the skin cold, and there may be hiccough. Patients who have been accustomed to take considerable quantities of beer or spirits frequently present, during the stage of *reaction,* a condition very similar to *delirium tremens.* In individuals who are naturally weak and delicate, *reaction,* although favourable in its progress, may be slow, so that complete recovery is not attained for several days.

*Treatment.*—The requirements are to keep up the action of the heart and lungs, and to maintain the temperature of the body, until the effects of the sudden shock to the brain and nervous system have passed away, but the treatment should differ with reference to the *presence or absence of bleeding* (*vide* p. 514, *general treatment of bleeding*). If there is no bleeding the person should be placed between blankets, bottles of hot water or hot bricks wrapped in flannel being placed near the feet and in the armpits, taking care that the heat is not sufficient to burn the person. Warm brandy (or other spirit) and water should be given frequently in small quantities, the brandy being diluted with an equal proportion of water. Until *reaction* has well advanced, *the patient must not be raised to an upright position.* After reaction is established, and the patient becomes feverish, purgatives (Recipes 1 and 2) and cooling medicine, as citrate of magnesia, will probably be required. The treatment of unfavourable symptoms of *exhaustion* consists in support by nourishing broths or beef-tea, and in allaying nervous irritability by sedatives, of which chloral (Recipe 64) is one of the best.

**CONCUSSION OF THE BRAIN**, or **BRAIN-SHAKE.**—This condition, commonly called 'stunning,' signifies sudden interruption of the functions of the brain, by a blow or other injury to the head, either direct or indirect. In the mildest form the patient experiences a sudden weakness and trembling in the limbs, cannot walk without staggering, and there is a ringing sound in the ears and dimness of sight. These symptoms soon pass away, after the person has rested for a time in a darkened room. In the *more severe* form of concussion the person falls, and lies motionless, pale and unconscious. The skin is cold and the pulse weak. The eyelids are closed, the pupils of the eyes contracted, and the arms and legs generally bent on the body. The breathing is feeble and sighing, and, if the patient is roused and questioned loudly, he opens his eyes and answers hastily, and again relapses into insensibility. *The two facts stated in the last paragraph mainly serve to distinguish concussion from compression of the brain* (*vide* p. 525), when the breathing is heavy and laboured, and the patient cannot be roused. After a variable time, ordinarily about an hour, the patient moves uneasily, vomits, and recovers his senses, but remains giddy, confused, and sleepy for some hours. In a *still more severe degree* of concussion, the patient is more profoundly insensible, the surface of the body pale and cold, the pulse not only weak but also intermittent, and the breathing drawn in sighs. If the patient cannot be temporarily roused, if the pupils of the eyes are insensible to light, and if the legs are not drawn away, when the soles of the feet are tickled, the condition is very unfavourable.

Concussion of the brain often leaves mischief which may be permanent and of serious import. There may arise an irritability of the brain, marked by hasty, violent temper, or by very speedy excitement after drinking spirits or wine; there may be defects of sight, hearing, smell, or speech, muscular weakness and nervous debility; or temporary or permanent insanity may result. These sequences are due in many cases to indiscretion on the part of the patient, who as soon as the symptoms of concussion have passed away, and while the brain is still irritable and enfeebled, returns to his former habits, and probably to brain work.

*Treatment.*—No case of concussion, or of partial concussion, is so trivial that it may be neglected with impunity. The patient should be placed on a bed or couch in a quiet, darkened room, the neck and chest should be freed from articles of clothing, the head should be slightly raised, and a cold wet cloth should be applied to the forehead. In more severe cases, when the surface of the body is cold, the patient should be placed between blankets, bottles filled with hot water and wrapped in flannel should be applied to the feet and armpits, and the legs, hands, and arms should be well rubbed. Stimulants must *not* be administered, but as soon as the patient can swallow, a little water may be given, or, if procurable, milk, broth, or beef-tea. If there is long-continued insensibility or imperfect rallying, an assafœtida injection (Recipe 105) should be used. Natural sleep should be encouraged. The after-treatment consists of perfect rest both of body and mind, and in maintaining the bowels freely open by aperients (Recipes 1 and 2), with a mild nutritious diet. Stimulants of all kinds must be avoided, and the person must return gradually to former occupations. If headache or feverishness comes on, or any impairment of the mental faculties is observed, a strong mustard poultice (or, if procurable, a blister) should be applied to the back of the neck, and the bowels should be still more freely purged. If unfavourable symptoms persist, it may be necessary to cut the hair close, and to apply leeches to the temples.

**CONCUSSION OF THE SPINE.**—Usually occurs from severe shakings, as happen on carriage or railway accidents, or from blows on the spine. Concussion of the spine is marked by more or less severe pain at the seat of injury, bodily prostration, weakness of the lower limbs, or difficulty of walking, numbness in the feet, and diminished sensation of the lower extremities. In more severe cases there may be difficulty of making water, and swelling of the bowels, due to their distension by gas. If the injury has been only shaking of the spinal marrow, and nothing has been torn or ruptured, these symptoms usually subside in the course of two or three weeks, and the patient recovers. In some instances permanent weakness of the lower limbs, or even complete palsy, with difficulty or inability of making water, results. The *treatment* consists mainly in keeping the patient in bed, in applying leeches to the painful part of the back, and in giving tonics and nourishing food.

Severe shakings consequent on *railway accidents* have resulted in a peculiar condition of the spinal cord, to which the term 'railway spine' has been applied. The rapidity of the movement causing the injury, the momentum of the person injured, the suddenness of its arrest, the helplessness of the sufferer, and the natural fear occasioned, are all circumstances in railway accidents greatly increasing the severity of the injury to the nervous system. A person is often unaware that anything serious has happened, feeling perhaps only violently jolted and a little giddy and confused. After a day or two, he becomes excited, cannot sleep, and feels bruised all over, or as if he had gone through some violent exertion. After another few days he finds he is unable to undergo any exertion, or to attend to business. The thoughts become confused, the temper irritable, the sleep disturbed, and there are often noises and singing in the ears. The senses of hearing, taste, and smell sometimes become perverted. There is also a loss of freedom of movement, and the gait becomes uncertain and 'straddling,' while one or both of the feet may be unusually cold. The first requirement is *complete rest*, both for body and mind, and cold lotions or ice should be applied over any part of the spine in which pain is felt. Internally, the bichloride of mercury, with quinine and bark, are perhaps the most satisfactory remedies.

A similar condition arises from fright, as during the bombardment of cities, from fires, or from lightning-stroke.

**COMPRESSION OF THE BRAIN.**—This results either from blood being effused beneath the skull, or from a piece or pieces of bone being detached or depressed, and driven down on the brain or its membranes, which the blood or other substance *compresses*. Both conditions may be the result of injuries. At a later period compression may result as the consequence of 'matter' formed within the skull as a sequence of an injury. When, after the symptoms of *Concussion of the Brain* (*vide* p. 522), or after severe injuries without such symptoms, the patient does not revive; or reviving, afterwards sinks into stupor, from which he cannot be roused; with heavy laboured breathing, accompanied by puffing movement of the muscles of the mouth, with one or both pupils of the eyes dilated, with the surface of the body becoming warmer, and the pulse quicker and full, and perhaps with bleeding, or watery discharge from the ears and nose, serious injury of the brain may be suspected. Stimulants must *not* be given, but a cold lotion may be applied to the head and purgative injections (Recipe 105) should be administered. The condition requires skilled advice, as the operation of 'trepanning' may be necessary.

The principal distinctions between *concussion* and *compression* of the brain are given below.

| CONCUSSION | COMPRESSION |
|---|---|
| Insensibility takes place immediately on receipt of injury. | Insensibility, although sometimes present from the first, generally comes on gradually. |
| Breathing feeble, intermittent, diminished in force, often sighing, never stertorous. | Breathing slow and laboured, often stertorous, and accompanied with puffing movement of the lips and cheeks. |
| Pulse small, thready, intermittent, sometimes quick. | Pulse slow, full, and bounding. |
| Pupils of the eyes generally contracted. | Pupils generally dilated. |

| Concussion | Compression |
|---|---|
| Skin sensitive to prick of pin, or to pinching. | Skin not sensitive. |
| Surface of body cold and pale. | Surface of body warm, moist, and of natural colour. |
| Patient can be roused so as to answer questions. | Patient cannot be roused. |
| Retching and vomiting are very constant symptoms. | Retching and vomiting absent. |

**DISLOCATIONS.**—A bone is dislocated, or, vulgarly, 'put out,' when the head of the bone slips from the socket in which it plays. Therefore the injury must be at a joint.

*Symptoms.*—1. Pain. 2. Deformity; there being an alteration of the normal shape of the joint; such as an unnatural prominence in one part, and a depression at another, with generally *shortening*, but in some varieties *lengthening*, of the limb. 3. Loss of the proper motion of the joint.

*Dislocations are distinguished from fractures* near the joint; *first*, by the absence of *grating* on movement of the injured parts; *secondly*, a fractured bone is more freely movable than natural, a dislocated bone is less so; *thirdly*, if a fractured bone is drawn into its proper place it will return as soon as the 'extension,' or pulling, is discontinued; but a dislocated bone drawn into its proper position will remain there; *fourthly*, by measurement of the *bone* supposed to be broken, which, if fractured, will be shortened, while the dislocated bone is of the natural length. Comparisons of the length should be made with the bone of the sound limb.

*Dislocations are distinguished from sprains* (*vide* p. 596) by pressing the swollen part steadily and firmly. If it be a dislocation the end of the bone is felt firm and hard; while the swelling caused by a sprain is soft and yielding. Also by the facts, that neither *lengthening* nor *shortening* are caused by the sprains; while natural motion of the joint, although painful, is possible.

*Treatment.*—The immediate treatment of any injury is given at p. 497. Dislocations must be 'reduced,' or returned into place. Sometimes this can be effected by placing the parts in such a position that the muscles will draw the head of the bone into the socket. Most dislocated bones may be readily returned into place by pulling the limb and manipulation, *immediately after they are put out.* But when any time has passed and the faintness usually caused by the accident is recovered from, a greater degree of force, or chloroform, are required to put the bone in place. Dislocations should, therefore, always be reduced as soon as possible, before the muscles swell or contract and fix the bone in its new position. When an hour or so after the accident has passed, or when all faintness has subsided, it would be wiser to delay any attempt to reduce a dislocation till assistance could be obtained, provided it could be available within twenty-four hours. The harm that ensues from the delay is more than compensated for by the great good secured by the use of chloroform or other anæsthetic. But if chloroform and surgical aid cannot be secured within a reasonable time, it will be better to make careful attempts to put the bone in place, even although the first effects of the accident have passed away. After reduction the limb should be kept at rest and fixed by bandages. Fomentations will usually be necessary to relieve inflammatory pain and swelling. When all pain and swelling has disappeared the joint may be *gently moved by another person,* in order to prevent the formation of adhesions which might eventually cause a stiff joint (*vide* p. 597).

Compound Dislocation is the term applied to those cases where an external wound communicates with the dislocated joint, and such injuries are always most dangerous.

**DISLOCATION OF THE LOWER JAW.**—This may be caused by a blow on the mouth, or from spasmodic action of the muscles, when a person gapes. The mouth is open and cannot be shut. Speech and swallowing are scarcely possible, the saliva dribbles away, and the chin protrudes forwards, so that the lower row of teeth project beyond the middle teeth of the jaw above. Sometimes one side

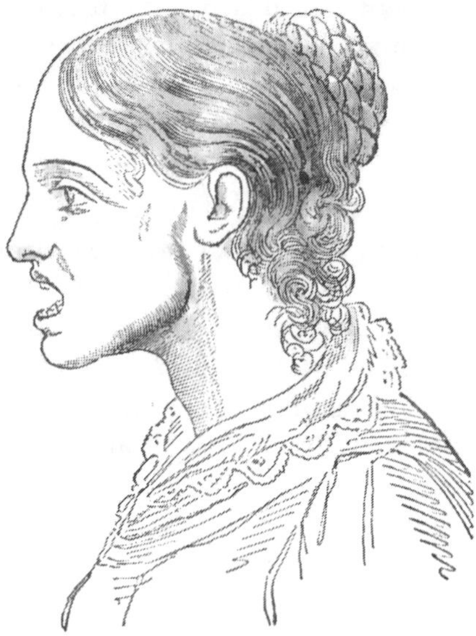

only of the bone is dislocated, and then the teeth are displaced laterally *away* from the side of dislocation.

*Treatment.*—Put the patient in a chair, with the back of the head against a wall. Then let the operator wrap a napkin or handkerchief round each of his thumbs. Place the thumbs thus protected on the *back teeth of the lower jaw*, on each side, the fingers clasping the under part of the jaw outside. Then press the thumbs firmly downwards and backwards, elevating the chin at the same time with the fingers. The jaw will generally return into its proper place with a snap, and, if the thumbs of the operator were not protected, they would probably be injured by the patient's teeth. Afterwards a four-tailed bandage, as described for a broken jaw (*vide* p. 559), should be worn for a week, during which time the patient should have only fluid food.

**DISLOCATION OF THE COLLAR-BONE.**—This usually occurs from falls on the shoulder. The dislocated head of the bone may be felt as a protrusion over the upper part of the breast-bone, and the arm cannot be raised. To restore it, the shoulder should be pressed *upwards, outwards,* and *backwards.* This may be accomplished by drawing back the shoulders with the hands, while pressing against the spine with the knee. If necessary the end of the bone should also be pressed *upwards* with the finger and thumb into its place. To retain it there, bandages should be applied as for *fractured collar-bone* (*vide* p. 560), but a pad should be also placed *over the end of the bone,* and the bandage should be broad, to keep the pad and bone in position. This should be worn night and day for five or six weeks; but in spite of every care, some deformity often results, as it is usually difficult to retain the bone in position.

**DISLOCATION OF THE SHOULDER-JOINT.**—The *humerus,* or arm-bone, may be thrown from its socket in several different directions, but most commonly it slips by the side of the socket, or below the socket, into the armpit. If the bone slips by the side of the socket, the arm is slightly shortened; if below the socket the arm is lengthened. A hollow is seen or felt under the tip of the shoulder, where the head of the bone should be, and the whole shoulder looks flattened. The elbow projects out from the side, and cannot be brought to touch the side. The head of the bone can be felt in the armpit, becoming more evident if the elbow is raised. There is also great pain, and numbness of the fingers, caused by the pressure of the dislocated head of the bone on the nerves of the arm. The patient leans over to the side of dislocation, and endeavours to support the elbow of the injured side with the opposite hand.

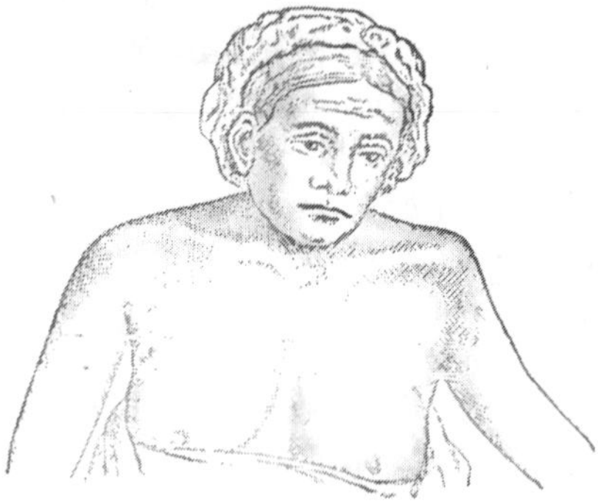

In addition to the above-mentioned signs (or without such features, if the dislocation is in other directions), the shoulder may be recognised as 'out of joint,' if the fingers of the injured limb cannot be placed by the patient, or by some one else, on the sound shoulder, while the elbow touches the side. In the natural state of the parts this can be easily done; and if it can be accomplished there is no dislocation. Again, the shoulder should be measured, by carrying a tape round the prominent bone at the tip, and under the armpit. If the shoulder is out, the injured side will measure about two inches more than the sound one. Thirdly, if there is a dislocation, a straight stick or rule will touch both the tip of the shoulder and the elbow at the same time, which it cannot do when the bones are in their natural places.

*Treatment.*—There are several methods by which this injury may be righted; *but if grating should be felt or heard on moving the injured limb, attempts at replacement should not be continued, as there is probably also fracture* (*vide* p. 561).

*First.* If the person is seen immediately. Put a cloth or shawl round the patient's body close under the armpit, and let some one hold the ends to steady the body. Then raise the arm gently to a right angle if possible. Then pull from above the wrist, steadily with moderate force, and the bone will probably slip into its place. If not successful the next methods may be tried.

*Secondly.* By the heel, or foot, in the *axilla* or armpit. The patient lies down on a bed, or on the floor, and the operator sits on the edge of the bed, or on the floor, at the patient's side. The operator then places his *unbooted* foot in the armpit, pressing upwards and outwards, at the same time grasping the hand and wrist, which he pulls

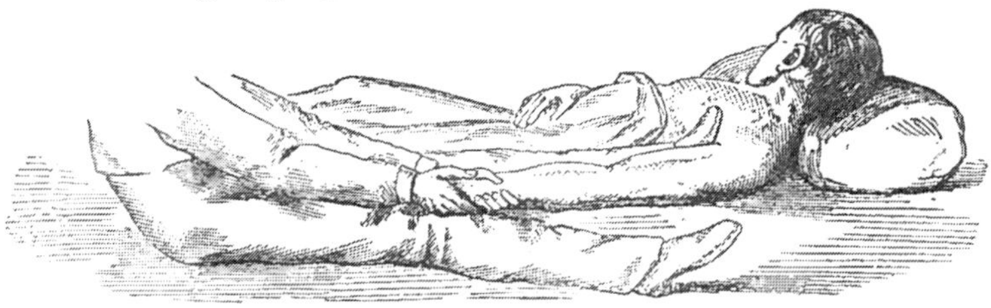

steadily towards him, gradually carrying the hand across the patient's body. When commencing to pull, he should tell the patient to make some change in his position, in order to take his attention away, by which the resistance of the muscles implicated in the dislocation will be lessened. The head of the bone will then probably pass into its place. The left foot should be used if the left arm is to be operated on, and *vice versâ.*

*Thirdly.* Have the patient seated on a chair, rest your foot on the chair, and place the bent knee in the armpit. The positions necessary are shown in the sketch accompanying the fourth method. Then depress the elbow with the hand, and at the same time raise the head of the bone with the knee, and it will probably glide into its place.

One or other of these methods will usually be successful in persons who are not very muscular, or when the shoulder has been dislocated a second or third time in the same person. But if not successful, or for muscular persons, the most certain plan is with the towels as described below, by which more force can be applied.

*Fourthly.* A long strong towel, or other piece of cloth, should have a slit made in the centre. Through this slit

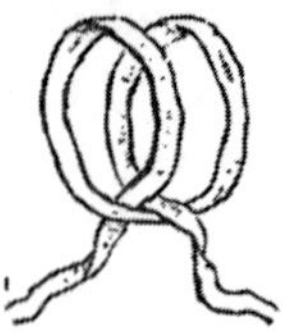

the hand and arm must be passed, until the towel presses on the chest below, and on the upper part of the shoulder above. Another long towel, or piece of cloth, must be fastened round the arm above the elbow. When fixing this, the knot called the *clove-hitch* should be used, as it does not tighten round the limb when pulled (*vide* sketch). The patient should then sit on a low stool.

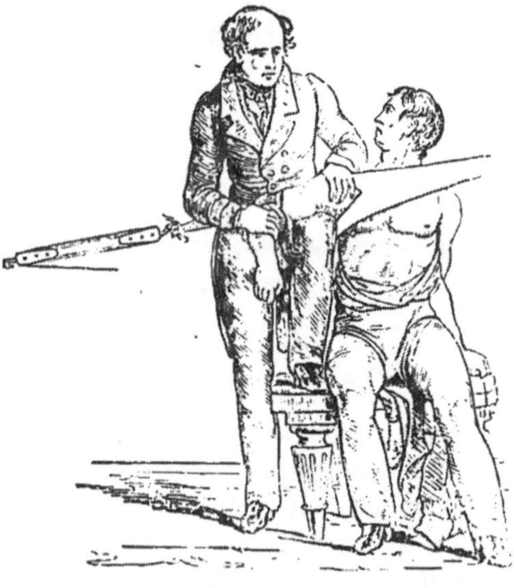

Then, let the chest towel be firmly held, while the arm towel is *gradually* pulled by assistants, the operator standing behind the arm. After the extension has been continued for two or three minutes the operator should lift the head of the bone with his knee, when it will probably pass into the socket. The positions necessary are shown in the preceding drawing.

A person who has repeatedly dislocated his shoulder, and the accident is always more liable to happen after having once occurred, may, if he have courage to bear a little pain, manage to reduce it himself. By getting his arm over the top rail of a gate, or over any other object affording similar purchase (which, should be first covered by some article of clothing), seizing one of the lower rails with the hand of the injured arm, letting the whole weight of the body hang over the other side of the gate, and then making some movement to change the position of the body while its weight still tells on the top bar, the bone will probably slip into its place. The principle is the same as when the heel is put into the armpit, and the arm pulled. The head of the arm-bone is moved towards the edge of the socket from which it has escaped, and the muscles pull it into its place. The position is shown above.

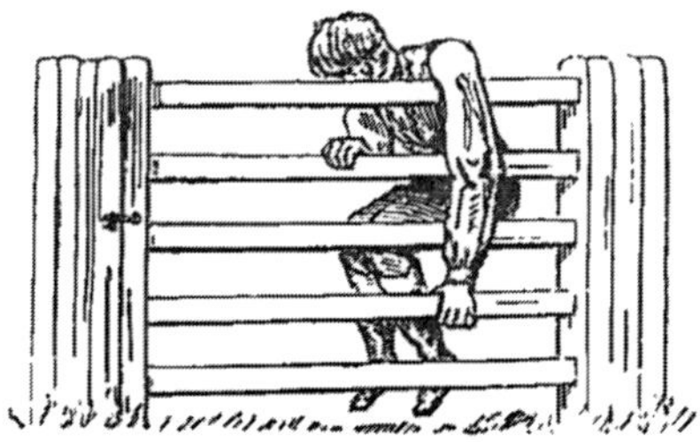

After a dislocated shoulder has been replaced, the *elbow and arm* should be put in a sling, and the arm should be confined for a fortnight to the side by a bandage passing lightly round the body. When the person begins to move about, the 'pin sling' (*vide* p. 464) may be used.

**DISLOCATION OF THE ELBOW.**—This may occur backwards, or to either side, and one or both bones of the forearm may be displaced. In complete dislocation there is much deformity and swelling, the joint being bent at a right angle, and remaining almost immovable, while the elbow protrudes, the end of the arm-bone can be felt in front of the elbow, and the thumb and outer surface of

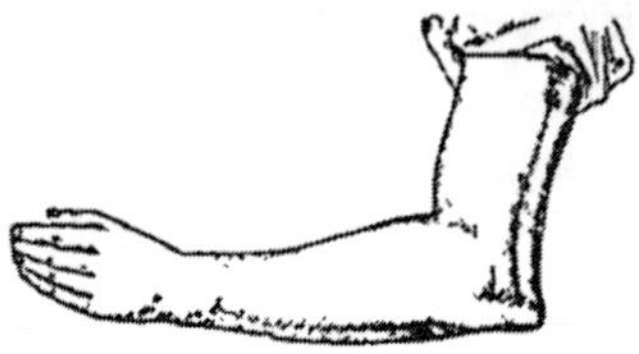

the wrist are turned forwards. In dislocation to one side there is more deformity on that side. In dislocation of one bone only the deformity is less. Dislocation of the elbow is chiefly to be distinguished from fractures about the joint by the absence of grating.

*Treatment.*—One person must take firm hold of and steady the upper arm above the elbow. Another must pull from the wrist. After extension for about two minutes, the elbow must be suddenly bent by the person holding the wrist, when the bones will resume their natural position. The arm should be kept in a sling for seven or eight days, after which the joint should be gently moved.

It often happens that in injuries of this joint one or other form of dislocation is combined with one or other form of fracture, especially of the bones forming the point, and side prominences of the elbow. This complicates the case; splints are generally required, and the services of a surgeon should be procured. Until professional aid is obtained, the best plan is to lay the elbow, bent almost at right angles, on a pillow, and apply a cold lotion (Recipe 83).

PARTIAL DISLOCATION OF THE ELBOW IN CHILDREN.—The forearm of children from a fall or drag upon the wrist, is subject to a displacement caused by the head of the smaller bone (or *radius*) slipping forward and lodging against the front part of the bone of the arm, where it may usually be felt. The arm thus injured hangs down, and the hand is supported by the other. The hand is also turned inwards and downwards. Attempts to move the hand give considerable pain. The position which the child thus injured naturally assumes, as the most easy posture, namely, supporting the injured forearm with the sound hand, gives an appearance at first sight very much resembling the characteristic posture assumed by persons with fractured collar-bone. But on feeling the latter bone it will be found there is no fracture there. To remedy this accident at once, take hold of the upper arm firmly with the left hand, and the patient's hand with the right hand, in such a manner that the back of the patient's hand lies in the palm of the operator's. Now bend the elbow-joint quickly, turning the forearm outwards, so as to bring the palm of the patient's hand to front his upper arm. A crack will probably be felt, and the child will be able to use the arm. A bandage should be applied, and the arm kept at rest in a sling for some days, as the bone is liable to slip again.

**DISLOCATION OF THE WRIST.**—This may be distinguished by the altered position of the hand, which is thrown backwards or forwards, or is twisted, if only one bone is dislocated.

*Treatment.*—Extension of the hand, and if the natural position is not retained the application of splints as for fractured forearm. Fractures of the lower end of the forearm are sometimes mistaken for dislocations, and it often happens that when the large, or under bone of the arm is dislocated, the small or upper bone is broken. In all cases of doubt, after extension, it will be best to apply splints as for fracture. (*Vide Fracture of the Forearm*, p. 565.)

**DISLOCATION OF THE THUMB AND FINGERS.**—These accidents are known by the deformity present, and in consequence of the strength and tightness of the ligatures fixing the joints such injuries are often difficult to treat.

*Treatment.*—If the dislocated bone does not return into

position by simple extension with the hand, a firm hold must be obtained by a piece of tape fastened as represented below, by the clove-hitch knot (*vide* p. 532). Then the

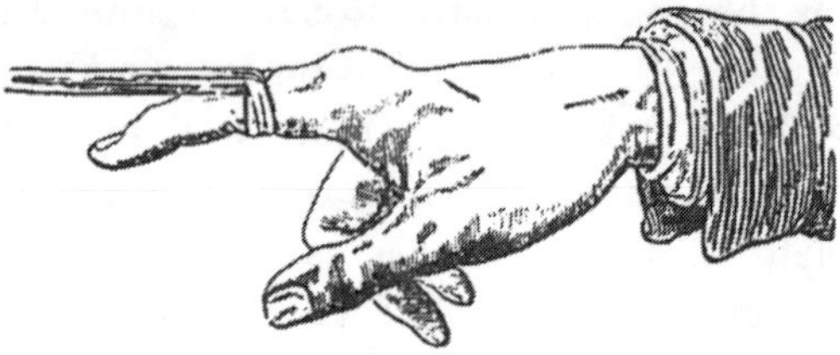

wrist must be held by one person, while another pulls the tape till the bone slips into its place.

**DISLOCATION OF THE HIP-JOINT.**—There are four principal varieties of this dislocation, but the dislocation *upwards* is the most frequent. The injured limb is from one inch to one inch and a half *shorter* than the other. The toes rest on the upper surface of the foot, or on the instep of the sound limb, the knee is turned inwards, and is advanced on its fellow, the hip generally appears flattened, but the dislocated head of the thigh-bone forms an unnatural prominence above and behind the situation of the hip-joint, the limb cannot be moved, and if force is applied to straighten the limb the patient's back becomes arched.

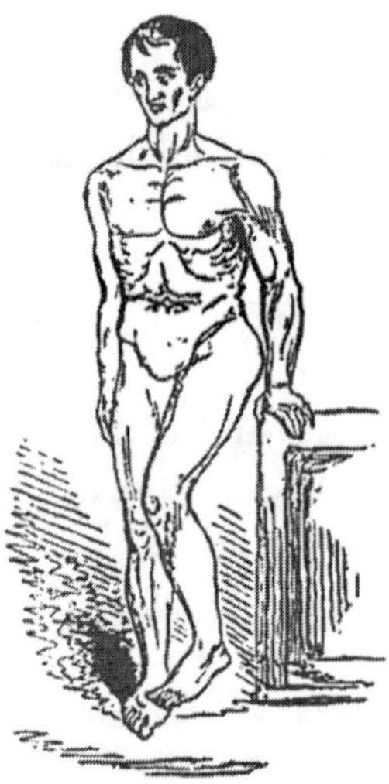

*Fracture* near the head of the thigh-bone is distinguished by these differences: In fracture the limb can be moved more freely; it is turned outwards instead of inwards; it can be drawn down to its natural level, but becomes again shortened as soon as the extension is discontinued; whereas a dislocated bone requires forcible extension to place the limb in its natural position, from which it does not again escape. The position of the limb, when the hip is dislocated upwards, is shown on the opposite page, and may be compared with *fracture*, p. 570.

To recognise and treat other, and less frequent forms of dislocation of this bone, so much special knowledge is necessary that no other variety is here described.

*Treatment.*—Dislocation of the hip is an injury urgently requiring treatment by a surgeon who may probably, when the patient is put under the influence of chloroform, replace the bone by manipulation, without the employment of force. Surgical aid being impossible, the following plans may be carefully tried. Either measure will be more likely to succeed if the patient can be put under the influence of chloroform. If chloroform is not available, 1 grain of tartar emetic may be given in an ounce of water every half-hour till nausea is produced, and which is attended with relaxation of the muscles.

*First.* Place the patient upon his back on the floor, with a pillow under the head. Then the operator should stand over him between his legs and opposite the knee-joints. The operator then clasps his hands below the knee of the injured limb, raises it, and places the ankle of the patient between his own thighs, the upper part of the patient's foot pressing against the operator's buttocks. He then lifts steadily, until the patient's body as far as the shoulders is raised from the floor, in which position it should be held for half a minute, or if possible a minute, when a click heard may denote that the head of the bone has slipped into its socket.

*Secondly.* Place the patient on his back on the floor, and, while he is firmly held by the shoulders, grasp the foot and ankle firmly, and by gradual extension parallel with the body, and rotation of the limb outwards at the same time, the head of the bone, if recently dislocated, will probably slip into its place.

*Thirdly.* If these methods do not succeed, more force must be used. A strong towel or sheet must be passed round the upper part of the thigh, and so adjusted that it does not interfere with or press on the private parts. This towel must be secured to a hook or ring in the wall, or to a tree. A bandage must next be applied over the thigh, as a protection to the skin, and then another towel or sheet must be fixed by the clove-hitch knot (*vide* p. 532) to the same part. When all is prepared extension must be firmly but gradually made, so as to draw the thigh across the opposite one a little above the knee. After a couple of minutes the knee should be gently turned, and the head or upper part of the thigh lifted up, when the head of the bone will perhaps return into its socket.

The position for the reduction of a dislocated hip is shown below.

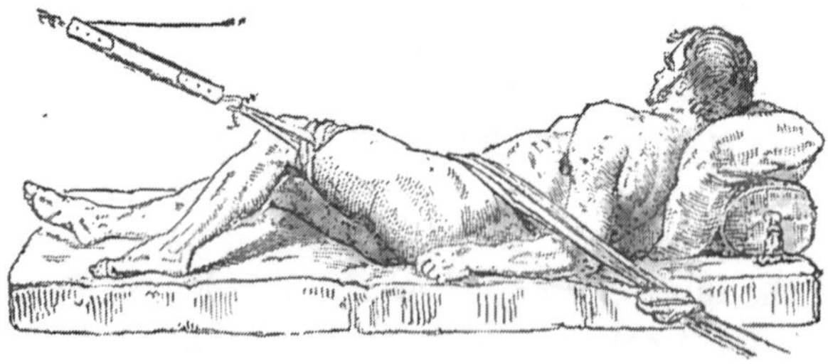

After the reduction of the hip the knees should be tied together, and the patient should be kept in bed. No movement should be allowed for three weeks, and then only gentle movement, for if this rule is not attended to, re-dislocation may occur. After such injuries it sometimes happens that the patient is unable to make water. Fomentations over the bowels will perhaps relieve this condition; otherwise the catheter must be passed (*vide* p. 493).

When no attempt can be made to reduce a dislocated

hip, or when attempts fail, the patient should lie on the back, and his thighs should be fastened together with a broad bandage.

**DISLOCATION OF THE KNEE-CAP.**—This bone may be dislocated either inwards or outwards, most frequently in the latter direction. In some cases it is half-twisted on its axis, so that its outer or inner edge rests upon the front of the lower extremity of the thigh-bone. A twisted knee-cap is the worst form of this injury, and it occasionally becomes so immovably fixed that it cannot be replaced. The symptoms are that the knee cannot be bent, and the bone may be felt in its new position, while there is a depression in the natural position of the bone.

*Treatment.*—It should be replaced by placing the patient on his back, straightening and well raising the leg, so as to relax the muscles in front, and then lifting the bone with the thumb and fingers into the middle of the joint, after which a splint should be applied loosely *behind* the knee. Then the patient must be put to bed, and fomentations should be employed to prevent inflammation. The person should not attempt to walk for a month, and then use a bandage round the knee, or an elastic knee-cap. The injury is likely to recur unless great care is taken.

**DISLOCATION OF THE KNEE-JOINT.**—The leg may be displaced from the knee, forwards, backwards, or to either side, but owing to the large extent of the opposed surfaces forming the joint, and to the strength of the ligaments, dislocation of the knee is always partial. In lateral displacement there is an unnatural projection of the inner or outer extremity (condyle) of the thigh-bone on the one side, and a projection of the inner or outer extremity of the leg-bone on the other, while the foot and leg are generally more or less twisted. Dislocations of the knee-joint, either forwards or backwards, are still more serious injuries, and are associated with much tearing of ligaments and soft parts surrounding the joint. In the backward dislocation the lower end of the thigh-bone projects in front, and the hollow at the back of the joint is occupied by the displaced head of the leg-bone. The dislocation forwards is rare, and is accompanied by much laceration of the soft parts, and often by rupture of the hamstring tendons.

*Treatment.*—The thigh should be fixed by being tightly held while the patient lies on his back. Then extension should be made by pulling steadily from the ankle. After the parts have resumed the natural position, fomentations should be applied, and the patient should be kept in bed for at least three weeks.

**DISLOCATION OF THE SEMILUNAR CARTILAGES OF THE KNEE-JOINT.**—The semilunar cartilages are two flat gristly structures of a horse-shoe shape, which are fixed to the margins of the upper surface of the leg-bone. One (usually the internal) or both may, in consequence of a sprain or twist, become detached and slip out of place, or a piece may be broken off. The symptoms are sudden, severe, *sickening* pain in the knee, and inability to walk. But the leg, though stiff and painful when the person is erect, can be generally moved when he lies down. After the accident the knee begins to swell, and remains swollen for some days. When the swelling subsides a painful spot is usually left, generally at the inside of the joint, where sometimes the displaced cartilage, or the piece broken off, may be felt or seen projecting, if it has not been properly replaced. If the patient is seen immediately, before the joint begins to swell, reduction of the cartilage may be readily effected by extending the leg, and pulling with some force from the ankle, when probably the cartilage will resume its place with an audible click. If this does not suffice, the leg when extended, should be suddenly bent backwards at the knee, until the heel almost touches the corresponding buttock, the other hand of the operator being placed on the front of the knee. Afterwards fomentations and rest for some time will be necessary. If the patient is not seen until the knee is swollen, fomentations and rest should be had recourse to, and the cartilages may gradually assume their natural position. But if a piece has been broken off, it may remain for months until eventually absorbed. The patient should not attempt to walk until all pain and swelling have ceased. This injury having once happened is very liable to recur from slight causes, and the person should wear a stout long bandage or a tight knee-cap for months afterwards. A bandage is better than a knee-cap, as it affords more support. If a knee-cap is used, it should be made of perforated india-rubber.

**DISLOCATION OF THE ANKLE.**—This is generally caused by jumping from heights, or from carriages in motion, and is nearly always complicated with fracture of the small bone of the leg above the ankle. The dislocation may be either inwards or outwards, and the swelling on either side will be the chief distinguishing mark. The dislocation outwards, involving fracture of the small bone on the outside, generally two or three inches above the ankle, is the most common variety. The shape of the limb will then be as opposite, presenting a hollow on the outer side at the site of the fracture of the small bone, the sole of the foot being turned rather inwards.

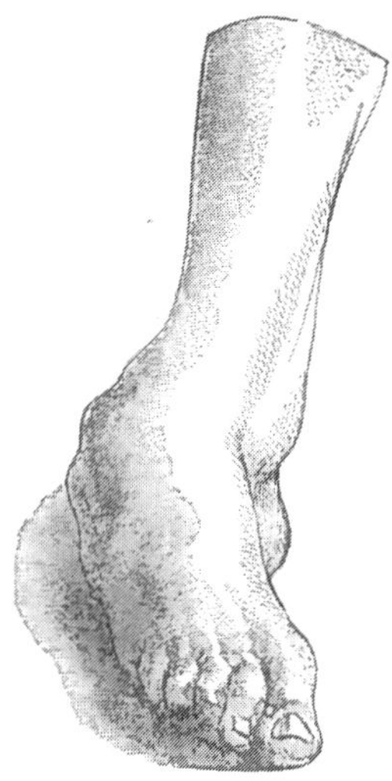

*Treatment.*—The person should be placed on his back, with the thigh raised and the knee bent. Then, while an assistant steadies the knee, the operator must grasp the instep with one hand and the heel with the other, and pull gradually and firmly till he has restored the parts to a natural shape. Then the limb should be bound up with splints on each side, as for a fractured leg; care being taken to keep the great toe on a line with the inner side of the knee-pan. The patient should lie on his back, although some surgeons prefer treating this accident by placing the patient on the side corresponding with the injury, the knee being bent. (*Vide Fractures of the Leg*, p. 575.) The splints should be retained for six weeks, and afterwards gentle movement of the joints should be made; but the person should not bear any weight on the limb for another month.

**DISLOCATIONS OF THE BONES OF THE FOOT.**—Such injuries are the result of great violence, are mostly attended with fractures, and will require the attention of a surgeon. Until this can be obtained the parts should be placed as far as possible in the natural position, perfect rest on a pillow should be enjoined, and fomentations applied.

**DROWNING.**—The injurious effects of submersion in water may be varied. If the water is warm, the principal hurtful effect will be the suspension of respiration, or suffocation; but if, as is often the case, the water be cold enough to extract heat from the body, a very powerful depressing action is added. Again, persons falling into the water may die from fright or syncope (*vide* p. 234); or they may be stunned (*vide* p. 522) if they fall from a great height. Those who sink at once are usually affected in one of these two ways. In the treatment of drowning, ARTIFICIAL RESPIRATION should be promptly resorted to and perseveringly continued. The following rules are those sanctioned by the Royal Humane Society:—

Send immediately for medical assistance, blankets, and dry clothing, but proceed to treat the patient INSTANTLY, securing as much fresh air as possible. Under no circumstances hold the body up by the feet.

The points to be aimed at are—first, and immediately, the *Restoration of Breathing*; and, secondly, after breathing is restored, the *Promotion of Warmth and Circulation.*

RULE 1. *To adjust the Patient's Position.*—Place the patient on his back on a flat surface, inclined (if possible) a little from the feet upwards; raise and support the head and shoulders on a small firm cushion or folded article of dress placed under the shoulder-blades. Remove all tight clothing about the neck and chest. Prevent unnecessary crowding round the body, especially if in an apartment.

RULE 2. *To maintain the Free Entrance of Air into the Windpipe.*—Cleanse the mouth and nostrils; open the mouth; draw forward the patient's tongue, and keep it forward; an elastic band (from a purse or pocket-book) over the tongue and under the chin will answer this purpose, or the tongue may be held by the fingers of a bystander wrapped in a handkerchief. Do not allow the body to remain on the back unless the tongue is secured.

RULE 3. *To imitate the Movements of Breathing.*

*First*—INDUCE INSPIRATION.—Place yourself at the head

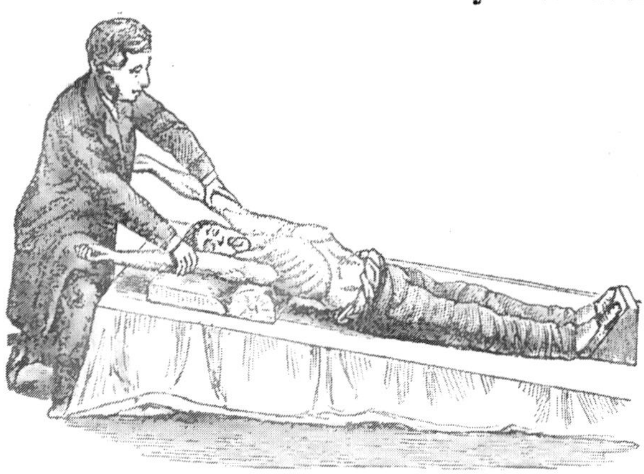

INSPIRATION

of the patient, grasp his arms, raise them upwards by the sides of his head, stretch them steadily but gently upwards for two seconds. [*By this means fresh air is drawn into the lungs by raising the ribs.*]

*Secondly*—INDUCE EXPIRATION.—Immediately turn down the patient's arms, and press them firmly but gently

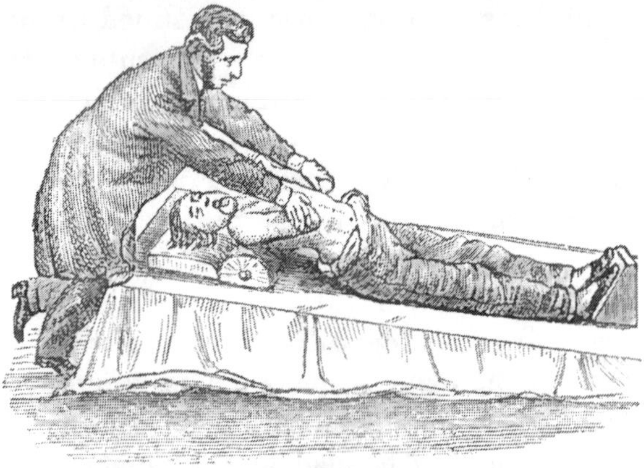

EXPIRATION

downwards against the sides of his chest, for two seconds. [*By this means foul air is expelled from the lungs by depressing the ribs.*]

*Thirdly*—CONTINUE THESE MOVEMENTS.—Repeat these measures alternately, deliberately, and perseveringly, fifteen times in a minute, until a spontaneous effort to respire be perceived. [*By these means an exchange of air is produced in the lungs similar to that effected by natural respiration.*]

RULE 4. *To excite Respiration.*—During the employment of the above method excite the nostrils with snuff or smelling-salts, or tickle the throat with a feather. Rub the chest and face briskly, and dash cold and hot water alternately on them. Friction of the limbs and body with dry flannel or cloths should be had recourse to. Should a galvanic apparatus be at hand, apply the sponges over the heart and back of the neck.

The efforts to restore life must be persevered in until

the arrival of medical assistance, or until the pulse and breathing have ceased for at least an hour. For appearance indicating death (*vide* p. 38).

When a spontaneous effort to respire is perceived, *cease* to IMITATE THE MOVEMENTS OF BREATHING, and commence TO INDUCE CIRCULATION AND WARMTH (*as below*).

TREATMENT AFTER NATURAL BREATHING HAS BEEN RESTORED.—*To induce Circulation and Warmth.*—Wrap the patient in dry blankets, and rub the limbs upwards energetically. Promote the warmth of the body by hot flannels, bottles or bladders of hot water, heated bricks, to the pit of the stomach, the arm-pits, and to the soles of the feet. When the power of swallowing has returned, a teaspoonful of warm water, small quantities of wine, warm brandy and water, or coffee should be given. The patient should be kept in bed, and sleep encouraged. During reaction, large mustard plasters to the chest and below the shoulders will relieve the distressed breathing.

**FOREIGN BODIES IN THE NOSE.**—Peas, beans, small stones, slate pencil, insects, &c., may be thrust into the nostrils by children, or may be accidentally inserted. They may be frequently discharged by compressing the clear nostril with the fingers, and then blowing forcibly through the obstructed nostril. If this does not succeed, snuff may be given to excite sneezing, or the nostrils may be syringed with warm water. These measures failing, a mustard and water emetic may be given, and when vomiting occurs the mouth should be stopped by the hand. A rush of fluid will then take place through the nose, and probably dislodge the foreign substance. If no effect is thus produced, a probe or piece of wire, bent into the form of a loop, or hook, may perhaps be passed *above* the substance so as to hook it down. Or it may sometimes be seized with a pair of forceps. Care must be taken not to push the foreign body backwards, and digging attempts *upwards* towards the head should be avoided. When a foreign body cannot be extracted, it will frequently work out if left alone. If a *leech* gets into the nose, a solution of 2 drachms of salt in 2 ounces of water, should be snuffed up or injected.

**FOREIGN BODIES IN THE EARS.**—The first thing is to examine the ear (*vide* p. 210), to make sure there is really anything inside, as well as to ascertain its size and situation. Unless the foreign body is something which might swell from moisture, as a pea, for instance, syringing with warm water (*vide* p. 210) should always be first tried. When ordinary syringing fails, the patient should lie with the head over the side of a couch, the affected ear being most dependent; so that gravity may be called into play, and the ear should be again syringed while in this position. The form of the canal of the ear is so peculiar, being curved and widest at each extremity, the shapes of foreign substances are so various, and some of them swell from moisture, that efforts to remove them by other means than a current of water should be most carefully undertaken. If syringing does not succeed, the best plan is the use of a wire loop. Take two pieces of fine flexible wire, double them, and then pass the loops into the ear, keeping them against the upper surface, then lower them gently until the foreign body is within one of the loops and then extract. The loop is less liable to injure the internal part of the ear than forceps. But in some cases the substance may be easily seized and extracted by a pair of thin forceps. In other instances a probe end, with a little cotton-wool attached, dipped in carpenter's glue, has been held firmly against the foreign substance, until the glue dries, or for about half an hour, when all was removed together. Great care must be taken not to injure the drum of the ear by pushing the foreign body, or the probe or wire used for its extraction, inwards—or by too forcible syringing.

Insects may be generally removed, or at least killed, and the pain they create therefore diminished, by pouring a little warm salad oil into the ear; or, if oil is not at hand, a saturated solution of salt and water.

After the removal of a foreign body from the ear, if much manipulation or syringing has been required, the ear is painful, and sensitive to cold, from which it should be carefully guarded by the use of cotton-wool for some days; otherwise inflammation or abscess might occur.

**FOREIGN BODIES IN THE EYES** may be often removed by raising the upper eyelid, drawing it down over the lower, and allowing the lids to separate themselves. Blowing the nose vigorously will sometimes effect removal. Otherwise, the eye must be opened, and the offending substance removed with the corner of a handkerchief, or camel's-hair brush, or a feather. But if the lodgment is under the upper lid, the eyelid must be turned inside out. This is done by placing a probe or knitting-needle on the middle of the eyelid *horizontally*, seizing the lashes with the fingers, and turning the lid back over the probe, when the inside of the lid will be exposed, and the substance, which generally lodges just above the margin of the upper lid, may be removed.

When *lime* has got into the eye, its effects are irritant and caustic, and the treatment should be prompt. The eye should be held forcibly open, and every particle gently picked away with a feather, the eye being frequently washed with vinegar and water, or lemon-juice and water, in the proportion of one-third of the former to two of the latter.

When a particle, as of metal for instance, is so firmly fixed in the *cornea*, or central part of the eye, that it cannot be readily detached, it should be left to separate by the natural process of inflammation which will be set up. If it be a piece of iron (as from a blacksmith's forge), the surface of the eye should be bathed with a solution of sulphate of copper (strength, 3 grains of the sulphate to 1 ounce of water). This may be applied with a camel's-hair brush, or with a syringe, and will tend to dissolve and loosen the iron. Sometimes particles of iron or steel may be removed by a magnet.

After the removal of any foreign body from the eye, light should be excluded, and a drop of salad oil placed in the eye will relieve the smarting usually present.

**FOREIGN BODIES IN THE THROAT AND GULLET.**—People are sometimes choked, and have been killed, by portions of food sticking in the gullet and preventing the air passing into the windpipe. As in the diagram below, showing a section of the parts, the windpipe (1)

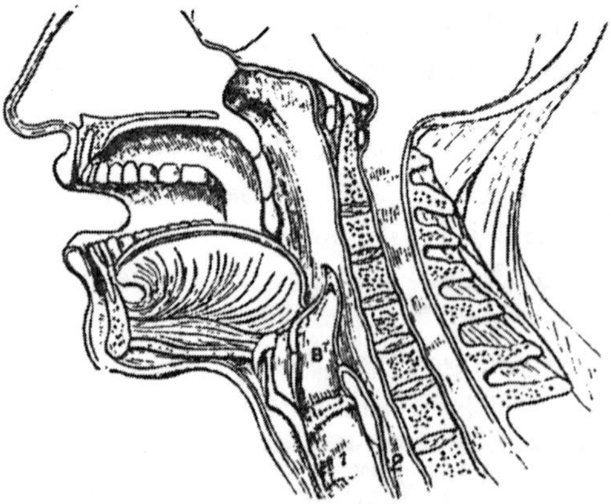


and the gullet (2) lie close together, the entrance to the former being protected by a little valve, A, the *epiglottis*. This remains open and upright except when the act of swallowing is performed, when it shuts down over the opening into the air-passage or windpipe, B, allowing the food to glide over it. When a person eats quickly or carelessly, pieces of food may pass beneath the valve into the windpipe, a circumstance popularly spoken of as 'going the wrong way.' Or a piece of food may lodge above the gullet and epiglottis, shutting the latter down, and thus producing suffocation. This may happen when masticating stringy meat. Two pieces may be attached like chain shot; one piece is swallowed while the other remains entangled in the teeth, and the connecting string shuts down the little valve at the top of the windpipe, and stops the breathing. The effects are spasmodic cough, protrusion of the eyes, blood or froth issuing from the mouth and nose, the person turning blue in the face and falling down insensible.

*Treatment.*—Place the patient where the best light falls from a window or lamp into the mouth, and then boldly and quickly examine the back of the throat and the base of the tongue, by passing the forefinger well down. Probably the foreign mass may be touched and hooked up if a hard body, or pushed down if a soft one, with the finger. This will be facilitated by directing that the tongue be put forward, well out of the mouth, and there retained, being grasped by the patient's own fingers covered with a handkerchief. This procedure mechanically draws forward the arches of the palate, and allows the operator to sweep his finger well across from one side to the other of the throat. If the finger does not reach the foreign body, a sharp blow on the back should be given with the flat of the hand. If the patient is a child, it will add force to the blow if the child is taken between the knees, so as to compress the belly; otherwise much of the impetus of the blow is lost by transmission to the yielding walls of the abdomen. Thus fish-bones, or other bones, or various foreign bodies lodged high up in the gullet may often be removed by the fingers. Or they may be, perhaps, brought up by the vomiting occasioned by passing the fingers into the throat in their search, or they may sometimes be dislodged by pressure with the fingers outside. Hard, angular, or pointed substances, such as false teeth and teeth-plates, should always, if possible, be got up; and in some instances they may be laid hold of with a long pair of curved forceps. But softer substances, when lodged low down, may sometimes be impelled onwards into the stomach by swallowing large pieces of food, or they may probably be ejected by an emetic (Recipe 54).

If these measures fail, a *probang* must be passed, to push the intruding substance into the stomach. This instrument is a long stick of whalebone, slightly bent, with a piece of sponge attached to one end, and a small hook to the other, as below. If such an instrument is not available, a substitute may be extemporised as follows:—Obtain a slip of whalebone or cane, and tie firmly to one end of it a knob of sponge about the size of a marble. The patient is made to sit with the head well thrown back,

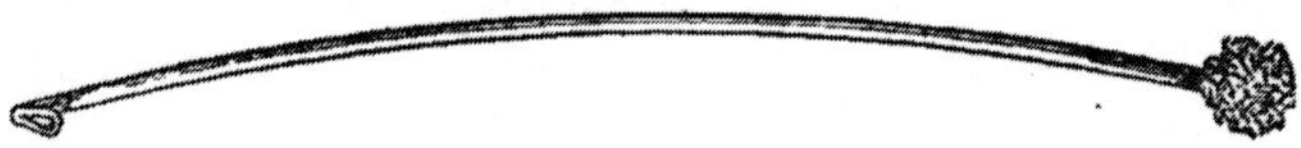

and the tongue should be put out, when the operator introduces the probang, sponge end first, into the throat *so as to touch the back part*, and then pushes it gently onwards and downwards towards the stomach, so as to displace and send before it the foreign mass into the stomach. Or the hooked end may be passed, under the hope of bringing the foreign body upwards. Or a number of loops of thread may be attached to the hook and passed down the throat, as foreign substances have sometimes been thus caught and brought up when other means have failed. But these operations can scarcely be performed except by a surgeon; although they should be tried, rather than a sufferer be left without attempts at relief.

*Needles swallowed*, if not easily removable, should be left alone: they will probably work out harmlessly through some part of the skin.

**FOREIGN BODIES IN THE WINDPIPE** cause difficulty of breathing and violent cough, and are sometimes expelled by the latter. If the patient is a child, he, or she, should be held up by the legs with the head down, and the back should be gently tapped. If an adult, the patient should be placed on a slanting board or a tilted table, as far as possible in the same position, and the back slapped. Coins and similarly shaped bodies have thus been got rid of. If these means do not succeed, and difficulty of breathing is urgent, nothing but a surgical operation will afford a chance of relief. Otherwise, if there are no urgent symptoms, the patient must be kept quiet, and the foreign substance becoming coated with mucus, or becoming softened, may be coughed up.

**FOREIGN BODIES IN THE STOMACH.**—When any foreign substance has passed into the stomach, as, for example, a coin, a marble, a piece of glass, or artificial teeth, the object is to allow it to pass through the intestines well enveloped in food, and as it passes on in fæcal matter. Therefore no purgatives should be given. The person should abstain from fluids, but otherwise the usual diet should be taken. A change of diet to rice pudding, cheese, and hard-boiled eggs with the view of producing hard consistent stools, enveloped in which the foreign body may pass without injury to the bowels, is sometimes recommended. But such changes of food often induce looseness of the bowels, and do injury. If metal has been swallowed, nothing acid should be taken, as it might dissolve the metal and produce poisonous compounds.

*Leeches* have sometimes been swallowed, giving rise to very unpleasant symptoms. A table-spoonful of salt dissolved in four ounces of water should be immediately taken, and repeated in half an hour, when the leech will be probably killed, or vomited up. If salt is not at hand, half a wine-glassful of sherry every ten minutes.

**FOREIGN BODIES IN THE SKIN.**—Splinters of wood, thorns, needles, fish-hooks, nails, &c., may be embedded in the skin. Splinters of wood or similar shaped substances should be, if possible, seized by forceps and dragged out.

To accomplish this, slight enlargement of the wound with a lancet may be necessary. Or they must be left a day or two and the part poulticed, when, becoming loose, they may be more easily extracted. Needles and fish-hooks in the person will be generally more easily extracted by pushing them out by the points, care being taken that they do not break. Needles introduced beneath the skin often travel to distant parts of the body, and therefore no operation should be undertaken for their extraction, unless the substance can be plainly felt.

*To take a tight ring from the finger.*—Hold up the hand for three minutes. Then wind a moderately broad piece of elastic round the finger, commencing at the nail. Still keep the hand well up; take the elastic off after five minutes, and if the ring will not come away repeat the procedure.

**FOREIGN BODIES UNDER THE NAILS.**—Thorns, splinters of wood, &c., must be extracted after gradually paring down the nail until the foreign body can be seized by forceps. If this cannot be effected after the nail is pared to the quick, the outside end of the splinter should not be wasted by fruitless picking at it, but the nail immediately above should be scraped as thin as possible; after which a small triangular piece may be cut from the top, when the splinter may be readily seized and drawn out. If all this cannot be accomplished, it will be best to poultice for a day or two, when probably the intruding substance will be loosened, and may be extracted.

**FOREIGN BODIES IN OTHER PARTS.**—Foreign bodies sometimes become impacted in the *private parts or fundament*, and may consist of substances which have been swallowed, as fruit-stones and fish-bones, or of articles introduced from without. As they cannot be extracted easily the assistance of a surgeon will probably be required.

**FRACTURED OR BROKEN BONES.**—These accidents

are spoken of as *simple fractures*, when there is no external wound leading from the surface of the skin to the injured bone. When there is such a wound they are called *compound fractures* (*vide* p. 580). Compound fractures are much more dangerous than simple fractures. When the bone is broken into several pieces it is called a *comminuted fracture* (*vide* p. 580). Fractures *implicating joints* are the most dangerous (*vide* p. 580).

*The usual symptoms of all fractures* are pain, swelling, alteration of shape, *grating* of the broken ends of the bone on movement, and more or less inability to move the limb. But sometimes, in children, bones are bent, not broken, when, although there will be no grating, the deformity or bent shape of the limb will sufficiently indicate the injury. For the signs distinguishing fracture from dislocation, *vide Dislocation*, p. 526. Fractures near the joints are distinguished from simple *sprains* (*vide* p. 596) principally by the presence of grating.

*Treatment.*—The *immediate* treatment after any accident is given at p. 497; of fractures at 499. *The after principles of treatment of all fractures* are to place and retain the fragments in perfect rest in their natural position until they have united.

*The surface on which the patient with a fractured limb* has to lie should be firm and level, and therefore no feather or very soft bed should be allowed. The lighter and cooler the method of fixing the limb, the less unpleasant will it be. The irritation when the part is thickly covered, and there is no escape for the perspiration, is often intolerable. It is also of importance to be able to undo the apparatus easily, to see the state of the limb, and to keep it clean with soap and water.

*In the treatment of fractured bones the following articles are required*:—Splints, bandages, pads, tapes, sometimes oiled silk, and simple ointment, or olive oil. Splints may be made of wood, or, except for the thigh, of gutta percha, of telegraph wire, of thick pasteboard, of newspapers, of bandboxes, or even of strong straw tied into a bundle. Bandages should be made of linen or calico (*vide* p. 493), or of old sheeting. Pads may be formed of pieces of blanket cut into the shape of the splints, or of cotton-wool, or tow, or of cocoa-nut fibre, chaff, or husks of grain in bags. Before attempting to treat a fracture everything required should be made ready. When adjusting splints, much care must be taken that there is no great pressure on prominent parts, as the bones of the ankle or elbow; otherwise blisters and sores will form. This is to be effected by making the pads fit the limb, or they may be fitted on the limb of another person, or on the sound limb. Before applying splints, the limb should be washed, dried, and dusted with violet powder or starch. Although frequent moving of splints when once applied is not desirable, it is still necessary to secure cleanliness, and to ascertain whether any wound is forming from pressure, or whether blisters have formed from the violence of the injury. It will, therefore, be necessary to move the splints with great care about the third day, when the limb will be probably found showing the discoloration described under *Bruises* (*vide* p. 515), and also presenting various blisters. These should be snipped at the most dependent part; the limb should be gently sponged and cleansed with warm water and carbolic soap; a little simple ointment (Recipe 86) or salad oil spread on lint or soft rag should be laid over the blistered part; and if pressure has occurred, the pads and splints should be carefully readjusted, so as to avoid it. Similar attention will be required in another day or two; and afterwards, the limb should be gently sponged every few days. If all this is done with care, no motion of the fractured parts need be entailed.

If there is great swelling of the parts, or much bruising, or escape of blood into the tissues (*vide* p. 580) apparent at first, broken limbs should not be bound on splints for the first three or four days. If limbs in such a condition are bandaged up tightly, much pain results, and, if the bandages are not slackened, serious injury or mortification may follow. It is best at first, if there is much swelling, to lay the broken limb in as comfortable a posture as possible, and as nearly as can be in its natural direction, and it may be lightly bound to a single splint merely for the purpose of keeping it steady. The arm, whether broken above or below the elbow, will lie most comfortably half bent on a pillow. The thigh or leg will rest most easily on the outer side, with the knee bent. It will always be proper to apply fomentation or lotion, or to use irrigation, while swelling continues (*vide Appendix, Cooling applications*), and as a rule it will be best to foment during the first two or three days, and then to gradually substitute a cooling application. Speaking generally, all fractures should remain in splints during one month, after which sufficient support may be obtained by a starch bandage (Recipe 112), or by plaster spread on strips of leather (Recipe 113).

In treating fractures of the lower limbs, and also sometimes for the arm, the use of a 'cradle' is necessary to keep the bed-clothes from pressing on the injured parts.

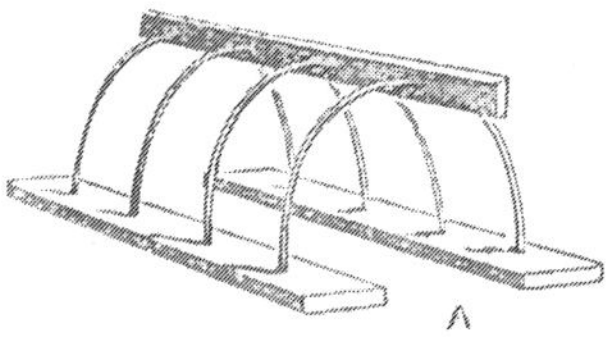
A

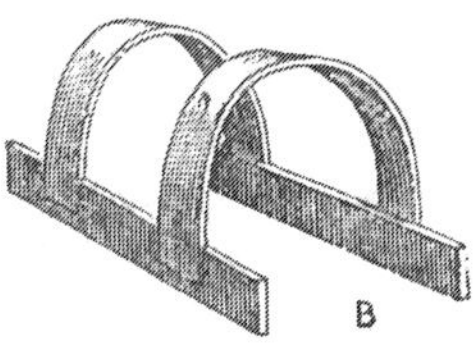
B

A 'cradle' may be constructed of some curved iron wires, passed through three slim pieces of wood, as in figure A. Or one may be made as figure B, by cutting a barrel hoop in two or three pieces, and nailing them to two pieces of wood.

**FRACTURE OF THE SKULL.**—If it be a simple fracture, or crack in the bones of the skull, nothing more will be required, beyond attention to the external wound, as mentioned under *Wounds of the Scalp* (*vide* p. 601). Such injuries are, however, generally attended by *concussion* (*vide* p. 522), and this state, if present, must be treated as there mentioned. If any portion of the bones of the skull is broken and *depressed* below the other part, the symptoms described under *Compression of the Brain* (*vide* p. 525) will be present; and the operation of trepanning may be required. For distinction between bruise and fracture (*vide* p. 517). When, after an injury to the head, there is bleeding or escape of watery fluid from the ears, or from the nose, in addition to insensibility and laboured breathing, *fracture of the base of the skull* has probably taken place, and the case generally ends fatally. In all injuries of the head there is special danger of inflammation of the brain, and therefore perfect rest from the first should be insisted upon, with a darkened room, low diet, cold lotion to the head (Recipe 83), purgative medicines (Recipes 1 and 2), and abstinence from all stimulants.

**FRACTURE OF THE SPINE.**—The fracture is usually partial, and frequently associated with dislocation of one bone, or of part of one bone. The symptoms are partly *local*, and partly *nervous*, depending on the nature and amount of injury which the spinal marrow has sustained. The *local* symptoms are pain, loss of power, and irregularity in the course of the spine at the seat of injury. Sometimes the bones of the spine, ordinarily felt as a succession of regular hard prominences in the back, are found to be unnaturally separated at the injured place, or one or more of the bones may be felt to be depressed *beneath the level* of those above and below. If the spinal marrow is so far injured that its functions are interfered with, there will be either partial or entire loss of both motion and sensation *below* the point of injury.

*If the fracture is situated about the loins,* the lower part of the body, the bladder, the rectum, and the lower limbs will be paralysed, the person being unable to move, or to make water, or to pass motions at will, both coming away involuntarily. The arms and upper part of the body remain unaffected. The patient may live for months or years, death eventually taking place from exhaustion, caused by bed-sores (*vide* p. 69), or from disease of the bladder (*vide* pp. 71, 74).

*If the injury is higher up, about the shoulder-blades,* the muscles of the chest will be also paralysed, and breathing will be carried on with difficulty. Under such circumstances the patient may live a few days, but the lungs soon become congested, and the person dies suffocated.

*If the injury is still higher, or at the lower part of the neck,* the arms are also paralysed.

*If the injury is still higher up, about the upper part of the neck* (above the origin of a nerve called the *phrenic*), death takes place instantly from cessation of respiration. Such cases are popularly talked of as 'broken neck.'

*Treatment.*—When the injury is in the lowest part of the back, much may be done to make the person more comfortable, and to prolong life. The sufferer should be placed, if possible, on a water bed, and kept perfectly clean. The tendency to bed-sores (*vide* p. 69) about the buttocks and back from pressure, and about the privates from irritation by urine, or by fæces dribbling away, should be held in mind, and the parts should be protected by variously shaped pillows, and by suitable coverings of oiled silk. As the person cannot make water, the urine accumulates in the bladder, until, that organ being filled to distension, it dribbles away; but the bladder remaining always full, the urine contained therein becomes offensive, ammoniacal, and doubly irritant to the inside of the bladder, and to the skin which it may run over outside. From the first, therefore, the urine should be drawn off with the catheter twice a day, and if a surgeon and the necessary instruments are at hand the bladder will probably be washed out daily. No medicine, except an occasional purgative, such as castor oil, will be required. But the rectum should be washed out every two or three days by an enema of soap and water (Recipe 104). When the injury is higher than the loins, very little can be done to alleviate the sufferings of the patient, and no medicine is of any use.

**FRACTURE OF THE BONES OF THE NOSE.**—This is known by the nose being flattened, and by the grating of the broken bones when the nose is raised to its natural position. The bones should be pushed into their proper place by passing a pair of forceps or piece of wood into the nostrils, and lifting up the fractured parts. If they do not remain *in situ*, a plug of oiled lint must be placed in the nostril. If the fracture is compound, that is, presenting an external wound, and any splinters of bone are loose, they should be removed with the forceps. Bleeding, if violent and protracted, must be stopped, as mentioned under *Bleeding from the Nose* (p. 510).

**FRACTURE OF THE LOWER JAW.**—This usually occurs at about the middle of one side of the part in which the teeth are placed, and is known by pain, swelling, inability to move the jaw properly, and irregularity of the teeth; the front teeth being drawn *down*, and the back teeth *up*, by the action of the muscles. The point of fracture may be easily felt, and the saliva dribbles from the mouth. On moving the jaw grating will be felt. If the fracture is compound, there will also be bleeding, from laceration of the gums, and probably one or more teeth may be knocked out or loosened.

*Treatment.*—If teeth are only loosened they should be

left, and may perhaps be secured in their places, by silver wire, passing round adjacent teeth. If teeth, or fragments of bone, are wholly detached, they had better be removed. Then the teeth should be brought into a natural line. Then a piece of gutta percha, or thick pasteboard softened by hot water, should be accurately fitted to the jaw (previously shaved, if necessary), and extending from ear to ear. The gutta percha should be about eight inches long, and should be split up the middle from each end to within an inch of the centre. When applied, the lower portion should be doubled on the upper, by which means there is a double support at the part most requiring it. The gutta percha must be secured by a four-tailed bandage, made by taking a yard and a half of calico roller about four inches wide, tearing each end longitudinally, so as to leave about eight inches in the middle, in which should be a slit for the reception of the chin. This slit should be about an inch from the anterior margin, so that the latter may not rise so high as to cover the lower lip, or get into the mouth. Two of the tails are then tied over the crown of the head, and two at the back of the neck; or the latter may be crossed and brought round and tied in front. The bandage may be rendered more secure by a circular one round the head above the ears, the two being secured by pins where they cross. The mouth is thus closed, and the patient must be fed

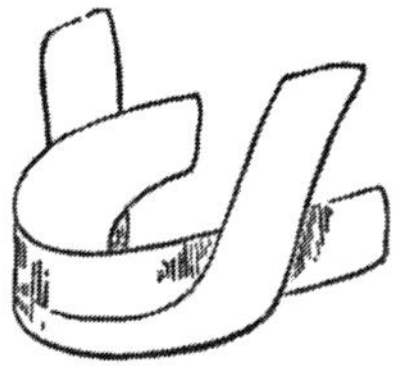

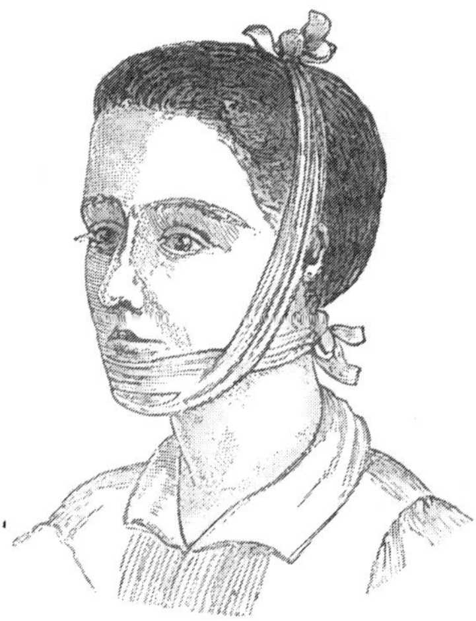

entirely on fluids for the first fortnight. The cure occupies about five weeks. Dribbling of saliva, and fœtid taste in the mouth, are a great nuisance to the patient. Frequently washing the mouth with carbolic solution (Recipe 119), or with myrrh gargle, is desirable.

**FRACTURE OF THE COLLAR-BONE.**—The person cannot raise the arm upwards towards the head; the broken part of the bone may be seen and felt prominent; grating of the broken ends occurs on movement of the shoulder; the shoulder is flatter than the other, and falls forwards and inwards; the person supports his elbow and forearm with the opposite hand and forearm. This accident frequently occurs to children.

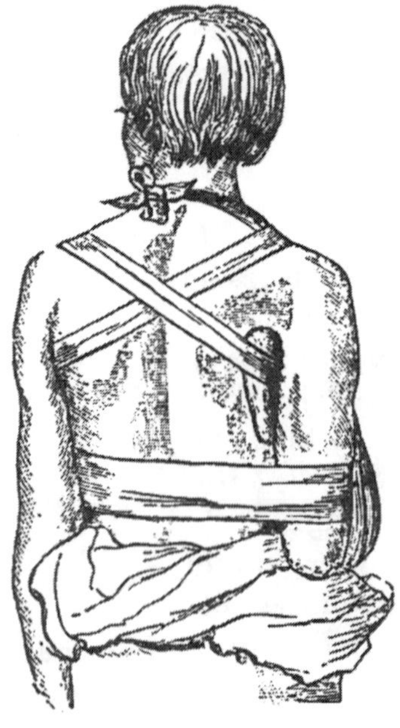

*Treatment.*—Place a big cone-shaped pad in the armpit, then bandage the shoulders so as to draw them well backwards. This is effected by a figure of ∞ bandage, passing several times round each shoulder and crossing behind. The arm must be then bound to the side by another bandage, with the elbow well back, and lastly *the elbow* must be supported by a handkerchief, used as a sling round the neck. Thus the shoulder is kept *up* by the sling, *out* by the pad, and *back* by the bandage, bringing the broken ends of the collar-bone into position. When the bandages are adjusted, they should be stitched in several places, as they are liable to slip. They should be tightened when they grow loose. They should be worn a month, after which plaster on strips of leather (Recipe 113) may be applied over the injured part. The preceding diagram represents a broken collar-bone bandaged.

It is difficult to keep this bone, when broken, at rest and in exact position, unless the patient lies on his back, with his arms confined to the side of the body, and keeps his head quite still. For ladies, when it is a matter of importance to prevent deformity, the recumbent posture in bed should be maintained three weeks, till union has fairly taken place. But such a position for days, for such an injury, would be to most people intolerable. With the bandages as above described, a broken collar-bone unites speedily and strongly, although some little deformity must be expected.

**FRACTURE OF THE HEAD, OR UPPER PART OF THE ARM-BONE.**—There are various kinds of fracture of this part, but the one now described is the most common. The arm is slightly *shortened*, and the broken end of the bone may be felt in the front of the armpit, while the round *head* of the bone is felt in its right place, and does not move when the elbow is turned. The shoulder, when compared with the other, will be seen to have lost its rounded form. Grating will also be felt when the elbow is pulled downwards, so as to restore the broken parts to their natural position. There is severe pain from pressure on the nerves. The following features distinguish this accident from dislocation. Although the shoulder loses its rounded form, it does not present the sharp angle of dislocation; the head of the bone is felt in its natural position; there is grating; the broken end is felt in the armpit; and the parts return to their unnatural position after becoming right by extension; none of which signs present in dislocation.

*Various other Injuries affecting the Shoulder Joint* occur, presenting symptoms very similar to fracture of the head of the arm-bone, or to some forms of dislocation (p. 529). In any case of doubt, it will be well to apply the crossed bandage as for fractured clavicle, and to keep the arm to the side, until the advice of a surgeon can be obtained.

*Treatment.*—If there is no reasonable doubt that the head of the bone is fractured it should be treated as follows. If, as often the case, there is great swelling, it will be advisable to put the patient to bed, and to use fomentations for a few days until the swelling subsides, before applying splints. Then, or at first, if there is no swelling, a well-padded splint should be prepared, about three inches wide, and long enough to reach from the armpit to the elbow-joint. Another splint of gutta percha or strong leather should be made by moulding the material, when softened by immersion in hot water, on the shoulder of some one of similar size, in the form of a cap. The tail of this splint should be nearly three inches wide, and long enough to reach to the outside of the elbow, where it should be well padded. When all is prepared, the limb must be first restored to the natural position by raising the arm parallel with the shoulder, and then by pulling or extension from the bent elbow. The splints should be secured by tapes above and below, taking care that the tapes do not cut the skin between the splints, which they will not do if the splints are broad enough. Then, a bandage should be applied, commencing from the hand, passing over the forearm, and then over the splints. This prevents swelling of the hand and forearm. Lastly, the *wrist and hand* should be comfortably supported by a sling, but the *elbow should be allowed to hang down*, its weight tending then to prevent the lower part of the bone being dragged upwards by muscular action. Splints should be worn for six weeks, after which plaster spread on leather may be applied across the shoulder, from near the middle of the chest to near the middle of the back; after which the joint may be gently moved.

**FRACTURE OF THE MIDDLE OF THE ARM-BONE** is easily detected from the deformity, the grating, the bone being movable at the broken point where it should be firm, the local pain, and the inability to use the arm.

*Treatment.*—The parts should be restored to their natural position by raising the arm parallel with the shoulder, and then by pulling or extension of the bent elbow. Then four carefully padded splints should be placed, one in front, one behind, and one at each side. These splints must be long enough to reach from the top to the bottom of the arm, and the *outside* one should be the longest, as it should rest above on the shoulder, and below on the outside of the elbow. Great care must be taken that this splint does not press too much on the prominence of the elbow—to be avoided by well padding opposite the hollow of the arm *above* the elbow. The skin of the armpit and the inside of the elbow is also liable to be frayed by the inside splint, which must be avoided by care and padding. Similarly the skin of the forearm may be blistered by the lower end of the front splint. The splints, when properly adjusted, must be secured by tapes tied round at the top and the bottom. Then a bandage should be applied from the hand upwards. The arm thus treated is sketched below. The wrist and hand should be supported by a sling and the elbow allowed to hang down.

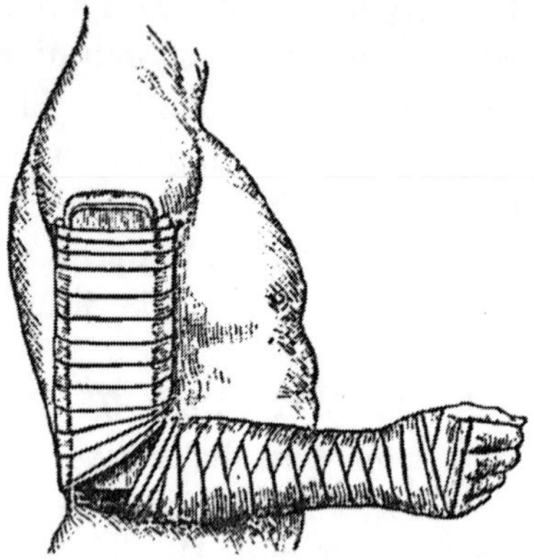

After about six weeks a starch bandage (Recipe 112) may be applied instead of splints.

**FRACTURE OF THE LOWER PART OF THE ARM** will be known by the elbow being drawn backwards, by its

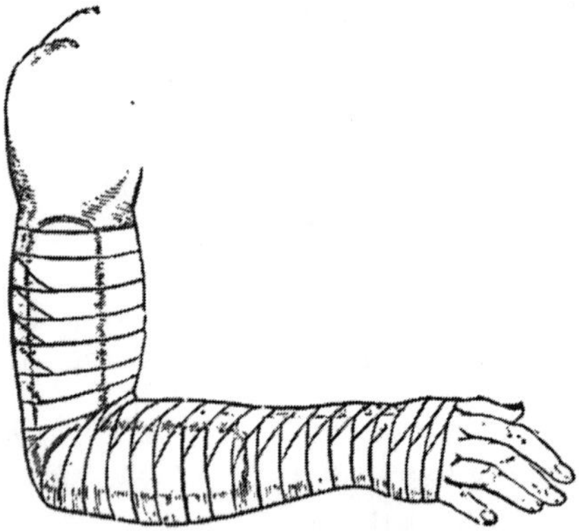

being restored to the natural position by pulling the hand, by its returning to the unnatural position if the hand is not pulled, and by the grating.

*Treatment.*—The parts should be brought into proper position by pulling from the hand, the elbow should be bent, and an angular splint made of gutta percha or leather softened in hot water applied on each side. The hand and forearm must be bandaged, and the elbow and forearm supported by a sling from the neck. The part thus bandaged is figured on opposite page. Splints should be worn for a month, after which the joint should be gently moved.

**FRACTURE OF THE PROMINENCES OF THE ARM-BONE.**—The prominences of the arm-bone on either side, just above the elbow, may be split off. The broken piece of bone forms a swelling towards the back of the joint, and there is difficulty in the motion of the joint. When these prominences are broken there may be much pain from injury of nerves. The injury should be treated as advised for fracture of the lower part of the arm.

**FRACTURE OF THE PROMINENCE OF THE ELBOW.** There is a depression at the back of the joint, above which the broken end of the bone will be felt detached from the body of the bone, and the person is *unable to straighten* the arm. This injury should be treated by placing the arm *straight*. A well-padded splint, long enough to reach from the middle of the forearm to the middle of the arm, should be placed *on the front* of the elbow, and secured by a bandage. The limb should be kept up on a pillow, otherwise the hand will swell. This injury does not unite by bone but by ligament, so that there may long be some imperfection of movement. After four weeks the joint should be gently moved.

*There are other Injuries of the Elbow Joint*, presenting symptoms of fracture, or of dislocation. The precise nature is difficult of detection; but in case of doubt keeping the arm *bent at right angles*, resting on an angular splint, will be the best plan, until the arrival of skilled aid.

**FRACTURE OF THE FOREARM.**—The two bones of the forearm may be both fractured in any part or only one may be broken. There will be pain, loss of power of turning the hand, grating on movement, and the arm will be misshapen; the more so if both bones are broken.

*Treatment.*—One person should hold the elbow and another pull the hand, *keeping the thumb of the injured limb upwards*. Then well-padded splints, a little *broader* than the arm, must be applied *from the fingers to the elbow* on each side, and the whole secured by tapes and bandages. The splints should not be removed, except to sponge and clean the arm, until after three weeks, when shorter splints may be substituted, and a little movement of the wrist allowed. During the whole time the arm should be supported in a sling. In two weeks the short splints may be left off, but some support in the shape of a starch bandage, or leather plaster (Recipes 112, 113), will be required for another week or two. The forearm bandaged is shown below.

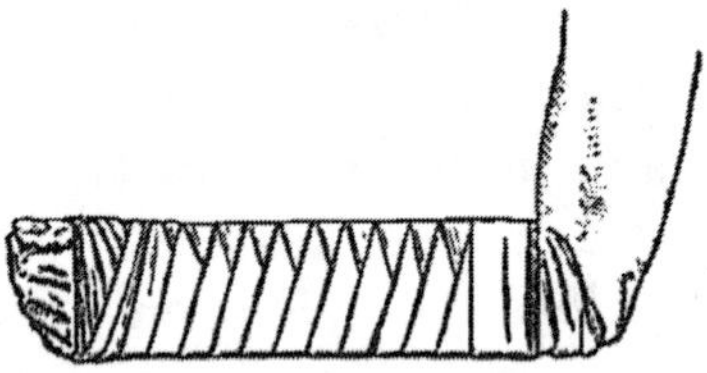

*In Children the Forearm is often Bent*, rather than quite broken. In such cases it must be forcibly straightened, during which, grating will be felt, and then splints are to be applied, and worn for three weeks. This injury is called 'green stick' fracture.

**FRACTURE OF THE FOREARM CLOSE TO THE WRIST.** This is an injury chiefly occurring to elderly persons and from which recovery is tedious. The limb is peculiarly bent, as in the accompanying sketch, and there is generally much swelling, while grating is felt on extension of the hand. The lower fragment of the broken bone forms a marked projection at the back of the limb, and leaves in front, just above the line of the wrist-joint, a corresponding depression. It is distinguished from dislocation by grating being felt when the hand is extended and slightly moved.

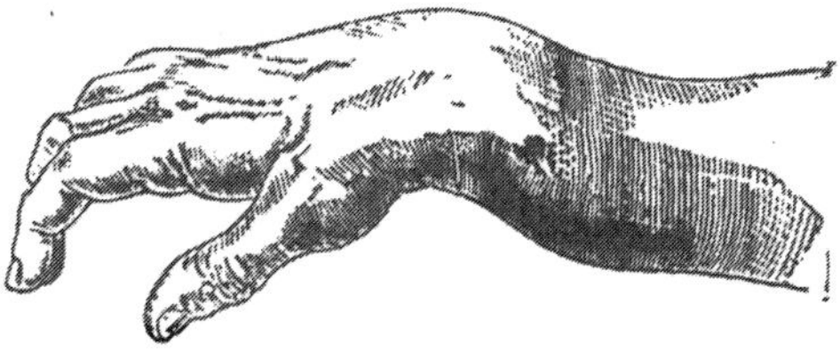

*Treatment.*—The thumb must be placed upwards, the elbow steadied, and the hand pulled until the natural position is restored. Splints should be applied, the inner one extending from the elbow to the palm of the hand, the outer one curved as in the accompanying diagram, and

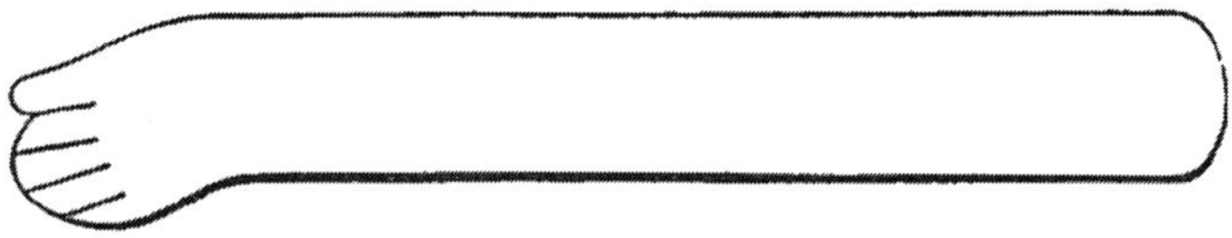

extending to the ends of the fingers. This position of the hand brings the fractured parts into better contact, when it should be secured by tapes and bandages round the splints. In this injury occurring to a person up to thirty years of age these splints should not be used more than three weeks, nor more than four weeks for an older person; after which they should be shortened so as to allow the fingers to be gently moved. In another week splints may be left off, after which the wrist should be gently moved daily, otherwise the joint is liable to become stiff.

*Other injuries about the Wrist Joint* occur, difficult of detection, involving often both the small bones of the joint, and the ends of the bones of the forearm. In the absence of surgical skill, when there is doubt, it is best to treat the case as for fracture of the middle of the forearm.

**FRACTURE OF THE BONES OF THE HAND AND OF THE FINGERS.**—These injuries are known by the attendant swelling pain and grating. The best method of treating fractures of the *bones of the hand* is by laying the extended hand on a wooden or gutta-percha splint, cut to the shape of the part. The *inner* or palmar surfaces of the bones of the hands are *concave*, and the splint should therefore be well padded, so that it may adapt itself to their form. Sometimes, in order to maintain the broken parts in better contact, a small splint is desirable on the back of the hand. Then, a bandage should be applied so as to keep the hand and fingers immovable. In some instances, the broken bones are brought into more natural position when the hand is closed. If this is the case, the injury may be treated by causing the patient to grasp a ball of tow, or other soft substance, about half the size of a cricket-ball, or so large as to permit the thumb and fingers meeting within an inch. The closed hand, with the ball of tow inside, should then be secured in such position by a bandage. The hand should be kept bound for about three weeks, and supported by a sling as noted below.

*When a bone of the finger is broken*, it may be treated by binding the finger to a narrow splint of wood or gutta percha, or, best of all, perforated zinc, which should reach to the wrist. If the injury is very severe, or several fingers are involved, it will be needful to lay the whole hand on a wooden splint cut to the shape of the hand, thumb, and fingers. The inner surfaces of the bones of the fingers are concave, and the splints should therefore be well padded. *In all cases of fracture of the bones of the hands or fingers*, the limb should be supported by a sling, so disposed as to raise the hand a little above the level of the elbow.

**FRACTURE OF THE RIBS.**—The ribs are liable to be broken by falls or blows, or by a crushing weight, as from a wheel passing over the chest. When the injury results from direct violence, the rib is generally broken at the seat of injury; when from crushing or squeezing, it breaks at the bend, or middle of the bone. The patient complains of severe pain on drawing a deep breath, and there is a grating sensation in the side, evident to the patient, and which may be felt on applying the hand flat over the part, unless the patient is very stout. Grating is also felt if the person coughs, and there is generally a short, hacking, frequent, but suppressed cough. If the fracture is near the spine, or the patient corpulent, detection will be more difficult. But if, after an injury to the chest, cutting pain is complained of, the treatment for fractured rib should be pursued. The principal danger from fractured rib is, lest the lung or its covering (the *pleura*) may be injured, when there may be spitting of blood, or *emphysema* (*vide* below), or pleurisy (p. 352), or pneumonia (p. 325).

*Treatment.*—Diminish motion of the chest, by passing a broad roller, eight inches in width, and about twelve feet long, tightly round the body, from the pit of the stomach to the armpit. The bandage will require shoulder-straps to maintain it in position. The patient should be kept in bed on spare diet, and if cough occurs, Recipe 57 should be given. The bowels must also be kept open (Recipes 1 and 2). Chloral may be given at night to relieve pain. The bandage should be worn for three weeks, after which leather plaster may be applied over the seat of injury. Pleurisy, or inflamed lung, caused by fractured ribs, should be treated as advised for such ailments (*vide* pp. 353, 327).

*Emphysema, or Air Entering Beneath the Skin.*—This sometimes results from the fractured ends of the ribs wounding the lungs. Emphysema forms a soft puffy swelling of the skin, sometimes extending to the neck, which crackles when pressed. For this complication, a pad of lint should be first placed over the seat of injury, and the bandage should be tightly applied over the pad. The necessity for perfect rest must be more especially enjoined; for the occurrence of *pleurisy*, or of *inflammation of the lungs*, is more likely.

**FRACTURES OF THE UPPER PART OF THE THIGH** are of various kinds, but the one described is the most common. It is marked by inability to stand, shortening of the leg, and turning out of the toes, the heel of the injured limb pointing to the instep of the sound member, as shown in the sketch. If the foot is drawn down to its proper length, and turned about, while a hand is placed on the hip, grating will probably be felt. This accident frequently happens to old people. The figure may be usefully compared with the drawing representing the aspect of the limb in dislocation of the same bone. (*Vide* p. 536.)

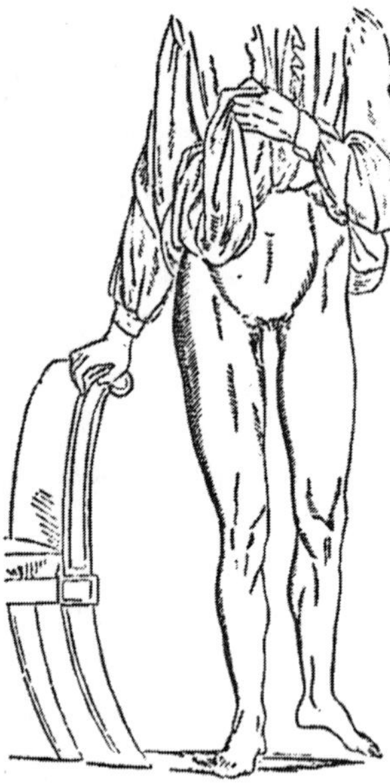

*Treatment.*—Unless the person is old and feeble, the limb should be bandaged, as detailed on next page for fracture of the middle of the thigh. If the patient is old and feeble, health would be sacrificed, and probably bed-sores formed by long confinement in bed, under the treatment by splints. The patient should be kept in bed for a fortnight, with one pillow under the whole length of the limb, and another rolled up under the knee. When pain and tenderness abate, which will be ordinarily in about a fortnight, the patient may be allowed to sit in a chair, and to use crutches. What is called 'ligamentous union' will take place, and although the leg will be shorter than before, it will be fairly useful, and the shortening may be remedied by a thick-soled shoe. This 'ligamentous union' consists in the junctions of the broken ends of the bone by a tough leather-like substance, but not by bony matter.

**FRACTURE OF THE MIDDLE OF THE THIGH.**—This accident is readily distinguished by shortening of the limb, by great swelling, and by grating when the ends of the bones are placed in contact by extension, or pulling from the foot; which also restores the natural shape of the limb.

In young children this fracture is often incomplete, the bone being only bent. In such cases there is no grating, and pulling the foot does not restore the natural shape of the thigh, which must be bent back with the hands into position, much in the same way as a stick would be bent.

*Treatment.*—For all cases of this kind, and for fractures of the upper part of the bone, up to fifty years of age, the long thigh-splint must be used. This is a narrow board

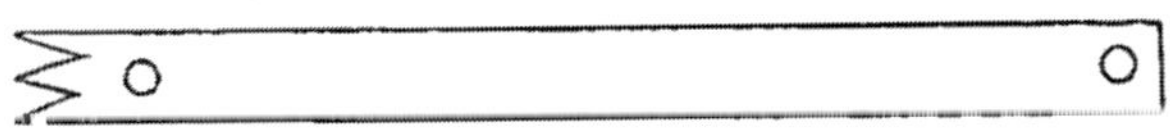

of a hand's breadth for an adult, but narrower and slighter for a younger person. It must be long enough to reach from just below the armpit to four inches below the sole of the foot. At the upper end must be a hole, at the lower end two deep notches with a hollow or hole just above for the reception of the ankle-bone. First the splint must be thoroughly padded, with layers of blanket or otherwise. Then the limb should be evenly bandaged from the toes up to the knee, and then gently extended to its proper length and shape by pulling the foot. Next, the lower end of the splint is to be fixed to the ankle, by passing a bandage round the foot, and through the notches of the board.

Next, the splint is secured to the limb by a bandage passing upwards. During all this time an assistant must keep the limb in proper position by pulling the foot. Lastly, this extension must be maintained by 'the perinæal band.' This band is formed of a large handkerchief or piece of silk, doubled cornerwise, and rolled round a long thin pad. This is placed between the legs, one end passing over the groin, the other under the buttock, and the ends are tied through the holes at the top of the splint. This mechanically pushes the foot down, and so keeps up the extension. A roll of broad bandage should also be passed round the

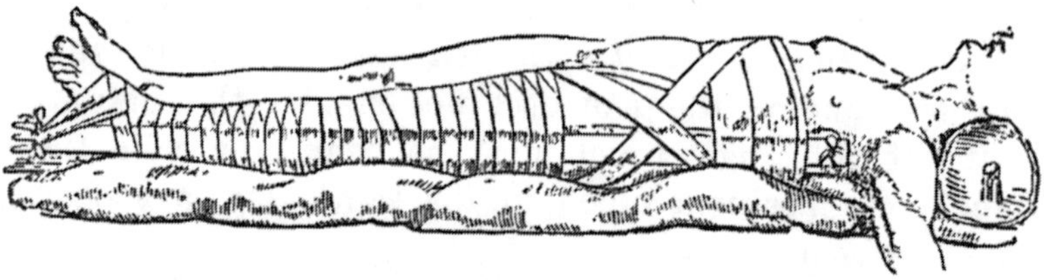

body and upper part of the splint, to keep the latter close to the person. The perinæal band is likely to gall, and constant attention must therefore be directed to this part; particular care being taken that it does not press on the privates, or become wet with urine. And as considerable pressure is exerted on the ankle, padding and manipulation are necessary at this part to prevent blisters or sores forming. It is also sometimes necessary to apply short splints, both on the inner side and on the front of the thigh, when the bones have a tendency to project in either direction. The figure above shows a thigh thus bandaged to the long splint.

It often happens that the bandage round the foot, notwithstanding careful padding, causes pain, or blisters from the pressure, which, when the band between the legs is drawn tight, is considerable. Or the band may cause soreness between the legs. Under such circumstances it may be necessary to continue the treatment without these aids, and this may be effected in the following manner. A fixed point, in the shape of a foot-piece, must be attached firmly to the foot of the bed, so that the sole of the foot of the injured limb may rest against it as the patient lies on his back. Then several long broad strips of plaster must be carried down the leg from the seat of fracture on the one side, round the foot-piece, and up the leg to the same point on the opposite side. By this means the pressure and extending force will be so diffused that the person will be scarcely sensible of it. But something is still wanting as the extending force, in place of the perinæal band. And this difficulty is to be overcome by tilting up the lower end of the bed about twelve inches from the floor, and placing blocks of wood below the feet of the bed. The patient then lies on an inclined plane, and the body having a tendency to slip towards the head of the bed, while the foot is fixed by the plasters to the immovable foot-board, the desired extension is thus maintained at the seat of the fracture, the body itself being the counter-extending force. As a further precaution, small splints should be applied round the thigh at the point of fracture. The best method of applying the foot-board is to procure a piece of wood, about half an inch thick, as broad as the sole of the foot, and in length sufficient to reach from the floor when the bed is tilted to the extremities of the toes of the patient as he lies with the heel downwards. The upper portion should be cut into the shape of a foot-piece, and the board should then be firmly screwed to the cross-piece of the bed. A little adjustment by cutting the latter, or the foot-piece, or by inserting a wedge between the two where they meet, will be necessary, in order that the upper part of the board to which the sole of the foot is bound may be perpendicular, and not participate in the tilt of the bed. To render it still more firm, a nail may be driven in the floor, in front of the lower end of the foot-board.

After any variety of fracture of the thigh it often occurs that the bladder is temporarily paralysed, and the person cannot make water. The passage of water should therefore always be inquired about, a few hours after an injury of the kind. If no water has been passed the bowels should be fomented (*vide Appendix*), and if this does not succeed the catheter must be used (*vide* p. 492).

However a fractured thigh is treated, the patient must remain in bed for five or six weeks, and must then go about on crutches, not putting his foot to the ground for another two or three weeks. In almost all cases some shortening of the limb occurs; and occasionally this is not apparent until the patient begins to walk.

When a fracture of the thigh happens away from home, a gun, a rifle, a broom-handle, or any long stick, wrapped in clothing, may be used as a temporary splint.

**FRACTURE OF THE KNEE-PAN.**—This generally results from spasmodic muscular action, as occurs from missing a step in coming downstairs. A sharp pain is experienced, accompanied by an often audible crack or snap. The person falls, and cannot stand. The knee cannot be straightened, and a hollow, or chink, is found between the broken parts a little above the knee.

*Treatment.*—The patient must be put to bed, and the limb extended on a light well-padded wooden splint or board reaching from the buttock to the heel, and having a hole at the end to receive the latter part, and a small piece, projecting at right angles from the end, to receive the sole of the foot. The heel end of the splint should then be raised about a foot and a half, which has the effect of relaxing the muscles, and so allows the broken parts to come into contact. The foot and leg must be lightly bandaged to the splint. Or the leg may be laid flat, the body of the patient being propped by a slanting board or bed-rest, in the semi-recumbent posture, which has a similar effect on the muscles. Or when one position becomes irksome, it may be exchanged for the other; or one may be maintained during the day, and the other at night, care being taken not to *lessen the angle* at the hip when changing posture, so that the muscles may be constantly relaxed. This may be readily accomplished by raising the body before lowering the foot, or by raising the foot before lowering the body. In some cases the broken parts of the knee-cap cannot be brought into satisfactory contact until both the heel is raised as above and also the body propped in the semi-recumbent posture. Whatever position is chosen, if there is much swelling and bruising, fomentation should be first used. Afterwards a bandage should be applied round the knee in the form of the figure of ∞, which will have the effect of bringing and retaining the broken parts together. A month at least should elapse before the patient attempts to move the knee. All movement should be made very carefully and gradually, as the union between the broken ends does not take place by bone but by the formation of a ligament, which may afterwards stretch. The person should go about on crutches, and wear an elastic knee-cap for some months. There is, notwithstanding all care, frequently permanent limping after this accident.

**FRACTURE OF THE LEG.**—May occur in any part of the leg, and one or both bones may be broken. When both bones are broken, the fracture may be generally easily detected by running the fingers down the shin, when an irregularity or prominence will be felt at the fractured part. There is also swelling, grating when the limb is moved, deformity, and when both bones are broken inability to stand. Sometimes the displacement of the bones may be masked, and the presence of fracture rendered doubtful by great swelling of the soft parts.

*Treatment.*—When there is great swelling, and the existence of fracture is not to be ascertained without subjecting the patient to great suffering, the limb should be as nearly as possible brought into a natural position, and then gently placed on a well-padded splint or on a pillow, to which it may be lightly tied by broad tapes. The person should lie on the side, so that the leg may be placed, with the knee bent, on its *outer* side. Then the limb should be well fomented for several days, or until the swelling subsides, when the broken bones, if not already in place, may be properly adjusted, or 'set,' and splints applied, as advised below. When this fomentation is desirable, it will be necessary to prevent saturation of the bed by placing an india-rubber sheet, or some oiled silk, or waxed cloth, under the part affected.

There are *two* positions in which a person with fracture of the leg may be placed, viz. *on the side* as above described, or *on the back*. Sometimes the nature of the fracture decides this point, the bones coming into better contact in one position than in the other. The position, however, may be ordinarily determined by the wish of the patient, some persons lying and sleeping more comfortably on the side, others on the back. *If it be determined to place the patient on the side*, splints should be first prepared wide enough to rather overlap the leg, long enough to reach from the knee to the foot, and provided with foot-pieces. If wooden

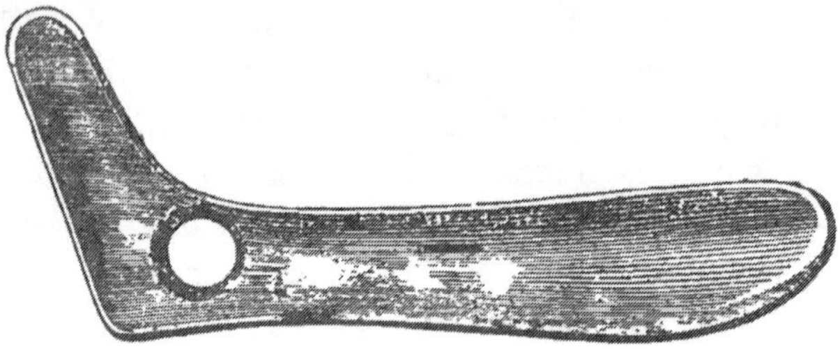

splints in the shape of the diagram are not available, they may be made of thick pasteboard, or of gutta percha, or they may be cut out of tin. The two first-named materials should be soaked in nearly boiling water, and moulded to the shape of the leg, by placing them for a short time on the corresponding leg of another person of about the same height. Then the splints should be well padded with cotton-wool, sewed in calico bags of the same shape as the splints. When all is ready, the knee of the patient should be fixed by an assistant holding it firmly with both hands, and the broken ends of the bone should be brought into position by steadily but gently pulling the foot, as shown in the sketch on p. 578. When under this operation the leg assumes the natural shape, the outer side should be gently laid upon one splint, and the other splint should be placed on the inner side; the whole to be secured by tape as shown in the figure. The leg being laid on its *outer* side, the knots must be tied on the *inner* side, and

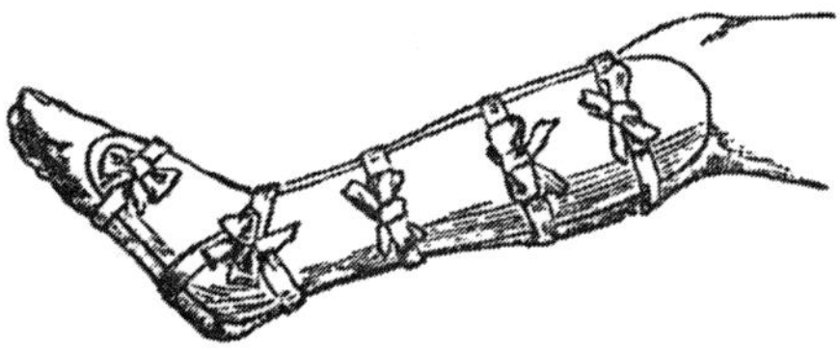

care must be taken that they are not, especially at first, drawn too tight, as the injured part will probably swell for a few days, and the pressure of the tape, especially on the shin bone, may produce blisters. To avoid this the splints should be rather wider than shown in the sketch. Knots are more easily loosened and tightened than a bandage, and further allow of the splint on the inner or upper side being lifted off, and the leg examined without disturbing the whole limb. After three weeks, if all swelling has disappeared, and the fractured part is firm, a starch bandage (Recipe 112) may be applied, and should be worn for a fortnight, after which it will be well to support the parts with plaster (Recipe 113) and a bandage for a week or two longer. The person may walk with crutches after the starch bandage is dry, being careful to rest no weight on the limb, until at least six weeks after the accident.

*When the person is to be placed on the back* it is desirable, although not positively necessary, that the leg should be laid on a splint with a *rectangular foot-piece* for the sole of the foot, as shown on next page.

If such a splint is obtainable, foot-pieces to the side splints are not so necessary, and the outside splint at least may be cut off above the hole for the ankle-bone. If a rectangular foot-piece is used, care should be taken that the ball of the heel, the ball of the great toe, and the ball of the little toe, *all* press against the pad of the splint, to which the foot should be securely bound. When the limb

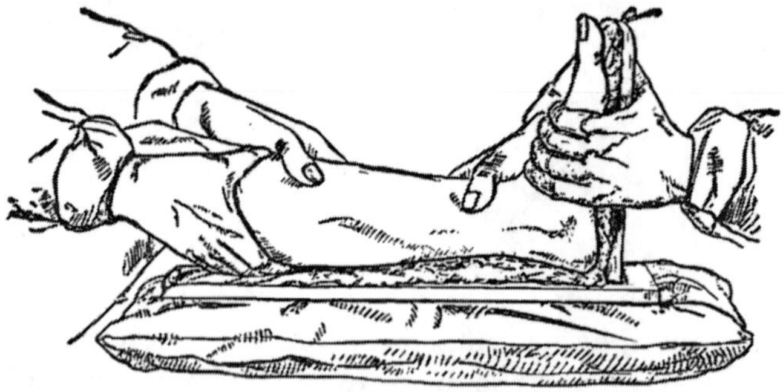

is brought into its natural position by extension of the foot as above described, the well-padded splints, reaching from knee to ankle, must be applied on each side, secured with tapes, and (if necessary) a bandage. The person

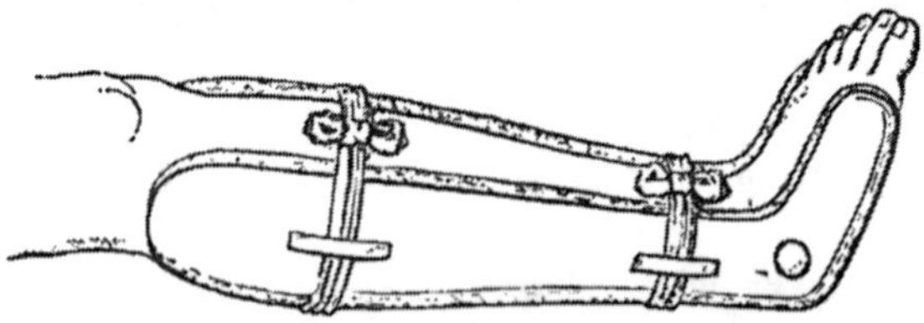

should be placed in bed, and the limb with the heel downwards, a small pillow being adjusted *under the hollow* of the ankle, to prevent the heel bearing the whole weight of the leg. Then, especially if there is no rectangular splint to which the foot may be bound, two bricks wrapped in cloth, or two bags of sand, should be placed on each side for the purpose of steadying the limb, and preventing it rolling round, to either side. Every endeavour should be made to keep the inner side of the ball of the great toe *in a line with the inner side of the knee-cap*, otherwise deformity will ensue. After about three weeks, a starch bandage or leather plaster may be applied, and the patient may move, but no weight should be borne on the limb for double that period.

**FRACTURE OF THE LEG IMMEDIATELY ABOVE THE ANKLE.**—One or both bones may be broken. In the second case the position of the foot is as sketched below.

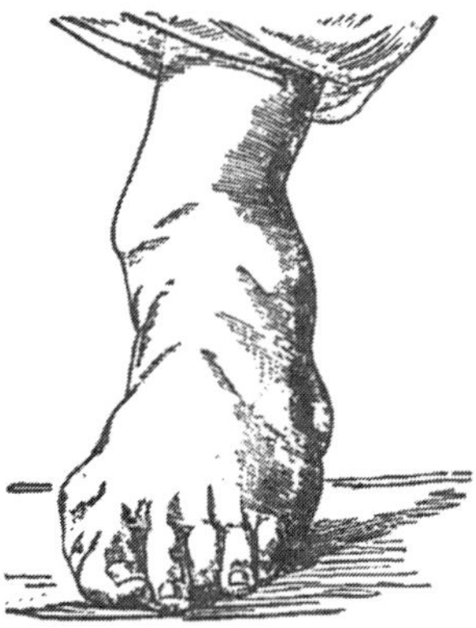

But often only the small bone (the one on the outside) is broken, when the deformity will not be so evident, and the swelling will be chiefly on the one side.

Fractures of this description should be treated with two splints, the patient lying either on the back or on the side, as for fracture of the upper part of the leg.

In treating cases of fracture of the small bone of the leg, or any injury near the ankle-joint, splints ought not to be used for more than a month or five weeks, for fear of stiff joint. At the end of that time the joint should be slightly moved daily, in order to secure mobility.

**FRACTURES OF THE FOOT.**—These injuries are difficult to detect and generally occur from great violence: the soft parts are frequently also much injured, and such cases necessitate surgical advice. Usually they do not require splints, placing the part as nearly as possible in the natural *position*, rest, fomentations, and lotions being the proper remedies.

FRACTURE, COMPLICATIONS OF.—1. *From rupture of blood-vessels, a quantity of blood may escape into the tissues of the limb.* If small it constitutes a bruise (*vide* pp. 515, 554) But it may be so large as to cause the limb to swell, and eventually abscess. In the absence of surgical advice, the injured limb should be kept at rest in an elevated position, and fomentations should be applied.

2. *Comminuted fracture.*—This is when the bone is broken into several small pieces. It is generally the result of direct violence, and the soft parts are usually a good deal bruised. The treatment is the same as for simple fracture, although there will be more trouble in keeping the parts in apposition, and much care must be taken to avoid pressure on the bruised parts, lest a wound results.

3. *Compound fractures.*—When there is an external wound communicating with the fracture it is called *compound.* Compound fractures are more dangerous than simple fractures, and are also more troublesome, as in addition to treating the *fracture* in the manner described, the wound must be cleansed and dressed daily, or more frequently, involving in every case different adjustment of splints and bandages in order to get at the wound easily without moving the fractured bone. When it is necessary to fix a limb with *compound fracture* on a splint, the seat of the injury should, as far as possible, be left uncovered by the baudage. If requisite, a second bandage may be applied over the first one, to retain poultices, dressings, &c. In this way local treatment may be used, without disturbing the position of the limb, and the progress of the wound can be watched, without causing unnecessary pain to the patient.

4. *Fractures implicating joints* are most dangerous, owing to the greater shock with which they are attended, and the risk of inflammation of the joint. They are also liable to be followed by some stiffness of the joint. Such cases require very careful treatment; at *first* absolute immobility of the injured bone and joint being the essential point, while inflammation is combated by fomentations. The *second* point is early *passive* motion of the joint, which should be gently moved by another person after the lapse of four weeks, in order that any adhesions which may have formed, may be broken down.

5. Other dangers from bad or compound fractures are inflammation of the veins, tetanus, and blood poisoning.

FRACTURED, TORN, OR CUT TENDO ACHILLIS.—The large thick tendon, thus called, which connects the heel with the great muscles forming the calf of the leg (and which are the main instruments in keeping the lower limbs erect and straight when we stand, and in throwing the body forward when we walk), is liable to be torn or cut. It may be torn in making a false step in walking, or running, or in coming downstairs, or when dancing. The tendon tears without warning, and the person drops to the ground with the sensation of a smart blow on the part. On attempting to rise he finds himself unable to rest the least weight on the foot, and a gap will be distinguished where the tendon is separated, into which the finger drops in passing it from the heel up the leg towards the calf.

*Treatment.*—This consists in putting the patient to bed and laying the leg on the outside with the knee much bent, and the *toes much pointed*, by which position the torn ends of the tendon are brought as nearly as possible together. This posture must be preserved for a fortnight, to give time for the production of the new substance by which the tendon is repaired. To secure this position it will be necessary to bind a piece of thin board, about four fingers wide, extending from below the knee-cap to beyond the toes, upon the *front* of the leg, taking care to have the board well padded so that it may not rub. The board must be confined by a bandage to the foot, and above to the calf. Or the same position may be secured by the patient wearing a slipper attached by a band fixed to the slipper heel, to a buckle and strap, fixed above the knee. Cold lotions may be applied. No bandage must be put on where the tendon is torn. After a fortnight or a little longer the gap mentioned above may be filled up with a firm substance. The person may then get up, the leg be straightened gradually, and a shoe with a very high heel worn, which may be gradually cut down till in some months' time the leg may be quite straightened.

When the 'Achilles tendon' is cut, which may happen

from the blow of a scythe or sickle, or sword, the case is more serious. The person is in the same condition as a beast which is 'houghed,' and cannot stand. When the wound has been brought together, by placing the limb in the position above described, the edges of the loose skin drop into the wound, so as to interfere with union. It is therefore necessary to nip up both edges of the cut skin, so as to make their *under* surfaces touch, then passing a needle and suture to keep them in such position. The limb must then be 'put up,' as described for simple rupture, and the stitches may be taken out on the third or fourth day. The wound should also be protected by plaster cut into long narrow strips, and applied *lengthwise* on the leg.

CRUTCHES.—Crutches should be just long enough to enable the person to raise the injured leg off the ground while he stands firmly on the other. The cross-bar should be oval-shaped and well padded, otherwise the pressure may strain the nerves of the arm. The ends of the crutch should be tipped with leather to prevent them slipping. If the state of the injured limb is such that the patient ought not to use it at all, support it with a bandage passed under the foot, the ends being brought up evenly in front and tied behind the neck. In this way a sort of sling is made, which assists the patient in keeping his foot from the ground.

**GANGLION.**—This is the term applied to a swelling of the membrane inclosing the tendons of the wrist. It may appear gradually, and it may arise suddenly, after a strain or twist of the part, and may attain the size of a marble or a small egg. Similar swellings also sometimes appear from blows or other injury, on the back of the hand, on the tip of the elbow-joint, on the side of the knee, and on the knee-cap. If the swelling is on the wrist, or back of the hand, and free from tenderness, it may burst by pressure with the thumbs, or by a blow with an unbound book. Then a pad made of a coin, or piece of lead wrapped in lint, should be bandaged on the part and worn for some weeks, to prevent re-formation. If there is any tenderness, the swelling should be first fomented and the part rested, in order to prevent inflammation. If on other parts of the body, blisters and other surgical treatment will probably be required.

**HANGING.**—Life may be destroyed at once, if the body falls any considerable distance, by dislocation of the neck. If the force of the fall does not cause this, pressure of the rope on the blood-vessels of the neck, preventing the flow of blood, may cause rupture of some vessel in the brain, when the person dies from apoplexy. Such cases, especially the first, are generally immediately fatal. Thirdly, the hanging person may die slowly from pressure of the cord on the windpipe, causing suffocation. If this occurs (and it depends on the position of the cord whether death takes place in this manner or by apoplexy) and the body be soon cut down, the person may possibly be revived by 'Artificial respiration.' (*Vide* p. 542.)

**LIGHTNING-STROKE.**—A person struck by lightning is suddenly, more or less completely, deprived of consciousness. But this may be either from fright, or from the electric fluid. If from fright, the condition quickly passes off, the person recovering as if from collapse, or shock (*vide* p. 520). Lightning may cause burns, sometimes of a deep and obstinate character, sometimes merely blistering, or redness of the surface. Occasionally arborescent marks are discovered, appearing as if trees or other objects had been photographed on the skin. Other affections caused by lightning are, fractured bones, wounds like stabs, partial loss of sight, smell, speech, hearing or taste, and paralysis, which may or may not be permanent. Usually, however, persons not killed on the spot, recover. The immediate treatment of persons struck by lightning should be as recommended for *Collapse* (*vide* p. 521). Burns, or other injuries inflicted, must be treated as recommended under the respective heads.

The following are useful rules concerning danger from lightning:—

1. Lightning always chooses the best conductors on its descent to the earth; consequently we should know what things are better conductors than man, and what are not such good conductors as man. Near the former we are safe; the latter should be carefully avoided.

2. It is dangerous to stand near any high object, such as a tree, spire, or large building, because its height is likely to discharge the electric fluid passing overhead, and it is not as good a conductor as a man would be; consequently the lightning, having been discharged by it, would pass through the man's body, which offers a better passage to the earth.

3. It is dangerous to stand near running water if no higher object than yourself be near, as water is an excellent conductor, and a man's height may be sufficient to discharge the lightning, in which case it would choose him as its conductor to the water.

4. It is dangerous to be in a crowd, as the vapour arising from a mass of people affords great attraction to the lightning.

5. It is very dangerous to carry jewellery or pieces of metal about the person—rings, brooches, keys, or watches—as they offer strong attraction to the lightning to take them on its downward course, but are not sufficient to carry it to the earth.

6. If you are driving on a carriage during a storm, do not lean back, but sit upright, as the lightning might run down the sides of the carriage.

7. Indoors the safest place is the middle of the room, as, if the house were struck, the lightning would run down the walls.

8. Mattresses and hearthrugs, &c., are non-conductors, and sitting on these you are comparatively safe.

9. A person lying on an iron bedstead is comparatively safe, as it is a better conductor than the human body.

10. If you are out walking during a storm and your clothes become wet through with the rain, you are free from danger, as wet clothes will conduct the electric fluid harmlessly over the body.

11. During a storm, a person is safer in the open, although a wetting may be experienced, than under trees, or in sheds, which may attract the lightning.

**PRIVATE PARTS, INJURIES OF THE.**—In the male, the testicles are liable to be injured by blows, or by the patient being thrown forward on the pommel of the saddle. The effect is swelling of the parts, accompanied by great pain and tenderness, with faintness immediately after the injury. At first a stimulant, as wine, or brandy and water, will probably be required. Afterwards fomentations and rest will in the great majority of cases effect a cure.

**POISONING.**—Poisoning by almost any agent is best treated by making the patient vomit at once. If the person can swallow, give a mustard or salt emetic (Recipe 54) and repeat every five minutes till vomiting occurs. If the person cannot swallow, endeavour to excite vomiting by tickling the inside of the throat with a feather. After vomiting, or immediately if vomiting cannot be induced, give the *antidote* as below, if available, in water.

**POISONS AND ANTIDOTES.**—The subjoined table affords at a glance guidance in cases of poisoning. The Indian poisons referred to on the next page are in italics.

| *Irritant Poisons* | *Antidotes* |
|---|---|
| Mineral acids, as vitriol or sulphuric acid, nitric acid, spirits of salts, hydrochloric acid . . . . | Magnesia, chalk, or whitewash scraped off walls; washing soda in milk or water. |
| Vegetable acids, as oxalic acid, tartaric acid, acetic acid, salts of sorrel, cream of tartar . . . | Chalk, whiting, whitewash, or soda in milk or water. |
| Alkalis, as potash, soda, ammonia, sal volatile, smelling salts . . | Equal parts of vinegar and water, lemon-juice, oil. |
| Alum . . . . . . . | Washing soda, smelling salts in water. |
| Antimony, as tartar emetic . . | Tincture of kino or catechu, magnesia, tannin or gallic acid. |
| Antimony, butter of . . . | Magnesia, washing soda, chalk. |
| *Arsenic* and its salts . . . | A mixture of oil and lime-water, soap suds, milk, flour and water, powdered charcoal in water, rust scraped off old iron. |
| Baryta and its salts . . . | Epsom salts, in water. |
| Copper salts, as blue vitriol, verdigris | White of egg in water, milk, wheat flower in water. |
| Iron salts, as sulphate of, or green vitriol . . . . . . | Soda, or smelling salts, in water. |
| Lead salts, as sugar of lead, white lead . . . . . . . | Epsom salts, or vinegar diluted. |
| Mercury salts, as corrosive sublimate | White of egg in water, wheat flour thick in water. |
| Silver salts, as nitrate of, or caustic . | Common table salt in water freely. |
| Zinc salts, as sulphate or acetate of . | Milk, soda, magnesia, in water. |

| *Narcotic and Deliriant Poisons* | *Antidotes* |
|---|---|
| *Aconite*, chloral, *dhatura*, hemlock, morphia, *opium*, *hemp*, fungi | Strong coffee or tea, motion and means to prevent sleep, artificial respiration. |

---

| *Other Poisons* | *Antidotes* |
|---|---|
| Prussic acid | Ammonia, sal volatile, smelling salts, hartshorn. |
| *Strychnine* | Powdered charcoal in water, chloral. |

**INDIAN POISONS.**—The principal poisons made use of in India are as below, and the prominent symptoms caused by each are contrasted.

| *Poisons* | *Prominent Symptoms* |
|---|---|
| ACONITE Vernacular: *metha-thelia, dakra, bish* | Numbness and tingling of the tongue and lips, burning of the throat, spitting, hawking, frothing at the mouth, vomiting, pupils dilated, but contracting on exposure to strong light, delirium, stupor, paralysis, insensibility, convulsions. |
| ARSENIC Vernacular: *sunkiah, saffed sumbhul.* | Faintness, nausea, violent vomiting and purging of material streaked with blood, burning in the throat, stomach, and fundament, thirst, cramp of legs, feeble pulse, cold skin. |
| DHATURA Vernacular: *kala* or *Krishna dhatura.* | Headache, faintness, dimness of sight, giddiness, thirst, excitement, voluble talking, laughter, fatuity, dilated pupils, insensibility, stertorous breathing, frothing at the mouth. |
| INDIAN HEMP Vernacular: *gungah, bhang* | Appears like a drunken person, fits of laughing alternating with intervals of stupidity, which gradually increase to insensibility. |
| OPIUM Vernacular: *offeem, umal* | Giddiness, drowsiness, stupor, succeeded by total insensibility and stertorous breathing, skin cold, face pallid, eyes closed, pupils contracted. |
| STRYCHNINE Vernacular: *koochla, koochla-bij* | Feeling of suffocation, difficulty of breathing, twitching of the limbs, locked jaw, convulsions, the body being bent back, features drawn into a characteristic grin. |

POISONING BY GASES, *as carbonic acid, carbonic oxide, sulphuretted hydrogen, &c.*—Persons going into pits, wells, drains, &c., are sometimes poisoned by unrespirable gases. The symptoms vary. In slight cases there is faintness and vomiting. In more severe cases there is more or less insensibility, and generally stertorous or snoring breathing, and sometimes convulsions. Removal to fresh air, stimulants, and in bad cases artificial respiration (*vide* p. 542) are required.

**POISONING OF THE BLOOD.**—Blood poisoning may occur under a number of varying circumstances. The blood is more or less poisoned in many diseases of which typhus and typhoid fevers are the type. But the term 'blood poisoning' is more conveniently applied to conditions in which a diseased or injured part secretes an unhealthy material, which may be absorbed into the system; or from which minute portions (called *emboli*) of *thrombi* or clots formed in the neighbouring veins may be transferred to different parts. The term is still more popularly applied to cases in which a sore surface of one person has come into contact with the diseased discharges of another person, or with those of some animal or insect.

According to the latest researches, when a poisoned wound is made certain blood cells known as *leucocytes* crowd to the spot, block up the avenues by which poisonous microbes seek to gain entrance, and engulf and destroy them. The poisonous microbes at the same time multiply with rapidity, endeavouring to destroy the blood cells and force a passage. This local war, which under the microscope is stated to be 'as realistic as one of Homer's battles,' is defensive inflammation. If the blood cells prevail there will probably be only a local abscess; if the poisonous microbes prevail, and gain access to the circulation, there will be blood poisoning.

When poisonous matter enters the system it may cause a condition known as *septicæmia*, which occurs more especially from the absorption of chemical products resulting from the decomposition of inflammatory material. Or it may cause a condition known as *pyæmia*, which occurs more especially from the circulation of some animal poison in the blood.

Thus 'blood poisoning' may result from bad forms of dysentery, when, deleterious matter being conveyed from the bowels, abscess forms in the liver (*vide* p. 323), being determined to that organ by peculiar anatomical configurations. Or it may result from putrid matter from the womb during puerperal fever (*vide* p. 630); or from unclean and lacerated wounds, especially from burns and scalds (*vide* p. 519); or from bad or compound fractures (*vide* p. 580); or from wounds inflicted by wild animals (*vide* p. 607); or from the circumstances giving rise to one variety of carbuncle (*vide* p. 113); or especially from wounds received during the manipulation of diseased bodies of living or dead animals. Blood poisoning is attended from the first with great depression; there are repeated shiverings, quick pulse, hot skin, dry tongue, sallowness of the surface, peculiar odour of the breath, thick ammoniacal urine, profuse perspirations, and the cessation of discharge from any wound. If *pyæmia* results soon after the first symptoms, sometimes in twenty-four hours, throbbing pain, or swelling in different parts, point to the localisation of the mischief by *abscess* which may form in the liver, lungs, skin, joints, or other parts. When blood poisoning occurs, the requirements are to support the strength by nourishing diet and stimulants, to give chloral to relieve pain, and to favour the formation of matter, where pain and swelling indicate its localisation, as detailed under *Abscess*, p. 41.

**RIDER'S BONE**, or **SPRAIN**.—This consists of rupture of fibres of the *adductor* muscle, situated at the inner part of the thigh. It may occur to those riding a great deal, without any extraordinary exertion. But it commonly results from violent efforts to grip the horse when making a jump; or to *football*-players. A snap is felt, followed by pain and tenderness on the inner surface of, usually, the right thigh, close to the trunk, and sometimes extending to the knee. There may also be bruise, coming on immediately, or not till some hours afterwards. The injury usually leaves some thickening or hardness of the tendons in the inner part of the thigh, which in some cases becomes almost like bone; hence the name 'Rider's bone.' Generally, the symptoms subside under rest and fomentations. If neglected, the hardness may become permanent, causing some lameness, and inability to ride far or fast. Supports are made for this condition, for which measurements round the body at the hip-bone, round the top of the thigh, and round the leg just above the knee are required, with intimation of which leg.

**RUPTURE.**—Technically spoken of as *hernia*; vulgarly as 'broken belly.' There are several varieties, but the most common appears in the *male* as a tumour in the groin; in the *female* as a tumour a little lower than the groin. This tumour is caused by the muscles over the bowels giving way, and letting some portion of the intestines escape outwards beneath the skin. The affection may come on gradually from natural weakness of the parts, but it more often happens suddenly during extraordinary exertion. A sudden sensation of something giving way is felt, and a soft elastic swelling appears. In the male, the rupture eventually makes its way into the purse. In the female, it remains as a smaller tumour in the groin. When a rupture has occurred, *the bowel may return or be returned into the cavity of the abdomen,* when it is said to be *reducible.* Or it may *remain down and cannot be returned,* when it said to be *irreducible.* Or, *it may be compressed and fixed by the ruptured muscular fibres through which it has passed,* when it is said to be *strangulated.* In the *first* result no symptoms present; but a rupture having once occurred, the tumour is liable to come down when the person stands or walks about; and although it may return when he lies down, or when pressure is made, there is always danger that *it may remain down and become strangulated.* A person with *reducible* rupture should avoid excessive exertion, and wear a truss.

A truss is composed of a pad connected with a circular metallic spring, and so arranged that the pad keeps the bowel from descending, the spring maintaining the pad in position, and allowing free movement of the body. A truss should be fitted to the person by the instrument-maker, under the supervision of a surgeon. But if obliged to send for a truss, the measurement of the body, one inch below the hips, should be given, and the side affected should be mentioned. Care should be taken that the spring is strong enough to control the rupture, and to ascertain this, after adjusting the truss, the patient should stand up, with his legs wide apart, and cough strongly. If the truss is not suitable, the rupture will come down. The truss and pad should be covered with leather, from which the skin is less likely to chafe.

If the truss chafes at first the skin should be bathed with alum water (Recipe 42), which will harden it. Wrapping a narrow thin calico bandage round the truss, which may be taken off and washed, is desirable for cleanliness, or a washable truss may be obtained. The truss should be put on *before* rising in the morning, and be taken off *after* lying down at night. The person should have two trusses, one for wearing when bathing, so that he may never be without the protection, and retain his truss in ordinary wear dry. It is generally desirable for a person, although only ruptured on one side, to wear a double truss, for there is often a weakness of the corresponding region on the opposite side, and with a truss upon one groin, a greater strain is thrown upon the other, which is therefore apt to give way. Unless a truss fulfils all the requirements as above, and unless it is used in the manner directed, it may do injury. Without a truss, a person with reducible rupture is in constant danger of life ; with a good truss, properly used, he is safe. If, when a rupture first appears, a truss cannot be procured at once, a figure of ∞ bandage (*vide* p. 109) with a pad over the rupture should be used.

*When the tumour remains down and cannot be returned, although not strangulated* (*vide* below), there is a colourless, elastic tumour often penetrating to the purse, which causes disorder of the digestive organs, with colicky dragging pains, flatulence, and constipation. It is also apt to become strangulated or inflamed, or to be injured by external violence. The requirements are to render the hernia reducible if possible, to prevent it increasing in size, and to treat dyspeptic symptoms. The patient should be kept in bed on spare diet and ice should be applied to the swelling. Aperients (Recipe 1, 2) and iodide of potassium (Recipe 21) should be given. The rupture, if penetrating to the purse, should be supported by a suspensory bandage or bag.

*When the tumour does not return*, symptoms of *strangulation* are very likely to commence. The patient first complains of flatulence, colicky pains, a sense of tightness across the belly, desire to go to stool, and inability to evacuate. Some fæcal matter may, however, be passed if any happens to be present *below* that part of the intestines which has become strangulated. To these symptoms succeed vomiting of the contents of the stomach, then of sour bilious fluid, then of material like coffee-grounds, and lastly of matters having the odour, and often the appearances, of fæces. The swelling becomes tense and incompressible and does not move when the person coughs. If this state continues the inflammatory stage sets in. The tumour, and eventually the whole surface of the belly, becomes swollen and painful. The countenance denotes anxiety, the vomiting is constant, the patient restless and desponding, the pulse is small, quick, and wiry, and there is constant hiccough. After a variable time the parts mortify, the tumour becomes dusky red, the pain ceases, and the patient, having probably expressed himself relieved, soon after dies.

*Treatment.*—Purgatives either given by the mouth or as enemata will do harm. Therefore, the feeling of a desire to stool, causing entreaty on the part of the patient for something to open the bowels, should not be complied with. *The great point is to return the protruding intestine into the cavity of the abdomen.* The bladder having been emptied, the patient should lie down with his shoulders raised, and with both thighs bent towards his belly, and placed close together. This relaxes all the muscles. Then the operator grasps the swelling with the fingers if small, with the palm of the hands if large, and *gently* compresses it. This will dispel wind, and other contents of the swelling, into the belly. Then the swelling may be raised by its neck, *gently* pulled forward, and again compressed. This should be continued for a quarter of an hour if the swelling is not tender and there is no hiccough; but for a shorter period if the reverse conditions present. Much force must not be used, as the tumour may be injured or pushed between the muscles, instead of back into its proper place. If this does not succeed, the patient should be either put into a hot bath, or chloroformed, and similar endeavours made while the person is in the water, or when he is insensible from the chloroform. If there is no hot bath, or no chloroform, or no one to administer it, and symptoms of strangulation are not violent, 40 drops of chlorodyne, or 40 grains of chloral, or, if available, 40 drops of laudanum in an ounce of water, may be given; pounded ice in a bag, or if not available the freezing mixture (Recipe 83), may be applied to the part, the *foot* of the bed being raised two or three feet from the floor, and the patient let alone for two or three hours, when the rupture may return, or it may be put back by repetition of manual endeavours as above. When successful, the tumour usually disappears with a sudden gurgling, the pain is relieved, and the vomiting stops. A pad should be carefully placed over the part, and the figure of ∞ bandage applied (*vide* p. 109). The diet should be fluid, until the bowels have acted naturally, and no aperient medicine should be given; but if the bowels do not act in twelve hours, an injection of warm water and soap should be used (Recipe 104). If symptoms of strangulation are urgent, and the swelling cannot be returned, a surgical operation of an important character affords the only chance of recovery.

Rupture is liable to be mistaken for *hydrocele* (*vide* p. 308), or for *varicocele* (*vide* p. 454), or *vice versâ*. The distinctive features are therefore contrasted.

| RUPTURE | HYDROCELE | VARICOCELE |
|---|---|---|
| Usually comes on suddenly. | Comes on gradually. | Comes on gradually. |
| Disappears when the person lies down, and reappears when he stands up. | Does not disappear when the person lies down. | Disappears when the person lies down. |
| If the fingers are pressed on the *external ring* when the patient is lying down, and he rises with the fingers still pressed on the part, a rupture does not return. The *external ring* is the part through which the rupture passes, and is about an inch above, but to the side of, the root of the penis. | Pressure with the fingers makes no difference. The swelling remains as before. | Pressure with the fingers does not prevent the reappearance of the swelling, which gradually returns when the person stands up. |
| The tumour commences above, or in the groin. | The tumour commences below, or in the purse. | Commences from below, or in the purse. |
| Tumour tense, or elastic; or 'gurgling' may be felt or heard inside. | Tumour smooth, affording a fluctuating feeling, like water in a bladder. | Feels like a bag of worms. |
| When the person coughs the impulse communicated by the cough is felt in the tumour. | No impulse or shake from coughing felt in the tumour. | No impulse or shake from coughing felt in the tumour. |
| The tumour is opaque. | Tumour is translucent; that is, light may be seen through it. | The tumour is opaque. |
| No pain or tenderness in the tumour, unless *strangulated*. | No pain or tenderness in the tumour. | Dull aching of the part. |
| The tumour does not obscure the testicle, which may be felt below it. | The tumour obscures the testicle, which is behind it. | The tumour does not obscure the testicle, which is below it. |
| No distinct separation between the tumour and the bowels. | Distinct separation between the tumour and the bowels. | Distinct separation between the tumour and the bowels. |
| Dangerous to life. | Not dangerous to life. | Not dangerous to life. |

**RUPTURE, INFANTILE.**—Infants are sometimes born ruptured, or may become ruptured from natural weakness of the parts, and straining when crying, or from costiveness. If a truss is used it is necessary to procure several, in order to have a dry truss every time one gets soiled; and, besides, if the child thrives, the old trusses in eight or ten weeks will be too small and useless. But a figure of ∞ bandage, if properly used, is quite sufficient.

A skein of Berlin or lamb's wool, of 35 to 40 threads, may be crocheted into a flat band about two inches wide, and looped at the end. Then return the rupture by pressure, and place the looped end of the skein over the seat of rupture. Then pass the other end round the body and through the loop, which must be carefully adjusted over the seat of rupture. Then carry the end down between the thighs, bring it up outside the thigh, and fix to the loop. A pad may be used if necessary, but usually none is required.

**RUPTURE AT THE NAVEL.**—Most frequently happens to children, and infants are sometimes born with it. It may also occur to adults, especially to females. In children it may result from inattention to the navel after birth, or it may occur suddenly during paroxysms of crying, or straining. In adults it may be caused by violent exertion, or straining. It is known by bulging of the navel, which may assume the size of an egg in children, but is much larger in adults. When the person lies on the back the swelling subsides, and the circular opening through which it presents may be felt with the fingers. As mentioned of rupture at the groin (*vide* p. 589) it may become *irreducible* or *strangulated.*

*Treatment.*—For children, a large piece of cork covered with lint (or sometimes a rupee or piece of lead, being heavier, answers better) should be fitted over the swelling, and retained in its position with strips of plaster and a light flannel bandage 2½ inches wide. Fits of crying should as much as possible be prevented, as the rupture always protrudes more on such occasions. The child should wear the pad and bandage constantly. As the child grows, the tendency of the tumour to increase will lessen, and, by continually using pressure as above, the tumour will gradually disappear. An adult should wear a pad and belt, especially if engaged in an occupation involving much exertion, or if subject to chronic cough, and should avoid straining at stool. If a rupture at the navel becomes irreducible or strangulated, the measures mentioned at pp. 590, 591 should be adopted. If strangulation cannot be thus relieved, a surgical operation is requisite.

**SPLEEN, RUPTURE OF THE.**—When the spleen is diseased or enlarged it is excessively tender, and a very slight injury will rupture it, sometimes without any external mark. Occasionally the spleen ruptures from a fall, or even from muscular exertion. When the covering or *capsule* of the organ is ruptured, blood escapes into the cavity of the bowels, and the symptoms are those of collapse (*vide* p. 520), the person becoming faint, complaining of great pain, and the pulse rapidly growing imperceptible. Such injuries are nearly always quickly fatal, and no medical treatment is of much utility. Perfect rest, and the administration of stimulants, are indicated; but stimulants must be given with caution, and only when the pulse can scarcely be felt: otherwise, the excitement of blood-circulation they cause will add to internal bleeding (*vide* p. 514).

Though death from ruptured spleen nearly always takes place in a few hours, rare cases occur in which life is prolonged for several days. In these cases blood is not poured out into the abdomen immediately, the injured person appears to be in no danger, and the spleen is thought not to be injured. After an interval of some days, however, sudden symptoms of syncope are manifested, the abdomen becomes distended with blood, and death occurs within a very short time. The reason for the delay in the occurrence of death after a rupture of the spleen, is that although the spleen is ruptured at the time of injury, the *capsule* or covering of the organ does not give way till some time afterwards.

**SPRAINS or STRAINS.**—The terms signify a violent stretching of the tendons, ligaments, or muscles of the part. But some of the fibres of the tendons about the injured part are often ruptured or torn. Sprains generally occur to the joints, as the ankles, wrists, or knees. But similar accidents may occur in other parts, the 'lawn-tennis leg' being strain or rupture of some of the muscular or tendinous structures of the calf. The symptoms of a bad sprain are severe pain, and often faintness, followed by swelling and discoloration, with subsequent weakness and stiffness. If the part is not kept at rest, or if the diet be intemperate, or the blood impure, or if the knee or some other large joint is injured, there may be inflammation and fever, which, if neglected, may lead to serious results. How sprains are distinguished from *dislocations*, and from *fractures* near joints, is mentioned at pp. 526, 553. A minor degree of sprain, arising from continued minor concussions, rather than from one violent wrench, is known as the 'lawn-tennis arm,' and may occur in the shoulder, elbow, or wrist.

*Treatment.*—The most essential measure is *perfect rest.* If serious, the injured part should be confined by pasteboard or gutta percha splints. If the wrist is injured, it must be constantly suspended in a sling. If the ankle, the patient must lie or sit, with his leg on a couch or stool. Warm fomentations generally give more relief than cold lotions, but in this the patient's feelings may be consulted (*vide Appendix, Cooling applications*). If a large joint is affected, and inflammation and fever are high, leeches should be applied (one for each year of the person's age up to thirty), and cooling medicines, as citrate of magnesia (*vide* p. 15), may be administered. Subsequently, friction with soap liniment. After some time (as an average, a fortnight in sprains of joints), gentle movement of the part by some one else, then moderate exercise, and the support of bandages will be required. After a sprain the part remains weak, and liable to injury for some time. In delicate children sprains are frequently the origin of disease of the joints.

For minor sprains arnica or hazeline may be used. Persons who meet with a strain—lawn-tennis players, for instance—are often desirous to be strapped up and allowed to play again. This may succeed in some instances, but it is a bad plan. A sprained part must have time to recover itself, and this it will not do thoroughly while the muscles are in action, even if supported by strapping. A sprain thus treated is more liable to recur. For the 'lawn-tennis elbow' an elbow-cap has been devised, but it is not recommended, as it obstructs the veins of the arm below.

**STIFF JOINTS.**—May be caused by injury or from disease. Stiff joints from injury usually occur after dislocations, or fractures near joints, or after sprains.

When an injury is followed by local swellings, as happens in most sprains, this swelling is produced by an effusion of fluid into the tissues, and the fluid effused is of an adhesive character. The result is as if liquid glue had been introduced among the weakened and tender parts; and, if the sticky effusion has been abundant, or if rest be too long maintained, the resulting adhesions may prevent free movement, or any movement, of the joint concerned. In order to prevent such adhesions early *passive movement* has been recommended after all injuries liable to be followed by adhesions. When they do occur and prevent movement of the joint, rupturing them by forcible movement is the only cure. When ruptured a snap is felt and heard. These are the cases in which 'bone setters' are sometimes successful. The surgeon knows that by forcible manipulation he is often as likely to do harm as good. Occasionally by risking dangers from which the educated surgeon shrinks, the bone-setter is successful.

The proper treatment of stiff joints is gentle *passive movement* (*i.e.* movement of the joint by some one else), and rubbing with soap and opium liniment, until the advice of a surgeon can be obtained. The propriety of forcible treatment depends *both* on the condition of the joint, and on the constitution and general health of the patient.

**TEETH, INJURIES OF THE.**—When a tooth is broken, any sharp point should be smoothed with a fine, sharp file, which will prevent injury to the mouth or tongue, and render the tooth less liable to decay commencing from the seat of injury. The part should be afterwards touched several times daily for a week with spirits of wine, which renders the tooth hard and insensitive. If a tooth is loosened so much as to shake about, it should not be removed, as with care it will probably again unite to the gum. It should be replaced in its natural position, and the person should be instructed to avoid moving it with the tongue. If it will not remain *in situ*, a fine piece of wire or silk, or a horsehair, should be passed round it and the adjacent tooth, so as to prevent motion. Teeth knocked out of the mouth, or drawn by mistake, being immediately returned to the socket, have taken root. These facts led to the replanting of teeth as an operation of dental surgery.

**URINE, RETENTION OF.**—Retention of urine signifies an inability to pass water, *not a stoppage* of the formation of urine. Urine still flows from the kidneys where it is secreted, into the bladder, but cannot escape from the latter organ. Retention of urine may arise from stricture (*vide* p. 419); from an enlarged prostate gland (p. 366); from a small stone lodging in the passage (p. 73); from paralysis of the bladder (p. 74); from hysteria (p. 305); from fracture of the thigh or spine (pp. 573, 557). It may also arise from injury, such as falling cross-legged on a gate or wooden bar, which may cause bruise, swelling, or worse injury of the parts about the passage. The symptoms and treatment of retention from the different maladies named are given under the respective headings. When retention occurs from injury, fomenting between the legs and over the bowels with a dose of chloral (Recipe 64) will generally afford relief. Otherwise, the catheter must be used (*vide* p. 493).

**WOUNDS AND CUTS.**—Wounds may be *clean cut* with a sharp instrument as a sword, or made *jagged and ragged* by a blunt instrument as a saw, or *bruised* as by a rough club or stick, or *punctured* by a sharp-pointed instrument as a bayonet.

In *clean-cut or incised wounds*, bleeding must be first checked, and then all dirt and *débris* removed. To arrest bleeding, a raised position, the application of cold water, and pressure with a sponge will often suffice. But if an artery is wounded, and the bleeding prove obstinate, measures must be adopted as pointed out under *Bleeding* (p. 505). The removal of dirt and foreign bodies from the wound may be effected by a stream of cold water, the sponge, and the forceps. Having stopped bleeding and removed dirt, clots of blood should be taken away, and the wounded part placed in such position as will best favour approximation of the cut edges, which must be brought together and maintained in position by long strips of plaster; one end of the plaster being first applied to that side of the wound where the skin is most loose, and each strip should slightly overlap its neighbour. But the strips should *never* be long enough to encircle a limb, as they would then act as ligatures, and cause swelling of the parts below. Then a pad of lint wet with water should be placed over the wound, and a bandage applied to retain all in position. For a slight clean cut wound collodion may suffice. The edges of the cut should be held together while the collodion is applied with a brush. The collodion quickly hardens and contracts, and the wound heals beneath. For large wounds, or wounds of loose parts, as the eyelids or ear, stitches will often be required. But stitches should never be used to *drag* the edges of a wound together, and they should be removed on the third day, or inflammation may result. In stitching a wound the needle should be passed deep enough to obtain a firm hold, but should not penetrate any tendon or muscle; and, as a rule, one stitch will be required for every inch of wound.

In Jagged, Lacerated, or Contused Wounds, while restraining bleeding and removing foreign bodies may be easily accomplished, it will often be impossible to approximate the edges of the wound, either by plaster or stitches. But this should be effected as far as possible. In many wounds the laceration is so great that it is necessary to abandon all attempts to bring the edges together. Poultices, and afterwards water dressing, will be best. For pinches of nails bathe with hot water.

When dressing wounds, everything likely to be required should be ready before the wound is uncovered. Clean-cut wounds should not be opened the day after they are dressed, but may be cautiously re-dressed on the third day. Care must then be taken that the support of one strip of plaster or of the fingers is always afforded, otherwise the union taking place will be broken through. In removing the plasters the *ends* should be first raised, and *both* ends should be lifted up at the same time, *from the outside to the centre,* so that no dragging may separate the edges of the injured part. Care must be taken to thoroughly clear away all discharge, lest it become offensive; and it should be recollected that a wound which is doing well has no bad smell. After the third day all wounds in India should, as a matter of cleanliness, be dressed daily unless they can be treated antiseptically as below.

Although thorough division of a part may have taken place (*e.g.* a finger, or a toe, or a portion of the nose or ear may have been completely severed), still an attempt to unite the divided parts should be made and success will frequently follow the attempt.

If the appliances are at hand, it would be better to dress clean-cut wounds *antiseptically*. The procedure is based on putrescence being fermentation due to germs from the atmosphere, which is prevented by the antiseptic dressing. But antiseptic dressing requires appliances, only to be found in the possession of a surgeon. Still, if the whole procedure cannot be carried out, it is advisable that, when possible, antiseptic solutions should be used. The wound and skin around should be washed with a solution of 10 grains of crystallised carbolic acid to an ounce of distilled water, and it should be covered with lint, moistened in a solution of 20 grains of the acid in 1 ounce of salad oil.

The neglect of cleanliness of wounds is frequently followed in tropical climates by the appearance of *maggots.* When the wound permits easy access to all parts of the injury, the maggots may be picked out with forceps, or destroyed by injections of black wash (Recipe 88), or, this not available, lime-water (Recipe 25). If maggots have penetrated into a sinus stretching away from a wound, the use of the knife to open up the part may be necessary.

WOUNDS OF THE SCALP may be either cleanly cut or jagged. If the scalp is detached from the bone it should be carefully cleaned and replaced. In addition to restraining bleeding, clearing away foreign matter and clots of blood, the scalp should be shaved for several inches round the wound, to afford space for plasters. Wounds of the scalp, however slight, should never be neglected, as they are liable to be followed by erysipelas; and for a similar reason stitches should, whenever practicable, be dispensed with. If it is positively necessary to apply stitches, plasters may generally be dispensed with, the wound being covered by a pad of cotton-wool, or lint smeared with olive oil, or, if available, carbolic oil (Recipe 119). Rest, an aperient, and simple diet are advisable.

PUNCTURED WOUNDS, *with which may be classed gunshot wounds and wounds of joints,* are the most dangerous—because deep-seated blood-vessels or nerves are often implicated; because the parts punctured must be also stretched and torn; in consequence of foreign bodies, as dirt, bullets, pieces of clothing, being often carried very deeply into the body; because there is often no free exit for matter formed; and because such injuries are more liable to be followed by lockjaw or tetanus. Punctured and gunshot wounds are attended with great shock to the system, so that brandy and water, or wine, will be required immediately after the accident. If a foreign body, as a bullet, a piece of cloth, &c., can be felt, it should be gently removed with the fingers or forceps. If faintness or loss of blood indicate wound of some important internal organ, or of a large artery, the case assumes a most serious aspect. But in all instances it will be best to apply cold-water dressing, to keep the patient lying on the wounded side, so as to favour escape of blood or discharges, to enforce perfect rest, and to give low diet. If the wound throbs and the sufferer becomes feverish, poultices, a purgative (Recipe 2), and cooling draughts of citrate of magnesia (*vide* p. 15).

**WOUNDS OF THE BRAIN.**—These injuries will be accompanied by *concussion* (*vide* p. 522) or *compression* (*vide* p. 525). Treatment accordingly, and Recipe 85 to any wound.

**WOUNDS OF THE LUNGS.**—There is difficulty of breathing and sense of suffocation, the countenance is pallid and anxious, and florid blood mixed with clots is coughed up. These symptoms may subside, or the patient may die from loss of blood; or, at a later period, from inflammation. In all such cases the only means to be adopted are keeping the person quiet, giving a stimulant in very small quantity at a time, and desisting altogether if the pulse becomes stronger. Under such measures, if the internal wound is small, the flow of blood may cease, and the patient recover. For the external wound, little more can be done than applying cloths wet with cold water.

**WOUNDS AND INJURIES OF THE BOWELS AND OTHER ABDOMINAL ORGANS.**—*Injuries of the muscles of the* *belly, the bowels, liver, spleen, kidneys, or other abdominal organs,* are marked by a fixed pain at the seat of injury, faintness and feeble pulse, or collapse (*vide* p. 520), from which death may result immediately. There are also other symptoms enumerated below, characterising injury of different organs.

BOWELS. The muscles of the bowels may be injured, but the *intestines* inside may not be touched. In cases of stabs or gores, the question is whether or not the intestines are injured. If the intestines appear through the wound, it may be seen whether or not they are injured. If they do not appear, the escape of fæces through the wound, the passage of bloody stools, and the vomiting of bile or blood, is evidence that the intestines are injured, and in such cases the collapse will be greater. If there is *no* reason to suppose the bowels are wounded, and they do not protrude, dirt and blood should be washed away with glycerine soap and lukewarm water, and as soon as bleeding has ceased (which probably will not be great), the edges of the wound should be brought together with long strips of plaster, cold lotion (Recipe 83) should be applied to the whole belly to prevent inflammation, and only fluid diets should be allowed. If there is reason to fear the bowels *are* wounded, or in all cases of punctured wounds such as by the horns of animals, a poultice should be applied. Also, in all cases it will be desirable to give a full dose of chloral.

*If from a wound the bowel protrudes* it must be carefully washed with warm water, cleansed from all impurity, and returned by pressure with the fingers. If the bowel itself is torn, the wound must be closed; if very small, by pinching up and tying; if large, by stitching it up. The edges of the wound should be *turned in,* so that the *outer* surfaces come into contact. Fine silk should be used, and small stitches taken. The ends of the thread should be cut close off, and the bowel then returned, as if it were uninjured. If the patient recover, the ligatures will drop into the cavity of the gut, and no ill consequences result. The external wound should be closed up by stitches and plaster. Ice should be applied to the abdomen afterwards. Chloral should be given twice daily, but no solid food for three weeks.

LIVER. If the liver is injured in addition to the general symptoms enumerated above, there will probably be vomiting, white stools, and jaundice. *Treatment* as for wounds of the lungs.

KIDNEY. There will probably be blood in the urine, frequent calls to make water, the testicle will be drawn up, and the person will be unable to stand erect. *Treatment.*—Both loins and bowels should be alternately fomented with hot water. The bowels should be kept moderately open by Recipes 1 and 2, and small doses of chloral (Recipe 64) may be given to relieve pain. Thirst may be allayed by iced milk and water; beef-tea, arrowroot, tea, and barley water may also be given. When the urine assumes a lighter colour it shows that less blood is being passed, and that improvement is taking place; and this may occur at the end of a few days, or be delayed for weeks. During convalescence *albumen* should be tested for (*vide Bright's Disease*, p. 101), and the patient ought to be kept to the house until all traces of albumen are gone.

SPLEEN. (*Vide* p. 595.)

BLADDER. There is a feeling as if something had given way, with violent burning pain. There is desire to make water, but inability to do so. The person is unable to stand or walk. Soon the symptoms are those of extravasation of urine (*vide* p. 420), and the *treatment* should be the same.

**WOUNDS OF THE THROAT.**—These wounds are generally made with the intention of suicide, and are dangerous, both from the importance of the parts injured and from the desponding condition of the patient. They may be clean-cut, or lacerated; they may be superficial, or deep; they may implicate arteries, veins, windpipe, or the gullet. If the air-passage only is cut, recovery often takes place; but if large blood-vessels are cut, death occurs from profuse bleeding.

*Treatment.*—Any arteries wounded must be twisted or tied (*vide* pp. 504, 505), and bleeding from veins, known by the blacker colour of the blood (*vide* p. 503), must be restrained by pressure with the fingers. The patient should be put to bed in rather a warm room, and as soon as all bleeding has ceased, *but not before*, the shoulders should be raised on pillows, with the head bent forward. The head should be retained in this position by tapes passing from each side of a cap, or of a bandage round the head, to another bandage placed round the chest. *No* plasters or sutures should be used. If the wound penetrates the windpipe, it should be covered with a loose woollen comforter, or cotton-wool. If the gullet is wounded the patient will probably require to be fed with a tube. Thirst may be relieved by sucking wet rag or ice. As these injuries are generally inflicted with a suicidal intent, it will be needful to have the patient watched, or he may repeat the attempt. If the patient is unruly, and tries to tear open the wound, he may be confined by a strait waistcoat (*vide* p. 160).

**WOUNDS OF THE EYES.**—Any protruded part should be gently and carefully pushed back with a probe; the patient should be placed in a darkened apartment, the lid should be kept closed by a covering of cotton-wool and a light bandage, and cold water should be used as a lotion. Purgatives should be administered and abstinence from stimulants should be enjoined.

[It will be advisable to obtain a solution of *atropine* (strength 2 grains to an ounce of water), a drop or two of which should be dropped into the eye twice daily, in order to dilate the pupil, and prevent adhesions from inflammation.]

**WOUNDS OF THE TONGUE.**—Are liable to occur, in connection with other accidents, when the organ gets accidentally thrust between the teeth. As a rule, it is best to leave wounds of the tongue entirely to nature, as it is difficult to introduce ligatures, and plasters are inadmissible. But sometimes wounds of the tongue bleed very freely, and may require twisting or ligature of an artery (*vide* p. 504); or the actual cautery (a red-hot iron wire) may be necessary to arrest the bleeding.

**WOUNDS OF THE PALM OF THE HAND.**—Sometimes give much trouble from the artery of the palm being injured (*vide* p. 507). After bleeding has stopped, the wound should be dressed with plasters.

**WOUNDS CAUSED BY THE BITES OF ANIMALS.**

CAMEL AND HORSE BITES are attended with much bruising of the parts, and a sharp tooth may wound an artery, as, for instance, the artery of the wrist. If this occurs, the flow of blood must first be stopped, as directed under *Bleeding* (p. 504). Afterwards, or at first if no bleeding, the wounds require washing with warm water, poulticing, and rest. At a later period simple dressing, or water dressing. (Recipes 85, 86.)

Dog and Cat Bites.—Are difficult to heal, from the wounds being punctured, contused, or lacerated. Such injuries should be washed with warm water, after which a bread poultice may be applied. If there is pain the parts should be fomented with hot infusion of poppy-heads (*vide* Recipe 81) previous to each change of poultice. When the wounds look clean and free from discharge, simple dressing, or water dressing should be used (*vide* Recipe 85). For the treatment of the bite of a mad dog, *vide Hydrophobia*, p. 301.

The idea that a person bitten by a dog will suffer from hydrophobia if the dog should *afterwards* go mad, is erroneous. The practice of killing a dog because he has bitten a human being, in order to prevent hydrophobia in the latter, is ridiculous and useless. If the dog goes mad *after* the infliction of the bite, there is no danger of hydrophobia.

Wounds from Scratches by a Cat.—These are best treated by well washing the part with warm water, then applying a poultice and afterwards a little simple dressing. Slight scratches, whether from the claw of a cat or from the tooth of a horse or dog, may be sucked, as the ready means of preventing future irritation.

Tiger or Bear Bites.—These injuries may involve deep-seated parts. The hand may be bitten to pieces; the chest may be seized, when the teeth or claws will probably penetrate the lungs. Or the thigh may be seized, and the large artery wounded. When such accidents occur, measures to arrest bleeding should be taken (*vide Bleeding or Hæmorrhage*, p. 504), after which the wounds should be thoroughly cleansed, and, if available, antiseptic lotion (*vide Appendix*, No. 119), or, if not, water dressing (*vide* No. 85) should be applied. If the injured person escapes with only superficial fang or claw wounds, poultices should be applied for the first few days, and afterwards water dressing, or, if available, oil and carbolic acid (*vide Appendix*, No. 119).

There is an impression that wounds from the teeth or claws of animals must be poisoned. This is not correct, and has arisen from the slow manner in which such wounds heal. Wounds from the teeth or claws of animals must be attended by laceration and contusion: conditions sufficient to account for slow healing. It is possible that the teeth or claws of a carnivorous animal, when inflicting a wound, may be impregnated with some deleterious material from rotting carrion, and so the blood may be poisoned (*vide* p. 587). But this is not usually the case.

**WOUNDS CAUSED BY SNAKES.**—There are in India 213 species of snakes, of which 33 are poisonous. Of the latter there are two varieties, the *Viperine* and the *Colubrine*. The *Viperine* poisonous snakes have stumpy tails, and triangular-shaped heads. The *Colubrine* poisonous snakes are hooded. Neither have the *loreal* shield, which is a crescentic-shaped scale, directly behind the nasal shield. Poisonous snakes have only two teeth in the upper jaw, and these are the grooved erectile poison-fangs. There are other teeth in the palate, but no other teeth in the jaw proper. The fangs of some species are perforated instead of grooved, and in addition there is an opening at the base, so that when the reptile bites, the poison is not only carried to the bottom of the puncture inflicted from the point of the fang, but it also escapes at the base.

*Symptoms.*—The bites of poisonous snakes, as a rule, show two marks thus ·· When there are more than two marks, ⁚⁚ it may be safely assumed that the reptile was not poisonous, or that the wound has not been inflicted by the poison-fangs. The parts most frequently bitten are the fingers, toes, ankles, and hands, and the person, if asleep, is aroused by the pain, which is of a stinging character, but not very severe at first. Faintness, sickness, loss of power in the legs, and perhaps vomiting, are the next *immediate* effects. Then the breathing becomes short and laboured, the pulse quick and intermittent, the powers of speech and swallowing are lost, the tongue protrudes, and frothy saliva issues from the mouth. Twitchings of the muscles also occur, followed by loss of power to move the limbs. The pain from the wound extends upwards towards the body; the absorbent vessels becoming inflamed, appearing on a fair skin as painful red lines stretching up from the wounded part towards the groin or armpit. Cold sweats and often convulsions succeed, and the patient, becoming insensible, sinks, sometimes in a few hours. More commonly, however, the case is prolonged several days, blood poisoning (*vide* p. 587) occurring. The wound becomes discoloured, the limb swells, blisters may form near the injured part, abscesses may occur in any part of the limb, and the glands of the armpit or groin (according to the limb injured) enlarge, inflame, and suppurate. Sometimes there is diarrhœa, at others bleeding from the snake-bite, or from scarifications made in the neighbourhood. In some cases there is also bloody urine, or bleeding from the nose, bowels or gums. The depressing effects of fear will aid the operation of the poison; and the symptoms will be more or less intense, according to the amount of venom inserted into the wound.

*Treatment.*—Although no antidote has yet been discovered, treatment may save life. But the measures indicated below, to be successful, must be applied *immediately*. If the bite is anywhere on the limbs, tie a tight bandage or string round the limb, a few inches *above* the wound. The ligature should be tight enough to arrest the circulation, which may be known by the part below becoming red, and then darker coloured. Then let the wound be *well* sucked; care being taken that the person performing this office has no sore on the mouth or lips; or, if a ligature cannot be applied (as, for instance, if the body is bitten), let the wound be sucked first. Afterwards, or previously if suction cannot be accomplished, make four or five punctures with a lancet, or sharp knife, a quarter of an inch deep, one across each bite and the others a quarter of an inch or so from the bite. (A surgeon would probably cut the bitten part out.) When puncturing care must be taken not to injure any *vein* which, if in the locality, will be recognised, blue and prominent underneath the skin. No *artery* is likely to be injured by the punctures, unless the bite were on the wrist close to where the pulse is usually felt, and this may be known by the beat (*vide Blood-vessels*, p. 502). Then encourage bleeding by, if possible, immersing the part in hot water, or otherwise by bathing with hot water. If the knife cannot be used, a live coal or stick, a red-hot iron wire, or a drop of nitric or carbolic acid, or a solution of permanganate of potash (5 grains to a tea-spoonful of water) may be passed into the wounds. If nothing of the kind is available suction should be continued.

The strongest stimulant at hand, whether brandy, whisky, rum, wine, sal volatile, or liquor ammonia (*eau de luce*) should be given at once. Eau de luce should be given in 30-drop doses, diluted in two table-spoonfuls of water; sal volatile in half-ounce doses; spirits in ounce doses, diluted with water, so that the stimulant used may be swallowed without difficulty. If wine is used, four-ounce doses should be given. Whatever stimulant is used, the dose should be repeated every fifteen minutes until the first depressing effect of the poison subsides. If the faintness is great cold water should be dashed on the face and head, and mustard poultices should be applied over the heart and stomach. During the whole time the patient should have plenty of fresh air, but he should be kept moderately warm, especially about the feet. At a later period poultices should be applied to the wound. If red lines form, stretching from the wound towards the body, they should be fomented. Fomentations and poultices must also be applied to any swelling about the armpit or groin; and if matter forms in such positions, it must be treated as an abscess (*vide* p. 41). As soon as the first effects of the poison pass away, the patient should have nourishment, soup, broth, or raw-meat tea.

When a ligature is applied, and no symptoms of snake-poisoning make their appearance in half an hour, the ligature may be relaxed; but if symptoms as above detailed present, it should be kept on until the part has been sucked, cut out, and bathed in hot water, after which the ligature serves no useful purpose and may do injury. But if the limb swells and grows a little cold, the ligature should be removed, even if the treatment has not been carried out.

If the person is not seen until the limb is swollen, the absorbent vessels are inflamed, and there is more or less insensibility, stimulants and poulticing afford the best chance.

**WOUNDS FROM SCORPIONS AND CENTIPEDES.**—The pain is at first like a prick from a needle, but in a few seconds it assumes an agonising form, as if many needles were being thrust into the part, and it also shoots up towards the body, reaching a climax in about ten minutes. The parts injured swell; frequently the absorbent vessels running from the sting are implicated, as evidenced by a red line seen in the skin; and the joint above the part feels stiff. Death from scorpion-sting has been recorded, but to a person in good health such injuries are not dangerous. The best applications are poultices made of equal parts of opium powder and ipecacuanha powder; or, if both are not available, of ipecacuanha powder alone; or a rag steeped in vinegar, or in sal volatile, should be laid on the part; or a strong solution of common salt and water may be employed; or the part may be rubbed with a cut onion, or with wet tamarind seeds. The inflamed red line of absorbent vessels should be fomented, and it will be advisable to give some aperient.

**WOUNDS FROM WASPS or BEES.**—When a swarm of wasps attack a person, the number of stings inflicted may induce serious illness. Or in delicate persons, or children, several stings may cause faintness, nausea, vomiting, and purging. Under such circumstances a stimulant will be first required. Then the stings should be extracted by pressing the tube of a small key over the part, when the sting, if left in the wound, will probably start out, or a watery fluid will escape, carrying with it some of the venom. Then the best application is sal volatile, or vinegar-and-water, or eau de Cologne; or, if these are not at hand, moist snuff or tobacco may be rubbed in. If the stings are numerous chloral may be required to relieve pain. If sickness persists, one drop of ipecacuanha wine in a spoonful of water every hour. At a later period soap liniment may be used to remove any remaining swelling of the skin.

In cases of stings *inside the mouth* or in *the throat*, the sting should be sought for, and extracted if possible. Ice should be kept in the mouth, and leeches should be applied outside. If danger of suffocation appears urgent, opening the windpipe may be required.

**WOUNDS FROM MOSQUITO-BITES.**—The effect of a mosquito-bite does not altogether depend on the introduction of the proboscis of the insect into the skin, for so small an object, although containing six lancets, would scarcely create the irritation often following. The fact is, that there is not only the wound, but also the discharge of an irritating fluid into the wound. A mosquito-bite usually rises into a white hard lump, which may inflame and become an obstinate sore if the individual be out of health. The best application is sal volatile; or a strong solution of carbonate of potash in water; or, if these are not at hand, vinegar. Or water alone may be well rubbed into the part, so that some may enter the wound made by the sting, and dilute the poison. Any sore afterwards forming must be treated in the ordinary manner.

After a mosquito has fed on an individual or animal affected by *filaria* (a microscopical worm found in the blood), the insect's stomach contains living examples of the parasite. The latter escape, when the mosquito dies, in the water to which it betakes itself; and the parasites may thus find their way with water into the human system. It is probable also that *filaria* may be directly conveyed from one person to another by mosquitos. The influences which *filaria* in the blood exert are not well understood; but it is possible they may have more connection with certain diseases, especially leprosy, than has been recognised. However this may be, enough has been proved to afford another reason why persons in tropical climates should seek protection from mosquitos; also another reason why care, as regards purity of drinking-water, should be systematically practised (*vide* p. 678).

**WOUNDS FROM LEECHES.**—In some parts of India small land leeches abound. They are about one inch long and very thin, looking like little withered sprigs, standing out from the bushes. When distended they are much larger. They are of a yellowish-brown colour, streaked with black, with one greenish line along the whole length of the back, so that they are not easily seen when hidden among green leaves or grass. By a muscular effort they throw themselves from trees on passers-by, and insinuate themselves through every aperture of clothing, or down the back of the neck. Their bites scarcely inflict any pain at the time, but they cause much after-irritation, and in persons in a bad state of health often occasion ulcers difficult to heal. The bleeding should first be stopped (*vide* p. 512), and then a cooling lotion should be applied (Recipe 83). Any ulcer forming must be treated on ordinary principles. When passing through marshes, 'leech gaiters' may be worn, which are very long, closely woven cotton stocking, passing over the socks.

**WOUNDS FROM FLEA-BITES.**—Flea-bites are recognised by small darkish red spots surrounded by a circle of a paler colour, which fades before the central puncture does. Flea-bites have been mistaken for eruptions accompanying different kinds of fever or *vice versâ*. The smallness of the spots, their uniform character with central puncture (seen more certainly through a glass), and their decided isolation are sufficiently characteristic. Vinegar and water is the best application, and cleanliness is the best means of preventing fleas swarming in Indian houses.

**WOUNDS FROM BUG-BITES.**—These insects cause an itching swelling, sometimes red, sometimes white, almost resembling the mosquito-bite. Vinegar-and-water is the best application. Taking furniture to pieces and placing the ends in boiling water is the best method of destroying bugs. Pouring turpentine occasionally between the joints is the best method of prevention.

**WOUNDS FROM LICE.**—Lice-bites present an itching, whitish swelling. Lice generally inhabit the scalp, laying their eggs (called *nits*) near the roots of the hair. A method of killing lice is washing the head with a solution of carbolic acid (one part of acid to fifty parts of water). Or carbolic acid and oil may be used together in similar proportions. But neither measure may suffice to kill the eggs. If lice still appear the head should be shaved, and a mixture of equal parts of pomatum and mercurial ointment may be rubbed on the scalp every other day for three days, an oilskin cap being worn in the meantime.

OTHER INSECTS AND REPTILES which may cause annoyance and injury are, certain *caterpillars* which leave hairs in the skin; *sand flies* (*pulex penetrans*) which cause bright red, itching papules; the *peepsa fly* of Assam, which attacks the hands and feet, causing a red blister with much itching. The *common house lizard* may also cause redness or even blistering. For all these injuries cold lotion, Recipe 83, or vinegar-and-water, are the best applications.

# CHAPTER IV.

## *PREGNANCY AND LABOUR*

**PREGNANCY.**—The pregnant condition lasts from 273 to 280 days, or about 40 weeks. The following table is for calculating the period of pregnancy.

| Nine Calendar Months | | | Ten Lunar Months | | |
|---|---|---|---|---|---|
| From | To | Days | From | To | Days |
| January 1 | September 30 | 273 | January 1 | October 7 | 280 |
| February 1 | October 31 | 273 | February 1 | November 7 | 280 |
| March 1 | November 30 | 273 | March 1 | December 5 | 280 |
| April 1 | December 31 | 273 | April 1 | January 5 | 280 |
| May 1 | January 31 | 273 | May 1 | February 4 | 280 |
| June 1 | February 28 | 273 | June 1 | March 7 | 280 |
| July 1 | March 31 | 273 | July 1 | April 6 | 280 |
| August 1 | April 30 | 273 | August 1 | May 7 | 280 |
| September 1 | May 31 | 273 | September 1 | June 7 | 280 |
| October 1 | June 30 | 273 | October 1 | July 7 | 280 |
| November 1 | July 31 | 273 | November 1 | August 7 | 280 |
| December 1 | August 31 | 273 | December 1 | September 6 | 280 |

The above 'Ready Reckoner' is used as follows. A woman has ceased to be 'poorly' on July 1, her confinement will be at soonest about March 31 (*the end of nine calendar months*); or at the latest on April 6 (*the end of ten lunar months*). Another has ceased on January 20; her confinement will be on September 30, *plus* twenty days (*or October 20 the end of nine calendar months*), at soonest; or on October 7, *plus* twenty days (*or October 27, the end of ten lunar months*), at latest.

SIGNS OF PREGNANCY.—1. *Morning sickness*, usually commencing about one month after conception, sometimes earlier. 2. *Cessation of the monthly flow* at the first month. which, however, in exceptional cases may not occur. 3. *Enlargement of the breasts*, generally after the first month; occasionally not till the third month; sometimes after the first few days. 4. *Dark appearance and soreness of the nipples and breast*, about the third month. Sometimes (usually at a later period) *oozing of milky fluid*. 5. *Enlargement of the abdomen*, about the third month. 6. *Quickening*, or movements of the child, felt about the fifth month, and often attended by fainty feelings. (It has been observed that if these movements are felt chiefly on the left side, there will be a male birth.) 7. *Pulsation of the child's heart*, which resembles the ticking of a watch under a pillow; heard first about the fifth month, and most distinctly at the centre of a line drawn from the hip-bone to the navel: sometimes on one side, sometimes on the other. 8. *Movement of the child*, which may be felt after the sixth month, on placing the cold hand over the lower part of the bowels. 9. *Variations in temper and disposition, capricious appetite, and 'longings,'* the woman often showing a desire for special, and sometimes improper, diet.

TREATMENT OF PREGNANCY.—Unless other ailments (*vide* p. 356), or unless any of the signs mentioned above, prevail to the extent of becoming serious inconveniences, pregnancy being a natural condition, the manner of living, if healthy, need not be altered. The diet should be ample, but simple, and the taste may be reasonably indulged. But the mother's blood yields nourishment to the unborn infant; therefore deterioration of the former must affect the latter, and capricious appetite should not be yielded to. Moderate exercise and exertion is not prejudicial, provided care is taken not to strain the body. If the pregnant woman is exposed to sudden strains, or to shaking, the womb may be excited to premature action, and *miscarriage* (*vide* p. 362) or other evils, such as *Cross Birth*, p. 628), are liable to occur. As the dangers of any disease are increased if it occurs during pregnancy, any unhealthy pursuit should be discontinued. It is especially deleterious for a pregnant woman to sleep in a badly ventilated apartment: for as the unborn child grows there is greater want of fresh air. The liability of pregnant women to be affected injuriously to themselves and unborn child by disgusting objects should be recollected, and such sights should be avoided. The clothing should be warm but easy. Stays may be enlarged by a gore of elastic in each side, and if there is a steel in front it should be removed. The breasts should have plenty of room, and if tender or irritable should be treated as directed at p. 360. In healthy pregnancies no medicine is required, excepting probably during the last few days, when it may be desirable to overcome constipation by castor-oil. Castor-oil is the best opening medicine during pregnancy, when powerful purgatives, especially those containing aloes, should be avoided. Neither should patent medicines, the composition of which is unknown, be taken during pregnancy, as they may contain drugs deleterious to that condition.

PRECAUTIONS PREVIOUS TO LABOUR.—Bath-rooms, water-closets, and drains, if any, should be well cleansed. Inquiry should be made where the sweeper takes refuse, and proper disposal of it should be insisted upon. The best ventilated room obtainable should be selected for the lying-in chamber, and it should not be kept too warm either before or after labour, as is generally the case in the cold season of northerly districts. The antecedents of the nurse should be inquired into. If there is the slightest suspicion of her having been recently (within four weeks) engaged with a scarlet fever patient, or with a blood-poisoning case, or with a woman suffering from puerperal fever, she should not be engaged. If she has been attending any other diseases, or burns or scalds, she should wash all over with 20 p.c. carbolic soap, and be given new clothing. Arrangements should be made for a supply of pure cotton wool, to be used instead of sponges if the latter are required during labour. If practicable, absorbent cotton, or artificial antiseptic sponges, and sanitary towels should be obtained. All these things, if used, should be burnt after labour. Plenty of ordinary napkins should be well aired and put ready to hand. Arrangements should be made that both hot and cold water should be ready; and if a first labour, and therefore likely to be long, some beef-tea should be prepared, and a drinking-cup obtained. A chamber utensil to receive the after-birth, and an enema syringe, should be in readiness. Other things which should be ready beforehand are, the bandages for the woman and child; a large square of flannel called the 'receiving flannel' for the child to be placed in at its birth; a waterproof sheet; a bed pan; the child's clothing; large and small pins; three or four ligatures to tie the navel-string with, as below; blunt-pointed scissors to cut the string with (*vide* p. 632); soft linen for dressing the navel (*vide* 633); glycerine soap and a fine sponge for washing the child (*vide* 633); cimolite powder and a puff; sound salad oil in a wide-mouthed bottle.

[The bandage for the woman should be made to fit at five months of pregnancy. It should be composed of strong unstarched calico, and reach from just below the breasts to a little below the hips. In length it should go round the woman's hips, with a hand's-breadth additional for overlapping. It should be narrow above, wider below, and gored so that it will be a little narrower at the lower part than a few inches above, to prevent it from sliding upwards. If a binder has not been prepared, the bandage used should be fourteen inches broad and a yard and a half long.

The binder for the infant should be of thin flannel, about five inches broad, and long enough to go twice round the body.

The ligatures for the navel-string should consist of sewing thread, as cotton is not strong enough, and tape is likely to slip. Each ligature should be composed of ten threads, loosely rolled into one cord, and all of one length, so that they may not tie unevenly.]

A lady writer gives the following as the layette of an infant in India. 8 day shirts; 8 night gowns; 4 monthly gowns; 4 day flannels; 4 night flannels; 2 head squares; 5 flannel bands; 4 robes; 1 hood and veil; 2 dozen diapers; 4 long petticoats; 6 pairs wool boots; 12 flannel pilchers; 4 cradle sheets; 4 pillow cases; 2 blankets.

**LABOUR.**—Labour is the common term for a confinement. If the birth takes place before six months, it is called an abortion or *miscarriage*, and when between six and nine months, *premature labour*. A full-time labour, as a rule, being a natural process, is attended with little danger to either mother or child. The signs of *approaching* labour are a sinking of the size of the belly; a feeling of comparative lightness; frequent desire to make water; perhaps griping, and a sensation of squeezing; and a mucous discharge, sometimes streaked with blood, and known as 'the show'; all or any of which may occur some hours, or even a day or two, before actual labour-pains commence. On the symptoms of *approaching* labour, *the patient's bed* should be prepared. A hard or horsehair mattress is preferable. On this, over the usual blanket and sheet there should be placed a piece of oiled cloth or india-rubber sheeting; then on this 'guard,' a blanket folded four times, then a sheet doubled in similar manner, which is called the 'draw sheet.' All this is to absorb discharges, and to prevent the mattress, on which the woman has to lie afterwards, becoming wet. After the labour is over, and the oiled cloth and extra blanket and sheet are removed, the bed should be quite dry. A long towel should also be attached to the foot of the bed for the purpose indicated below. *The woman's dress* should consist of garments which may be easily removed after the labour. The best plan is for the woman to be undressed, with the night-dress rolled above the waist, so that it may not be soiled. A loose sheet should be spread over her, to be taken away with the 'guard' and 'draw sheet.' *If the bowels* have not acted within six hours, an enema (Recipe 104) should be administered. Emptying the bowels facilitates the action of the womb, and prevents discomfort; for the contents of the bowel may be forced into the bed during labour.

The *commencement of labour* is denoted by pains in the lower part of the belly, gradually settling in the loins and back, then passing to the thighs, and known as 'bearing down pains.' After such pains the waters generally break. There is also often shivering and vomiting. The patient may at first sit, or walk about, which accelerates the labour, and she should, if necessary, relieve the bladder and bowels. In a variable time, the pain returns at lessening intervals, while they increase in duration and violence. The patient should now take to the bed, and the position most convenient, both for the attendant and the woman, is for the latter to lie on her left side with the hips near to the edge of the bed, and the knees drawn up towards the belly, and a pillow may be placed between the knees. When violent pains occur, the patient should hold her breath, place her feet against the footboard of the bed, or against some person sitting at the foot, and pull hard at the towel (recommended to be) attached to the foot of the bed (*vide* above). This assists the expulsatory efforts of the muscles concerned. The time of labour varies from six to twelve hours, being generally longest in those having a first child. In ninety-five cases out of a hundred the head of the child first emerges, the rest of the body soon following. The main objects of care are: *First*, to support the *perinœum*, or that part of the person of the mother exposed to pressure as the head passes, which otherwise might be torn and lacerated. This support is afforded by applying the hand covered with a napkin in a moderately firm yet yielding manner. *Secondly*, to free the child's mouth from discharge or mucus. *Thirdly*, to see that the womb contracts as soon as the child is born. To secure this, when the head is born the hand of an attendant should be placed over the womb, making moderate pressure, which should be maintained until the *after-birth* comes away; or until the womb is well contracted, when it may be felt in the lower part of the bowels in the shape of a *round hard ball.* If the womb cannot be thus felt, bleeding may occur. *Fourthly*, to divide the navel-string (as described at p. 632).[1] During the labour, thirst may be relieved by cold water or cold tea, or, in prolonged cases, beef-tea may be taken; but solid food may cause vomiting. Sleep during the intervals between the pains should not be interfered with; and the face and hands may be sponged with cold water. As soon as the child is born, 6 or 8 grains of quinine should be given, which will tend to prevent malarious fever occurring, and assist in securing contraction of the womb.

In from ten to twenty minutes after the child is born the *after-birth* comes away, but it is sometimes longer, and the cord must not be pulled to hasten its progress. The after-birth is attended with renewal of pains, and if the interval between the birth of the child and the after-birth is long, it is accompanied by clots of blood. In other cases a more fluid bloody discharge occurs, which is of no consequence to the extent of a few ounces, but which, if profuse, amounts to *hœmorrhage* (*vide* p. 628). In some cases the after-birth presents at the orifice, but does not

[1] For the general treatment of infants after birth, *vide* Chap. V.

pass out. It may then be *twisted round*, and gradually extracted.

[The above refers to a straightforward labour; but sometimes labour is preceded for some days or hours by 'false pains.' Such pains are felt in the bowels, and not in the back; they are of a *straining*, and not of a *grinding* character, they are not accompanied by any 'bearing-down' efforts, and they come and go at *irregular* intervals. False pains are usually caused by intestinal irritation, and may generally be removed by castor-oil, followed by an opiate, as Recipe 64.]

Treatment after Labour.—When the after-birth is removed, the abdominal bandage (*vide* p. 617) should be applied. To do this, roll the binder up, and while the patient is on her back pass it under the small of the back, and let someone standing on the opposite side draw it out. The patient is not to give assistance. Draw the binder comfortably tight, and fasten with safety pins, pinning at the top first. It must act as a broad belt, and not like a cord. If the womb cannot be felt as a round hard ball, a napkin may be doubled into a pad, and placed over the womb underneath the bandage, by which pressure is exerted more directly on the organ: and the infant should be put to the breast, which also tends to insure contraction of the womb. The pad may be removed next day, but the bandage should be worn during the whole time the patient remains in bed. After adjustment of the bandage all soiled clothing should be taken away; the parts should be wiped dry, and a dry warm napkin applied; the night-dress should be brought down smoothly under the hips; and the woman should be allowed to turn round and go to sleep, or to lie still for an hour and a half, or for a longer period should any bleeding have occurred. It should be recollected that nothing is more likely to give rise to bleeding than permitting a patient to sit up soon after her confinement. There is often some loss of blood, so that a slight appearance of the kind need not excite alarm, especially if the womb can be felt hard, round, and firm. If the womb cannot be so felt, and if considerable bleeding occurs, the woman should be treated for *Bleeding after Delivery* (*vide* p. 628).

If after the birth of the child the mother is much exhausted, strong tea, *not too warm*, is the best stimulant After the woman has well rested, and perhaps slept a short time, the private parts should be washed with milk-and-water, and another dry napkin applied. Usually at this time, some bloody discharge, or clots of blood, may be found. This washing should be repeated several times daily, until after four or five days, when 1 ounce of vinegar to 10 ounces of tepid water may be substituted for the milk and water; or glycerine soap may be used. As a female after confinement is susceptible to cold, care should be taken to prevent draughts, although it is *essentially necessary* that the chamber be maintained cool and airy. Excitement from visitors should be avoided. None but the husband and the necessary attendants should be admitted for the first five days; and especial care should be taken that no one approaches the chamber from whom the occupant could incur the chance of contracting infectious disorder, to which lying-in women are peculiarly liable.

*The patient should pass urine* within six hours after delivery, and this should be done as nearly as possible in the horizontal posture. Or if it cannot be made in such position, the patient may turn on the hands and knees. If there be still difficulty, the lower part of the bowels and the private parts should be fomented with hot water. Owing to the distensible state of the belly, the patient will often wait longer than proper if not reminded to make water, and the consequences may be inflammation or paralysis of the bladder (pp. 70, 74).

*The state of the bowels after delivery* is of great importance. On the evening of the second or morning of the third day, if the bowels have not been opened, a table-spoonful of castor-oil, or a dose of senna tea, should be given. If there is reason to suspect accumulation in the lower bowel, as often occurs during the later days of pregnancy, and is known by the passage of hard round lumps, an enema of warm water should be administered. If the patient does not suckle her child, purgatives will be the more necessary for the relief of the breasts. In the latter case saline aperients, as Recipe 2, or citrate of magnesia (*vide* p. 15), which is a milder laxative, will be found most useful.

*Diet.*—Until the milk has come, and the period of milk fever (*vide* p. 629) has passed, the mother, *if in good health*, should live on gruel, tea, toast, and arrowroot. Afterwards the *diet* may be regulated a good deal by the inclinations of the patient. Good soup or beef-tea may be given on the third day, as there is no advantage in keeping a woman who has had a 'good time' on too low a diet. If there is decided disinclination for food, there is probably something wrong. On the fifth or sixth day, solid food may be given. Wine or beer is better delayed till the person gets up. *If the mother has been previously in feeble health*, it will be desirable for her to be supported by nourishing food, as soups and beef-tea, from the first.

*Attention must also be directed to the discharge called lochia*, popularly 'the cleansings.' The passage of this is accompanied by more or less 'after-pains,' generally felt about half an hour after delivery. During their presence the discharge increases, and black clots of blood may be expelled; especially when rising in bed to take food or make water. After-pains are, within certain limits, salutary; they prevent bleeding, diminish the size of the womb, and expel its contents. The application of the child to the breast often brings on or aggravates the after-pains. Unless very severe, no medicine should be given; but if troublesome, an opiate, as chloral (Recipe 64), may be administered, and the bowels may be fomented. At first this discharge is in black clots, or more or less red like blood; then thin and watery, changing colour to greenish-yellow, and at last appearing like soiled water. It has a peculiar odour, more powerful in some instances than in others. The quantity and duration vary a good deal. In some patients it ceases with the after-pains a few days after delivery. In other instances it does not cease till the end of a month. Its continuance is a sign of weakness, either general or local, and is a reason why extra caution and time in getting about should be taken, with additional attention to frequently washing. As this secretion is necessary, the *sudden* interruption is generally attended with evil consequences, such as suppression of milk, or fever.

*In ordinary cases the breasts remain quiescent* for about twelve hours, or longer in first confinements, but soon after begin to enlarge, with stings of pain, their substance becoming heavier and more tense. This depends on what nurses call the 'draught,' or the rush of blood to the breasts, to be converted into milk. There may be *shivering*, and the woman may be feverish. This usually subsides with the flow of milk. If *shivering* occurs the woman should be treated as directed under *milk fever* (*vide* p. 629). If simply feverishness, without shivering, attends the secretion of milk, saline purgative (Recipe 2) and citrate of magnesia draughts (p. 15) should be given, while the breasts may be fomented, and they may also be *gently* rubbed with salad oil every four hours; the greatest pressure being made when the hand is passing from the base of the breasts towards the nipple. Unless some bleeding occurs, and the child is put to the breast, as recommended at p. 621, to secure contraction of the womb, the breasts should not be interfered with in first confinements for five or six hours, when the infant may be applied. But if the breasts become rapidly full, as sometimes happens in persons who have borne children, or if the infant is restless and does not sleep (as mentioned at p. 634), it may be applied at an earlier period. If the breasts are flat and limp, frequent application of the child is not desirable, as fruitless sucking renders the nipple hot, irritable, and tender. If the nipples are short and badly formed, or the breasts swell so much as to prevent the child seizing the nipples, they should be drawn out by a breast pump; or a larger child or a grown-up person should suck them first. Or the cut bottle (*vide* p. 95) or the heated bottle (*vide* p. 98) may be used. The first milk is a watery fluid with yellow streaks in it. It is called *colostrum*, and acts as a purgative to the infant (*vide* p. 635). After twenty-four hours the milk becomes whiter, opaque, and has a sweeter taste.

Each time the child is about to suck, the nipple should be cleaned with soft rag and plain water; and again when the child ceases sucking. This is desirable because even a very little milk drying about the nipple may turn sour and irritate the part; or it may be received into and disorder the infant's stomach. The nipples and breasts should also be washed with warm water and soap morning and evening. By such care the chance of sore nipples and bad breasts (*vide* pp. 94, 96, 97) will be avoided. During the first week the mother should give suck while lying down. She can turn to one side, and, supporting herself on her elbow, let the nipple fall into the mouth of the infant. But afterwards the semi-erect posture should be taken, from which the infant swallows best. Both breasts should be equally used. For times of suckling, *vide* p. 635.

*The mother should remain in bed till the twelfth day*, and afterwards recline on a couch. She may be shifted from one side of the bed to the other, and soiled sheets may be then taken away and clean ones introduced, but she should not get up, even to have the bed made—especially if there has been much bloody discharge—for the womb requires time to recover its normal size and condition. Debility, pain, and continued discharge, often spoken of as 'a bad getting up,' are among the least penalties consequent on imprudence after confinement. A too early return to the duties or pleasures of life often lays the foundation of chronic inflammation, or displacement of the womb. It is a mistake to suppose that women in the lower walks of life, or native women, attend with impunity to their avocations a few days after confinement. Those who have any tendency to womb affection should remain *recumbent* for a full month. If bloody discharge occurs after getting up, it is a warning to go to bed again. Throughout the whole period ventilation must be carefully attended to, no charcoal fire should be allowed in the room, and the immediate removal of soiled linen is essentially necessary.

*When the mother resumes her dress*, the corset should be so arranged as to prevent pressure upon, and give support to, the breasts. She must remember that her milk will be affected by any indiscretion either in food or habits, and that unless her health is maintained her infant will certainly suffer. Nursing women are especially liable to latent scurvy (*vide* p. 381), so that vegetables and milk should always form part of the dietary. There is no valid reason why potatoes should not be taken, against which there is a popular impression. A little malt liquor may generally be used with advantage; but women when nursing usually require *more fluid*, not *extra stimulation* from fermented drinks.

The foregoing relates to natural and straightforward confinements, but other circumstances may arise, which are now briefly noticed.

1. The Labour may be Tedious and Long.—This occurs to weakly females, the pains being feeble, or ceasing usually after the waters break. If four hours elapse without pains, assistance should be sought. In the meantime nourishing soup, and chloral (Recipe 64), should be given, and after rest and sleep the pains may probably return.

2. Cord round the Neck occurs once in about 12 cases. Frequently it is not of much consequence, as when the cord is round the child's neck it is usually long. It should be loosened by gentle traction, and the shoulders should be allowed to slip through the loop. Or, if the cord is long, it may be slipped over the child's head. In some cases it has been necessary to *saw* the cord through, to prevent the child being strangled. When so necessary, the cord should be *sawn* through with the finger-nail, and *not cut*, or it will bleed profusely.

3. Presentation of the Breech.—This occurs once in 60 cases, and the labour is tedious, because the infant, being doubled at the haunches, requires a larger space. As a rule no interference is required until the breech and feet are born, when the case becomes converted into *presentation of the feet* (*vide* No. 5).

4. Twin Births.—This occurs about once in 70 cases. The presentation generally varies, the first being the head, and the second a foot case, or the reverse. After the birth of the first child, the presence of a second is known by the slight reduction in size of the womb. Sometimes the after-birth of the first child comes away before the birth of the second, sometimes not till afterwards, and attempts should not be made to remove it, as there may be only one after-birth for both infants. After the birth of the first, the womb should be stimulated to contract by keeping up a grasping movement of the fingers and thumb on the lower part of the bowels. Sometimes the birth of the second child follows that of the first in ten minutes, but on other occasions not for some hours. Under such circumstances the woman should rest until pains return, and she may drink a little cool tea or arrowroot; the precaution being taken to examine frequently, lest bleeding may be going on. The second labour is usually quicker than the first, the soft parts having been already dilated. After the birth of the second child and the passage of the after-birth especial attention must be paid to the contraction of the womb. The womb should be pressed with the hand until it can be grasped as a firm hard ball, and the bandage should be applied (*vide* p. 621).

5. Presentation of the Feet.—One or both feet may come first, which happens once in 100 cases. The birth is generally safe for the mother, but not for the child, which is apt to suffer from the circulation of the cord being obstructed by pressure. Footling cases should not be hastened in the early stage, as the longer the buttocks are detained the greater will be the dilatation of the parts, and the birth of the head will be more easy. When the breech is expelled, the cord should be examined,

and, if the pulsation of the cord has ceased, the birth of the shoulders should be hastened by pulling the body steadily down during the next pain. The toes of the infant turned to the back of the mother is the most favourable position for the birth of the head; and when the breech is expelled, if the toes are turned forward, the assistant should seize the breech in both hands, and during the next pain endeavour to turn the child round. If circulation is restored in the cord after the birth of the shoulders, there is little cause for anxiety for the safety of the child; but if there is no pulsation in the cord, it is necessary to assist at every pain, and hasten the delivery of the head by pulling the shoulders down. The head being born, the assistant should examine the cord, and, if it pulsates, the child should not be separated for a few minutes until it begins to cry. If there is no circulation in the cord, the infant should be treated as detailed for *still birth* (p. 637).

6. PRESENTATION OF THE FACE.—Instead of the top of the head, the face may present, which happens once in about 230 cases. When it occurs, the labour is protracted. The child is seldom in danger, but the head and face are swollen and disfigured, and unless the mother is prepared, the appearance may give a severe shock. In the absence of medical aid, it will be best to wait patiently for the natural termination.

7. PRESENTATION OF THE HAND, *or 'cross-birth.'*—Presentation of the hand, or the elbow or shoulder, occurs once in about 230 instances. The assistance of a medical man is urgently required, as the operation of turning the child will probably be necessary.

8. BLEEDING OR HÆMORRHAGE.—Bleeding may occur either *before* or *after* the birth, but does not happen to an alarming extent more than once in 300 cases. Bleeding occurring *before* the birth generally depends on the after-birth being seated over the mouth of the womb, so that, as the latter dilates, the vessels of the after-birth are torn. This kind of bleeding may occur at any time after the sixth month of pregnancy, but is more frequent between the eight and ninth month. In every case of bleeding during pregnancy, absolute rest is necessary; the patient's room should be well aired, her food should be farinaceous, her drink toast and water, or weak cold claret and water, and cold applications should be made to the privates. When bleeding happens during the last months of pregnancy the person should obtain medical advice, and the presence of a surgeon during labour.

Bleeding *after* delivery may happen *immediately*, before or after the expulsion of the after-birth, or it *may come on some hours or even days* after the confinement. *When bleeding occurs immediately after delivery*, it depends on feeble contraction of the womb. When the after-birth separates, loss of blood to some extent is the natural consequence; nor is the woman injured by a moderate loss, such as eight to ten ounces. But if the quantity exceeds such amount it produces fainting, the woman being pale, cold, and gasping for breath. The womb will be found soft, and to induce it to contract, firm pressure should be made over the lower part of the bowels, and if possible the womb should be firmly grasped in the hand through the skin. Cloths wet with cold water should be applied to the privates, iced or cold water given to drink, and the child should be put to the breast. Cold water may be suddenly poured on the bowels from a height of two or three feet; and if a syringe is at hand, cold water may be injected into the passage. Twenty grains of ipecacuauha may be given in a wine-glassful of water; or if not at hand, two-thirds of a wine-glassful of vinegar in four ounces of water; one-third of a glassful being given at intervals of a quarter of an hour three times afterwards. No stimulants should be given, and the person should not be raised into the upright posture, which might bring on fatal fainting.

*When bleeding occurs some hours or days after delivery*, it may depend on relaxation of the womb; or on the retention of some part of the after-birth, or of a clot of blood, preventing perfect contraction; or it may arise from fright or excitement. Cold wet cloths externally, and the injection of cold water, are the means of relief.

9. Convulsions may occur before, during, or after labour. All clothing should be loosened, the patient should be allowed plenty of fresh air, and the face should be sprinkled with cold water. To prevent the tongue being bitten, a piece of soft wood should be held between the teeth. If the head is hot, cold applications should be used to the forehead. An injection (Recipe 105) should also be given.

10. Laceration of the Perinæum.—The necessity of supporting the *perinæum*, or that portion of the person of the mother exposed to pressure, as the head passes, has been mentioned at p. 620. But in first labours, notwithstanding support, some amount of tearing often occurs. This is of little consequence, as it quickly heals, and no treatment beyond cleanliness is required. But in exceptional cases the tearing may be greater; and if the wound exceeds an inch, the patient should be kept in bed with her legs tied together, the wound being frequently cleansed until healing occurs. Occasionally the rupture extends to the anus, when a surgical operation is required.

11. Emphysema, *or entrance of air into the tissues of the neck*, may occur during labour. As a consequence of the straining, air escapes from the lungs, and penetrates the neighbouring structures. It is distinguished by puffy swelling of the parts, which crackle when pressed. A cold lotion (Recipe 83), or vinegar and water, should be applied.

12. Milk Fever, or *Weird*.—In ordinary cases, the milk flows from twelve to eighteen hours after delivery; but the patient may, especially if exposed to chill, suffer from shivering, heat of skin, quick pulse, with pain and soreness of one or both breasts, the milk being delayed. When a woman after confinement takes a shivering fit, she should be attended

to instantly; hot bottles to the feet, warmer clothing, and Recipe 50 being the requisites to induce perspiration. For, although shivering is often merely the prelude to the secretion of milk, it may be the forerunner of milk fever; or of the still more dangerous puerperal fever; or of inflammation or abscess of the breast. The bowels should be well opened by castor-oil, chill guarded against, and hot fomentations applied to the breasts. If the breasts become swollen, knotty, and hard, they should be gently rubbed with salad oil, and the infant should be put frequently to them. If matter forms it must be treated as *Abscess of the Breast* (*vide* p. 96). Fever under such circumstances is sometimes accompanied by an eruption of small vesicles on the body, attended by itching, and profuse perspiration. This is called *miliary fever*, and sometimes occurs independently of any disorder of the milk or breasts. It is favoured by too warm beds or too warm rooms.

13. Puerperal Fever.—This is a very dangerous fever, sometimes occurring after confinements. It depends on poisoning of the blood from the absorption of putrid matter retained within the womb (*vide* p. 587). When a woman shortly after labour is seized with shivering, and this is followed by a hot and sweating stage with feelings of relief, when the breasts swell, and when the discharge or 'cleansings' are passing freely, it is the *Milk Fever* or *Weird*, as described above. But when, after perspiration, no relief is experienced, when the breasts become flabby and smaller, when the discharges lessen or cease altogether, and when the pulse remains above 120 beats in the minute, there is reason to fear puerperal fever. Such fear will become certainty if prostration of strength, difficulty of breathing, and suppression of milk come on. Pain and tenderness of the bowels are very frequent and prominent symptoms. There is bilious vomiting, thirst, and profuse perspiration. The tongue and breath are foul, the face sallow, and there is probably diarrhœa, marked by the passage of hard lumps of fæcal matter. At a later period *pyæmia* (*vide* p. 587) may occur, and one or more of the joints may become swollen and painful. Puerperal fever is highly contagious, and may be carried by attendants from one lying-in woman to another. The first thing necessary is to act on the bowels and skin. Recipe 1 should be given, followed after four hours by a purgative draught, Recipe 2. An injection composed of two ounces of castor-oil and ten or twelve ounces of soap and water should also be given. Citrate of magnesia draughts (*vide* p. 15) should be taken every four hours. Injections of warm water (with, if possible, 20 to 30 drops of Condy's fluid added) should also be thrown up the private parts. The belly should be covered with hot linseed-meal poultices. Great attention should be paid to the ventilation of the room, and disinfectants should be freely used (*vide Appendix*, No. 118). The diet should be strong soups and broths.

14. Malarious post-partum Fever.—At a later date than that on

which either *milk* fever or *puerperal* fever occurs, women after delivery are, in the tropics, liable to attacks of ordinary ague and fever to which the above term has been applied. This has been guarded against in the direction, at p. 620, to give quinine as soon as the child is born. If it occurs, it does so after milk has been secreted, the secretion of milk is not checked, and there is no tenderness of the bowels as in puerperal fever. It should be treated as ague (*vide* p. 251).

15. PHLEGMASIA DOLENS, or *milk leg*, is a painful swelling of one or both legs, beginning generally in the thigh, and extending downwards to the leg. It may come on from one to five weeks after delivery, with shivering, fever, thirst, quick pulse, nausea, furred tongue, and pain in the loins. The swollen part is hot and tender, and presents a pale, shining appearance, while the power of moving the limb is nearly lost. Such cases generally do well, although recovery is tardy; and the limb may be stiff years afterwards, with tenderness, perhaps the feeling of a cord beneath the skin down the inner part of the thigh, and swelling of the leg. The swollen part should be continually fomented with poppy-head infusion; saline purgatives (Recipe 2) should be given; and saline mixture (No. 50) to act on the skin and urine, while pain may be relieved by chloral. When pain and fever subside, the swollen parts should be gently rubbed twice daily with brandy and salad oil in equal proportions; iodide of potassium (Recipe 21) should be given, and the limb should be enveloped in flannel. Generous diet, wine, and tonics will be necessary.

86. PUERPERAL MANIA.—Occasionally attacks women shortly after child-birth, or at the period of weaning, especially when there has been *over-nursing* (*vide* p. 655). It may commence with a little feverishness, or it may follow convulsions or puerperal fever. It is often characterised by loquacity, laughing, singing, obscene talk, sometimes a tendency to murder the child, and it often terminates in melancholia. If there is any hereditary family tendency to insanity, recovery may be delayed indefinitely; but, in most instances, a few weeks restore the patient. In the majority of cases there are fæcal accumulations in the lower bowels, for which aperients and injections are required. The infant should be artificially fed. Tonic medicines, nourishing diet, and cheerful surroundings are necessary, and bad cases may require special restraint against homicidal or suicidal tendencies. As the disease is liable to recur, and as debility favours an attack, a woman who has once suffered from puerperal mania should never nurse again.

# CHAPTER V

## *THE MANAGEMENT AND FEEDING OF INFANT*

TREATMENT AFTER BIRTH.—As soon as the child [1] is born, any froth hanging about the child's mouth should be wiped away, and the head placed in a position that it may not be covered with bedclothing or other substance. Then, provided the child cries (which it probably will do unless stillborn, p. 637), the cord should be tied and cut. Two ligatures (*vide* p. 618) should be tied rather tightly round the cord, one at the distance of two and a half inches above the child's navel, the other rather more than three inches above the navel. Then the cord should be divided, ***between the two ligatures,*** with blunt scissors. Do not hurry this operation, as it may be delayed until all beating has ceased in the cord, by which the child receives more blood, and is probably more vigorous. When the child is separated from the mother, a warm blanket or piece of flannel should be ready to receive it (*vide* p. 617), and care should be taken lest the child slip out of hands and be injured. To guard against this, the back part of the infant's neck should be seized in the space between the thumb and first finger of one hand, while the thighs are grasped with the other. Warmth is at this time of importance, as the infant has just passed from the temperature of the mother's body into a probably much colder atmosphere, but the eyes must be guarded from glare.

[1] For the treatment of the mother, refer to Chapter IV., PREGNANCY AND LABOUR, p. 614.

As soon as a warm bath can be prepared, the body of the infant should be immersed in warm water, of the temperature of 97° Fahr., and if a thermometer is not at hand, the elbow will afford the fairest test of the degree of heat, the hand not being sufficiently sensitive. Then the greasy substance adhering to newborn infants should be washed off. This will be found adhering to the armpits, groins, eyebrows, or other places where the skin is loose. Glycerine or Castile soap and a very soft sponge will suffice for this purpose, but care must be taken that neither the soap nor the soiled water gets into the infant's eyes, which may excite ophthalmia. The infant should not remain in the bath more than three or four minutes, whether the body is free or not from the greasy substance. Any remaining deposit will separate at future washings, and its adhering for a few days will do no harm. It should be recollected, when washing the infant, that its bones are soft and unable to sustain the weight of the body. It should therefore be allowed to rest on the bath, and not be held up by one arm. After the washing it should be put on a soft pillow on the nurse's knees, and be gently dried with soft warm towels, and then enveloped in a thin flannel wrapper. Some advise powdering the body of the child after washing, but as the only benefit is to secure dryness of the skin, this procedure, provided due care be taken, may be dispensed with.

Treatment of the Navel.—The navel-string next demands attention. The string with which the navel-cord is tied should be cut off near the knot, and the knot should be examined to ascertain that it has not slipped (which it may do from the escape of a jelly-like substance from the cord), and that there is no oozing of blood, in either of which cases another ligature should be applied. Then a piece of old, oiled soft linen rag should be doubled, and cut in a circular shape, four or five inches in diameter.

In the centre of this a circular hole should be made, through which the tied cord is to be drawn. The latter should be then folded in the cloth, and the mass laid on the belly of the child, in which position it should be secured by the belly-band (*vide* p. 618). After the binder is applied, two or three fingers should pass easily beneath it; the object being, not to impede breathing, but simply to maintain a slight pressure over the navel, which at this period is the weakest part of the infant's body. In order to provide against rupture of the navel (*vide* p. 594) the bandage should be used for four months, and even then not be left off should there be any prominence of the part. The rag mentioned above should be removed, and new oiled rag applied daily. In five or six days the end of the navel-string will come off, leaving a depressed sore below, which ordinarily quickly heals. But if the string does not separate in this time, it should not be pulled or interfered with, but allowed to drop off by the natural process.

Medicine for Newborn Infants.—Many nurses are in the habit of dosing a newborn infant with castor oil, treacle, or some other substance. But this is seldom necessary, and may be injurious. The infant should be allowed to sleep for a time (which it most usually will do), the eyes being protected from strong light, and the body from draughts or cold. From this slumber it should not be waked under the idea that it will require nourishment or physic. In five or six hours the infant will probably awake crying, and may be put to the breast, which will encourage the flow of milk, and tend to secure contraction of the womb. Or should there be no inclination to sleep, which may arise from the infant being cold, it may be put to the breast at any earlier period. The milk first secreted contains natural aperient qualities, and the child should take this milk instead of the dosing referred to. It is only in cases where the first milk of the parent is not obtained, owing to the child being put to a wet-nurse, or in cases of premature birth when no milk is secreted, or from the first milk failing to be sufficiently purgative, that the administration of any medicine is desirable. Then half a tea-spoonful of castor-oil is the best aperient. The bowels of a newborn infant contain a dark secretion called *meconium*, which generally passes a few hours after birth, often with the first flow of urine; and which, unless removed, may give rise to diarrhœa. But in the great majority of instances the first milk is quite sufficient to effect this; and medicine may do harm by exciting an artificial appetite. If on the third day the stools are still black instead of yellow, half a tea-spoonful of castor-oil may be given.

Food for Newborn Infants.—The practice of feeding an infant immediately after birth is not to be approved. An infant requires little, if any, nourishment until ten or twelve hours after birth. There is a sufficient secretion from the mother's breasts to serve the scanty wants of the child. In second confinements the mother will frequently supply milk within twelve hours. If not, or in first confinements when the milk is later in coming, the infant may be fed every three hours with milk-and-water, proportioned and sweetened according to the directions at p. 648. After the mother's milk appears, the infant should obtain nourishment from this source alone. When suckling the mother should lean over and support the breast, allowing the nipple to fall into the child's mouth. During the first ten days it will be advisable to suckle the infant when it awakes; for the next twenty days every two hours by day, and every three hours by night. Frequent suckling during the first month is also better for the mother's breasts, as it maintains them constantly relieved; the distension of the breast from retained milk being a cause of inflammation and abscess. After the first month the intervals between suckling should be gradually extended to four hours. By care and firmness the habit of not suckling from 10 P.M. to 5 A.M. may also be acquired, to the great comfort of the mother. Often, when an infant cries, it is from thirst not hunger, and it may be soothed by a tea-spoonful of boiled and cooled water. The infant should be applied alternately to each breast. Sometimes a child, from some inexplicable reason, prefers one breast, and the mother, to avoid contention, concedes the point; or, in consequence of a cracked or sore nipple, the mother puts the child more to one breast than the other, the result being distension by retained milk, and often abscess.

CLOTHING.—The clothing of infants should be light, loose, and warm—especially the latter—as the innate power of generating heat is at a minimum in the new-born infant. Thin flannel fulfils these requirements better than any other texture. The garments should fasten in front, and the skirt should attach to the bodice. Sleeves and armholes should be so made that twisting the child's arms into unnatural positions may not be necessitated. Infants are frequently caused pain by their tender arms being thrust through narrow apertures, and from their skin being fretted by rough and tight garments, or by the incautious use of pins, which has been known to excite convulsions (*vide* p. 149).

WARMTH.—For warmth it is desirable that the child should lie with the mother or nurse at first; care being taken that it is not overlain, or smothered with pillows. After the first three weeks the infant should sleep alone.

CLEANLINESS AND DRYNESS.—Cleanliness and dryness are of great importance. The bath at bedtime is most useful, as it cleanses the skin, equalises the circulation, and induces languor, the precursor of repose. The urine of the infant is very frequently passed, and the bowels are often moved, and if the discharges are permitted to remain, they irritate and inflame the skin. Napkins, which should never be of waterproof material, should be changed whenever soiled, never dried and used again, and they should be fastened with a safety pin. 'Cimolite,' or white fuller's-earth, is the best application for chafing. Wet bibs are likely to give the infant cold on the chest. No soiled clothes should be allowed to remain in, and no wet clothes should be dried in, the nursery.

OCCASIONAL MALADIES AND CONDITIONS AFTER BIRTH.—After the birth of an infant, various circumstances may give rise to uneasiness.

1. BIRTH, STILL.—If the child is born apparently dead, or 'still-born,' and does not cry, it may present either of the following appearances: *First, the face may appear flushed and livid, the skin red, and the cord tense and pulsating.* The first thing is to wipe out the back of the mouth with a finger covered with a handkerchief, so as to clear it from sticky mucus or fluid; then tie one ligature round the cord upwards of three inches from the navel. Then place the second ligature round the cord an inch or so below, but do not draw the knot tight. Now divide the cord between the ligature tied tight above and the ligature laid loosely below. The latter is not to be tied tightly until a tea-spoonful of blood has escaped. This will often be followed by breathing, the child beginning to cry. If respiration does not take place, the child's body should be sprinkled alternately with cold and warm water, the limbs and spine should be gently rubbed, slight pressure should be made on the chest over the heart, and, lastly, artificial respiration should be tried (*vide* p. 542). *Secondly, the face may be pale, the features collapsed, the lips blue, the jaws fallen, the limbs cold, while no pulsation is felt in the cord.* Before the cord is tied and divided, warm and cold water should be sprinkled on the breast; the back of the mouth should be cleared; the face and buttocks may be tapped with the corner of a wet cloth; the nose and back of the mouth may be tickled with a feather; and if none of these means excite breathing, artificial respiration should be tried. While artificial respiration is being tried, a hot bath should be prepared (temperature 97° Fahr.), in which, after the cord is cut and tied, the child may be immersed. Infants have been recovered after upwards of two hours spent in such endeavours.

2. BREASTS, SWOLLEN.—In some infants, a few days after birth, the breasts are found swollen, and a whitish fluid is observed on the nipple. The swollen part should *not* be squeezed, which may probably cause a 'gathering,' but it should be frequently washed clean, after which salad oil, or, if much inflamed, a bread poultice, is the best application.

3. COLD IN THE HEAD is common, some infants sneezing immediately they are born. To avoid this, infants should be kept out of draughts.

4. CLEFT PALATE.—This means that the roof of the mouth is split. When this occurs to any extent the child cannot suck, and therefore cannot be fed in the ordinary way, as the food passes into the nostrils instead of down the throat. The infant must be placed in a semi-erect posture, and fed with a spoon, and the food must be tilted suddenly down the throat. The milk will then be swallowed without passing into the nostril. But, as soon as possible, nipples provided with artificial tongues or palates should be procured. With care an infant with cleft palate may be well nourished, and at two or three years of age the defect may be remedied by surgical operation.

5. CONSTIPATION. *Vide* p. 138.

6. CYANOSIS.—In exceptional cases this condition may be present. The whole surface is preternaturally dark and cold to the touch. It depends on an organic defect in the heart, and is incurable, although the child may live for some years.

7. HEAD, ALTERATION OF SHAPE OF.—From pressure during birth the shape of the head may be altered; the face may be disfigured; or bluish swellings may be raised on the scalp. This need not excite apprehension. The head or face will gradually assume its natural shape, and swellings about the scalp seldom require more than bathing daily with milk-and-water (*vide* p. 517).

8. LOCK-JAW AND TETANUS. *Vide* p. 441.

9. NAVEL-STRING, BLEEDING FROM THE.—Arises from the cord being carelessly tied, or from tapes being used, which are liable to slip. The proper treatment is placing another ligature below the first. Or the bleeding may come on when, after six or seven days, the navel-string separates. To stop this bleeding, pressure should be applied by placing the finger on the part for a few minutes. If this does not succeed, alum (20 grains to an ounce of water) may be applied with a camel's-hair brush.

10. NAVEL, ERYSIPELAS OF. *Vide* p. 221.

11. NAVEL, ULCERATION OF THE.—In some cases the navel remains red or ulcerated, presenting 'proud flesh,' and the irritation may give rise to convulsions. This is generally easily cured by the use of alum wash (Recipe 97) and simple dressing under the bandage.

12. NAVEL, RUPTURE OF THE. *Vide* p. 594.

13. NINE-DAY FITS. *Vide* p. 145.

14. OPHTHALMIA.—The eyelids stick together after sleep, the edges are red, the eyes are closed when exposed to light, the lids swell, and matter is discharged. This is often caused by uncleanliness, or from soap getting into the eyes during the first washing, or by the infant,

from lying in bed with the mother, getting perspiration or sour milk into its eyes, or by exposure of the infant to too strong a light, as from a blazing fire. The *treatment* is perfect cleanliness, frequently bathing the eyes with milk-and-water, smearing the lids with salad oil to prevent them sticking together, and keeping the child in a darkened room.

15. POMPHOLIX, or BLEBS. *Vide* p. 398.

16. RUPTURE. *Vide* p. 589.

17. SPINA BIFIDA.—This is a malformation of the spine, with protrusion, in the form of a tumour on the lower part of the back. The part should be protected from pressure, and it may gradually solidify.

18. SUFFOCATION OF INFANTS.—The danger of suffocation of infants is referred to under 'Warmth' at p. 636. Even the close wrapping of a child's head in a shawl to protect from cold may effectually smother it, without any convulsive struggle as indication of what is taking place. The mother should never go to sleep while suckling, as, the child's face being pressed on the breast, and both being asleep, the child may be slowly suffocated. To keep a child quiet a bag of wash-leather or of linen containing sugar is sometimes thrust into its mouth, which may also lead to suffocation.

The superstition that cats suck the breath of infants is not well founded. They may lie on the face, or accidentally draw some article of clothing over the face, and so cause suffocation. The moral, however, is the same: never to leave an infant in a room with the door or window open, or a cat therein.

19. THRUSH, or WHITE MOUTH. *Vide* p. 446.

20. TONGUE-TIE.—If the infant sucks and protrudes the tongue at all over the lower lip, it is not *tongue-tied*, even although for some days it may not suck vigorously. 'Tongue-tie' depends on the fold of membrane (or *frænum*) beneath the tongue being too far forward, and it may be seen in some cases extending nearly to the tip of the tongue, which cannot be raised by passing a finger under it, while the milk flows out of the mouth. The method of relief is the division of this structure for a quarter of an inch or less with a sharp pair of scissors. The snip with the scissors should be directed *downwards* towards the jaw, not upwards to the tongue, to avoid cutting a blood-vessel passing through the part, from which, when cut, a troublesome bleeding has proceeded. The operation is not advised in the absence of a medical man, unless in very bad cases; and the infant must be fed with a spoon, if possible with the mother's milk—or, if not obtainable, with milk-and-water (*vide* p. 646).

21. URINE, ACIDITY OF.—Infants sometimes expel urine frequently, although only a few drops at a time. This usually depends on *irritability of the bladder* caused by acid urine. The small amount passed quickly dries on the diapers, and there is no evidence by wetting of urine having passed. But the urine is highly coloured and leaves a stain which may

be mistaken for blood. Two or three grains of citrate of magnesia (*vide* p. 15) should be given twice a day.

22. Urine, Retention of.—Sometimes infants make no water during the first twenty-four hours. When this is the case, and the infant appears in pain, crying, and drawing up the legs, a warm bath, or fomentation over the lower parts of the bowels, will prove successful.

23. Vomiting.—Some infants vomit *immediately* after suckling, the milk returning *unsoured*, or without evident cause. This probably depends on a copious supply of milk, which the infant takes too fast or in too large a quantity. A finger should be placed near the orifice of the nipple, to prevent too rapid flow.

24. Red Gum, and Jaundice.—Red or yellow gum is the term popularly given to discolorations of the skin, which may occur to infants two or three days after birth. But all instances of discoloration of the skin are *not* jaundice, as the surface is often discoloured from the blood being congested in the skin, probably from the effects of cold, or owing to pressure from protracted labour, and such discoloration requires no treatment. When jaundice occurs the child's skin is yellow, the whites of the eyes are yellow, the urine is dark, staining the clothes yellow, and the stools are white. If the eyes are yellow, and if white linen is stained yellow by the urine, there is jaundice. It is due to the liver being engorged, from the lungs not acting properly at first. As a rule no medicine is required, the first milk of the mother being sufficient to open the bowels of the infant. In bad cases, when the whites of the eyes are yellow, and the bowels constipated, half a teaspoonful of castor-oil may be given. It is some days before the skin loses the yellow tinge.

Examination of Infants.—It is often difficult for a mother to know exactly when her infant first becomes ill, or even in some cases to be sure that it is really sick. It is often difficult to decide whether a fit of crying is due to bad temper, to passing discomfort, or to disease.

The *general demeanour and expression* are instructive. A flushed or a pale face, disinclination to play, drowsiness by day and restlessness at night, and unusual fretfulness, are signs of approaching illness; and may signify probably ague, or other maladies soon to be declared by their distinct symptoms.

The *cry of an infant* is often very characteristic of the malady from which the child is suffering. The cry of passion is a furious one; the cry of sleepiness is a drowsy one; when roused from sleep there is generally a sobbing cry; a shrill cry denotes hunger or thirst, and is often accompanied by movements of head and hands, as if seeking the breast; the cry of teething is fretful and intermittent; an infant with earache will cry in short, piercing tones, putting the hand to the affected ear, and perhaps rolling the head. If after giving a baby suitable nourishment or a drink of water it still keeps up a continued cry, there is probably pain in the ear. Bowel complaint causes a straining cry, with drawing up of the legs; in bronchitis the cry is gruff and husky; in inflammation of the lungs it resembles a moan; in croup the voice is hoarse, and the breathing sounds as if drawn through muslin; in inflammation of the brain the cry is often a piercing shriek at intervals, alternating with moaning. It should not be forgotten that crying may arise from a pin pricking, or a tight string, or a rough fold of clothing.

*When necessary to examine a child,* as to the existence of tenderness in the bowels, for instance, it is useful to bring the child suddenly before a bright light, as one of the apparently greatest pleasures of an infant consists in gazing at such an object. It almost always ceases to scream, and continues quiet while thus attracted, when the bowels may be examined by gentle pressure with the fingers. If the pressure causes the child to cry out, with frowns or contractions of the countenance, there will probably be some condition affecting the bowels.

*A child should never be roused from sleep in order to give medicine.* If a child, especially an infant, sleeps, it may be accepted as an indication of a mild form of disease or of a diminution of serious symptoms. With regard to the administration of medicine to children, if they are old enough, appeal to their reason, for if children are deceived they will soon become suspicious, and future trouble will be entailed. If too young to be reasoned with, and children will not take medicine, they should be compelled. Let a refractory child be laid across the knees, the hands, *nose*, and feet being tightly held. Then by means of a medicine spoon, or other spoon, pour the dose into the mouth, and it must be swallowed. Medicine should be made as palatable as possible for children, as giving nauseous doses excites a child, the passion probably doing more harm than the medicine forcibly administered does good.

The average weight of an infant at birth is 7 lbs., and the average length 18 inches.

It may also be mentioned that tears are not shed by infants until they are from three to four months old; and that the eyes of infants are blue up to the sixth or eighth week of age.

FEEDING OF INFANTS. PROPER FOOD, MILK.—Although a tropical climate is not so fatal to infants of European parentage as once supposed, still an amount of carelessness as regards food, which in England would give rise to minor maladies, will in India become the cause of fatal diseases. But with care as regards feeding, and under good hygienic conditions, there is no reason why European-born children should suffer in the future from passing the first years of their life in the tropics. At the time of birth the digestive organs of the child are in an immature state, and it is only gradually that their power becomes developed. For the first few months no saliva is secreted, there are no tears, and the stomach and alimentary canal are comparatively short. The teeth do not appear until the lapse of several months. All conditions pointing to feeble digestive capacity, and evidencing that the food must be specially adapted to the digestive powers. Of such food there is only one kind, namely, milk.

Women should Suckle their Children.—It is in accordance with nature that a *healthy* woman should suckle her offspring. The avoidance of this duty often reacts injuriously in various ways on the system of the mother. As nursing, generally speaking, prevents conception up to the tenth month, so it prevents the ruin of the mother's constitution by too rapid child-bearing. Moreover, it is advantageous to the breasts that their natural functions should be carried on, and may probably prevent the future development of breast diseases. But there are certain conditions of system, as a consumptive tendency, which forbid nursing, and the remarks apply only to healthy females. Notwithstanding the extreme desirability of *healthy* females suckling their children, there are a large number of Englishwomen in India unable to undertake this duty. In addition to those suffering from actual disease, or weakened by former attacks, there is a more numerous class who are debilitated, to a greater or less extent, by heat, malaria, and the relaxing nature of the climate. It is shown (*vide* p. 665) that the above influences lead to degeneration of the blood. And this is especially apparent in the weaker system of the female, particularly when child-bearing, parturition, and suckling are superadded as causes of debility. It may be broadly stated that, as a result of residence in India, the majority of European women are physically unable to nurse after the second or third confinement. On the first occasion they may be equal to the task, and should, when possible, nurse. But with every desire to fulfil such duties they find their strength unequal to the strain. Persistence in nursing after the appearance of the symptoms detailed at p. 655 is followed by gradual or sudden cessation of the secretion of milk.

QUESTION OF SUPPLEMENTING MOTHER'S MILK BY HAND-FEEDING.—When the mother finds her milk inadequate to supply the wants of the child, the question arises whether the mother's milk cannot be supplemented by hand-feeding. Many mothers are averse to delegating the duty of suckling to other women. In the minds of some people there is an objection to their children being suckled by a native female; but although the mother who bears a child may impress constitutional peculiarities on it, milk cannot subsequently do so. Others, again, may be unable to bear the expense of a wet-nurse or 'dhai'; or a suitable wet-nurse is not procurable. Such circumstances must sometimes lead to *supplementing* the milk of the mother by hand-feeding. But it is a practice which cannot be recommended. It is a fact that whenever the milk is not *sufficient* for the wants of the infant, it is also more or less *deficient* in qualities on which its nutritive properties depend; and it is therefore unsuited for use. The limited supply shows that the constitution of the mother is unequal to the tax, and milk of the best quality cannot be secreted by a person whose constitutional powers are failing. The sooner these facts are appreciated and acted upon, by the employment of a wet-nurse, the better it will be for both mother and child. But if from any cause a wet-nurse cannot be obtained, it will be advisable, on the appearance of the symptoms detailed at p. 655, for the mother to leave off suckling *immediately*, and to trust to hand-feeding. The child should then be fed as mentioned at pp. 646, 648.

COMPOSITION OF MILK, AND THE SELECTION OF A WET-NURSE.—One hundred parts of milk contain nearly 90 parts of water, the remaining being solid constituents, as *caseine*, or cheesy matter, sugar, fat, and various salts. The milk of women is liable to certain natural changes at different periods of suckling. The first milk differs from that afterwards formed in containing slightly purgative principles, the utility of which is referred to at pp. 625, 635. Until the end of the first month the amount of sugar is less than afterwards, and the *caseine* or *nitrogenous* matter is presented in a more easily digestible form than subsequently. From the eighth to the tenth month sugar is in excess. Caseine is most deficient during the tenth and eleventh months, and most abundant during the first two months. During the first month there is also more butter, or fat, and salts than at any other period.

From the above it is evident that when *selecting a wet-nurse* one of the requirements should be, that the milk should have commenced about the same date as that of the mother. The general health of the woman should be attentively considered; her teeth should be good and her breath sweet; and freedom from piles, from enlarged spleen, and from any skin disease must be ascertained. If either the woman or her husband has suffered from prolonged sore-throat, she should be rejected, as it is probably venereal. The condition of the child should be examined, and the mother of a weak, puny, badly nourished infant should be rejected; especially if there are sores about the buttocks, privates, or corners of the mouth, which are also probably venereal. No woman who has suckled any other than her own child should be engaged, unless the child is seen, for a woman may contract disease of the breast from one child, and convey it from her breast to another. It should also be ascertained that there is no epidemic disease where the woman comes from, as small-pox, scarlet fever, or measles. The condition of the woman's breasts should be examined, which should be round, prominent, with veins visible, and affording a rather hard, knotty feeling. It is not necessary that the breasts should be large, as those of a moderate size often furnish most milk; but it is important that the nipples should be well developed and projecting, and free from sores. A little milk should be procured, which should present a bluish-white colour, and possess a sweet taste. If tested with test-paper (*vide* p. 288) it should afford an alkaline, not an acid reaction; and if examined under a microscope, all globules should be seen floating about separate and free, and not massing together. Allowed to stand a few hours, it should give a thin film, resembling cream. Dropped in water, healthy human milk should form a cloudy mixture, and not sink in thick drops. The goodness of the milk may also be judged of by observation of the nurse's child. If it sucks heartily, the milk is most likely good; if it sucks laboriously, desists, and cries, the reverse is probably the case. Inquiry should be made as to whether the woman has been 'unwell' since nursing, for if so the milk is never good, and will probably soon stop altogether. Although the age of the wet-nurse's child should as nearly as possible correspond with that of the infant requiring wet-nursing, the age of the wet-nurse herself is not so important a matter. A woman from twenty to thirty years old is advisable. Native women commence having children at an early age, and cease to do so proportionally early; and neither a very young girl nor a woman approaching the termination of her child-bearing era is desirable. The woman should be of temperate habits, not addicted to over-eating or to drink, or to smoking opium or hemp. In certain parts of India, a moderate indulgence in tobacco-smoking must be permitted, as some women—Bheels, for instance—will rarely take service if debarred from the customary pipe. Cleanliness, equanimity of temper, cheerfulness, and an open, frank disposition are to be greatly desired. Lastly, the association of the woman with her friends and relatives should, if practicable, be stopped. If she becomes 'unwell,' or pregnancy occurs, the child should be taken from her. When a change of aymahs has to be made, the woman should not be told until a successor is at hand; as the tidings, perhaps exciting the woman, may influence the milk, and so injuriously affect the child.

The possibility of *deception* should be held in view. A woman by drinking largely, and by allowing the milk to accumulate, may present the appearances of breasts well supplied with milk, while in reality the daily amount secreted is not sufficient for a healthy child. Such deception may be suspected when a thin feeble-loooking woman appears with overflowing breasts. The only sure method of detection is applying a child to empty the breasts and watching the rapidity of the reaccumulation of the milk. It should also be ascertained that a child shown by a wet-nurse is not a borrowed one.

WET-NURSING FROM BIRTH.—The milk of a healthy woman is too rich for the delicate stomach of the infant during the first two or three days of its existence. It should therefore be fed artificially for the first seventy-two hours, in the manner detailed at p. 648; and on the first three or four applications of the child to the 'dhai,' it should be permitted to take only a small quantity of milk. If a wet-nurse confined at the same time as the mother of the child were available, the precautions as above would not be required; but this can rarely be the case. It is in instances of the kind, when the child does not take the first milk from the mother, that some aperient dose (*vide* p. 634) may be necessary for the infant.

It occasionally happens that, from some unexplainable cause, the milk of one woman disagrees with a child while that of another woman suits. Such exceptional case may be suspected when, after regulating the diet of an apparently healthy 'dhai,' and after any costiveness of the bowels of the woman has been removed by castor-oil, the child still does not thrive. Under such circumstances a change of nurses may be necessary. But alterations of the kind are often attended with much trouble and expense, and therefore should not be made on insufficient grounds. Very frequently when an *aymah's* milk disagrees, the reason may be found in the fact of the woman on becoming an *aymah* being able to indulge in a richer diet, while leading a more lazy life. Owing to the anxiety of parents that the nurse of their child shall be strong, too much or too rich food is often provided, the result being a change in the character of the milk, which therefore disagrees with the child. The fact of a child not thriving so well as could be wished cannot be immediately accepted as a reason why artificial feeding should be substituted, but must be regarded as indicating some dietetic error requiring amendment, and the desirability of some employment for the woman. Or, the child may not thrive from the fact of the woman surreptitiously suckling her own infant. Or, there may be a superabundance of thin poor milk, which is suggestive of its soon ceasing altogether (*vide* p. 655).

After ten days, it is desirable to teach the infant the use of the bottle. A tea-spoonful of goat's milk with four of water may be given once a day. This is *not* for nourishment, but as a *precaution* against interruption of the nurse's duties from sickness or otherwise, when it might be difficult to get the child to take the bottle.

HAND-FEEDING.—If the mother cannot suckle, and if a wet-nurse cannot be procured, *hand-feeding* must be adopted. Many, having known a successful instance of hand-feeding, regard it as generally applicable, but experience and statistics show the reverse. *However carefully conducted, it is a most fertile source of infantile disease and mortality.* Hand-fed children, although increasing in weight, and often *looking* fat and well, have not the harder flesh and stamina of breast-fed infants. They are more liable to diarrhœa, convulsions, rickets, and other maladies, and they do not recover from ailments so rapidly as the breast-fed. Human milk being the natural food of an infant, it will be preferable to somewhat relax the rules for the selection of a wet-nurse, rather than incur the risk of injuring the infant by other varieties of milk. Any ordinary healthy woman's milk is better for a child than the milk of a quadruped.

When hand-feeding is indispensable, it is expedient to modify the milk so as to make it resemble as much as possible that of a woman. The best substitute for delicate children is ass's milk, as in some respects it more nearly resembles that of woman, particularly in the high proportion of sugar and large amount of water it contains, although there is a great deficiency in solid matter. It is for this reason better adapted for the delicate stomachs of children reduced by illness than for the wants of a vigorous growing child. In India goat's milk is perhaps most desirable, which, although containing more solid constituents and less sugar than human milk, is more like the latter than most samples from the cow. The latter fluid contains more caseine, fat, and salts than either, and less sugar than ass's or woman's milk. Analysis of milk, however, varies, and different samples secreted by the same animal furnish somewhat different results, which must be influenced by feeding and the health of the animal. Hence it happens that sometimes goat's and at other times cow's milk agrees best with an infant. As a rule for India, goat's milk may be said to be the most suitable, and it is often the most conveniently procured.

Whatever animal is selected, it should be kept and fed for the purpose, as both the Indian cow and goat are very promiscuous and dirty feeders when hungry. It is best to see the animal fed, as servants may give inferior food. Grains from breweries should not be used, or the milk may cause diarrhœa. At the commencement of the rains, when green grass becomes plentiful, if the animal eats much of it a similar effect may be produced. The animal should be kept very clean, and should *not* be allowed to drink dirty water. The vessels in which the milk is received and kept should be scrupulously clean, put in a cool place away from sewers and smells, and protected from flies. The child's food should *never* consist of milk taken from two animals, even of the same class.

Supposing a child to be fed on ass's milk from its birth. For the first few days it should be given in the proportion of two-thirds milk and one-third water. After the first four or five days the quantity of milk may be gradually increased, until at the end of a fortnight ass's milk may be given pure. Ass's milk, being so rich in sugar, requires no addition of this kind. If cow's or goat's milk is used, it should be given for the first ten days mixed with one-half the quantity of water. After this period the amount of water may be gradually diminished, until at the end of the fourth month goat's milk may be given pure, and cow's milk almost pure. At the end of the fifth month cow's milk may be given pure. Both goat's and cow's milk, being comparatively deficient in saccharine matter, require the addition of sugar. 'Sugar of milk' is preferable, as it is not fermentable like other sugars, and is therefore less liable to turn acid on the stomach. If sugar of milk cannot be procured, pure white loaf sugar is best. Moist sugar should never be used, as it is certain to ferment in and disorder the stomach. Much harm is done by rendering the food too sweet. The desideratum is to form a compound resembling human milk. A moderate 'mawkish' sweetness is all that is required. The palate of the mother should be accustomed to the taste of good human milk, and the food prepared accordingly. A little variation in the sweetness or otherwise of an infant's food will make all the difference as to the food agreeing with the child or not. The *temperature* of an infant's food should be, as nearly as possible, that of the mother's milk; or, at least, it should not be below 96° Fahr. or above 98°. In addition to the above precautions, it will be desirable to test for acidity with litmus paper (*vide* p. 288). Woman's milk is slightly alkaline, and stall-fed cow's milk is often slightly acid. When this is the case a few tea-spoonfuls of lime-water (Recipe 25), may be added. It will also be desirable, when the infant vomits clotted material, to render cow's milk less rich in *caseine.* This is effected by exposing the milk to a gentle heat, in a wide open vessel, when a film of caseine forms on the surface, which may be removed with a spoon. Or sometimes cow's milk suits best if let stand for two or three hours in a tall glass, then dipping out the upper third, and using the lower two-thirds.

If the motions of a child fed on cow's milk contain specks of white undigested caseine or curds, a little barley-water added to the milk may correct this. Or, if the child is upwards of three months old, a *very little* farinaceous food, as Brighton biscuits, may be added, which, mingling with the curds, mechanically divides it, rendering it more digestible. This is a different thing from feeding on farinaceous food, which is highly objectionable (*vide* p. 652). Or the milk may be temporarily peptonised by Fairchild's powders, which have the property of rendering curds more digestible. Infants' milk may be peptonised as follows. Into a clean nursing-bottle pour ¼ pint of milk, ¼ pint of warm water, and ¼ of a Fairchild Zymine Peptonising Powder; place the bottle in water as hot as the hand can bear for *twenty minutes*; add a little sugar of milk to sweeten, and boil quickly; if this be not done a slightly bitter taste is developed.

Importance of Fresh Milk.—Milk given should be perfectly fresh, and not in the slightest degree soured, either by weather or by dirty vessels. Perfect cleanliness of the latter, and of the feeding-spoon or nursery bottle, cannot be too much insisted upon; and to secure this they should be washed in hot water containing a few grains of carbonate of soda, both before and after use, and be kept immersed in a similar mixture till again wanted. Sour milk, or soiled vessels, often cause bowel complaints. The least atom of stale milk sticking to the tube, or cork, or bottle will turn sour fresh milk touching it, and cause vomiting and diarrhœa. The crevices of corks are liable to hold atoms of decaying milk, and therefore a wooden stopper should be used. A ready method of turning the milk sour is allowing it to be in the bed, warmed by contact with the child's body. More milk than a child requires for the meal should never be put into the bottle. A grain of carbonate of soda added to the milk will prevent it turning sour for some time—a plan which may be adopted on a journey.

IMPORTANCE OF PURE WATER.—This is dwelt upon at p. 678. But further precaution is required where infants are concerned. The water should be filtered and afterwards boiled. It should then be allowed to cool, and, when required for use, should be heated to the proper degree.

GENERAL RULES FOR FEEDING.—A child should be fed from a bottle, and not from a cup; for the act of sucking, when feeding from the bottle, promotes the flow of saliva, mixes it with the food when the saliva appears, and thus assists digestion. Of various bottles 'the British feeding-bottle' may be recommended, as the infant using it cannot suck in air; or, still better, the Burroughs & Wellcome 'thermo-safeguard feeding-bottle,' which is graduated in ounces, thus enabling the nurse to estimate the exact quantity of food to be given. A strong thermometer embedded in the glass registers the temperature of the food. But the use of long tubes attached to bottles is not advised, as there is danger of some particle of the food remaining in the tube which will turn sour, in which case it will permeate the whole mass of food taken at the next meal and cause stomach and bowel troubles. The plain black rubber nipple is the best, and can be used upon any bottle having a heavy lip or rim. As a rule the food should be warmed by dipping the bottle in hot water, and not over a fire. An infant should be fed slowly in the semi-erect posture with the head slightly raised; and it should never be played with or dandled immediately after feeding; but it should be placed on its right side or back and kept quiet. It should be fed regularly every two or three hours during the day, and two or three times during the night; in the latter months of infancy, less frequently. The mother or nurse should always put the nipple to her lips the last thing before feeding the infant, and make sure that the nipple is clear and all is right.

The above are general rules for feeding an ordinarily healthy child. But it may happen that, from accidental causes, such as overloading the stomach, or from some deviation in the quality of the milk, temporary modification in the feeding, *generally in the way of further diluting the milk*, will be advisable. Both *over-feeding* and *too thick food* must be guarded against. It should be recollected that an infant quite as often cries from repletion as from hunger. If the child's stomach is overloaded, it will produce flatus, hiccough, indigestion, vomiting, diarrhœa, or other disorders. An infant under one month old will probably consume about two and a half pounds avoir. *per diem*, or from two to five ounces at each meal; at three months old about three pints daily; but no definite quantity can be directed for a child of any given age.

CONDENSED OR SWISS MILK.—While infants take readily to such food, on account, probably, of the sweet taste, and also grow plump, they are not in reality strong when so fed. A slight ailment renders them prostrate to a much greater degree than when fed on fresh animal milk. Still it may be necessary, on board ship, or when making long journeys, to use such food. Then for infants up to a month old a tea-spoonful of condensed milk to a teacupful of warm barley-water is the proper strength. After about six weeks it would be desirable to add to it some malted food as mentioned below. If on opening a tin of condensed milk gas escapes, it is bad.

WHEN A CHILD MAY BE FED WITH OTHER FOOD THAN MILK.—When a child is first given other food, it should only be used as an addition to the natural food, milk, and not as the main means of support. *Farinaceous* foods, as sago, arrowroot, rice, tapioca, gruel, often selected on account of their supposed lightness, are digested with difficulty by the infant, for they contain starch, which has no existence in milk. Such food excites eructation and vomiting, intestinal irritation, and diarrhœa. And not only are these farinaceous articles of food hard of digestion, but when reduced to their ultimate elements, as they must be in that process, they differ much from milk, the only natural food, and are thus rendered the most unsuited for the nourishment of the body. Food has two uses—one to afford matter for the growth of the body, the other to give material for the maintenance of the animal heat—and a child is not nourished in proportion with the bulk of the food swallowed. Health, and even life, cannot be long supported except on a diet in which the elements of nutrition and the elements of animal heat bear a certain proportion. In milk these are combined in the proportion of one to two. In arrowroot, sago, and tapioca, the proportion is one to twenty-six, in wheat-flour one to seven. Thus the child fed on farinaceous food is actually starved to death, for it is forced to supply from its own tissues the nitrogenous elements essential to the maintenance of life. This is a frequent cause of atrophy, diarrhœa, and convulsions.

From the above it is evident that a child should not be fed on other food than milk until some indication appears of the development of the digestive organs. The first sign is teething. As a rule, until the first teeth appear, no other food than milk should be allowed. After this period some kind of 'malted food' may be given cautiously, in small quantities, and at first only once in the day. These 'malted foods'[1] are really farinaceous, but the starch has been so treated by chemical process that the work of digestion has been partially performed.

It is not well to continue the use of 'malted food' too long. If we habitually rear children without putting them to the necessity of digesting their food, we shall evolve beings of weak digestion—Nature's revenge on organs not used. The proper use of malted food is as an aid to digestion at the period of transition from milk to other diet, and in cases of ailing children; but *not* as an ordinary food or as a substitute for milk, for without milk children are liable to become latently scorbutic.

After about a month ordinary farinaceous foods may be combined, those containing wheat-flour being, for the reasons above stated, the best; such as 'tops and bottoms,' or cornflour, or rusks, or Robb's biscuits, or prepared barley or soojee, sometimes one, sometimes another, agreeing best with the child. It will also be advisable to add a grain or two of salt to each meal. Animal food should not be given until two of the back teeth have appeared. As a preparation for animal food, especially for debilitated children, the following is advisable. Four ounces of milk, half an ounce of cream, a tea-spoonful of arrowroot, the yolk of an egg nearly raw, half a pint of warm water. For the first animal food, nothing is better than beef-tea in which sago has been boiled. Gradually the child may be accustomed to take chicken or mutton broth, eggs, rice, and dhall, and fine mince. Potatoes should be avoided, as unless very soft and mealy, lumps may be swallowed, which will irritate the bowels.

WEANING.—The propriety or otherwise of weaning a

[1] The Kepler Extract of Malt may be recommended.

child in India must be considered with reference both to the condition of the child and of the mother or nurse (*vide* Over-nursing). Speaking generally, weaning should not be commenced until the child has attained the age of twelve months, and then only provided the child is strong and healthy. If the child is not in good health, suckling should be continued until the child has cut at least twelve teeth. A good rule is, if dentition is backward delay the weaning; although suckling may be supplemented by some of the malted foods mentioned above. Weaning should not be commenced when a tooth is irritating, not in the autumn, the season of diarrhœas, and not when there is cholera about. When weaning is determined on, it should be a gradual process, and should be begun at night. The better way is to separate the child, and if it cries, it may be soothed with some tepid water. It will probably get very little sleep; but by the second night, if the mother has not yielded, half the work will have been done. The third night the child will probably sleep, or it will be satisfied with water. Too mixed diet should not be given after weaning, various articles being tried singly in succession for a few days, in order to ascertain which is most suitable for digestion. Milk-and-water thickened with baked flour or with well-baked bread, 'pish-pash,' or weak broth, suits most infants. No meat should be given for some weeks, and allowing a bone to suck is not recommended, as it will probably lead to a little meat and the daily demand of the child for more. When meat is given, it should be very finely minced.

The mother's breasts ordinarily give no trouble when weaning is performed gradually, but if necessary the dispersion of the milk may be assisted by a poultice of parsley leaves, by saline aperients (Recipes 2, 4, 6), by rubbing the breasts gently with soap liniment, or, if procurable, with belladonna liniment, and by abstinence from much fluid to drink. Drawing the breasts is not recommended, as it favours the continued secretion of milk.

Over-nursing.—The first signs are a dragging sensation in the back when the child is at the breast, and an exhausted feeling afterwards, often described as a 'sinking at the pit of the stomach,' and in exceptional instances there may be an *excessive secretion* of thin poor milk. In these cases, there is a constant oozing and loss of milk, which keeps the clothing wet, while the child suffers from its innutritious, watery character, and the mother from the amount of the discharge. These symptoms are accompanied or quickly followed by loss of appetite, constipation, or diarrhœa, sleeplessness, pain in the left side, often pain at the top of the head, or brow-ague, or throbbing of the temples, with giddiness, and depression of spirits, singing in the ears, disorders of the sight, palpitation of the heart, and a short dry cough. The monthly discharge may reappear, and may be irregular or excessive, with constant 'whites.' In extreme cases, the countenance grows pale and sallow, the body wastes, and there may be night perspirations and swelling of the ankles. When such symptoms appear it is useless attempting to support the strength by more generous diet, by ale, porter, or stimulants, as is often tried. The woman should cease suckling, otherwise Nature will take the case in her own hands, and the secretion of milk will stop—not, however, until the constitution is probably permanently impaired by the persistent drain which has been maintained. When *puerperal mania* appears long after a confinement, it is almost invariably in women debilitated by over-nursing.

When Children should be allowed to Walk.—The bones in a child's leg are soft, half cartilaginous, and easily bent. People who urge children to walk prematurely are often responsible for lasting injury. Long before soft bones ought to have any strain put upon them, infants are frequently made to stand and walk, so that the legs, especially if there is any rickety or scrofulous family taint, become bent. When children are a year old they should be encouraged to creep, but not to walk till after eighteen months.

## CHAPTER VI

### *THE PRESERVATION OF HEALTH*

THIS section is suggestive of the course to be followed to secure the preservation of health in the varying circumstances of residence and exposure in a tropical climate. Hence something of the following will be familar to those who have paid attention to sanitary demands. But to render the treatment of the subject such as will prove useful to all, the reader must be assumed ignorant of the topics to which the following pages refer.

The European is more or less rapidly—in these days much more suddenly than when so many doubled the Cape—transported from a climate where the mean temperature is low to one in which it is some twenty degrees higher (82° Fahr.), where the sun's rays are vertical, where the rainfall is violent, and instead of being spread over the greater portion of the year is practically confined to certain seasons, and where changes of temperature, both seasonal and daily, may reach 50°. The three great divisions of the year into hot, cold, and rainy seasons are found to be more or less correct throughout the whole Indian peninsula. But, consequent on periodical rains, mountains, sea coasts, rivers, jungles, varying soils, and sand tracts, most localities are found to possess a different climate, which is further influenced by cultivation. Thus local climates in India are more varied than at first would be supposed, and are consequently more or less inimical to the constitution of the European who sojourns therein.

It cannot be too much impressed on Europeans in India that the diseases incidental to the climate may be often escaped, or at least modified in severity, by attention to ordinary sanitary principles and to personal hygiene, especially by those newly arrived in the country. The Anglo-Saxon race is, perhaps, above all others endowed with a resisting power against the evil effects of adverse climatic influences; and this power may be materially assisted by care, and by avoidance of evident causes of disease. Improved habits of life and public sanitary measures of recent years have already increased the value of both European and Native health in many parts of India (*vide* p. 680).

In a hot climate the European must defend himself against three principal climatic enemies, and these are—HEAT, so-called MALARIA, and, paradoxical as it may appear, COLD. Keeping these three causes of disease prominently in mind, he must next look to the quality of the WATER he drinks; to the securing of a proper amount of SLEEP; to the quality and quantity of the FOOD he eats; to the amount of fermented LIQUOR he consumes; to EXERCISE; to CLOTHING; to the BATH; to the HOUSE he lives in; to the CONSERVANCY of his premises and neighbourhood; and to the CONDUCT OF THE PASSIONS. These subjects are now considered separately.

**HEAT.**—Heat will induce disease both *directly* and *indirectly*. *Directly*, as when an *immediate* fever or sunstroke is the result of exposure to the direct rays of the sun; or *indirectly*, as when *heat syncope* or fainting, *heat asphyxia* or suffocation, are excited by the sultry atmosphere of the Indian dog-days, or by the hot and vitiated air of crowded hospitals or barracks, *without any direct* exposure to the sun. *Long-continued heat* also acts still more *indirectly*, causing insidious blood-deterioration (*vide* p. 665).

Heat acting *directly* interferes with or suspends some of the most important natural functions of the body. Heat is continually produced within the body by chemical changes connected with respiration and nutrition, and this heat is regulated by evaporation and perspiration from the surface, and by the excretions. If anything prevents the latter opposing forces acting, natural heat accumulates in the body; which also, if unprotected by evaporation, absorbs heat from the hotter external atmosphere. Heat thus accumulating beyond a certain point causes paralysis of the nerves supplying the heart, or the muscles of respiration, or the brain. The hot dry atmosphere of Upper India is better tolerated than the hot damp atmosphere of Southern India, although the temperature is lower. For hot dry air favours evaporation, and this tends to keep the body cool, while in damp air evaporation decreases, and the natural cooling power is thus greatly diminished. But in any district the heat is too great, and too long continued, to be withstood with impunity, unless under precautionary measures. Hence the desirability of avoiding as much as possible exposure to the direct rays of the sun during the summer season, when, if practicable, the European should remain under the shelter of a roof between the hours of 9 A.M. and 4 P.M. Infants and children should be indoors by 7 A.M., for by that time the comparative coolness of the morning air is gone. Much of the fever and digestive ailments occurring to children is due to exposure to the sun. But such avoidance of exposure is not always in the power of every person. Work must be done and the sun must be braved. The surveyor or engineer must sometimes be abroad at such seasons looking after his works; the soldier must attend to the calls of duty, whether by day or by night; the doctor must obey the demands of his patients; the traveller pressed for time must proceed, whether the vertical sun shines fiercely or the frost of Upper India appears colder than that of Europe. On such occasions protection of the *head*, *back*, and *bowels* is the principal means by which exposure may be rendered less inimical. Therefore the adoption of a suitable headdress is a *sine quâ non*. But a material suitable for a headdress which will admit of compression without injury, and yet resume its shape, which possesses the characteristics of strength, durability, and lightness, is still a desideratum.

Thin leather is perhaps the only material, certainly the material more easily obtainable, most fulfilling the indications required. A low-crowned helmet, constructed of two layers of thin leather, is perhaps the most efficient headdress. The summit of the crown should be sufficiently elevated not to touch the top of the head. Where the helmet fits the head laterally, the separation of the two layers should be about a quarter of an inch. If the space is wider, as in many pith or wicker-work hats, the hot wind is allowed to pass in excess to the head, the hair and scalp are maintained dry by the immediate evaporation of the perspiration secreted, the head grows hot, and the person is thus predisposed to *coup de soleil*. On the other hand, if the headdress is so made as to admit of but very moderate ventilation, the head is maintained moist, a desideratum in all districts where the hot winds blow. The ideas prevalent, that the hair is injured by maintaining it wet with perspiration, and that baldness is thereby produced, are erroneous. Only a little extra cleanliness and care, with brush and comb, is necessitated. Sunstrokes will seldom occur when the head is *wet*, but when *dry* there is danger.

The *puggree*, or turban, should be some thin cotton texture, at least seven yards long, and, when doubled twice, eight inches broad. This may be wrapped according to fancy round the helmet, taking care that the greatest number of layers are over that portion where the helmet comes in contact with the head. But this is not the only use of the turban. When travelling, it should be worn as a 'cummerbund,' or protection to the bowels and loins at night. Thus the turban would defend two vitally important parts at that period of the twenty-four hours when each most requires defence, viz. the bowels by night and the brain by day. Also, when halting by day in the shade, with (as often is the case) a hot wind blowing, and converting the surface of the body into a kind of tatty, it is advisable to wind the turban round the bowels. This simple precaution will prevent chill, which otherwise may be the cause of bowel complaint. And for this use the turban is recommended to be sufficiently broad to reach over the whole bowels, and to be long enough to pass round the body several times. The protection of the head may be still further secured by wetting the 'puggree' with water before going into the sun, or by placing inside the hat a wet handkerchief, or green leaves, of which the best is plantain leaf. And the protection of the bowels may be rendered more certain by the habitual use of a flannel belt over the parts. This, with the addition of the turban, at the times and under the circumstances indicated above, will reduce the chances of bowel complaint, at least from cold, to a minimum.

The best and most simple belt is a piece of hemmed flannel of the ordinary breadth, and long enough to pass round the body, from the right hip to the left hip, where it may be pinned. This secures a double flannel over the bowels.

The *protection of the spine* is scarcely of less importance, for there is a species of *coup de soleil*, known as *heat asphyxia*, in which the origin of the evil is referable to the spinal cord. That part of the spine just below the neck, from which the nerves of respiration pass to the chest, becomes congested by the heat, the nerves become paralysed, the chest ceases to expand, and the person dies suffocated. Many cases recorded as sunstroke are, in fact, heat-suffocation. *A priori*, allowing the puggree to fall over the back would appear the most facile method of accomplishing the object. But there are several objections to this. The weight of the puggree hanging down becomes irksome to the wearer, who, when the puggree lies close to the coat, cannot move his head with freedom. On wind blowing, the puggree moves its position, and ceases to afford the desired shelter. The floating ends are also liable to entangle in adjacent objects, sometimes flapping round the wearer's face, and perhaps obscuring vision at a critical time. What is required is an immovable protection for the spine, which may be put on and off with the clothing. This is to be obtained by placing a pad about seven inches long and three wide from the collar of the coat to about the lower angle of the bladebone. This pad should be constructed of cork shavings—a material which, while acting as a non-conductor of heat, is light, and sufficiently soft not to occasion inconvenience even if lain upon. The shavings should be stitched, so that the position of the pad cannot alter. The thickness of the pad should be about three inches.

*The protection of the whole body from direct heat* is also necessary. For short distances there is the 'chatta,' or umbrella. Yet this can scarcely be used on horseback, when actively employed, or when in pursuit of game. But it should be recollected that what keeps out cold will, to a certain extent, also keep out heat. Or, stating the case scientifically, what is a bad conductor of heat *from* the surface of the body will be a bad conductor of heat *to* the surface of the body. Hence it is not advisable that the clothing of Europeans in India should be so thin as the majority of persons would suppose. Light it should certainly be, but the texture should be such as, while not inconvenient from weight, will yet afford some protection to the surface of the body. For the equestrian, even in the hottest weather, nothing will be better than cord breeches and flannel shirt, with overcoat of flannel or cotton. When less active exertion is anticipated flannel is also still desirable (*vide Clothing*, p. 688).

*Exposure to indirect heat* must be guarded against by

ventilation of dwelling-houses, especially of sleeping-apartments. And this should not be done by rule and measure. The number of cubic feet available as breathing-space is a fallacious method of gauging the capabilities of a sleeping-chamber. Except in the coldest weather of the coldest part of India, and in some positions and localities during the rains and unhealthy season, some doors or windows defended by chicks should always remain open. The sleeping-cot need not be placed in a draught, but to one side, so that ventilation may be secured without danger of chill. The punkah, thermantidote, and tatty are also useful in guarding against the effects of heated atmosphere. In many parts of India the punkah is always grateful by day, while the thermantidote and tatty will aid in reducing the temperature of the whole house. But they should be so placed that the wind passing from them does not blow directly on the person, as various diseases not unfrequently result from sitting too near or sleeping in front of these contrivances; and the thermantidote hole should be lower than it is usually made, by which the cool air is distributed more equably over the room. The night punkah is also very necessary in some districts where the oppressive sultriness forbids sound and refreshing sleep. But this may become a source of danger. The punkah-puller may sleep when, the wind from the punkah ceasing, the European becomes drenched in perspiration. The punkah-man, suddenly wakening, commences a vigorous pull, and rapidly cools the sleeper by the evaporation thus produced, the result being chill and its consequences. Or, while cooled by the action of the punkah on one side, the other half of the body in contact with the bed is wet with perspiration. The sleeper turns, and the process of evaporation, as above described, commences, with perhaps similar result. There are many parts of India where, from the extreme oppressiveness and sultriness of the night at certain seasons, the punkah cannot be dispensed with, and the lesser of two evils, viz. the chance of chill and its consequences, must be chosen, instead of the certainty of the debility and destruction of health attendant on continued sleepless nights. But in the more northerly districts the night-punkah may often be dispensed with, and in other localities generally favoured with the sea breeze, it is scarcely required, except perhaps for a short time during the most sultry weather.

Sleeping in the open air, or even in the verandah, would at least secure due breathing-space, but it is a practice which cannot be generally recommended. In the early part of the night the person, unable to bear clothing, either designedly or unknowingly throws off everything. Towards morning there is a considerable fall of temperature just at the period when during sleep the least animal heat is produced, and when the vital powers are less than at any other part of the twenty-four hours. The person so indulging often awakes chilled, and probably gets so-termed malarious fever. In the so-called malarious and damper portions of the peninsula such indulgence should never be permitted, as in addition to the morning fall of temperature chills from land winds and sea breezes, or from heavy dews, are liable to occur, and any check to the perspiration from such causes may excite liver disease, dysentery, or fever. Moreover, malaria is supposed to be more powerful during the hours of darkness. But there are parts of India where sleeping in the open air during the very hot weather is permissible, if not more advisable than subjection to the uncertain action of punkah, thermantidote, or tatty. In those countries of Western India where the hot winds blow steadily in one direction by day, where heated, if not hot, winds continue far into the night, and where comparatively little atmospheric moisture exists, the cot may safely be used in the compound, with some chance of refreshing sleep. It is not advisable, however, to sleep anywhere in the moonlight (*vide* p. 335).

*Long-continued heat* acts injuriously on the person of a native of a temperate climate, producing blood deterioration or *anæmia* in various ways through the nervous, circulatory, and respiratory systems, which is briefly explained below.

Even in a temperate climate a season of extraordinary heat causes languor, debility, and loss of appetite. This it does by a depressant effect on the nervous system. There is, therefore, as the starting-point of tropical heat blood deterioration, that approach to the condition which results from extraordinary heat in temperate latitudes. The greater portion of the waste of the body is passed off by the lungs, liver, skin, and kidneys; in the breath, bile, sensible and insensible perspiration, and urine. The atmospheric oxygen taken in by the lungs unites in the delicate tissues of those organs with the carbon of the blood, which it thus cleanses of noxious or effete matter, returning it to the external atmosphere in the shape of carbonic acid. In a temperate climate a full-grown man thus gives off with the breath about 8 ounces of carbon every twenty-four hours. But the atmosphere of the tropics is, from the heat, more rarefied than in a cold climate, the result being that a given bulk of air must contain less oxygen in the former climate than in the latter. And as, generally, comparatively less exercise is taken in the tropics (owing to the small amount of cool suitable time available, and to the lassitude induced by heat), it follows that the breathing is less accelerated by motion, resulting in a diminished bulk of air being inspired, and hence again a smaller amount of oxygen. As a necessary consequence of these two distinct manners in which the supply of oxygen is curtailed, the carbon breathed out from the lungs in the shape of carbonic acid is diminished in quantity. In other words, the higher the temperature and the less the exercise, the less carbon is exhaled from the lungs. Then, owing to the greater heat, and the consequent increase of evident perspiration and invisible evaporation from the skin, there is a smaller quantity of urine, so that there may not be sufficient water to hold in solution all the effete material which should be passed off by the urine. The skin, debilitated by excessive action, although pouring out more water, eliminates less solid matter. The lungs, kidneys, and skin thus acting imperfectly, some other organ must perform compensating work, or the blood must become charged with noxious carbonaceous material. Doubtless, if persons entering the tropics accommodated their living to the altered circumstances in which they are placed, such results might be to a great extent prevented. But often people coming to India continue to live as before, or even take more rich food, or, in consequence of thirst, or under a mistaken idea of 'supporting the system,' more fermented drink than they had been accustomed to consume in Europe. But the effete matter not required for the nourishment of the body must be removed from the system, and so the liver has an additional strain put on its capabilities. As a consequence the liver may become congested, or even more seriously diseased; or, failing to perform its functions, the bowels may be compelled to compensating action in the form of attacks of diarrhœa. Such vicarious work does not, however, long suffice; more or less effete carbonaceous material remains in the blood, and by such retention the blood becomes depraved and deteriorated, and is, in fact, in a semi-poisoned condition. The red globules of the blood decrease in number; the skin becomes pasty, pale, or sallow; the circulation is languid; the nights are restless, and there is a predisposition to a variety of ailments, as boils, skin, spleen, liver affections, or fever. In some constitutions there is also a disposition to the accumulation of fat in the heart and elsewhere; a condition physiologically explainable by the want of oxidation or destruction of material, which becomes converted into fat in the body instead of carbonic acid in the lungs. There is also loss of appetite, which, consequent on the diminution of the demand for carbonaceous or combustive material, is erroneously attributed to the debilitating influence of climate, and an attempt is made to neutralise this by artificial provocatives, which, while affording temporary relief, in reality pave the way to further deterioration. As a secondary result the *nervous system* becomes more implicated; the mental faculties are less vigorous, lassitude and fatigue are felt on the least exertion, and the daily avocations are performed with difficulty. Such a debilitated condition (or *anæmia, vide* p. 46) may occur in those predisposed by constitution, temperament, and habits within even a few months or years; or it may be deferred for a much longer period. It is true we occasionally see Europeans who have lived on the Indian plains for many years without loss of health or vigour. But these are exceptional instances, and only illustrate the inherent power against climate possessed by some constitutions. As a rule, the climate *per se* does, sooner or later, debilitate the European, rendering change to some cooler latitude imperatively necessary, and this debilitation will the sooner occur the less careful as regards diet and exercise the person may be. (For remarks on *Diet* and *Exercise*, *vide* pp. 683, 687.)

The insidious and debilitating effects of *continued heat* may be guarded against and delayed, *first*, by avoidance of exposure to *direct* heat—for the person who has suffered from sunstroke is the more liable to become affected by continued residence in a hot climate; *secondly*, by moderation in diet, especially as regards liquor; *thirdly*, by daily exercise short of fatigue; *fourthly*, by periodical change to Europe, or at least to some Indian hill station. A short periodical sojourn at some hill station, and a change to a European climate every six or seven years, would prevent many persons suffering from the effects of hot climates as here described. Those deferring such measures, after warnings of constitutional failure, frequently find a very long period necessary for the recovery of their strength. But the common error of expecting Indian hill climates to *cure* disease should not be entertained. As a rule, it is only those cases of ill-health when no specific disease exists which are benefited by change to the hills. But when lassitude, debility, loss of appetite, exhaustion after little exertion, and loss of energy and inclination for the daily avocation are the principal symptoms, the climate of the Indian hill ranges, particularly of the Himalayan stations, will generally prove most beneficial. Every mile the traveller advances from the plain into the hill ranges is eloquent of that change of climate which will soon effect a change of health. Vegetation, animal life, and even the appearance of human beings alter gradually but distinctly. As elevation is attained the air feels lighter, then crisp and exhilarating; the immediate relief experienced being a foretaste of that amelioration which soon takes place when the European is removed from the oppressing effects of a heated rarefied atmosphere affording a minimum proportion of oxygen, and in which he is frequently unable to take sufficient exercise. Also, innumerable impurities existing in the atmosphere of low levels are not found in the air of mountain regions. By such change the appetite and digestion are improved, the vital powers are stimulated, and the physical vigour is regained. Residence in the hills may, moreover, be regarded as exerting a sanitary effect not only on the body, but also on the mind; the freedom from the harass of daily work and the change of scene and society tending to raise and exhilarate the spirit, depressed by the continued influence of the climate of the heated plains. Much care, however, is necessary to guard against chill consequent on the lower temperature of the hills. The colder air checks the action of the skin, and the blood being driven within on internal organs, any weak part suffers from the strain. Although there is a comparative immunity from cholera, sunstroke, dysentery, and malarious fevers in the hills, there is usually a greater liability to bronchial affections, lung disease, rheumatism, and diarrhœa, while heart and kidney affections are usually made worse. Children are especially liable to throat or chest affections, or to diarrhœa; from which they may never have suffered on the plains. Warmer clothing should be put on *before* ascending a mountain, not *after* the ascent is made. However warm the hill climate may appear to persons fresh from the plains, the change of temperature involved, if made without care, is fraught with danger.

The hill stations may be divided sanitarily into *extra*-tropical and *intra*-tropical mountain climates, those in the Himalayehs belonging to the former class, the remainder to the latter. All hill climates, whether within or without the tropical line, are characterised by a summer season from ten to fifteen degrees cooler than that of the plains, by heavy monsoon rains accompanied by much mist and damp (rendering Mahableswar and Matheran, in the Bombay Presidency, uninhabitable during this period), by glorious autumnal weather, and in the *extra*-tropical stations by a winter season much colder than that of the plains, with usually heavy falls of snow about the month of January. On the *intra*-tropical ranges of hills the cold season is much less severe, and the changes of temperature are much less than on the Himalayehs, where the thermometer is influenced by cold winds from the snowy regions to the north. The Neilgherry Hills especially, from their altitude, their proximity to the equator, and their nearness to the sea, offer a cool climate, famed for evenness of temperature and consequent salubrity. The climate of most hill stations is, however, modified by neighbouring physical conditions, and the same mountains, or even the same station, may afford localities differing much in climatic respects. An account of the hill stations of India would therefore be a lengthy task.[1] All have excellences and defects; and many invalids have something special or peculiar in their ailments or constitution. The *intra*-tropical stations are preferable when there is tendency to chest affections or to incipient organic disease. When the ailment is simply debility from heat or from continued work, or convalescence from some malady which has merely left debility as a result, *any* hill climate, almost at any time, will prove beneficial.

Mal des Montagnes.—Some persons cannot ascend a mountain without suffering from troubled sleep, fatigue on slight exertion, muscular pains, quick pulse, hurried breathing, palpitations, giddiness, and perhaps nausea. It results from the oxygen of the blood being suddenly diminished *consequent* on a sudden move into a more rarefied atmosphere. Some individuals never become acclimatised to the mountain air. In others the effects are transient. An invalid known to suffer from *mal des montagnes* should not be taken to the hills.

**CHANGE TO EUROPE.**—Caution should be observed with regard to the more radical change to Europe, as a rapid journey to the British Isles is certainly not advisable for all Anglo-Indian invalids. In these days of quick transit, under the idea that the change home is all that is necessary, the tropical invalid too often rushes into the cooler climate of Europe or of the British Isles, the sudden change being in most instances as likely to do harm as good. The tropical invalid, especially if his malady is of long standing, or if he is organically diseased, cannot endure these sudden changes with impunity; and although it is often right that, as a last resource, they should be tried, they can only be attempted with a chance of success under the greatest care as regards regimen and protection from cold. It is doubly injurious for a person suffering from any predisposition to organic disease to return home in the winter. Invalids, especially with dysentery or 'liver,' should not reach England till after the vernal

[1] This has been attempted in the author's work entitled 'Health Resorts for Tropical Invalids; in India, at Home, and Abroad.'

equinox, for the gales at that time are often bitterly cold, and are apt to induce chill and consequent congestion of internal organs. Many would do better by sojourning for a period in Egypt, or Algiers, or at one of the Mediterranean or Continental 'health resorts,' most of which (like Indian hill stations) have excellences and defects peculiar to themselves. Such characteristics are fully set forth in books; [1] but a competent medical opinion is also desirable.

The subject of change of climate may be appropriately concluded by the hope that the time will come when all passenger ships will be better provided for the comfort and care of sick passengers. It is most painful to see a debilitated patient 'sent home,' as it is called, for the sufferings on board ship are manifold and continuous. Cabins with extra attendance, and good sick-cookery, would be a great boon to helpless invalids, especially when suffering from dysentery, diarrhœa, or lung disease. Such invalids ought to be in a cabin alone, not only for their own sake, but for that of others. To breathe constantly, in a confined and badly ventilated space, the same atmosphere as persons so affected is dangerous to the healthy, to whom disease may be propagated.

**MALARIA.**—*For an account of Malaria and its principal presumed characteristics, vide* AGUE, p. 252. Whether we regard malaria as a specific poison or entity, or as something yet undiscovered, or whether we deny its existence, there is no doubt that certain diseases do arise in certain localities, and that such diseases may be lessened, or even altogether prevented, by known agencies, the principal of which are indicated in the following remarks. In the uncertainty which exists whether or not there is such a poison as malaria, or whether or not that which is called malaria is really the operation of the various conditions

[1] The author's 'Health Resorts for Tropical Invalids.'

of climate and place by which we are surrounded, it is satisfactory to know that in using most of the precautions advised against malaria we are also protecting ourselves from such more recognisable evils as damp, cold, chill, bad air, and fatigue.

The measures to be taken to guard against the presumed effects of malaria—generally malarious fevers, or spleen disease, or malarious cachexia—are principally based on the avoidance of those localities in which residence or travelling is shown by experience to be most frequently followed by malarious maladies. But when necessitated to remain in, or pass through, malarious districts, the night air is to be as much as possible shunned. Wearing a silk handkerchief around the mouth and nose, or, better still, the charcoal respirator as sold, is a good plan when moving through very malarious districts. An efficacious form of respirator may be readily constructed by placing layers of charcoal, on cotton wool, between pieces of silk. Or keeping the mouth shut habitually and breathing through the nose, which, like a respirator, not only tends to prevent the entrance of malaria, but of all other atmospheric impurities, the convolutions or cells of the internal nostrils acting as a kind of filter, or entangling impurities which are afterwards expelled. Habitations or tents should never be placed to leeward of suspicious marshy surfaces. If obliged to sleep in unhealthy places, as malaria is supposed to be destroyed by fire, it will be well to keep large camp-fires burning. Also doors, windows, or tent *purdahs* should be closed, especially towards the malarious or damp locality, and particularly if wind comes from that direction. In some places safety from malarious fevers can only be secured in the autumnal season by closing all doors, the punkah or thermantidote being then necessary to procure sleep. Several writers state that mosquito curtains act as preservatives from disease. This, however, is not sufficient in the malarious districts of India. Unnecessary fatigue must be avoided. When either the body or mind is more than ordinarily fatigued, so-called malaria is more likely to produce bad effects. Similarly, depressing passions, as anger, grief, and prostration after intoxication, render the body more liable to malarious affections, as in fact to any other disease. The use of alcoholic liquors is not, however, to be entirely forbidden. When journeying by night through reputed malarious districts—which during the monsoon and after this season comprise nearly the whole of India—two or three table-spoonfuls of brandy not too much diluted will be beneficial. The stimulus thus afforded will give temporary support and lessen fatigue by preventing too rapid waste of tissue. The quantity is not sufficient to induce subsequent depression, while the advantage of local stomachic and slight general stimulation is obtained. It is worth mentioning that a stiff glass of brandy-and-water will sometimes cut short an incipient attack of ague. It must, however, be taken at the very commencement of the cold stage, otherwise it will be prejudicial.

Coffee is useful as a prophylactic against malaria, but is more adapted for general use during unhealthy seasons than for occasional consumption when passing through feverish districts. Coffee infusion is invigorating, and does not induce subsequent depression, the effect being confined to the first nervous stimulation. An infusion of unroasted coffee is a more powerful remedy against malarious influences than the roasted berry, and it may therefore be taken in malarious localities and seasons.

Tobacco-smoking in *moderation* may prove beneficial. Tobacco, like tea, coffee, and alcohol, restrains the waste of animal tissue, while it also exercises a tranquillising influence on those accustomed to its use. The wholesale denunciation of tobacco is neither in accordance with theory nor experience. But, as with alcohol, excess will, by the subsequent depression and nervousness so induced, predispose to those maladies against which moderate use may afford some preservative influence.

The diet of persons residing in malarious countries should be nourishing and liberal. Experience displays in a striking degree the prophylactic influence of a sound dietary against malaria. Where the inhabitants are poorly nourished, malarious disease, especially large spleen, abounds, and the manner in which natives of the country improve under better conditions of diet and living is a sanitary fact. Any scorbutic taint in the system, the result of food deficient in some requisite vegetable constituent, renders the individual more liable to malarious disease, and a due proportion of vegetable diet is therefore necessary. In malarious countries the stomach should be invariably fortified before going abroad in the morning by a cup of tea or coffee and a biscuit; and if a long journey is contemplated, a good meal is advisable. An early-morning meal has been supposed in some mysterious manner to prevent the noxious influence of malaria. But the benefit resulting is consequent on its rendering the system less liable to be affected by the chilly morning air, for the temperature of the body rises after food, although only in a small degree.

Quinine should be used as a prophylactic, once or twice a day, during the malarious seasons (*vide* p. 18); or a larger dose, as 6 grains, may be taken previous to passing through a malarious locality; or Recipe 76 may be obtained, which is a very efficacious pill for general camp use. If any constitutional idiosyncrasy, as referred to at pp. 7, 18, prevents quinine being used, the person should take 3 or 4 drops of the *Liquor arsenitis potassæ* instead: to be taken *after*, and not before, meals as advised for quinine (*vide* Recipe 75). Or Burroughs & Wellcome's arsenious acid tabloids, containing one-fiftieth of a grain of arsenic, may be similarly used.

Care should be taken not to drink water from wells in which leaves or other decaying matter have fallen. If necessitated to use such water, it should first be boiled and then filtered. It has been stated that water may hold malaria in solution, and that the poison may thus be introduced into the system.

It has been remarked that malaria is more powerful during the night than during sunlight. Whether this is correct or not, it is a fact that the human system is more likely to become impressed by any cause of disease during the relaxed condition of sleep than when awake and in action. It is also ascertained that individuals who have suffered from malarious fever may experience a relapse from exposure to cold. Hence the necessity of using, both by day and night, tolerably warm clothing, and especially flannel, than which no substance is better adapted to preserve the surface of the body from sudden changes of temperature, so often occurring in India, and especially during the night. It is asserted that malaria not only enters the system by the lungs and stomach, but may be also absorbed through the pores of the skin. When we recollect that every square inch of the skin contains upwards of 3,000 pores, and that thirst may be immediately relieved by immersion in water, which passes *into* the body through these pores, in the same manner as perspiration passes *out*, the theory that the skin may absorb malaria (if there is such an entity) seems plausible. As a protection against this danger, equally as against sudden vicissitudes of temperature, flannel is the best material, whether by day or by night.

Malaria is presumed to be heavier than atmospheric air. Examples are numerous where those living in lower stories suffered from fever, whilst residents in the same locality living in upper rooms retained their health. The damp and mist of night, or rather the descent of dew, has been presumed to retard the rise of malaria, and this mist is frequently only observable a few feet above the ground. Hence the desirability of sleeping in upper rooms in malarious seasons or localities, in order to escape the possible concentration of malaria near the surface of the ground, and the certain damper atmosphere.

Other *personal hygiene*, or *general sanitary* regulations tending to preserve from the effects of malaria, are:—Avoiding the cold bath when liability to febrile attacks is present, or when the body feels cold, and a warm glow does not occur after the bath. Avoiding unnecessary exposure to colds and chill. Attention to the disposal of bath-room water, which should not be allowed to sodden the ground in the neighbourhood of the house. Care not to live under rotting chuppers or thatch. Not to permit garden ground in the vicinity of the dwelling to become sodden by *over-irrigation*, as it then becomes a fertile source of damp, if not of malaria, although harmless when only sufficiently watered to assist the growth of vegetable life. Taking advantage of the power forest trees are said to possess in preventing the passage of malaria from one locality to another; and which should, therefore, be planted between inhabited places and adjacent swamps and marshes. For if trees do not protect from malaria, they modify and protect from cold damp winds. The *Eucalyptus globulus*, or Australian blue gum-tree, and the common sunflower, possess power in absorbing the malaria and damp of marshy places. Taking care that the locality is well drained. Periodical escape from the unhealthy Indian plains to one or other of the hill Sanitaria, where, from the absence of great heat, the constitution quickly becomes reinvigorated, and is thus better enabled to withstand what malaria may be present in the atmosphere of the mountains.

**CHILL** or **COLD** is in India a most fertile source of disease; fever and ague, or at least secondary attacks of fever, rheumatism, dysentery, diarrhœa, croup, and many other complaints arising from this cause. *A priori*, it would appear that taking cold in so hot a climate would be far from probable; but, in fact, the reverse is the case. *The heat renders the surface more impressionable* to falls of temperature, and it has already been shown (p. 657) how rapid and extended these may be. Of all the vicissitudes to which the climate of India is liable, none interfere more with health than the rapid changes of temperature, so that the Indian cold season has been spoken of as one of 'masked malignity,' especially to the old resident. There are old residents with a skin so debilitated by heat that they cannot stand five minutes in a draught without shivering or falling into a paroxysm of fever. Even those who attribute diseases to germs entering the system admit that a temporary depression caused by chill may give germs already in the system the necessary opportunity of developing themselves, when they would have been destroyed by inherent vital power had the chill not interfered. But chill is quite enough to excite disease without germs. The heat induces people incautiously to divest themselves of garments after exertion, and to sit in draughts for coolness, by which the blood is driven from the surface into the internal organs; whereas when in a state of perspiration, if the clothes cannot be changed, evaporation should be limited and chill prevented by putting on some other garments, and by avoiding draughts. In these or other ways persons constantly expose themselves to chill, with the almost inevitable results, a common cold, feverishness, or some worse disorder. A similar effect may be produced from the action of tatties, from the punkah, from the thermantidote, or from sudden breezes springing up and playing over the sleeping person. The advice given many years ago to the writer by an old Anglo-Indian, which may well be repeated, was never to lose sight of the blankets brought from Europe, which so many dispose of as no longer necessary; the fact being that protection from cold is even more necessary in India than in a cooler climate. It should be remembered that there is a considerable morning fall of temperature; that least animal heat is produced during sleep; and that the inherent power to withstand disease is then at a minimum. Hence the desirability of an extra covering being at hand, which may be drawn over the person in the early morning. It has certainly been questioned whether chill and cold in a tropical climate will excite *per se* an attack of ague; but experience has shown that it is quite sufficient to *re-excite* attacks of fever in the person who has once suffered from the disease. Whenever, as so often occurs in the autumnal and winter seasons, cold nights and hot days characterise the climate, then, without suitable protection by change of clothing, there will be danger of disease—fever, dysentery, or diarrhœa—and more especially so when the atmosphere is also damp. Chill is also a fertile cause of liver inflammation and abscess (*vide* p. 318). In short, exposure to cold, and especially to *damp* cold, is the most prolific source of disease in the tropics; meaning by cold, not a lowering of the temperature to the standard of temperate regions, but those sudden alterations from a very high to a lower standard so common, especially about the monsoon seasons, in India. The methods of protection from chill are so apparent that further remarks must be superfluous; while observations on the material for clothing will be found under that heading, p. 688. The brevity, however, with which this subject is treated must not be accepted as an index of its importance; for some authors have not hesitated to question the existence of malaria, attributing all so-called malarious diseases to chill alone. The author regards chill as 'The King of Causes of Disease.'

**WATER.**—Many diseases may be introduced into the system through the medium of water. Ague has been known to occur apparently from the use of impure water. Spleen disease may originate from similar cause. The introduction of the guinea-worm into the system is, probably, always by water. Dysentery and diarrhœa are excited by water containing either animal, vegetable, or mineral impurities. Dyspepsia will occur from a similarly impure fluid. Stone in the bladder, Derbyshire neck, or 'goitre' are other results of the continued use of bad drinking-water. Both cholera and typhoid may be propagated by contaminated water. Milk mixed with impure water has been the cause of outbreaks of disease. Intestinal worms may be propagated through the medium of water. The introduction of worms into the blood by the agency of mosquitoes and water is referred to at p. 612. When the filthy habits of many Indians as regards drinking-water are borne in mind, the European will find a *personal* supervision of his own supply the more incumbent. Drawn from a well generally uncovered, containing all kinds of impurities, and on the verge of which, or even in which, Natives wash themselves and their clothes; or taken from a tank in which men and women and animals drink, bathe, wash, wallow, and otherwise defile, the water next passes into the Bheestee's mussack, a receptacle made of untanned hide, kept when not in use in a dirty hovel, and probably never cleansed until rottenness from age and use renders its opening and repair positively necessary. Such water, if the European did not vigorously protest, would be daily given him to drink. Even vigorous protests would only result, as a rule, in the addition of another odour or taste to the fluid, by straining through a dirty cloth. Even should the water brought be seemingly unexceptionably pure and tasteless, it may still contain atoms deleterious to health. That the invisible germs of cholera, the ova of guinea-worm, or the spores of other maladies may exist in water will not create surprise when it is recollected that a single drop of water may contain five hundred millions of living infusoria, a number approaching that of the whole human species existing on the face of the earth. Hence the necessity of insisting by frequent personal supervision on drinking-water being boiled, then allowed to cool, and afterwards filtered. Boiling will not only destroy most organic impurities, but will also cause the deposit of inorganic salts or material held in solution. Neither does the double process destroy the taste and pungency of the water, which is restored during the time it is filtering by the reabsorption of air by the fluid. But all filters become in time foul and dirty, and, if not periodically cleansed, may be a breeding-ground for the germs they are designed to prevent.

Filters may be constructed in the form of three common 'gurrahs' placed one above the other, on a tripod stand, the two upper ones filled with layers of sand and charcoal, the lower one empty to receive the water straining through small holes in the bottoms of the others. If this kind of filter is used, an inverted cover with a small aperture drilled in it should be placed on each 'gurrah' to prevent the entrance of dust or mosquitos, and interference from birds, squirrels, &c. Or, what is preferable, a magnetic filter may be purchased, either sufficiently small and portable for camp use, or large enough to filter any amount of water. For travelling, the porous stone bottle is a good filter. Placed in a 'gurrah' of water, the fluid quickly finds its way into the interior of the filter, and drinkable water is obtained. A small portable syphon carbon filter may be useful on journeys. The home-made 'gurrah filter' of sand and charcoal will require changing at least *monthly*; others according to size and capability, which may be approximately ascertained when purchased. But much obviously must depend on the impurity of the water.

*How to purify a filter.*—Every two or three months (according to the kind of water) air should be blown through, and if the charcoal is in the block form it should be well brushed. Then six or eight ounces of Condy's fluid should be poured through; and an hour afterwards four gallons of distilled water (or, if not procurable, of the purest boiled and filtered water obtainable) in which an ounce of pure hydrochloric acid has been mixed. Then more pure water. Sponges should be washed in hot water every few days.

Condy's fluid is useful for purifying water when other means are not practicable. Eight drops, added to a gallon of water, will purify it, and render it more fit for household purposes. Condy's fluid is of a purple colour. When added to impure water the colour becomes brown, which forms a means of roughly testing the purity of water.

It is not always that there is any choice of water supply. If so, tank water should be avoided, as such places are liable to innumerable contaminations, especially if in the neighbourhood of villages. Surface and marsh water must always be rejected. Water from a well constantly being drawn is often the most satisfactory. But probably water from a swift-flowing river is best, as the motion of the stream and the exposure to the air tend to maintain the water good, notwithstanding the numerous impurities which find their way into rivers. Among the sanitary improvements of recent years is the introduction into many towns (especially in the Western Presidency, where the physical features of the country are favourable) of water supply from distant hills, rendering the inhabitants and travellers independent of the old sources of wells, tanks, or streams—a sanitary measure which more than any other tends to the preservation of the public health.

As a result of the heat of the climate, and of the consequent constant evaporation from the skin, Europeans are more thirsty, and require more to drink, than in their own country. But the practice of drinking largely, even of water, is not commendable. Thirst should be striven against, otherwise a habit of drinking deep draughts is contracted, which weakens the digestion and debilitates the skin, by the increased perspiration following excessive drinking. To allay thirst, there is no better beverage than cold, but not ice-cold, water. The evil effect of swallowing cold water when the body is heated (which often causes skin eruptions) is popularly recognised, but it is not understood that whatever harm a large quantity of cold water may do a smaller quantity of iced water may effect. If ice is placed on the back of the hand for a short time, the skin becomes pale, then reddened and hot. That which can be seen on the skin happens in the stomach, and hence taking ice-cold drinks congests the coats of the stomach and favours dyspepsia. With this condition, thirst returns in a double degree, and the relief gained by successive draughts is too dearly purchased. Neither should the injury to the teeth be ignored.

Many persons are under the impression that by drinking aerated water they will escape the ills so often the consequence of impure water. This, unfortunately, is not the case; for soda-water manufacturers in India are sometimes not particular what kind of water they use. It may contain lead, or oil from the machine; and if filtered, which is often neglected, the water aerated is seldom, if ever, boiled. Greater safety will be secured by supervision of the drinking-water than by the use of the so-called soda-water of the shops. Similarly, when it is mentioned that there are infusoria which retain vitality in boiling water, enough will have been said to dispel the popular delusion that the addition of liquors to bad water will render it less injurious.

**SLEEP.**—Not to sleep in comfort in India is to prepare the system for disease. Yet there are many hindrances to the European obtaining that refreshing slumber which is so desirable. During certain months, when the nights of the monsoon season are moist and 'muggy,' the European, after a restless night, arises tired, languid, and unrefreshed. In the fierce hot weather of Upper India, heated winds blowing almost to dawn, often accompanied by dust and sand, produce similar restlessness, and thirst. Then there are mosquitoes, which, although apparently insignificant, are capable of preventing, or at least disturbing, the slumbers of most Europeans. There are also the various noises which so frequently render the Indian night hideous. In addition, dinner taken late tends to produce restless nights. One or two nights of disturbed sleep would not much signify to the average robust European; but when the causes are in operation for months, the frame becomes debilitated, and is therefore placed in a condition favourable to disease. And, as before stated, malaria or chill is most powerful during the hours of darkness, or when the individual is most debilitated and distressed by vainly tossing throughout the night on a sleepless couch.

The measures to be adopted to secure comfortable sleep in India resolve themselves into protection from the causes of restlessness mentioned above. Protection from heat is to be obtained by sufficient ventilation of sleeping-rooms, by the judicious use of the punkah, or other artificial means of cooling the atmosphere (*vide* p. 663). By sleeping in upper rooms when practicable, where, at some elevation from the ground, air is often in motion, while all below is stagnant. By sleeping in some localities and seasons in the open air (*vide* p. 664). Protection from mosquitoes may be secured either by the mosquito curtains, or by the punkah, or to some extent by an elevated and breezy position. Protection from malaria has already been considered (*vide* p. 671). Protection from thirst is to be attained by avoiding improper diet and late dining, by keeping the mouth shut, and by putting a chlorate of potash tabloid in the mouth when retiring. It is much better to sleep on a hair mattress, or on a wire bed, or on a 'charpai' than on anything softer. It is also desirable that, especially for children, the head of the bed should point to the north; for there are electrical currents constantly passing from north to south, with which our nervous systems are in some mysterious manner connected, and which it is not well for the body to oppose. Sleeping in the day should be avoided, especially after a meal, as it tends to induce liver disease.

**DIET.**—Vegetable food is, generally speaking, better adapted to a tropical climate than animal food; not that it is quicker or easier of digestion, for it is slower, but because it is not so apt to cause plethora. Such considerations should induce the European, especially when newly arrived, to partake sparingly of animal food, which is not required to the same extent as in a temperate climate. It has been explained (p. 665) that carbonaceous material (of which meat, milk, eggs, fatty substances, contain a large proportion), taken into the system, is removed chiefly by the liver or the lungs, and that in a hot climate the lungs are less, and the liver more, instrumental in this process. Hence (as one means of avoiding disease of the latter organ) the necessity of caution as regards quantity of food taken. But following the example of some classes of the Natives, and abstaining from meat diet altogether, is not desirable. The custom of ages has habituated the Hindoo to taking large quantities of rice with pulses or corn; but a European would not digest this diet. Its bulk alone would prevent perfect digestion, even if aided by the large amount of condiments taken by the Native; which, in the unaccustomed stomach of the European, would also induce indigestion.

It can scarcely be necessary to lay down rules of diet, but some cautions may be added. Of all things, the most necessary is neither to eat too much, nor from too many dishes. The more simple the food, the better and longer will the stomach prove a good servant, rather than, as occurs when dyspepsia becomes confirmed, an irritable master. Avoid also eating too quickly, and masticate the food thoroughly, applying to the dentist for aid if the state of the teeth does not permit the grinding of the food. Also let all food taken be, although simple, of the best quality obtainable. The last remark especially applies to milk, in which the germs of various diseases may be conveyed, usually through the admixture of foul water with the milk. As regards the use of tinned foods, any which appear, when opened, wet, pappy, or emit a faint or putrid odour, or gas, should not be eaten.

Injury sometimes results from old 'tinned' provisions becoming impregnated from the 'sauder' (which contains lead) used to seal the cases. For symptoms of lead-poisoning, *vide* pp. 134, 344). It is advisable for all preserved provisions for tropical climates to be packed in glass capsules.

*The protection of food from the myriads of flies* abounding in India is urgently necessary; for no one can tell on what filth a fly may have previously settled, or what germ of disease it may not convey.

*Attention should also be given to the meat*, by which several maladies, and especially tape-worm, may be conveyed into the system.

As Indian butchers are not particular as to the meat they sell, it is well to know the characteristics of good meat. It should present a somewhat marbled appearance, from intermixture of streaks of fat with the muscle, a sign that the animal has been well fed. The colour of the flesh should neither be very pale nor very dark. If pale and moist, it indicates the animal was young or diseased; if dark and livid, it shows that the animal, in all probability, was not slaughtered, but died with the blood in it. Both lean and fat should be firm to the touch, not moist or sodden, nor showing white jelly-like spots, and the fat should be free from bleeding or dark spots. Fluid or juice exuding from the meat should be small in quantity, of a reddish tinge, and should be slightly acid, if tested with test-paper made for the purpose. The little bundles or fibres into which the meat is divided should not be large and coarse. The odour should be slight and not disagreeable even if chopped in small pieces and washed with water, which brings out the odour; or if a knife is thrust into the meat and smelled.

Bad meat is usually sodden and flabby, with the fat dirty or yellow-looking and the smell unpleasant or sickly.

The importance of looking to the condition of the cooking pots and pans used in India must not be forgotten.

The utensils used are copper, and, when properly lined with tin, are harmless. But the tin wears off, and exposing the copper may lead to copper-poisoning, the symptoms of which are usually pain in the bowels and diarrhœa, and, if much copper is taken into the system, also vomiting. If the cooking-pots are not properly *clean*, as well as not properly tinned, the chance of copper-poisoning will be increased, in consequence of the formation of *verdigris*, by the action of the acids and fats in the food remaining in contact with the metal. Cooking-pots used every day should be tinned at least every month, and examined periodically in order that it may be ascertained if the tinning is required more frequently. After tinning bran should be boiled in them before they are used for food. But these are not even sufficient precautions. Lead is cheaper than tin in the Indian bazaars, and the tin-workers will sometimes employ an alloy of tin and lead instead of the former metal. The symptoms of lead colic, or poisoning, and paralysis, are noted at pp. 134, 344. Either copper or lead, or both, may be taken into the system with the food daily, in very minute quantities, for an indefinite period. The characteristic symptoms of poisoning by either metal may not present in the unmistakable manner which results from large doses; but many cases of anomalous illness are either altogether due to, or are aggravated by, these often unsuspected causes.

**LIQUOR.**—It would be well if all, for at least some months after entering the tropics, would refrain from anything more powerful than a little claret and water, and perhaps a glass of sherry daily. Spirits should be shunned as poisons. Beer of good light quality is less deleterious, but is not necessary. As a rule, no beer, wine, or liquor should be taken excepting at meals. In the hot weather it is desirable that none should be taken till after sundown. It should be fully understood that in

India fermented liquors of any kind should only be taken for their tonic, *not* for their stimulating, effects. Physiological science and experience alike teach us that the condition of system most favourable to the development of zymotic poisons is set up by the presence in the blood of organic matter in a state of change, decomposition, or fermentation. Hence the blood of the intemperate charged with alcohol is in the condition *par excellence* favourable to attacks of such maladies as fever, cholera, and sunstroke. The liver also is liable to become affected from indulgence in spirituous liquors. Neither does the heart escape. One ounce of alcohol raises the pulse three beats per minute, or, in other words, causes the heart to beat, while its effect lasts, at the rate of 4,300 beats more than natural in the twenty-four hours. The heart cannot be made to do this extra work without suffering. The bad effects of the same agency on the brain might be portrayed with even greater force. But the loss of memory, the impaired intellect, the miserable thoughts, the imbecility, the loss of physical energy, so frequently resulting from *chronic alcoholism*, need not be dwelt upon here (*vide* p. 163).

Although so strongly condemning the practice of constantly using alcoholic beverages, the opposite extreme of teetotalism is not recommended. As a rule, Europeans in tropical climates require some amount of fermented drink as part of their daily *sustenance*. This is particularly the case with the old resident, and during the hot season when the heat destroys the appetite, and exerts its depressing and deteriorating influence on the system. When the quantity of solid food is not sufficient to supply the waste of tissue, and to counteract the 'wear and tear' of body—which it often is not during the exhaustion and loss of appetite caused by intense heat—an additional supply of wine may be taken with advantage. But this can only be safely used *for its tonic effects*, and *not for the temporary stimulation* it affords. It is the use, and not the abuse, of fermented liquors which is so much required. Moderation, instead of excess, is the great desideratum. But what moderation may be it is difficult to decide, so much depending on age, sex, temperament, habits, and occupation.

From experiment it appears that the body of a strong healthy man is capable of *appropriating* in a temperate climate 2 ounces of alcohol daily, as a *maximum.* If more than 2 ounces is taken, it may be chemically detected in the urine and breath. In a tropical climate, the power of appropriating alcohol is lessened. Approximately, 2 ounces of average brandy contain upwards of 1 ounce of alcohol; of sherry about 8 ounces, of champagne 14 ounces, of claret 16 ounces, of bottled beer 18 ounces, contain 1 ounce of alcohol. It will therefore be understood that the limit of appropriation of alcohol by the system may be reached by very moderate indulgence in wine or spirits. And there is every reason to believe that the limit of *benefit* to the system from alcohol is arrived at long before the limit of *appropriation.* But liquor, wine, and beer are made from many things, and many drinks sold in the Indian bazaars contain specially deleterious principles.

**EXERCISE.**—A due amount of exercise in India is even more necessary to health than in England. As a rule, the most healthy people are those who take exercise regularly. The circulation of the blood is thus equalised, and the tendency to congestions, particularly of the liver, is often checked; the bowels are excited to healthy action, and effete material no longer required in the system is thereby expelled; while more air being inspired as a result of quickened respiration, more oxygen is introduced into the system, and more carbon expelled (*vide* p. 665). There is, however, a very general feeling of languor, the effect of heat, which prevents many people taking that amount of exercise which is desirable. Walking, riding, shooting, badminton, are the best exercises—cricket, boating, tennis, rackets, involving for many too great a strain on the circulatory and muscular systems. Bicycle and tricycle riding on most machines tends to round the shoulders and contract the chest. Healthy as such exercise otherwise is for the young and strong, with unimpaired condition of circulatory organs, it becomes a dangerously severe exertion for persons who, advanced in life, have any heart or arterial imperfection; especially if they mount after a meal.

Whatever exercise is taken, it should not be sufficient to induce exhaustion. Fatigue carried beyond a moderate stage subjects the blood to a decomposing process through the infiltration into it of substances which act as poisons. Many persons feel fatigued during the day after exercise in the early morning, and this may be accepted as a sign that it does not agree with them. Weak and delicate persons should avoid exercise before breakfast, especially if they are employed during the day. Extremes of exercise should be avoided during seasons of epidemic, as fatigue tends to predispose the system to epidemic diseases. Children should not be wakened to be sent out. They should go to bed early, and will then wake early. And they should have a little milk and bread before going out.

**CLOTHING.**—The quality of dress in India depends on the season and the part of India in which the wearer is located, and on the duties to be performed. Clothes do not keep us warm by excluding air from our bodies, unless they are impermeable, as india-rubber textures. The textures most permeable to air keep our temperature most equable, air being a bad conductor of heat. Wool, being very permeable to air, is a non-conductor of heat, while linen and cotton are rapid conductors. An object covered with wool is less susceptible to changes of temperature than one covered with linen or cotton, which is the reason why ice is kept under blankets. Wet clothes in which the air is replaced by water keep us less warm than dry clothes, because water is a better conductor of heat than air. Hence the ease with which we get chilled in wet clothes. Evaporation also takes place more rapidly from cotton than wool, because wool does not absorb moisture so readily as cotton. If a piece of flannel is stretched over a glass of water so that it just touches the surface of the fluid, scarcely any moisture will be taken up by the flannel. Linen or calico so placed will quickly become saturated. This is another reason why chills more quickly occur with linen or cotton than flannel clothing. Perspiration penetrates at once to the external surface of the linen, and is acted upon by the atmosphere. With a woollen garment perspiration is more retained by the texture, and absorbed more gradually, and thus not so quickly evaporated from the surface. When the body is heated, a profuse perspiration wets the clothing, evaporation follows, causing chill, checking the perspiration, and so originating numberless cases of illness; and this is much less likely to occur when wool is used. Even when there is no perspiration visible, insensible perspiration is always occurring, and this passes through wool, in the form of vapour, to a much greater extent than through vegetable textures, which retain it on or near the surface. Wool is really cooler than vegetable fabrics, for heat is most felt when the skin cannot exhale freely through the clothing. The exhalations from the skin are the means provided by nature for cooling the body and maintaining an equable temperature; and wool is most pervious to such exhalations. Another advantage attributed to wool is the fact of its being a non-conductor of electricity. A woollen garment has the merit also of affording more protection to the back (the necessity of which has been already dwelt upon at p. 661) than either linen, silk, or cotton, which, although *looking cool*, afford no protection in this respect. Persons who say they cannot wear flannel next the skin may do so at first over very thin silk; but if the thin, flexible woollen clothing now manufactured is procured it will not irritate the most sensitive skin. It may be here remarked that there is no other special advantage to be derived from various advertised wool clothings which is not obtainable from good Welsh flannel. It would be well if all clothing were woollen, but underclothing is of more importance as regards health than external clothing, and this should consist of flannel next to the skin. It is one of the best safeguards against fever, dysentery, and various disorders, and it should be remembered that it is as useful to women as to men. But the resident in the south will not at any period of the year require the warm woollen clothing necessary for those residing during the cold season in the northern provinces, when the skin, irritable from prolonged heat, has to encounter the dry and piercing cold of the winters. Neither will the man devoted to office-work want the strong durable material desirable for the classes employed in outdoor occupation. Generally, light tweeds are the most useful external wear in India; but every person should possess warmer clothing, which may be required at any time. During the rains, especially with children, much care is required. Flannel clothing should be insisted upon, and jacket and trousers should be made in one, so that the dress cannot be kicked off. Lastly, clothing should be changed after exercise, and not allowed to dry on the body; or, if it cannot be changed, some other garment should be put over it to limit evaporation and so prevent chill.

**BATHING.**—The daily bath is an essential requisite in Indian life, and when the excessive action of the skin is recollected, and that in every square inch of skin there are some 3,000 perspiratory pores, the necessity of attention to this organ becomes sufficiently apparent. But besides these little tubes there are large numbers of small glands, secreting an oily substance, which is conveyed through other minute orifices to the surface of the skin, which it thus insensibly lubricates, while freeing the body of material no longer required in the system. It is therefore not only external impurity but also internal waste which finds its way to the surface, to the extent of about 10 grains per hour, which has to be removed. If this oily secretion and the perspiration are left undisturbed, the pores become blocked up, a safety-valve of health is closed, and some malady is almost certain to ensue. In India, moreover, there is at all times a greater action of the skin than in temperate climates, and if more attention is not paid to this organ the health will very soon suffer. The bath is, therefore, an essential part of the ordinary daily routine, if only as a matter of cleanliness. But it also may be regarded as a general tonic, imparting or maintaining vigour and energy, and fortifying the system against the influences of climate. Whether cold, tepid, or warm water is used, must be decided by the effect produced. There are many persons who after a cold bath feel a pleasurable glow over the whole surface. To these the cold bath cannot fail to be beneficial. On the other hand, there are numerous individuals who after a cold bath feel depressed, languid, and as if shrivelled, and whose cutaneous surface does not answer the shock of the cold water by any reaction. If this occurs, or if the fingers become at all cold or white after bathing, cold water must be abandoned, and tepid or even warm water substituted. Women who have miscarried should avoid too cold baths; neither are they advisable immediately before or during the monthly period. Some persons will bear a cold bath in the warm weather but not in the cold season. The extreme of too hot water must be guarded against; otherwise gradually the habit of bathing in very hot water will be contracted, to the enfeeblement of the skin and weakening of the system. A child's bathing water should be not cold enough to drive the blood from the surface, and not warm enough to induce the child to stay in the water. Bathing in 'chunamed' baths is not recommended, as the water there is often very cold, and the shock may be too great. Many persons have with truth dated the origin of fever or 'liver' to an imprudent plunge. Where there is a large lake or river, free from crocodiles, leeches, or other dangerous living things, bathing may be safely indulged in, with necessary precautions against the sun. When thus bathing, the body should be a little warm, not chilly, and the plunge should be made at once. The best time for bathing is a couple of hours after a meal. Bathing should be avoided when suffering from fatigue; and on leaving the bath, although the person may feel invigorated, too violent exercise should not be taken. Sea-bathing is not often practicable in India, but in many cases of debility sea-water may be beneficially used. For temperature of baths, *vide Appendix, Baths.*

**HOUSES.**—Europeans in India seldom have much choice of a house, the number in up-country stations being generally exceeded by the number of residents. And the majority of these Indian bungalows are not what is requisite for health or comfort. Although affording sufficient space, they are frequently not at all raised from the surface of the ground. Sometimes there is only an earthen flooring. They are mostly constructed of porous material, as inferior or sunburnt bricks and mud, and they are in many localities covered with an old, sometimes rotting, 'chupper,' or thatch. As a consequence, during the monsoon—especially in those parts of the country where the rains are heavy and the atmosphere saturated with moisture—damp rises from below, and damp permeates into and percolates through the walls, while not unfrequently the vitiated atmosphere caused by a mouldy, rotting thatch is recognised by the sense of smell. Most Indian bungalows in up-country stations have been originally built hurriedly, and as cheaply as possible. The majority of occupants being but temporary sojourners, few have cared to expend money on dwelling-houses. Many of the best houses have attained their dimensions by periodical additions to small temporary erections.

It is impossible to frame rules for the construction of a dwelling-house adapted for Europeans and suitable for every part of India, as the material available and the climate differ in various parts of the country. *Speaking generally*, a dwelling-house in India should be elevated four or five feet from the earth, by which greater freedom from damp and greater coolness are secured, and the entrance of snakes or other noxious living things is rendered more unlikely. The walls should be of masonry, as thin as compatible with strength. The idea that very thick walls prevent heat is a mistaken one, as massive walls, thoroughly heated by the sun's rays, do not cool during the night. The best material for floors is smoothly hewn stone of a non-porous description, Venetian tiles, or wood where there are no white ants. 'Chunam' is liable to break, to require constant repairs, and unless thickly covered it feels cold, while thick coverings harbour dirt and insects. But almost anything is preferable to the ordinary beaten earth floor, from which not only damp but bad air rises; for the atmosphore does not end where the earth begins, but permeates it in all directions. For the roof there is nothing better than well-fitting tiles, which should be large and heavy enough to prevent crows displacing them. Instead of lath and plaster ceilings, 'chuts,' made of whitewashed cotton cloth, are commonly used. To this there is no objection, provided the chuts are well secured, so as to prevent ingress into the space between the roof and ceiling of sparrows, bats, or pigeons. Similar care must be taken that all apertures between the wall and overhanging roof are well stopped; otherwise birds, squirrels, rats, bandecoots, and cats will find their way into the interior. Such intruders dying in the roof give rise to much trouble and to disagreeable effluvia; while the noise they make, especially at night, is anything but pleasant or conducive to repose. As a rule, Indian houses should possess chimneys and fireplaces. Such apertures tend to the ventilation of the apartment, and fires may be advisable on account of damp, while in the northerly districts fires are always acceptable, if not actually necessary, during the cold weather. Verandahs cannot be dispensed with, and their breadth can scarcely be too great. Doors and windows should be furnished with chicks opening in frames—serviceable alike for keeping out glare and insects. A sufficiency of light is a desideratum not always secured. For if the original construction admits sufficient, it is often shut out, under the idea of promoting coolness. The great importance of solar light is referred to under *Anæmia* and *Scurvy* (pp. 47, 381), both being diseases to which deficiency of light predisposes. Lastly, the colouring of the inner walls should be a neutral tint, instead of the glaring whitewash so often seen.

As regards *site*, the first thing to look for is natural drainage, and therefore a slight elevation of the ground will be the preferable locality. But the surface of some districts is so flat that this desideratum cannot be secured—so level, that good drainage is not even possible—and where this is the case elevation of the dwelling-house is the more requisite. The windward position to any marsh, pond, or native village, a gravelly soil, a dry substratum of soil, the absence of rocks or hills, which would radiate heat on the house, the facility of procuring water for garden purposes, the proximity of trees, not overhanging the house, but affording shade in the immediate neighbourhood, are all desiderata which should be if possible secured.

*The position* of the house is to be determined as far as possible by the direction of the prevailing wind and the diurnal sun-line. But as these do not generally correspond, that position should be taken which will secure the greatest amount of perflation by the prevailing breeze, through the front and back, and the minimum of sunshine passing directly into the house, in similar directions.

*Space.*—The space in European barracks found necessary for the soldier is 90 superficial feet and 1,800 cubic feet per man in the dormitories, and private houses should not give less. In European hospitals 120 superficial feet and 2,400 cubic feet are allowed, showing the greater necessity of fresh air and ventilation in the sick-chamber. But no artificial ventilation and no amount of cubic space will obviate the necessity of natural ventilation, and this is only obtained by open doors and windows. In the hot season, it is necessary to close the doors and windows during the day, to prevent the entrance of hot air; but on the approach of sunset doors and windows should be thrown open for the free admission of air throughout the whole dwelling.

The impurities found in air are mentioned at p. 732. At present, we are only considering the gaseous and organic emanations from the lungs and skin of persons resident in a house, and particularly of the occupants of a sleeping-room. The principal object of breathing is to maintain the blood in a state of purity, and to render it capable of affording to all parts of the body the materials necessary to maintain nutrition and vitality. When an adult is in a state of rest every breath conveys about 1 pint of air into the lungs, or 18 pints every minute, or 57 hogsheads in 24 hours. By the process of the circulation 8 pints of blood every minute, or 24 hogsheads every 24 hours, meet the air in the delicate tissues of the lungs, where the blood parts with the carbon or effete material it has received from the tissues, and takes the oxygen it receives from the air. The air when it leaves the lungs is composed principally of carbonic acid, which is a poisonous gas, and will neither support life, nor even the flame of a candle. But other matters besides carbonic acid are constantly thrown off by the lungs, and by the skin, viz., watery vapour, and microscopical atoms of organic matter. When the air of an inhabited room is thus vitiated to the extent of ·7 per 1,000 cubic feet of air, the vitiation becomes perceptible to the sense of smell. Persons sleeping under such circumstances wake in the morning unrefreshed and suffering from headache. They lose their appetites, become enfeebled, and more liable to various disorders. If the contamination of the air is still greater, some form of fever, probably typhus, will be excited. If the air is excessively charged with the products of respiration, and with emanations from the skin, those breathing it must die, as occurred in the Black Hole of Calcutta when, in 1756, out of 146 prisoners confined, 123 expired in one night. It may be stated as an axiom that the most ordinarily impure external air is less deleterious than that arising from overcrowding, or want of ventilation in dwellings, and especially in sleeping-apartments.

**CONSERVANCY.**—Persons cannot be too particular regarding conservancy. Otherwise, the sweeper will remove bath-room refuse and deposit it in any corner. Hence it may become the cause of disease, probably of *enteric* fever (*vide* p. 240). All bath-room refuse should be first disinfected by dry earth (*vide* p. 736) and then taken away and buried. It should also be recollected that Indian cattle and sheep will greedily devour human ordure, especially in the hot season, when grass is scanty. In this manner the germs of certain maladies—tapeworm, for instance—may be conveyed, with flesh food, into the human system (*vide* p. 483).

**CONDUCT OF THE PASSIONS.**—There is a proverb,

borrowed from the Persians, that 'the proper devil of mankind is man,' and it is a fact that the state of health of Europeans in India depends much on the control exerted over the enemy within. Moderation in all matters, whether in eating or drinking, business or pleasure, is one golden rule; another, equally important, being the endeavour to avoid those fits of irritability to which the European, fretful from heat of climate, and often annoyed by the not understood, dilatory, or otherwise objectionable conduct of the Natives, is apt to give way. It is a fact that ague at least not unfrequently follows, in persons predisposed to the affection, fits of passion, or other mental excitement. The *mens sana* is even more than ordinarily desirable in India, as a security for the *corpus sanum.*

**MANNER OF LIFE DURING EPIDEMICS.**—When epidemic disease, as cholera, for instance, occurs, it will be best not to make any decided change in the manner of life. Caution as regards diet, exposure, fatigue, and local sanitation will be advisable, but any sudden change of habit which may tend to unsettle the system should be avoided. Neither should spasmodic sanitary measures be attempted at such times, as the disturbance of masses of filth during an epidemic season may be followed by increase of disease. Fear of disease should be guarded against, if not altogether dispelled, by the recollection that even during the worst epidemics immunity is the rule, and not attack.

# CHAPTER VII

## *THE MANAGEMENT OF THE SICK-ROOM*

APPEARANCE OF THE SICK-ROOM.—The whitewashed walls of an Indian bungalow are not conducive to the repose demanded by a patient. The best colour for the sick room is a uniform neutral tint, such as light green, buff, or slate colour. The windows should be so arranged as to admit, except in some diseases of the eye and brain, abundance of light, or at least as much as is agreeable to the patient. Light is a stimulus to the body, and the mistake is often made of shutting out the light too much. The windows should not be surrounded by woollen curtains, a plain green blind, or 'chick' tempering the light sufficiently, and, if necessary, cutting off outside objects from the patient's view. All hangings and curtains, particularly woollen textures, should be avoided, as they may become harbourers of the germs of disease. For the same reason carpets should as much as possible be dispensed with, although it is advisable to have something to deaden the noise where the most traffic occurs. Each morning carpets or mats should be quietly taken out, and be thoroughly shaken and aired. The floor should be wiped with a damp cloth. If a chunam floor is broken up, it will absorb not only fluid and moisture, but probably also disease germs. Therefore any holes in the chunam floor of a sick-chamber should be repaired immediately. A wooden floor, if not polished, requires even greater care and cleanliness than the chunam floor. The porous brick flooring and the 'rammed earth' floor sometimes found in bungalows are in every way objectionable. *Leeping* or smearing an earthen floor with wet cow-dung, of which the Natives are so fond, is, from concealing dirt and the attendant damp, less desirable than simply sweeping. If a patient with a contagious disorder must be treated on an earthen floor, it will be advisable to slightly scrape the floor every day. In cholera, fresh dry earth should be placed around the bed. The less furniture in the sick-room, the more air there will be for the patient, and therefore furniture not required for use had better be removed. Cushions and covers should also be dispensed with. Beds having iron frames are less liable to harbour either the germs of disease or insects. The bed-head should if practicable point to the north, for the reasons given at p. 683. But it should not face a window so as to expose the patient's face to the light; it should not be side on to a wall; at least ten inches should intervene between the bed-head and a wall; and it should not be in any position, as between windows and doors or fireplaces, exposing the patient to a draught. The room should be made bright and cheerful by flowers, pictures, books, or other things pleasant to the patient. Such objects should not, however, be intruded on his attention, and if they create disgust, or excitement, or feverishness, they should be quietly removed.

Aspect of the Sick-Room.—When practicable, it will be most frequently advisable to take the coolest room. Unless in the cold weather of Northern India, when cold north-east winds often prevail, the room which admits the greatest amount of perflation by the prevailing breeze, and the minimum of sunshine passing directly on it, will be the apartment best suited for an invalid.

Cleanliness of the Sick-Room.—This can never be thorough when carpets are nailed down so that they cannot be removed to be shaken and aired. In fevers the bed-linen *under* the patient should be changed at least once a day. The upper sheet, if not soiled, may be used next day after airing as the under one. The pillow cases should also be changed daily. Patients suffering from contagious diseases should have the whole of their bedding changed every day (*vide* p. 703). Bath-rooms, closets, or cupboards should not be made the repository of unnecessary articles, and used clothing or bed-linen should never be put in such places. These things should be immediately disinfected (*vide Appendix*, No. 122).

CONSERVANCY OF THE SICK-ROOM.—Unless required for inspection, the dejections should be received in a utensil charged with some disinfecting agent and buried (*vide Appendix*. No. 126). When the dejections are preserved for inspection, they should be put in an outhouse, and not in a room or bath-room adjoining the sick-chamber. Great care should be taken that urine does not come into contact with the chunam floor of the bath-room usually found in Indian bungalows. The absorption of fluid by a broken chunam floor has been referred to (p. 697); but there is an additional reason why urine should not be permitted to come in contact with chunam. If this occurs chemical action takes place, and ammoniacal odours are emitted. This will happen even when the chunam floor is not broken up, but much more quickly and powerfully when holes exist.

DEODORISATION AND DISINFECTION OF THE SICK-ROOM. *Vide Appendix*, Nos. 118 to 125.

DIETETICS OF THE SICK-ROOM.—Although we now know better than to starve persons because they are sick, yet the sick cannot take the same food as the healthy. When a person has fever (the majority of diseases being thus accompanied), the appetite for solid food is gone, and therefore all nourishment must be given in a liquid form. Milk is an article which all may take in almost any illness; and in some cases of bowel complaint, milk diet alone is often taken with benefit (*vide* pp. 194, 244). If good fresh milk cannot be obtained, preserved milk may be tried. Cold milk is sometimes more agreeable than warm. It may require the addition of limewater when there is acidity of the stomach or gastric disease present, and it may be necessary to give the milk in small quantities, repeated often, and in this way, when ice-cold, it may be administered to irritable stomachs with the best effect. Cold water, and sometimes even ice-cold water, is a most beneficial drink, which patients may take as often as they wish, provided too much be not taken at any one time. Tea is often comforting to sick people, and may be given without harm if sufficiently diluted with milk. Other fluids suitable for invalids are beef tea, chicken, veal, or mutton broth, chicken jelly, bread jelly, flour and milk, Liebig's raw-meat soup, gruel, &c. (*vide Addendum*). Raw eggs beaten with milk are frequently useful, and *occasionally* arrowroot and other farinaceous foods.

When the appetite returns, and a desire for solid food is felt, much care should be taken for some days. Boiled fish, chicken or mutton, with bread and dry toast, will generally be the best diet. Vegetables are not recommended. Jelly, blanc-mange, light puddings made of tapioca, sago, or rice, may be given, and an egg for breakfast, or in the evening. But generally all preparations made from wheat flour, oats, grits, barley, are to be preferred in recovery from fevers, to tapioca, cornflour, rice, sago, or semolina. As a rule no stimulants need be given until the stage of convalescence, when two or three glasses of good port or claret may be taken daily. In instances when disease assumes a tendency to sinking, stimulants must be administered freely; but no general rules can be laid down (*vide* Enteric Fever, p. 245). When food is given to either the sick or convalescent, only a little should be brought at a time, and that in a tempting form, and frequently. A large basin of beef-tea or bread and milk is often refused, when a small quantity offered in a tempting manner would be taken. But the patient should not be too much pressed to take food, especially when it is apparent that he has no desire for it. Particular care should be taken that the patient is not neglected at night. Weak patients are often not able to take food till nearly forenoon, and an egg or beef-tea given during the night will probably prevent this; for there is a want of staying-power in sickness, which is particularly felt during the night. If food is declined the patient should be asked if there is anything he prefers, and if reasonable it may be provided, for the food most relished is generally that most needed. Food offered should always be fresh; it should never be left in the sick-room, and no cooking should ever be allowed in the sick-chamber.

When during convalescence the appetite is bad, tonics are generally desirable. To most invalids in India a large amount of quinine, or perhaps of arsenic, will have been given, so that more of these remedies will probably not be desirable (*vide* p. 267, small type). Under such circumstances, if the malady has been one affecting the bowels, acids may be taken with advantage, such as Recipe 34. If the malady has been fever (excepting enteric), malarial fever, ague, influenza, or neuralgic affections, an infusion of the Indian plants *chiretta* or *kreat*, may be taken, which possess tonic and anti-periodic powers. An infusion may be made by pouring a pint of boiling water on three ounces of dried chiretta and standing for half an hour. Dose of the stained infusion, one to two ounces. A concentrated tincture has been prepared called *kreat halvira* which is an excellent tonic after the maladies named above; also exerting a preventive influence against so-called malarious diseases. It is a safe tonic for children. Dose for an adult, from one to two drachms in a little water. For children according to table of proportions at p. 6.

NURSES, DUTIES OF.—The nurse must remember that *she is not* to diagnose the case, but to repeat all symptoms to the doctor, and leave him to draw his own conclusions. If a nurse wishes to serve a doctor, she must, in his absence, use her five senses to detect anything that can add to his knowledge of the case. There are no such things as 'trifles' in nursing. Nothing is beneath notice, and the more minute the observations the better. Among the prominent duties of the nurse are, to see to the cleanliness of the patient, to make provisions for his food, to note the quality, the time at which it is taken, and the quantity; to note the temperature as directed; to see that the excretions are preserved or measured as directed, or otherwise to notice their appearance; to note the periods of sleep, the expressions used by the patient, and any change in his appearance or demeanour.

NURSING OF HELPLESS PATIENTS.—The patient's strength should be saved; he should not be permitted to excite himself or to exert himself unnecessarily, and he should never be waked to take medicine. When patients are weak or have been a long time in bed, there is a tendency to faint when they are raised into an erect posture. Therefore such patients should be removed from the horizontal position as little as possible. When *washing* patients the points to be secured are not to tire and not to chill. Washing should be done after food, and part of the person should be washed at one time. When *beds or clothing require changing*, a time should be chosen when the patient is least exhausted, as half an hour after food.

*A patient's bed may be changed* by bringing another bed alongside, and sliding the patient from one to the other, or lifting him in a sheet. The new bed should be placed by the side of the old one, but sufficiently distant to allow a space between the two for attendants to move freely. Then, the patient being carried feet foremost over the foot of the old bed, so as to clear it, he should be carried head foremost over the foot of the new bed, the attendants walking along the sides of the bed, and lowering the patient steadily into the proper place. Or, if there is space, the bed-heads may be placed end to end, and the patient may be lifted out of the first and over it into the second.

*Changing the Sheets of Helpless Patients.*—Roll up, lengthways, half of the dirty sheet, and push the roll under the side of the patient. Then roll up one half of the clean sheet, and spread the other half over the side of the bed from which the dirty sheet has been removed, and, tucking it under the mattress, place the roll alongside the roll of the dirty sheet. Then gently raise the patient, and turn him over the rolls of sheets, or draw the rolls under him. Then take away the dirty sheet and unfold the clean one. When the patient can be raised, it may be convenient to roll the sheets from the head towards the foot of the bed. The patient should be raised into a sitting posture, the dirty sheet should be rolled, and the clean one spread down to the buttocks. Then the patient should lie down, and, the legs and buttocks being raised, the dirty sheet may be drawn away, and the clean one brought down.

*Changing the Clothes of Helpless Patients.*—This should be done without uncovering or raising the person. The dress should be taken from over each arm, and then drawn out from under the body. The arms should be placed in the sleeves of the clean garment, the body of which should be placed over the patient's head, and drawn down without lifting the shoulders. A 'divided dress' has been invented which is very convenient.

*Position of Helpless Patients in Bed.*—Every sick-bed should be provided with a rope, and transverse handle hanging above it, by which the patient will often be able to slightly raise himself, and so materially assist his nurses. Or a substitute for the rope and handle is a long towel fastened to the foot of the bed. When pillows are used to raise a patient in bed, they should not be piled one on top of the other under the patient's head, as this has only the effect of raising the head and pressing the chin forward on the chest, a position irksome to the patient, and which obstructs the breathing. The pillows should be placed under the patient's back as well as his head, commencing at the small of the back, and rising gradually to where a pillow is placed for the head. When the upper part of the body is raised, there is a tendency for the patient to slip downwards. A foot-board with a pillow for the feet to rest against will prevent this, but often the patient cannot bear his feet against the board. Under such circumstances a pad, or an air or water cushion, either horseshoe-shaped or circular, with a hole in the centre, may be put under the buttocks of the patient, and tied by two tapes to the head or sides of the bed, and thus a fixed obstruction will be opposed to the buttocks slipping down.

*Feeding Helpless Patients.*—When necessary to give food, drink, or medicine to a patient, the head, and, if possible, the upper part of the body, should be raised. For fluids, a feeding-cup should be employed. Where this is not provided, a spoon, a glass, or a mug may be used. When the latter are used they should be only half-filled. If too full, the fluid is sure to be spilt.

*The Bed-pan for Helpless Patients.*—The bed-pan should be used with great care, and with as little disturbance as possible to the patient, especially when injury necessitates its use. There are two kinds of bed-pans—the circular and the slipper. When the circular bed-pan is used, the patient will have to be lifted by two or three attendants, and the pan slipped under him. With the slipper bed-pan the patient should be raised at one side, and the thin end introduced under the buttocks.

QUIET IN THE SICK-ROOM.—None but the attendants required should be admitted. A patient is often unwilling to talk, and excitement always does harm. Asking unnecessary even if sympathising questions, whispering, walking on tiptoe, rustling garments, or creaking shoes, and all unnecessary noise, both inside and outside the house, should be avoided.

TEMPERATURE OF THE SICK-ROOM.—In a temperate climate, unless in some particular forms of disease, the temperature of the sick-room should range between 65° and 70° Fahr. But in India it will frequently be much higher, and the use of punkahs, or even of tatties, although often undesirable, cannot always be dispensed with. Whatever the temperature may be, every care should be given to maintain it *equable*, especially when dealing with affections of the chest. During the spring and autumnal seasons in the more northerly parts of India, there is a great difference of temperature between the night and day, particularly apparent in the early morning; when extraordinary care should be taken to prevent a patient being chilled. At page 676 chill is mentioned as a fertile source of disease in India, and the liability to take cold in a hot climate is insisted upon. As such is the case with persons in health, the sick must be doubly susceptible.

VENTILATION OF THE SICK-ROOM.—The amount of air required for breathing; the impurities in air; the disease germs which arise from the sick; and the necessity of ventilation to remove or destroy these germs, are detailed at pp. 694, 732. In Indian bungalows the entrance of fresh air into the apartment and the exit of foul air from the room are only to be obtained through the doors and windows, and in many parts of the country at some seasons of the year the hot winds forbid opening doors and windows during the day. Much, however, may be done by the arrangement of doors and windows in different parts of the house, so that fresh air from *outside* the house may enter the chamber; and for this nearly all houses require different arrangements. The purity of a sick-room may be judged of by noticing whether there is any perceptible odour on entering the room. A better test is placing a wide-mouthed bottle in the room for some hours, and then pouring a little clear lime-water (Recipe 25) into it, and shaking it. If the air is impure, the fluid will become more or less milky in appearance.

VISITING THE SICK-ROOM.—Visitors should be guided by the medical attendant as regards time of interview and subjects mentioned. They should not make a noise, nor speak in whispers, nor walk about on tiptoe. They should avoid talking about the patient and asking questions. If there is any breeze, visitors should remain on the side of the bed to which the air approaches. The mouth should be kept closed, as the penalty of breathing with the mouth open may be infection, which is much less likely to occur through the nose (*vide* p. 671).

# APPENDIX

## *PRESCRIPTIONS*

**The** prescriptions to be made up from the small medicine case to accompany this volume, or from articles procurable in the bazaars, are placed *first* under the following headings, and are separated by a double line from the prescriptions to be procured from chemists. For the peculiar action of these medicines *vide* page 8. The *first* prescriptions are those referred to in the *large* type of the preceding chapters ; the *others*, to be procured from chemists, and are those referred to in the *small* type.

### Aperients and Purgatives

**The above terms sufficiently denote the action of these kinds of medicines. But many have influence on different internal organs, and are therefore of use under different conditions.**

1. Take of Podophyllum resin . . . grain, one sixth.
   „ Compound Rhubarb Pill . . grains, two and a half.
   „ Extract of Hyoscyamus . . grain, one and a quarter.

Mix well, and make into one pill. To be coated tasteless.

The pill may be taken at night, and, if not acting sufficiently, Recipe 2, or citrate of magnesia (*vide* p. 15), or some mineral water, or a Seidlitz powder, may be taken in the morning. Ordinarily one of the pills will be sufficient, although some will require two, or even three.

This pill is carried ready-made in the medicine case designed to accompany the volume. It should be supplied in a tasteless capsule which quickly dissolves in the stomach. It is as good a pill for general use as can be devised. It is therefore referred to in the foregoing chapters for maladies for which nothing could be better suited. But it is sometimes recommended (as indeed are various other prescriptions) as a substitute for medicine which could not be included in the medicine chest, or procured except from a chemist's. *But no pill yet devised will suit all people at all times.* If, therefore, anyone consulting this book possesses a recipe which experience has shown acts satisfactorily, such recipe may be used when this prescription is recommended. Otherwise, Recipe No. 1 not answering, Recipe 7 may be procured for ordinary use, and Recipes 9, 10, 13, 14, for occasional use.

2. Take of Sulphate of Soda . . . drachms, six.
   „ Tincture of Ginger . . . minims, twenty.
   „ Water, distilled . . . ounces, two.

Mix well, and make a draught. An aperient, which may be taken alone, or used in the morning to assist the action of pills taken overnight. If a quicker action is required, the draughts may be taken three or four hours after the pills. The quantity of sulphate of soda may be increased by one or two drachms if the above prescription is not sufficiently powerful; or if too strong, the amount may be diminished.

3. Take of Sulphate of Soda . . . drachms, six.
   „ Quinine . . . . . . grains, twenty.
   „ Sulphate of Iron (the *Hera-Kusees* of the bazaars) . . grains, fifteen.
   „ Water, distilled . . . ounces eight.

Mix well, and make a mixture. Dose—two table-spoonfuls every four hours. A tonic and aperient. Useful in affections of the spleen, and for amenorrhœa; also for thread-worms.

---

4. Take of Sulphate of Soda . . . drachms, six.
   „ Dilute Sulphuric Acid . . drachm, one.
   „ Infusion of Roseleaves . . ounces, eight.

Mix well, and make a mixture. Dose—two table-spoonfuls every four hours. A cooling aperient with astringent action. Useful in miscarriage, menorrhagia, epistaxis, and in other cases where loss of blood occurs.

5. Take of Sulphate of Magnesia . . drachms, six.
   „ Tincture of Digitalis . . . minims, eight.
   „ Camphor Mixture . . . ounces, two.

Mix well, and make a draught. An aperient and sedative. Useful in asthmatic attacks with constipation.

6. Take of Bicarbonate of Magnesia . . grains, ten.
   „ Bicarbonate of Soda . . . grains, eight.
   „ Compound Senna Mixture . . ounce, one.

Mix well, and make a draught. An antacid and aperient. Useful in dyspepsia and liver affections.

7. Take of Euonymin . . . . . grains, twelve.
„ Extract of Hyoscyamus . . grains, eighteen.
„ Extract of Gentian . . . grains, eighteen.
„ Extract of Belladonna . . grains, three.

Mix well, and make into twelve pills. Dose—one, two, or three occasionally. A good vegetable aperient for liver.

8. Take of Blue Pill . . . . . . grains, five.
„ Calomel . . . . . . grains, five.

Mix well, and make into two pills. A strong purgative; for use only as prescribed in preceding chapters.

9. Take of Blue Pill . . . . . . grains, five.
„ Compound Extract of Colocynth grains, five.

Mix well, and make into two pills. A moderate purgative; for occasional use.

10. Take of Compound Extract of Colocynth grains, five.
„ Compound Rhubarb Pill . . grains, five.

Mix well, and make into two pills. A mild purgative; for occasional use.

11. Take of Calomel . . . . . . grains, five.
„ Compound Jalap Powder . drachm, one.

Mix well, and make a powder. A strong purgative, producing watery stools. Used in dropsical affections.

12. Take of Podophyllum resin . . . grain, one and a half.
„ Compound Extract of Colocynth grains, thirty.
„ Ipecacuanha Powder . . grains, four.

Mix well, with a little gum, and divide into twelve pills. Dose—one twice a day. In liver affections, and for constipation.

13. Take of Extract of Aloes (Glacial) . grains, fifteen.
„ Powdered prepared Castile Soap grains, fifteen.
„ Extract of Glycyrrhiza . . grains, fifteen.
„ Ipecacuanha Powder . . grains, two.

Mix well, and make into twelve pills. One or two for a dose. A mild aperient, and a good dinner pill, taken a quarter of an hour after dinner.

14. Take of Pill Aloes and Myrrh . . grains, three.
„ Blue Pill . . . . grain, one.
„ Extract of Taraxacum . . grains, two.
„ Extract of Stramonium . . grain, one half.

Mix well, and make into two pills. Useful in asthma,

15. Take of Sulphate of Iron . . . scruple, one.
 ,, Extract of Aloes (Glacial) . grains, fifteen.
 ,, Powdered Rhubarb . . . scruple, one.

Mix well, and make twelve pills. Two for a dose. A good aperient for weakly constipated persons, and for delayed monthly courses.

16. Take of Powdered Rhubarb . . . ounce, one.
 ,, Powdered Ginger . . . ounce, one half.
 ,, Carbonate of Magnesia . . ounces, three.

Mix well in a mortar. This is known as 'Gregory's Powder.' Dose—half a tea-spoonful to a tea-spoonful, in a little peppermint water. For indigestion and acidity of the stomach. It may be used for children from two to three years old in ten- or twelve-grain doses, when a mild purgative is required. It may be given at night, and be followed by a tea-spoonful of castor-oil in the morning.

## Alteratives

Alteratives are medicines given to alter the condition of the blood, or the secretions of the kidneys, liver, and bowels.

17. Take of Compound Ipecacuanha Powder (*Dover's Powder*) . . grains, ten.
 ,, Quinine . . . . . grains, three.
 ,, Ipecacuanha Powder . . grain, one.

Mix well, and make a powder. To be taken at bed-time. For dysentery, diarrhœa, and liver affections. It may be necessary to omit the ipecacuanha powder if it causes nausea or sickness.

18. Take of Compound Ipecacuanha Powder (*Dover's Powder*) . . grains, two.
 ,, Quinine . . . . . grain, one.

Mix well, and make a powder. Dose—one night and morning for a child two years old. For a child one year old, half the quantity. For a child six months old, one quarter. For infantile diarrhœa with fever.

19. Take of Bromide of Potassium . . drachm, one.
 ,, Water, distilled . . . ounces, six.

Make a mixture. Dose—two table-spoonfuls three times a day. For nervous affections. (*Vide* note to Recipe 21.)

20. Take of Bromide of Potassium . . drachm, half.
 ,, Spirits of Nitrous Ether . . drachm, half.
 ,, White Sugar . . . . drachm, one.
 ,, Water, distilled . . . ounce, one and a half.

Mix well, and make a mixture. Dose—a tea-spoonful every second hour for a child from one to two years old. Two tea-spoonfuls after two years old. For nervous affections and convulsions of children.

---

21. Take of Iodide of Potassium . . drachm, one.
 „ Water, distilled . . . ounces, eight.

Make a mixture. Dose—two table-spoonfuls three times a day. For syphilitic diseases, and various other morbid deposits.

*Note.*—Iodide and bromide of potassium as in Recipes 19, 20, and 21, after being taken for some time (days in some persons, weeks in others), may produce symptoms of cold in the head, sore-throat, or an eruption of pimples on the body. When this occurs the medicine should be stopped.

22. Take of Bicarbonate of Magnesia . . grains, fifteen.
 „ Oil of Aniseed . . . drops, two.
 „ Water, distilled . . . ounce, one and a half.

Make a mixture. Dose—one tea-spoonful occasionally for an infant from six months to one year old, with flatulence or 'wind on the stomach.' At less than six months old, half a tea-spoonful. Useful also for the sickness of pregnancy, when the whole may be taken.

23. Take of Calomel . . . . . grains, two.
 „ Extract of Opium . . . grain, one quarter.

Mix well, and make into a pill. Dose—one every three or four hours. Used when the specific action of mercury on the system is required.

24. Take of Blue Pill . . . . grains, two.
 „ Extract of Opium . . . grain, quarter.
 „ Ipecacuanha Powder . . grain, quarter.

Mix well, and make a pill. Dose—one every three or four hours. In dysentery or bad diarrhœa.

Calomel and blue pill contained in the two last recipes are preparations of mercury, and it should be a rule, before prescribing any preparation of mercury, to inquire if there be any peculiarity of constitution permitting very small doses of mercury to affect the system; for it occasionally happens, owing to some constitutional idiosyncrasy, that even one dose of calomel or blue pill will produce salivation, and to such persons no preparation of mercury can be safely given. If ever calomel is given to children, it should be held in mind that it produces in children unnatural-looking stools having a greenish slimy appearance, and care must be taken that more mercurials are not administered with the view of correcting the condition they induce.

25. *Lime-water.*—Place one quart of pure cold water in a glazed earthen vessel, and add half an ounce of quicklime. Cover, let it stand for three hours, and pour off the clear liquid for use. The bottle in which it is kept should be provided with a stopper, as access of air spoils lime-water. For the same reason it should be made fresh every second or third day. Dose—from one to three ounces, several times daily, with a child's food. Useful in teething, diarrhœa, indigestion, cholera, dysentery.

26. Take of Powdered Rhubarb . . . scruple, one.
„ Sulphate of Soda . . . scruple, one.
„ Aromatic Spirits of Ammonia drachm, one half.
„ Peppermint Oil . . . drop, one.
„ Water, distilled . . . ounces, two.

Make a draught. For acidity, and in the sickness of pregnancy.

27. Take of Solution of Potash . . . drachm, one.
„ Tincture of Hyoscyamus . . drachms, two.
„ Tincture of Cinchona . . drachms, two.
„ Infusion of Buchu . . . ounces, six.

Make a mixture. Dose—two table-spoonfuls three times a day. For chronic affections of the bladder.

28. Take of Bicarbonate of Soda . . drachm, one.
„ Tincture of Hyoscyamus . . drachms, two.
„ Decoction of Pareira . . ounces, six.

Make a mixture. Dose—two table-spoonfuls three times a day. For chronic affections of the bladder.

29. Take of Salicylic Acid . . . grains, forty.
„ Hydrochlorate of Morphia . grain, one.

Mix well, and make into eight pills. One every four hours. For acute rheumatism.

30. Take of Bicarbonate of Soda . . drachms, two.
„ Colchicum Wine . . . drachms, two.
„ Spirits of Nitrous Ether . . drachms, two.
„ Water, distilled . . . ounces, eight.

Make a mixture. Dose—two table-spoonfuls three times a day. For gout or rheumatism.

31. Take of Benzoic Acid . . . drachm, one.
„ Carbonate of Ammonia . . drachm, one.
„ Water, distilled . . . ounces, eight.

Make a mixture. Dose—two table-spoonfuls three times a day. For chronic cystitis, urinary disorders, and rheumatism.

32. Take of Bicarbonate of Soda . . drachms, two.
„ Tincture of Rhubarb . . ounce, half.
„ Tincture of Ginger . . . drachm, one.
„ Spirits of Chloroform . . drachm, one.
„ Water, distilled . . . ounces, six.

Make a mixture. Dose—two table-spoonfuls three times a day. Useful in jaundice.

33. Take of Extract of Taraxacum . . drachms, two.
„ Dilute Muriatic Acid . . drachm, one.
„ Infusion of Gentian . . ounces, eight.

Make a mixture. Dose—two table-spoonfuls three times a day. Shake the bottle before using. Useful in jaundice and for liver affections.

34. Take of Dilute Nitric Acid . . . drachm, one.
„ Dilute Hydrochloric Acid[1] . drachm, one.
„ Tincture of Ginger . . . drachm, one.
„ Water, distilled . . . ounces, eight.

Make a mixture. Dose—two table-spoonfuls three times a day. In affections of the liver and dyspepsia. Also as a tonic, after dysentery and fevers. After taking this medicine the mouth should be well washed. [1] Hydrochloric acid is also called *muriatic* acid.

35. Take of Bicarbonate of Potash . . drachm, one and a half.
„ Water, distilled . . . ounces, eight.

Make a mixture. Dose—two table-spoonfuls three times a day. For fever and certain affections of the urine. Also sometimes useful as a lotion for external use in skin diseases.

36. *Effervescing Draughts.*—Dissolve twenty grains of Bicarbonate of Potash in two ounces of water, and add fourteen grains of Citric Acid when about to be taken.

Or, dissolve seventeen grains of Bicarbonate of Soda in two ounces of water, and add ten grains of Citric Acid. For acidity of the stomach.

Or, dissolve two drachms of Bicarbonate of Soda in eight ounces of water, and place in a bottle. Dissolve one drachm of Tartaric Acid in four ounces of water, and place in another bottle. Dose—two table-spoonfuls of the Soda Mixture with one table-spoonful of the Acid Mixture. Useful in fever, and in the sickness of pregnancy.

*Effervescing Mixture with Chloroform.*—Add to the Soda Mixture given in the last para. twenty minims of Chloroform. *Shake well before using.* For sickness and indigestion of pregnancy, also for sea-sickness.

37. Take of Bicarbonate of Potash . . drachm, one.
„ Nitrate of Potash . . . drachm, half.

Take of Tincture of Ginger . . . drachm, one.
„ Water, distilled . . . ounces, eight.

Make a mixture. Dose—two table-spoonfuls three times a day. For indigestion or rheumatism, attended with scanty, high-coloured urine.

## Antispasmodics and Sedatives

Antispasmodics are stimulating medicines usually combined with sedative or soothing agents.

38. Take of Strong Tincture of Ginger . drachm, one.
„ Aromatic Spirits of Ammonia drachm, one.
„ Spirits of Nitrous Ether . . drachm, one.
„ Brandy . . . . . ounce, one.

Mix. Dose—one tea-spoonful in a glass of water hourly, or every two hours. For a child six months old, three or four drops; one year old six or seven drops; two years old, ten or twelve drops, in a little water. For diarrhœa and cholera. To be kept in a well-stoppered bottle.

---

39. Take of Chloroform . . . . drachm, one.
„ Aromatic Spirits of Ammonia drachm, one.
„ Chlorodyne . . . . drachms, two.
„ Brandy . . . . . ounce, one.

Mix. Dose—one tea-spoonful in water every two, three, or four hours. For diarrhœa and cholera. This and Recipe 38 should be taken in as much water as will dilute the compound, so that it may not be unpleasantly strong to swallow. Shake the mixture before using.

40. Take of Prepared Chalk . . . drachm, one.
„ Aromatic Spirits of Ammonia drachms, two.
„ Tincture of Opium . . . minims, forty.
„ Camphor Mixture . . . ounces, eight.

Make a mixture. Dose—two table-spoonfuls three times a day. For dyspepsia and diarrhœa.

41. Take of Extract of Conium . . . grains, three.
„ Extract of Indian Hemp . . grain, one quarter.
„ Camphor. . . . . . grain, one.

Make a pill. Dose—one three times a day. For asthma and spasmodic bronchitis.

## Astringents

Astringents are medicines which, acting on different parts of the system, diminish the secretions of various organs. They also when applied locally, contract the mouths of small bleeding blood-vessels, and prevent the continuance of loss of blood.

42. Take of Powdered Alum . . . drachm, one.
„ Water, distilled . . . ounces, eight.

Make a mixture. Dose—two table-spoonfuls every four hours. For miscarriage, menorrhagia, chronic dysentery. Also used as an external application for ulcers &c.

---

43. Take of Dilute Sulphuric Acid . . drachms, two.
„ Tincture of Ginger . . . drachm, one.
„ Water, distilled . . . ounces, eight.

Make a mixture. Dose—two table-spoonfuls every four hours. For miscarriage, or bleeding from the lungs, also for dyspepsia. After taking this medicine the mouth should be well washed out.

44. Take of Acetate of Lead . . . grains, three.
„ Tincture of Opium . . . drops, five.
„ Water, distilled . . . ounce, one and a half.

Make a draught. To be taken every three or four hours. For bleeding from the lungs.

45. Take of Dilute Sulphuric Acid . . minims, twenty-five.
„ Tincture of Opium . . . drops, eight.
„ Water, distilled . . . ounce, one.

Make a draught. To be taken three times a day. For bleeding from the lungs, or for bleeding from the stomach. Useful also in diarrhœa and cholera. The dose for a child six months old is half a tea-spoonful; at a year old one tea-spoonful. A tea-spoonful contains nearly one drop of laudanum (or tincture of opium); and one small drop of laudanum for each year of a child's age is the ordinary dose. Any preparation containing opium must be given with great caution to children, on account of their susceptibility to the drug. The dose should not be repeated oftener than every four hours.

46. Take of Gallic Acid . . . . grains, five.
„ Water, distilled . . . ounces, two.

Make a draught. To be taken three times a day. For bleeding from the lungs or stomach, or in scurvy, diarrhœa, and dysentery.

47. Take of Acetate of Lead . . . grains, three.
„ Extract of Opium . . . grain, quarter.

Mix well, and make a pill. One to be taken three times a day. For bleeding or hæmorrhage. Also in diarrhœa and dysentery.

48. Take of Compound Chalk Powder with Opium . . . . } grains, five.
 „ Bicarbonate of Soda . . grain, one.
 „ Powdered Alum . . . grain, one.

Make a powder. To be taken every night, or, in bad cases, every night and morning. For infantile diarrhœa and dysentery. Forty grains of compound chalk powder with opium (*Pulvis Cretæ Aromaticus* [*vel compositus*] *cum Opio*) contain one grain of opium. Therefore five grains of the compound chalk powder contain one-eighth of a grain of opium. The powder may be given to a child of one and a half to two years old. Half the powder at one year old ; a quarter at six months.

49. Take of Dilute Sulphuric Acid . . minims, twenty.
 „ Tincture of Catechu . . minims, forty.
 „ Syrup of Ginger . . . drachms, two.
 „ Water, distilled . . . drachms, ten.

Make a mixture. Dose—half a tea-spoonful for a child six months old ; one tea-spoonful for a child one year old ; two tea-spoonfuls for a child eighteen months old. For diarrhœa, and after dysentery.

## Diuretics and Diaphoretics

Diuretics are medicines which, acting on the kidneys and urinary passages, increase the quantity of urine. Many of the same medicines also act on the skin, increasing perspiration, and are therefore termed diaphoretics.

50. Take of Nitrate of Potash . . . drachm, one.
 „ Spirits of Nitrous Ether . . drachms, three.
 „ Water, distilled . . . ounces, eight.

Make a mixture. Dose—two table-spoonfuls three times a day. For fever and rheumatism, and to increase flow of urine.

51. Take of Spirits of Nitrous Ether . . drachm, one.
 „ Aromatic Spirits of Ammonia drachm, half.
 „ Ipecacuanha Wine . . minims, twenty.
 „ White Sugar . . . . drachm, one.
 „ Water, distilled . . . ounce, one and a half.

Make a mixture. Dose—half a tea-spoonful every third hour for a child six months old ; a tea-spoonful for a child one year old ; two tea-spoonfuls for a child two years old. For fever in children when the skin is dry. If the stomach is irritable, the ipecacuanha may be omitted.

52. Take of Nitrate of Potash . . . scruples, two.
    „ Spirits of Nitrous Ether . . drachms, two.
    „ Wine of Colchicum . . . drachms, two.
    „ Water, distilled . . . ounces, eight.

Make a mixture. Dose—two table-spoonfuls three times a day. For rheumatism.

53. Take of Nitrate of Potash . . . scruples, two.
    „ Spirits of Nitrous Ether . . drachms, two.
    „ Tincture of Cantharides . . drachms, two.
    „ Water, distilled . . . ounces, eight.

Make a mixture. Dose, two table-spoonfuls every three hours. In cholera, when no urine is secreted.

## Emetics

Emetics cause the stomach to contract on its contents, and to expel them through the gullet and mouth. The emetics in common use are mustard, ipecacuanha, tartar emetic, and sulphate of zinc. *Ipecacuanha* is the best of all emetics, especially the wine for children. For the proper doses *vide* p. 15.

54. Take of Mustard Flour . . . . table-spoonful, one.
    „ Common Salt . . . . tea-spoonful, one.
    „ Warm Water . . . . ounces, ten to twelve.

Mix, and let the patient drink it all. This emetic should act within five or eight minutes. For children a tea-spoonful of mustard and a quarter of a tea-spoonful of salt in half a tumbler of warm water. It is desirable to promote the action of emetics by copious draughts of warm water, which, filling the stomach, also diminish the disagreeable sensations accompanying vomiting when the stomach is empty.

## Expectorants

Expectorants are medicines which, acting on the air-passages leading to the lungs, and also, in some degree, on the general system, facilitate the passage of fluids secreted in the lungs and in the tubes leading to the lungs, in cough, catarrh, bronchitis, and asthma.

55. Take of Aromatic Spirits of Ammonia . drachms, two.
    „ Spirits of Nitrous Ether . . drachms, four.
    „ Tincture of Ginger . . . drachm, one.
    „ Water, distilled . . . ounces, five and a half.

Make a mixture. Dose—two table-spoonfuls every two or three hours. For asthmatic attacks and chronic bronchitis.

| | | |
|---|---|---|
| 56. Take of | Camphorated Tincture of Opium (*Paregoric*) . . . . | drachms, three. |
| ,, | Aromatic Spirits of Ammonia . | drachms, two. |
| ,, | Water, distilled . . . | ounces, eight. |

Make a mixture. Dose—two table-spoonfuls every two or three hours. For asthmatic attacks and chronic bronchitis.

| | | |
|---|---|---|
| 57. Take of | Camphorated Tincture of Opium (*Paregoric*) . . . . | drachms, three. |
| ,, | Ipecacuanha Wine . . . | drachms, one. |
| ,, | Spirits of Nitrous Ether . . | drachms, three. |
| ,, | Water, distilled . . . | ounces, seven. |

Make a mixture. Dose—two table-spoonfuls every three or four hours. For catarrh, bronchial and lung affections. Useful in smaller doses for children with cough, bronchitis, inflammation of the lungs, and croup. The dose for a child one year old is one teaspoonful, increasing half a tea-spoonful for every year of age.

---

| | | |
|---|---|---|
| 58. Take of | Camphor . . . . . | grain, one. |
| ,, | Powdered Ipecacuanha . . | grains, three. |

Mix well with a little gum, and make into a pill. May be taken every two hours for asthma.

| | | |
|---|---|---|
| 59. Take of | Tartar Emetic. . . . . | grain, one. |
| ,, | Camphorated Tincture of Opium (*Paregoric*) . . . . | drachms, two. |
| ,, | Water, distilled and boiling . | ounces, twelve. |

Make a mixture and allow it to cool. Dose—two table-spoonfuls every two or three hours. For bronchitis, pleurisy, laryngitis, and pneumonia.

| | | |
|---|---|---|
| 60. Take of | Camphorated Tincture of Opium (*Paregoric*) . . . . | drachms, three. |
| ,, | Ipecacuanha Wine . . . | drachms, two. |
| ,, | Tincture of Scilla . . . | drachms, one. |
| ,, | Bicarbonate of Soda . . | scruples, two. |
| ,, | Water, distilled . . . | ounces, eight. |

Make a mixture. Dose—two table-spoonfuls every three or four hours. For bronchial affections, especially when there are also dyspeptic symptoms or acidity. Useful for children in smaller doses, for cough, bronchitis, or croup. The dose for a child one year old is one tea-spoonful; increasing half a tea-spoonful for every year of age.

61. Take of Carbonate of Magnesia . . grains, twenty-five.
„ Peppermint Oil . . . drops, two.
„ Water, distilled . . . ounce, one.

Make a mixture. Dose—a tea-spoonful three or four times a day. In hooping-cough, for a child one or two years old. Before using, the bottle should be well shaken. Also useful for the sickness of pregnancy, when the whole may be taken at once as a draught.

62. Take of Sulphate of Zinc . . . grains, two.
„ Camphorated Tincture of Opium (*Paregoric*) . . . . } minims, sixty.
„ Water, distilled . . . ounce, one and a half.

Make a mixture. Dose—a tea-spoonful three times a day. For a child from one to two years old, for hooping-cough.

63. Take of Extract of Conium . . . grains, three.
„ Water, distilled . . . ounce, one and a half.

Make a mixture. Dose—a tea-spoonful three times a day. For a child from one to two years old with hooping-cough. Shake the bottle before using.

## Opiates

Opiates are medicines which relieve pain and induce sleep. Of these the principal are opium, morphia, chloral. In large doses they are poisons, and must be administered with caution.

64. Take of Chloral . . . . . grains, twenty.
„ Water, distilled . . . ounce, one and a half.

Make a draught. (*Vide Chloral*, p. 10.)

---

65. Take of Hydrochlorate of Morphia . grain, one.
„ Rectified Spirits of Wine . . drops, ten.
„ Water, distilled . . . ounce, one.

Make a draught. To be taken when a strong opiate is required, as in obstruction of the bowels, and in tetanus.

## Tonics

Tonics impart 'tone' or strength to the system, and are useful during convalescence from exhausting maladies, and in most debilitated conditions. Tonics act without stimulating the system, and are thus different from 'stimulants.' One variety of tonics—namely, preparations of iron—owes its virtues to its power of supplying a deficient element of the blood (*vide* p. 24).

66. Take of Quinine . . . . . . grains, twenty-four.
„ Sherry Wine . . . . . ounces, two.
„ Water, distilled . . . . ounces, eight.

Make a mixture. Dose—two table-spoonfuls three times a day.

67. Take of Quinine . . . . . . grains, twenty-four.
„ Lemon Juice (fresh) . . drachms, two.
„ Water, distilled . . . . ounces, eight.

Make a mixture. Dose—two table-spoonfuls three times a day.

68. Take of Isinglass . . . . . . drachms, two.
„ Sugar, white . . . . . drachms, two.
„ Brandy . . . . . . half a wine-glass, or
„ Sherry . . . . . . one glass.
„ Nutmeg . . . . . . a pinch.
„ Boiling Water . . . . ounces, four.

Make a draught. A good stomachic tonic in diarrhœa.

---

69. Take of Quinine . . . . . . grains, twenty.
„ Dilute Sulphuric Acid . . drachm, one.
„ Tincture of Ginger . . . drachm, half.
„ Water, distilled . . . . ounces, eight.

Make a mixture. Dose—two table-spoonfuls every three or four hours.

70. Take of Citrate of Iron and Quinine . scruples, two.
„ Water, distilled . . . . ounces, eight.

Make a mixture. Dose—two table-spoonfuls every three or four hours. Wash the mouth after taking the medicine. For a child one year old, two tea-spoonfuls; two years old, a dessert-spoonful. It should be recollected that any iron medicine colours the stools black.

71. Take of Tincture of Iron (*Steel Wine*) . drachms, two.
„ Water, distilled . . . . ounces, eight.

Make a mixture. Dose—two table-spoonfuls three times a day. For anæmia and debility. Wash the mouth after taking the medicine. *Neutral solution of peroxide of iron* (known as liquid dialysed iron) may be substituted for those objecting to the taste of steel wine. Or the solution, being almost tasteless, may be taken in eight- or ten-drop doses on a lump of sugar. *Carbonate of Iron* is a good remedy for those objecting to the taste of the tincture. It may be taken in five- to ten-grain doses, in water; or as a powder mixed with sugar, or alone; or, being almost tasteless, it may be sprinkled on the food. Iron lozenges may be procured from the chemists.

72. Take of Sulphate of Iron . . . grains, twelve.
„ Dilute Sulphuric Acid . . drachm, one.
„ Water, distilled . . . ounces, six.

Make a mixture. Dose—two table-spoonfuls three times a day. For anæmia and debility.

73. Take of Sulphate of Iron . . . grains, nine.
„ Sulphate of Quinine . . grains, twelve.
„ Dilute Sulphuric Acid . . drachm, one.
„ Sulphate of Soda . . . ounce, one.
„ Sugar, white . . . . drachms, two.
„ Water, distilled . . . ounces, twelve.

Make a mixture. Dose—two table-spoonfuls two or three times a day. For painful menstruation with constipation. As a tonic aperient, in affections of the liver or spleen.

74. Take of Syrup of the Iodide of Iron . ounce, one.

Dose—thirty drops three times a day in a wine-glassful of water.

75. Take of Arsenical Solution . . . minims, forty.
„ Water, distilled . . . ounces, eight.

Make a mixture. Dose—two table-spoonfuls three times a day after meals. Arsenical solution is also called *Liquor Arsenitis Potassæ*. As a tonic; also used for the cure of ague, and in skin disease.

After arsenic has been taken for some time (varying with different people from days to weeks), it produces certain effects. These are colicky pains in the bowels, diarrhœa, watering, itching, and irritation about the eyes, the whites becoming 'blood-shot,' and the eyelids feeling stiff. These effects show that the system has been brought under the influence of the medicine. In order to avoid pain in the bowels and to prevent the arsenic passing away with diarrhœa, arsenic should be taken a quarter of an hour after meals.

76. Take of Sulphate of Quinine . . grains, twelve.
„ Sulphate of Cinchonidine . grains, twelve.
„ Arsenious Acid . . . grain, one quarter.
„ Carbolic Acid . . . . grain, one and a quarter.
„ Camphor . . . . . grain, one and a quarter.
„ Powdered Capsicum . . grains, five.

Mix well with a little gum arabic, and make into twelve pills. One night and morning, or every three or four hours. For use as a tonic, and preventive of fever in malarious districts.

## Hot Applications

77. *Bran Poultice.*—Make a linen or flannel bag of the size requisite and fill loosely with bran. Pour boiling water on till thoroughly moistened. Put it into a coarse towel and absorb excess of moisture. Then place it on the part, and cover with a dry towel.

78. *Bread Poultice.*—Put half a pint of scalding hot water into a basin. Add as much crumb of bread as the water will cover. Let it steep five minutes. Then drain off the water and spread the moistened bread on a piece of linen, and apply. In India, *atta* or flour must often be substituted, bread not being always available. If *atta* is used it will be necessary to stir it, to mix it well with the water.

79. *Linseed Meal Poultice* is made in a similar manner by scalding finely powdered linseed meal.

*Powdered Charcoal* is also used for poultices when an application to a gangrenous wound is required. It should be made of equal parts of linseed meal or bread and powdered charcoal.

When applying a poultice, cover the surface with a little butter or oil, which will prevent the poultice sticking to the skin when removed. Poultices should never be allowed to remain on after they have cooled, as they become clammy, unpleasant, and injurious.

80. *Fomentation.*—This is managed by some pieces of flannel of the required size, and containing four or five folds, soaked in water so hot as to be grateful to the patient. The hand is not a fair guide to the heat necessary; neither is the thermometer, as some persons bear without flinching heat to the skin which would be painful to others. Beneath the part to be fomented should be placed a waterproof sheet or oil-cloth. Then the flannel should be wrung nearly dry (by twisting it in a towel), applied to the part, and covered with a thick, warm towel. Another fold of flannel should be in the water in readiness, and the flannels should be changed before they feel cool to the patient. This should be effected quickly, so that the patient may not take cold, and care should be taken to dry the parts after the fomentation. Sometimes, instead of poultices or fomentations, it will be more convenient to use spongiopiline, which is composed of felt with an impervious covering. Or 'Iceland Moss poultice,' which only requires steeping in hot water.

81. *Poppy Water for fomentation.*—Steep half a dozen bruised poppy-heads and the contained seeds in as many pints of boiling water, and, after half an hour, strain the infusion. It is employed instead of plain water for painful affections, and may be used to make poultices.

82. *Dry Fomentations.*—This may be effected by flannel bags filled with camomile flowers, hops, bran, or even sand. The bag thus filled should be heated and then applied to the part, another being substituted when it becomes cold.

## Cooling Applications

Hot applications are most useful to hasten a 'gathering,' but in the commencement of any local inflammation it will often be proper to use cooling applications, and thus endeavour to check the 'gathering.' As it may be sometimes difficult to decide whether the use of hot or cold applications will be best, the sensations of the patient should be consulted, which are generally a safe guide. Thus, if shivering or pain follow the application of cold, it should be cautiously changed for *warm* applications, *gradually* made hotter. The application of cold may be effected by the following means:—

1. *Evaporating Lotions.* (*Vide* Recipes 83, 84.)—A piece of linen, *not doubled*, should be dipped in the liquid and laid on the part affected, but no covering should be permitted over this. To secure evaporation and the resulting cold, exposure to the air is required. The piece of linen should be frequently freshly wetted, or the lotion may be dropped upon it from a sponge. In the absence of a lotion, iced water may be used. Or a lotion may be made by mixing two ounces of spirits of wine and two ounces of vinegar in a pint of cold water.

2. *Ice in a Bladder or India-rubber Bag.*—Ice roughly pounded, or shaved with a cucumber grater, placed in a bag, will produce intense cold. Or, if ice is available in small quantities, it may be mixed with an equal bulk of salt. *Ice Poultices* are made by placing lumps of ice on a thick layer of linseed meal. Sprinkle more meal lightly over and cover with another cloth. Fold in the edges to prevent escape of the meal, and apply the thick side. The exclusion of air prevents quick melting of the ice, and the thick layer of meal prevents a high degree of cold.

3. *Irrigation.*—Expose the part, beneath which india-rubber cloth or oil-cloth should be placed. Then a vessel containing cold water should be suspended on the bedpost, or from a hook in the wall, or from a stand as here figured, so that the receptacle may hang directly over the part to be 'irrigated.' Continuous dripping of the water may be accomplished by hanging over the edge of the vessel a thin strip of lint previously well soaked. Capillary attraction will cause the fluid to drop more or less rapidly, according to the size of the strip of lint. The exact point on which the dripping occurs should be varied from time to time by altering the position of the hanging vessel.

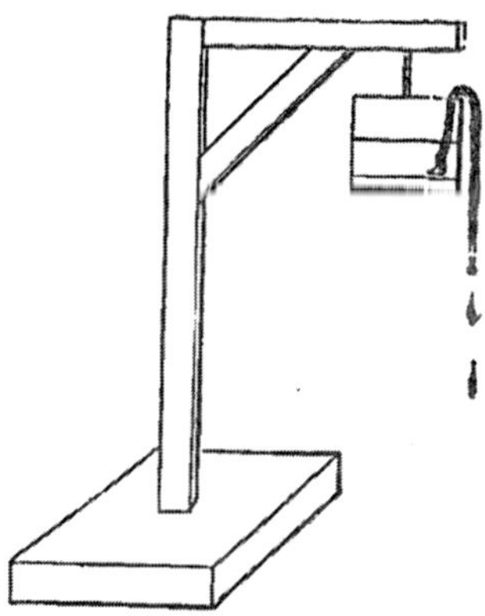

IRRIGATION STAND

83. Take of Nitrate of Potash . . . ounce, half.
 „ Hydrochlorate of Ammonia . ounce, half.
 „ Common Salt . . . . ounce, half.
 „ Water . . . . . ounces, twelve.

Make a lotion. Either this or Recipe 84 may be used when cooling lotions are required. The materials may be procured in Indian bazaars. *Vide* pp. 21, 26. If greater cold is required, equal parts of the ingredients may be mixed roughly in a very small quantity of water, then placed in an india-rubber bag or bladder, and applied to the part. This forms a good substitute for ice.

---

84. Take of Acetate of Lead . . . drachm, one.
   „ Rectified Spirits of Wine . ounce, one.
   „ Water, distilled . . . ounces, twelve.

Make a lotion. To be applied as mentioned under 'Evaporating Lotions,' p. 723.

### Soothing Applications

85. *Water Dressing.*—This consists of a double fold of lint or linen soaked in water and applied to the part. Over this a covering of oil-silk, gutta-percha tissue, or bladder should be laid. Warm or cold water may be used, and the dressing should be changed three times a day. It is often advisable to use carbolic acid lotion (No. 119) instead of water.

86. *Simple Ointment.*—Mutton fat, two parts; olive oil, one part; yellow beeswax, half a part. Melt in a saucepan, and stir while cooling. This forms a healing ointment, which may be medicated in various ways by other agents (*vide* Recipes 95, 96). If practicable, *lanolin* should be used instead of mutton fat. Lanolin is made from wool oil, is absorbed readily by the skin, and does not become rancid.

87. *Carron Oil.*—Equal parts of linseed oil and lime-water (*vide* Recipe 25) should be taken together. For burns and scalds. If no linseed oil, use olive or salad oil.

---

88. Take of Calomel . . . . . grains, thirty.
   „ Lime-water (*vide* Recipe 25) . ounces, ten.

Mix well, and make a lotion. 'Black Wash,' so called from the dark colour the mixture assumes, is chiefly used for venereal sores.

89. Take of Tincture of Opium . . . drachm, one.
   „ Tincture of Aconite . . drachm, one.
   „ Chloroform . . . . drachm, one.
   „ Soap Liniment . . . ounce, one and a half.

Mix for a liniment, and mark Poison. This liniment may be rubbed on the skin with a piece of sponge or lint for neuralgic pains.

90. Take of Tincture of Opium . . . drachm, one.
   „ Tincture of Aconite . . drachm, one.
   „ Chloroform . . . . drachm, one.

Mix for a liniment, and mark Poison. This liniment may be rubbed on the skin with a piece of sponge or lint for neuralgic pains. It is much stronger than Recipe 89. It should not be used when any injury of the skin exists, or for the mouth; or for children.

N.B.—*Solidified liniments* are made by chemists. They may be sent by post, and they possess the advantage of not running away from the hand when used like fluids.

91. Fill a small phial two-thirds full with powdered camphor, and fill up with rectified spirits of wine or sulphuric ether. With this solution the part affected by neuralgia should be lightly rubbed by means of a sponge or lint fixed to a piece of stick. A minute suffices to produce almost entire loss of sensation, but this effect does not last long.

### Stimulating Applications.—Ointments

92. Take of Flour of Sulphur . . . ounce, one.
„ Nitrate of Potash . . . drachm, half.
„ Soap, or Glycerine . . . drachm, one.
„ Mutton Fat . . . . ounces, four.

Mix thoroughly after melting the fat over a fire. For itch.

---

93. Take of Tincture of Opium . . . drachms, two.
„ Carbolic Acid . . . grains, twenty.
„ Mutton Fat . . . . ounce, one.
„ Olive Oil . . . . ounce, one.

Melt over the fire, and stir while cooling. A good stimulating ointment for ulcers.

94. Take of Red Iodide of Mercury . . grains, sixteen.
„ Mutton Fat . . . . ounce, half.
„ Olive Oil . . . . ounce, half.

Mix the fat and oil by melting over a fire, and then rub the iodide of mercury thoroughly into the fat and oil in a mortar. For enlarged spleen, 'Derbyshire neck,' and enlarged glands generally.

95. Take of Powdered Gall Nuts . . grains, eighty.
„ Extract of Opium . . . grains, thirty.
„ Simple Ointment (Recipe 86) . ounce, one.

Mix thoroughly in a mortar. A good application for piles.

96. Take of Acetate of Lead . . . grains, thirty.
„ Simple Ointment (Recipe 86) . ounce, one.

Mix thoroughly in a mortar. A good ointment for scorbutic ulcers.

### Lotions

97. Take of Powdered Alum . . . grains, twenty.
 „ Water, distilled . . . ounces, eight.

Mix well, and make a lotion. Useful for eye and ear affections, for ulcers and skin diseases.

---

98. Take of Sulphate of Zinc . . . grains, eight.
 „ Water, distilled . . . ounces, eight.

Mix well, and make a lotion. For eye and ear affections.

99. Take of Bicarbonate of Soda . . drachm, one.
 „ Water, distilled . . . ounces, eight.

Mix well, and make a lotion. For eczema and other skin diseases.

### Stimulating and Astringent Gargles

100. Take of Alum . . . . . drachm, one.
 „ Water, distilled . . . ounces, eight.

Mix, and make a gargle. For sore-throat, ulcerated mouth, and scurvy. Also as an injection.

101. Take of Tincture of Ginger (*strong*) . drachm, one.
 „ Water, distilled . . . ounces, eight.

Mix well, and make a gargle. For relaxed throat.

---

102. Take of Gallic Acid . . . . scruple, one.
 „ Brandy . . . . drachms, four.
 „ Water, distilled . . . ounces, six.

Mix, and make a gargle. For salivation, ulcerated mouth, and scurvy.

103. Take of Sulphate of Zinc . . . grains, thirty.
 „ Water, distilled . . . ounces, eight.

Mix well, and make a gargle. This and the three preceding gargles are useful in salivation, ulcerated mouth, and relaxed and sore throats.

### Injections or Enemas

Previous to giving an injection the bed and clothing should be well protected. Then the tube of the injection syringe should be warmed and oiled, and the instrument should be filled so that air may not be pumped in. 'Lynch's safety enema syringe' is to be recommended, being light, portable, suitable for travelling, and by which air cannot be pumped in. The patient should lie on the left side, with the knees drawn up, and the passage should be opened by the finger and thumb placed on each side of it. The tube should be *gently* introduced, in the direction of the bowel, which is *towards the left hip bone.* The instrument should be worked slowly, and not too forcibly. Two drachms may be injected if the patient is an infant; from one to five years, one to three ounces; from ten to fifteen, four to six ounces; above that age, eight to twelve ounces. For children, an india-rubber bottle furnished with a gum elastic pipe screwing on to the mouth is the best kind of instrument, as fluid can scarcely be injected too forcibly from it. If an injection syringe is not available, a substitute may be improvised by tying a piece of tobacco pipe, or other tube, into a bladder containing the injection. The contents must then be squeezed out of the bladder through the tube.

*Injection of the Female Privates.*—A female syringe should be employed, and when using the syringe the patient should lie with the hips raised on a pillow, in which position the injection flows over all the affected parts, and she should remain in such position for at least five minutes. It is also *essential* that the parts should be *first* washed out with tepid water. A cane couch and utensil beneath are required.

*Injection of the Male Privates.*—A glass syringe three inches long with a smooth round nozzle half an inch long, should be used. The patient, having passed water, puts the nozzle into the orifice and holds the head of the penis with the left thumb and fingers. The piston is then pressed down with the right forefinger, while the syringe is held with the thumb and other fingers. The nozzle is then withdrawn, the patient still nipping the penis to prevent escape of the injection. After two minutes on relaxing the hold of the penis the injection is forcibly discharged.

104. Take of Starch or Soap . . . drachms, two.
" Water, warm . . . ounces, ten.

Mix well, and make an injection.

105. Take of Asafœtida . . . . drachm, one.
" Soap . . . . . drachm, one.
" Castor Oil . . . . ounce, one.
" Water, warm . . . ounces, eight.

Mix well. A stimulating injection.

---

106. Take of Castor Oil . . . . ounce, half.
" Spirits of Turpentine . . ounce, half.
" Croton Oil . . . . drops, four.
" Soap . . . . . grains, thirty.
" Water, warm . . . ounces, eight.

Mix well. A purgative injection. For apoplexy.

107. Take of Sulphate of Zinc . . . grains, twenty.
„ Tincture of Opium . . minims, thirty.
„ Water, warm . . . ounces, eight.

Mix well. Useful for 'whites' and womb diseases.

*Nutrient Enema.*—A good nutrient enema may be made with two eggs, four ounces of beef tea, four ounces of port wine or two of brandy, beaten up in a pint of water, thickened with arrowroot, at temperature of 100° Fahr.

*Digested enemas* are useful when the patient cannot take food. Eight ounces of beef tea, the yolk of an egg, and a tea-spoonful of raw arrowroot should be mixed and warmed in a covered jar to 100° Fahr. Then fifteen grains of pepsin and ten drops of strong hydrochloric acid should be added separately. The whole should stand, at the same temperature, for one hour. Then, while the mixture is stirred, small quantities of bicarbonate of soda should be added so long as it occasions effervescence. This imitates the process of digestion, and the material is injected into the bowel in a state in which it may be easily absorbed.

Previous to giving a *nutrient* or *digested* enema, if a natural motion has not been lately passed, the gut should be washed out by an injection of warm water. The quantity of nutrient or digested enema given should not exceed four or five ounces. Neither should injections of the kind be given more frequently than every four hours, as the gut soon becomes indolent and does not absorb. After injecting, a towel should be placed against the orifice for some minutes to prevent escape of the enema.

## Irritating, Rubefacient, or Blistering Applications

108. *Turpentine Stupe.*—Saturate a piece of lint or a piece of flannel with spirits of turpentine. Place this on the painful part and cover with oiled silk or a dry cloth. Retain it on the part for an hour, or until it is too painful. It produces redness of the skin, but does not blister.

109. *Mustard Poultice.*—Mix flour of mustard with lukewarm water into a thick paste, and spread thickly over a piece of linen of the size required. A piece of muslin should be placed between the mustard and the skin to prevent the mustard adhering to the skin, and in delicate people to prevent too great action of the mustard. Then apply it on the part for twenty minutes, or less if very painful. On removal the skin should be sponged with warm water and cotton wool applied. *For children* the mustard should be diluted with half flour, it should be guarded by muslin, and it should be removed in eight minutes. A good substitute is 'Mustard Paper.' One leaf immersed in water half a minute and applied to the skin will have the same effect as a poultice, and save the patient from the disagreeable smell and acrid vapour arising from a poultice. When used for children it should be guarded by muslin.

110. *Blisters.*—Cantharides plaster is spread thinly on a piece of sticking-plaster, leaving a margin which, when the blister is applied to the skin, adheres, and maintains the whole in position. The blister begins to smart in about two hours, and may be taken off in six or eight hours. But the time necessary to produce a blister depends on the sensibility of the person's skin. When the blister is taken off, all the raised blebs should be snipped at their most bulging parts with sharp scissors, and the water allowed to drain out, but none of the raised skin should be removed. Then the part should be dressed with Recipe 86, or with salad oil spread on linen or lint. In six hours this should be taken off, when other blebs will have formed. These must be snipped and the water drained out. Then the place should be dressed twice daily with simple ointment. If, after blisters, boils form near the part, they should be fomented and poulticed. There is also a *blistering tissue* made, but it does not keep well in India. No kind of blister should be applied to children except under medical advice.

111. *Iodine Paint*, called 'Liniment of Iodine,' is sometimes used instead of mustard or blisters. It should be lightly applied with a feather or brush every day, or less frequently after the first three or four days, so as to maintain an irritation of, but not to blister, the skin. Iodine paint acts more energetically on some sensitive skins, and therefore must be used with caution. The ordinary effects are, after a second application, itching and smarting, which soon subsides. After several applications the upper layer of the skin becomes loose, and may be rubbed off. If too much paint is applied, blisters may form.

### Applications for Injuries

112. *Starch Bandage.*—Make a very thick solution of starch, soak a bandage in it, and apply it to the part, winding fold after fold until four or five folds cover the limb. While applying the bandage smear it thickly with starch. Then let it dry, when it forms a firm support or shell. It should be applied with firmness, but not too tightly. It is useful as a support after the splints are removed from a fractured limb.

113. *Leather Plaster.*—This is adhesive plaster spread on leather. It is useful for fractures as a support after splints are taken away.

## Baths

Judiciously used, warm baths are remedies of great utility, but improperly used they do injury. The effect of a hot bath is to relax the muscles, to diminish the force of the heart's action, and to produce faintness. In weakness of the heart this danger is exaggerated. It is, therefore, necessary to watch a person placed in a warm bath, and while in the bath the reclining position should be assumed, which renders fainting less likely. The time which a person should remain in a warm bath must be regulated by the effect. Faintness requires removal; the person should lie down, and be dried in that position.

*The temperature* for baths is, cold, 60° to 75°; tepid, 85° to 92°; warm, 92° to 98°; hot, 98° to 115°. But the skin of infants will suffer from a degree of heat innocuous to an adult. Infants have been scalded to death in too hot baths. The temperature for children should not exceed 96° to 98° Fahr.

*The complaints for which warm baths are most useful* in adults are those accompanied by great and spasmodic pain, as gravel, rupture, stoppage in the bowels, and rheumatism. In children warm baths are chiefly required in convulsions, croup, pain in the bowels, restlessness from teething, flatulence.

When necessary to put the *feet of insensible patients* in a hot bath, this may be accomplished by drawing the person over the foot of the bed until the knees bend and the feet hang down.

*A method of applying heat* when a hot bath is not advisable is wrapping the patient in a blanket wrung out of hot water, and covering with dry blankets, in which the patient may remain twenty minutes, and must then be dried with warm towels.

*Modified Turkish baths* are often beneficial to tropical invalids, who, without organic disease, suffer from prolonged residence in the East. The patient should leave the hot chamber as soon as perspiration occurs, and should take a tepid douche, instead of the plunge into the cold bath. The mistake usually made is staying too long in the hot room.

*A Medicated Bath* is one in which some substance, to act as a medicine through the pores of the skin, has been mixed with the water. Substances thus used are salts, acids, soda, sulphur, &c.

114. *Nitro-muriatic Acid Bath.*—

Take of Muriatic Acid . . . three parts.
,, Nitric Acid . . . two parts.

Mix the acids slowly, then add slowly five parts of water. Wait till the heat produced by the mixture of the ingredients subsides, and bottle. One ounce of this solution should be added to each gallon of water, and the vessel for the bath should be wood or earthenware. The patient should remain in the bath fifteen minutes, the temperature being maintained at 98° by the gradual addition of hot water. On coming out of the bath the body should be rubbed with coarse towels. The Acid Bath is used in chronic liver and spleen affections. For children, half strength. When using strong acids care must be taken, as they burn anything they come in contact with. Muriatic is also called *hydrochloric* acid.

115. *Dry-Cupping.*—This means the application of the cupping-glasses, without the following use of the scarificator. Several glasses may be applied, which causes a rise of blood to the surface. If cupping-glasses are not at hand, dry-cupping may be accomplished by tumblers, which should be first exhausted of air by the introduction inside of a little cotton wool tied on a stick and saturated with spirits of wine or brandy, and then lighted. Care must be taken that the glass is not sufficiently heated to burn the skin. To take the glass off, the finger nail should be insinuated between the edge of the glass and the skin, when the glass will become loose. After dry-cupping no application is required; the parts will recover their natural appearance in a few hours. If it is desired to maintain the irritation caused by dry-cupping, hot fomentations should be used.

116. *Massage.*—Massage is methodical shampooing, and consists of rubbing, stroking, and kneading, principally in the direction of the veins, or from below upwards. It stimulates the skin and superficial vessels, promoting the flow of blood and lymph and the absorption of effete matter, thus exciting appetite to supply the place of removed material. It also increases the muscular strength and promotes sleep. In these ways it in some degree proves a substitute for exercise. There is nothing mysterious in massage, which is efficiently performed by many Indians. Heart affections, disease of blood-vessels, albuminuria, gastric ulcer, consumption, disease of joints, contra-indicate the employment of massage. Systematic massage, combined with strict isolation of the patient and feeding, is known as the 'Weir-Mitchell treatment,' and often much benefits hysterical, nervous, and debilitated persons.

117. *Leeches—how to apply them.*—The leech has three teeth, and makes a triangular wound. The Indian leech, being smaller than the European, does not take so much blood. Leeches should be kept in a cool place, in a jar of water with mud at the bottom, the mouth of the vessel being covered with muslin. The water should be changed every two or three days. There is often trouble in getting leeches to fix. The part to which they are to be applied should be cleansed with a cool moist cloth, so as to leave it damp. If they do not bite readily, the part may be moistened with a little sugar and water, or milk. If this does not answer, the skin may be slightly scratched with a sharp needle till the blood comes. Sometimes rubbing a refractory leech in a dry towel, or placing it for a moment in warm water, will cause it to bite. To

apply leeches in one circumscribed spot, put them all in a wineglass, which is to be turned down over the part. If required over a large surface, they must be put on singly; they should be held lightly by the tail, wrapped in a piece of wet cloth, so that they may not be inconvenienced by the heat of the hand. If the leech does not fix soon, it is better to return it to the water for a time, trying another in the meantime. More leeches than the number to be applied should be obtained, as often some will not bite. It is advisable, if possible, particularly with children, to apply leeches over some bone, against which pressure may be exerted to stop the bleeding, if necessary. A rule with regard to children is to employ small leeches. Two little leeches may be used instead of one large one, the bites of the former rarely bleeding so much after their removal. When applied, they should not be disturbed or torn off, as the teeth may be left in the wound. They should be covered with a light cloth until, having filled, they will fall off in about three-quarters of an hour. Then the leech-bites should be fomented with hot water, if it is wished to encourage the flow of blood, otherwise they should be covered with dry lint. A little salt should be sprinkled on the leeches after they drop off, which causes them to disgorge the blood, otherwise they probably die. They should then be returned to clear water, which should be frequently changed.

Leech-bites will generally stop bleeding without interference; if not, the measures noted at p. 512 should be adopted.

## Disinfection

The impurities in air may be suspended, or gaseous matter. The universal diffusion of suspended material is proved by the atoms which become visible in a ray of sunlight. These are atoms of the local soil; spores, germs, pollen, decaying débris from the vegetable world, decaying tissue, cells, germs of animalcula and of disease, particles of carbon, fibres of hair, cotton, wool, and other fabrics from various sources. Noxious gases arise from sewers, from decaying animal and vegetable matter, and from the respiration and skins of animals, and all such gases are charged with inconceivably minute particles of decaying matter, and with living germs, either animal or vegetable, or of disease. There are also present in air vital bodies, known as *vibrios* and *bacteria*, which, brought into contact with dead organic matter, increase hourly by myriads; this being in fact the process of putrefaction.

The simplest form of *contagion* is when a disease is communicated by the conveyance of a palpable, minute poisonous matter from the sick to the healthy, either directly or through the medium of clothing, food, animals, &c. But the poisonous matter of many diseases may be transmitted through the atmosphere by the agency of invisible *germs* generated by the sick, or from the discharges of the sick ; or even, as there is reason to presume, spontaneously—or certainly localised—under various unsanitary conditions and favouring atmospheric influences. The appearance of vegetable growths or of insects in unexpected places often creates surprise ; but the germs must have been wafted to such places through the atmosphere. The unexpected appearance of disease is explainable in a similar manner. Disease germs are most abundant where sick people are congregated. Germs may be breathed into the lungs, or be taken with food or drink, or be absorbed by a sore. They may multiply, and grow with rapidity within the body ; they poison the blood, and they excite disease similar to that from which they originate. All persons are not alike, or always in the same degree susceptible, to contagion by contact, or to infection by germs. A weakened, fatigued, or chilled person will become affected more easily than a robust vigorous man ; the intemperate sooner than the temperate ; the hungry and poverty-stricken before the well-fed, well-clothed, and well-housed. Similarly, all germs (as is the case with seeds) are not prolific. The great majority are destroyed by the oxidising influence of the atmosphere before they find a suitable ground for their development. Disease germs may or may not be associated with bad smells.

*Disinfection* means not only the removal of bad smells, but the more important operation of rendering innocuous all germs, or decomposing or diseased matter from which germs may arise. Two classes of agents are in use. One class are simply *deodorants*, and only act by overpowering one odour by the substitution of another, and do little good. They may be pleasant as deodorisers, and therefore not to be altogether condemned, but they fail as disinfectants. Under the head *deodorants* are the fumes from burning brown paper, tar fumes, vinegar, acetic acid, ammonia, roasted coffee, pastilles. Agents can only be termed *disinfectants* when they destroy, or at least render harmless, noxious emanations. Under this head may be classed extreme dry heat, charcoal, quicklime, carbolic acid, sulphurous acid, nitrous acid, Condy's fluid, nitrate of lead, sulphate of iron, chloralum, &c. But there are some agents which act both as *deodorants* and as *disinfectants*, the principal of which are Condy's fluid, carbolic acid, chlorine gas, chloride of aluminium, nitrate of lead, and izal.

Deodorants and disinfectants should never be permitted to take the place of ventilation and cleanliness. If dirt and filth are not removed, and if fresh air is not admitted, neither disinfectants nor deodorants will do good. They simply hide the dirt, and conceal the want of pure air, instead of destroying the evil arising from it. The poison of all infectious diseases may be *best* diluted and destroyed by fresh air.

The method of using some of the principal disinfecting agents is now given.

118. *Condy's Fluid.*—Is a dilution of strong solution of *permanganate of potassium.* May be placed in saucers, or cloths soaked in it may be hung up in apartments where there are contagious maladies. Furniture, clothing, utensils, the hands of the attendants and of the sick, may be washed in one part of Condy's fluid to fifty of water. As Condy's fluid is odourless it is preferred by many to carbolic acid preparations, but it is not so powerful, and its use must be limited by the fact of its leaving a brown stain on linen. It should not be used at the same time as carbolic acid, as they are chemically opposed. Messrs. Burroughs & Wellcome prepare compressed tabloids of permanganate which may be used as a *disinfectant* for foul discharges in the sick-room. Three tabloids, 2 grains each, dissolved in an ounce of water is the proper strength to use for this purpose. These pellets are useful for travellers, who find themselves occupying rooms requiring both ventilation and disinfection.

119. *Carbolic Acid.*—In its *pure* state it is a white crystalline solid, which burns everything it comes into contact with. The *commercial* acid is a thin, tarry fluid, possessing a strong odour and poisonous properties. The *powder* is made by treating a certain quantity of sawdust with a certain proportion of the acid. The *pure* acid is used for surgical purposes, the *lotion* most generally applicable for ordinary sores, boils, abscesses, and ulcers being ten grains of acid (or drops if the acid has liquefied) to one ounce of water; and it is recommended that this lotion be used, if available, instead of plain water when water dressing No. 85 is required. For foul ulcers, from ten to thirty grains to an ounce of water; for sore throat with fœtid breath, or for a mouth-wash, two grains

to one ounce; if used with a spray apparatus, twenty grains to the ounce; for inhalation, fifteen grains in a pint of hot water; as an injection for the male or female privates, one grain to an ounce; as an ointment for ulcers or skin diseases, five grains to an ounce of simple ointment. *Carbolic oil* is often useful, and should consist of twenty grains or drops of acid, to one ounce of salad or olive oil. When the *commercial* acid is diluted by fifty parts of water, it may be used for washing furniture, clothing, utensils, hands of attendants and of the sick, the heads of children, in skin affections, and as a wash for the mouth. In consequence of the poisonous properties of carbolic acid, the disinfecting powder is safer as a domestic disinfectant. It may be employed for scrubbing floors or furniture; it may be put in water, in the proportion of half a pound to the gallon, to form a solution for steeping infected clothing in; and it may be placed in vessels used for receiving the discharges of the sick. It is also very useful for disinfecting urinals, water-closets, &c.

120. *Chlorine Gas* would be best if it were not, unless largely diluted, irritating to the eyes and lungs. It may be obtained in various ways. Chloride of lime (popularly bleaching-powder), moistened with water in a saucer, gives off small quantities. If a quicker effect is desired, a little *dilute sulphuric acid* may be added. Chlorine gas may also be obtained by adding a little *dilute muriatic acid*, gradually, to half a tumblerful of Condy's fluid. Both these methods are convenient, and sufficient for a sick-room. When required in larger quantities, as for the disinfection of a sick-room during the absence of the occupant, chlorine gas may be generated from the following combination: common salt, four ounces; binoxide of manganese, one ounce; sulphuric acid, one ounce; water, two ounces. Mix the salt and manganese roughly, and place in a basin; then add the sulphuric acid *gradually* to the water, and pour over the powder. If the basin is placed on a box of hot sand, the formation of gas will be more rapid.

121. *Disinfection of the Air of Rooms.*—Ventilation and cleanliness being accorded the first places, the following agents may be used as most conveniently procurable. Baskets containing charcoal, which has the property of absorbing sewage gases, especially sulphuretted hydrogen, may be hung in the room. Quicklime, which absorbs carbonic acid, may be used, placed in a saucer. Chlorine gas may be obtained and used as mentioned under No. 120. Carbolic acid, one ounce mixed with a pound of sand, may be placed in saucers about the room. Cloths damped in carbolic acid solution, or in Condy's fluid, may be hung about the room, unelss in cases where there may be an objection to a damp atmosphere. The isolation of the patient may be rendered more certain by suspending outside the door a sheet moistened with a solution of carbolic acid or Condy's fluid. One or more of the above means may be used (excepting carbolic acid at the same time as Condy's fluid, *vide* No. 118). Charcoal

in bags, chlorine gas, and carbolic acid solution or powder, are probably the most efficacious, and the most easily procurable.

122. *Disinfection of Clothing, Bedding, Carpets, Tents, &c.*—Any material used by patients with infectious diseases should, if it can be spared, be immediately burnt. Otherwise articles of the kind should be immersed in solution of Condy's fluid or of carbolic acid, whichever may be available; and of the strengths given under Nos. 118, 119. This should be accomplished *immediately*, the things not being allowed to lie by, even for a few hours. A large vessel containing the disinfecting fluid used should be kept near the sick-room, for the reception of all bed and body linen. After soaking for three hours the articles should be boiled for half an hour in clean water, afterwards thoroughly washed with soap, and then exposed for three days to the sun and air. If disinfectants are not available, the time of boiling, of washing, and of exposure to the air should be doubled, or fumigation with sulphur may be used (*vide* No. 129). Where it can be carried out, clothing, bedding, &c., are best disinfected by being exposed for one hour or more to a dry heat of from 240° to 250° Fahr. For this purpose it would be well if public ovens were provided. The hair or other material of mattresses should be 'teased out' before being treated by disinfectants, washing, or heat. Disinfecting powder should be sprinkled on any soiled spots which may not demand immediate removal of the article. The final washing of infected clothing should be effected separately, as diseases may be conveyed by clothes prepared in a laundry where infected clothing has been 'got up.'

123. *Disinfection of Utensils.*—Utensils used by the sick, such as cups, spoons, forks, plates, &c., should be *immediately* immersed in some disinfecting fluid, of the strength mentioned under Nos. 118, 119; Condy's fluid is preferable, as carbolic acid might leave an unpleasant taste.

124. *Disinfection of the Hands of Attendants.*—Two basins, one containing Condy's fluid or carbolic acid solution, and another containing plain water, should be kept ready, so that attendants may wash *first* in disinfecting fluid, and then with soap and water *immediately* on the hands being soiled by infectious discharges. The strength of the solution should be as mentioned under Nos. 118, 119. If blood or thick discharges have dried on the hands, they should be scrubbed with sand.

125. *Disinfection of the Body of the Sick.*—The sick person should use water, for washing purposes, in which either Condy's fluid or carbolic acid (*vide* Nos. 118, 119) has been placed. When strong enough, benefit may often result from the use of disinfecting baths similarly medicated.

126. *Disinfection of Discharges from the Sick.*—Discharges should be soaked up with rags which may be burnt; sponges or pocket-handkerchiefs should not be used. Discharges from the bowels, or vomit, or urine, or expectoration, should be received into vessels charged with dis-

infectants. For this purpose four or five ounces of carbolic acid powder or six or eight ounces of a solution of commercial carbolic acid in water (strength, four ounces to the gallon), or six or eight ounces of a solution of sulphate of iron (strength, a pound to the gallon)—and which will probably be most easily procurable—should be placed in the close-stool, previous to use, and a smaller quantity in cups used for expectoration. The disinfected mass should be removed as soon as possible, and buried three feet deep, at some distance from any tank, well, or water. Otherwise, if not totally disinfected, it may infect the water and those drinking it. If thrown on the ground the material dries, and the germs of disease may be wafted to different places (*vide* p. 733).

The only safe disposal of material of the kind, whether arising from disinfecting clothing or utensils, or hands, or discharges from the sick, is burial in the earth, the oxidising powers of which render it innocuous. For this reason two or three inches of loose earth should be put daily around and under the cots of native cholera patients, so that it may receive any falling discharge. Thin wide gutta-percha placed under the breech of the patient prevents the discharge soaking into the bed, and, if kept clean and frequently changed and disinfected, is a great additional safeguard.

127. *Disinfection of Animals.*—Dogs and cats should not be allowed in rooms tenanted by patients with infectious disease, as they may convey contagion. If such animals have been exposed to contagion, they should be well washed with carbolic acid solution.

128. *Disinfection of Water-closets, Privies, &c.*—Dry earth is the best agent for ordinary use in privies attached to Indian houses. A handful of common dry earth placed over human excrement will prevent bad smell, and the mass may be taken away and used as manure, or be buried. But when infectious disease is present, or where water-closets are connected with sewers, disinfectants should be used. Water-closets, privies, cesspools, and drains can be disinfected by copperas (sulphate of iron). For the disinfection of a cubic foot of filth, half a pound of copperas dissolved in a couple of quarts of soft water is sufficient. The addition by each individual using a privy or water-closet of two-thirds of an ounce of copperas to such privy, or one-third of a pint of the above solution to such water-closet, will keep it wholesome. Carbolic acid can be used after the addition of copperas till the place smells strongly of it. It may be diluted by being shaken up with twenty times its volume of water, and if poured from a watering-pot with rose-nozzle over the sides of a recently emptied privy or cesspool will do great good. Sawdust or sand strongly impregnated with carbolic acid may be used for this purpose. All water-closets and privies should, when epidemics of cholera or typhoid may be expected, be disinfected, whether they be offensive or not. It is well at such periods to avoid using any such conveniences which have

not been disinfected, especially if, as at hotels and railway stations, they may have been used by persons from infected localities. Manure-heaps or accumulations of filth, which it is inexpedient to disturb during epidemics, or which cannot be moved, should be covered, especially if to leeward of dwellings, with coarsely powdered charcoal to the depth of two or three inches, or with freshly burnt lime, or with fresh dry earth if charcoal or lime cannot be obtained.

*To test the air of privies*, lay a piece of turmeric paper between two pieces of glass, so that half the paper hangs down. If the air is not pure, the part of the paper exposed turns reddish-brown after a few minutes, while the non-exposed part remains yellow.

129. *Disinfection of Rooms after Removal of the Sick.*—The room should be disinfected by burning brimstone in it in the proportion of four ounces to every 100 cubic feet. The cubic space may be calculated by multiplying the height, length, and breadth together by feet. The brimstone should be placed on an iron plate, which should be suspended over a lamp or charcoal fire (the whole supported, for protection, over a tub of water). Or the brimstone may be set fire to by putting live coals upon it. This causes sulphurous acid gas to be given off, which is a strong disinfectant. Doors, chimneys, and windows must be shut whilst this is being done, and clothes or carpets belonging to the room should previously to further disinfection (*vide* No. 122) be spread out on ropes during the process. The room should be kept closed for four hours. No disinfection of the kind is thorough if a man can live in the room whilst it is going on. After disinfection, the furniture, flooring, and all woodwork should be washed with solution of Condy's fluid, or with carbolic acid solution of the strength mentioned under those heads. If the walls are papered, the paper should be well wetted with the disinfecting solution and removed. If the walls are colour-washed, the wash should be all scraped off. If the floorings are earthen, or broken chunam, they should be dug up. The doors and windows should be thrown open and kept open for two or three days.

130. *Disinfection of the Dead Body.*—When a patient dies from infectious disease, the body should be washed with solution of carbolic acid (one part of acid to fifteen of water) and placed in the coffin as soon as possible. The body should be surrounded and the coffin filled up with charcoal, and chlorine gas may be generated in the room.

# ADDENDUM

## *DIETETIC PREPARATIONS FOR THE INVALID*

Barley Water.—Wash two ounces of pearl barley well with cold water, and reject the washings. Then boil in a pint and a half of water for twenty minutes in a covered vessel, and strain. The liquid may be sweetened and flavoured with thinly cut lemon-peel, which may be introduced during the boiling.

Beef Tea.—Mince finely one pound of lean beef, place it in a preserve jar, and pour upon it one pint of cold water. Stir, and allow it to stand for about one hour. Then place the jar with its contents in a saucepan of water, let it simmer gently over the fire for an hour, and strain. The liquid which runs through the strainer contains a quantity of fine sediment, which is to be drunk with the liquid, after flavouring with salt at pleasure.

Beef tea prepared as above is very nutritive, and possesses an agreeable meaty flavour. Beef tea should not be subjected to prolonged or violent boiling, as it then becomes a soup or broth, from the most nutritious portion (the gelatine and albuminous material) being, during the boiling process, incorporated with the solid rejected residue. The liquid thus loses in flavour and nutritive power.

Beef Tea, Savoury.—Mince finely three pounds of lean beef, and add one onion, half-a-dozen cloves, one small carrot, a little celery seed or essence, a little thyme and parsley, half a teacupful of mushroom ketchup, three pints of water, and salt and pepper according to taste. Prepare as directed for beef tea.

Beef Extract.—Cut up a pound of the best beef into small pieces, and put them into a good-sized pickle-bottle with a wide mouth. This is corked loosely, and placed in a kettle of water and kept boiling for two hours. If the bottle be now removed, it will be found to contain a considerable quantity of fluid, which may be poured off, the beef also being subjected to slight pressure to make it yield more. In this fluid we have a highly concentrated article of nourishment, which may be given, after seasoning, either pure or diluted, according to the state of the stomach.

Bread.—Obtaining good bread is very often a difficulty in India. Soda and baking powders, which contain an alkali, are objectionable, because they neutralise the gastric juice. So is, very often, the *mussallah* used by native bakers instead of yeast, which is not unfrequently sour. *To procure yeast or barm* is the difficulty in making good bread, which may be overcome, at least in the cooler weather, as follows: Put half a breakfast-cupful of good hops into a saucepan with two quarts of cold water, and boil slowly for some hours, until it is reduced to little more than one quart. Let this decoction get cool, then add half a breakfast-cupful of sugar, stir till the sugar is dissolved, then bottle and cork. Let the bottle stand in a cool place for three days, when yeast will be formed.

*To make bread*, take six pounds of flour, three table-spoonfuls of yeast, and one quart of lukewarm water. Put the yeast and water into the centre of the flour, mix, and cover with a cloth for five or six hours, till it rises. Then add as much tepid water as will make the whole into dough, also a dessert-spoonful of salt, and knead properly. Cover, and let the mass stand till it ferments, which is known by its cracking on the top. Then divide into loaves and bake. Double the propörtions of articles named will make better bread.

*To make unfermented bread.*—Take flour, one pound; bicarbonate of soda, forty grains; powdered white sugar, one teaspoonful; muriatic acid, fifty drops; water, half-pint. Thoroughly mix the soda and the sugar with the flour in a large basin with a wooden spoon. Then add the acid to the water, and gradually add the mixture to the flour, sugar, and soda, stirring well all the time. Divide into two loaves, and immediately put them in a quick oven.

Bread Jelly or 'Pap.'—Steep stale bread in boiling water

and pass through a fine sieve while hot. This may be flavoured with sugar or mixed with milk. It is suitable for children and invalids with weak stomachs.

BROTHS are made by boiling the materials chosen for two hours, and straining through a wide sieve. Pearl barley, rice, vermicelli, or semolina may be added. The bones of the meat may also be broken up, and used in the preparation of broth.

CHICKEN, VEAL, or MUTTON TEA may be prepared in the same manner as beef tea.

CHICKEN JELLY.—Cut up a chicken, and put the pieces into a jar; pour over it a tea-cupful of cold water, tie down closely with a piece of bladder, and boil the jar in a saucepan of water for six or eight hours. Strain the liquid, and when cold remove the fat. A nourishing jelly remains.

FLOUR AND MILK.—Fill a small basin with flour, tie a cloth over the mouth, and boil it slowly in a saucepan of water for eight or ten hours. The inside portion of the flour becomes incorporated into a hard mass. After removing the outer sodden part add one grated table-spoonful of the flour to a pint of milk, and boil. This preparation is often advisable in dysentery and diarrhœa.

IMPERIAL DRINK.—Take half an ounce of cream of tartar, the juice of one lemon, and two table-spoonfuls of sifted white sugar. Put the whole in a jar, and pour over them one quart of boiling water. Cover till cold. A useful drink in fevers.

LEMONADE.—Pare the rind from a lemon thinly, and cut the lemon into slices. Put the peel and sliced lemon into a jug, with one ounce of white sugar, and pour over them one pint of boiling water. Cover the lid closely, and let it stand till cold. Then strain and pour off the liquid.

LIEBIG'S RAW MEAT SOUP.—Take eight ounces of recently killed meat, and mince fine. Place the mince in twelve ounces of distilled or pure water, add four drops of strong muriatic acid (also called hydrochloric acid) and half a salt-spoonful of salt. Stir well, and allow it to stand one hour, then strain through a fine sieve or cloth. When all the fluid, which is of a red colour, has run through, add eight or ten ounces more water. It should be made fresh once daily and given cold. This preparation is often taken and retained when other foods are refused or vomited, as it presents a form of sustenance requiring very little aid from digestion. It is very useful in cholera, in fevers, and in the wasting diseases of children. A patient may be usually given as much as he will take.

Linseed Tea.—Place one ounce of bruised linseed and two drachms of bruised liquorice root into a jug, and add one pint of boiling water. Let it stand, lightly covered, for three hours near a fire. Strain the liquid, which may be flavoured as mentioned for barley-water. Useful as a drink in urinary affections.

Milk and Suet.—Boil one ounce of finely chopped suet with a quarter of a pint of water for ten minutes, and press through flannel. Add a drachm of bruised cinnamon, one ounce of sugar, and three-quarters of a pint of milk. Boil again for ten minutes and strain. A wine-glassful or more may be taken at a time. It is nutritive and fattening, and, if there is no diarrhœa, is useful in the atrophy or emaciation of children.

Oatmeal Gruel.—Mix thoroughly but gradually one table-spoonful of groats with two of cold water, and add one pint of boiling water, stirring all the while. Boil for ten minutes, continuing the stirring. Sweeten with sugar and add, if desired, a little sherry or brandy. Milk may be used instead of water. This is also a nourishing food, containing more nitrogenous matter than preparations of arrowroot.

Oatmeal Porridge.—Mix a large table-spoonful of oatmeal with two table-spoonfuls of cold water. Stir well, and pour into a pint of boiling water in a saucepan. Boil and stir well for ten minutes, and flavour with salt or sugar as preferred. Milk may be used instead of water. If the boiling is continued for half an hour, the porridge then turned out into a soup plate, and cold milk poured over it, it will become semi-solid. Oatmeal porridge is beneficial when constipation exists, but should not be used if there is tendency to diarrhœa. It is a nourishing food, but sometimes causes acidity or water-brash.

Panada.—Take the white part of the breast and wings of a boiled or roasted chicken, and pound in a mortar with an equal quantity of stale bread. Add the water in which the chicken has been boiled, or beef tea, until the whole forms a fluid paste; then boil for ten minutes, stirring all the time.

The under side of cold sirloin of roasted beef, or cold roasted leg of mutton, may be used instead of chicken.

RICE WATER.—Well wash one ounce of rice with cold water. Then steep the rice for three hours in a quart of water kept at a tepid heat; afterwards boil slowly for one hour and strain. It may be sweetened and flavoured as barley water. A useful drink in dysentery and diarrhœa.

TAMARIND DRINK.—Take a quarter of a pint of tamarinds, and pour over them a quart of boiling water. Sweeten as required, and cover till cold. A useful drink in fevers.

TAMARIND WHEY.—Boil a pint of milk, and while it is boiling add two table-spoonfuls of tamarinds. Strain, and sweeten to taste. A cooling and slightly laxative drink.

WHITE-WINE WHEY, OR 'POSSET.'—Boil half a pint of milk in a saucepan, and while it is boiling add a wine-glassful of sherry. Strain, and sweeten as agreeable. A useful drink in colds and mild febr[illegible] [illegible]tacks.

# INDEX